Amyotrophic Lateral Sclerosis

Amyotrophic Lateral Sclerosis

Edited by

Robert H Brown Jr MD DPhil
Professor of Neurology
Harvard Medical School
Director
Cecil B Day Laboratory for Neuromuscular Research
Massachusetts General Hospital East
Charlestown
MA 02129
USA

Vincent Meininger MD
Professor of Neurology
Féderation de Neurologic Mazarin
Hôpital de la Salpêtrière
Paris
France

Michael Swash MD FRCP FRCPath
Professor of Neurology
St Bartholomew's and the Royal London
School of Medicine and Dentistry
(Queen Mary and Westfield College)
The Royal London Hospital
London
UK

Kindly sponsored by Rhône-Poulenc Rorer

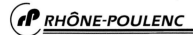

Rhône-Poulenc Rorer

MARTIN DUNITZ

© Martin Dunitz Ltd 2000

First published in the United Kingdom in 2000 by
Martin Dunitz Ltd
The Livery House
7-9 Pratt Street
London NW1 0AE

Tel: +44-(0)20-7482-2202
Fax: +44-(0)20-7267-0159
E-mail: info@mdunitz.globalnet.co.uk
Website: http://www.dunitz.co.uk

A CIP catalogue record for this book is available from the British Library

ISBN 1-85317-421-1

Distributed in the United States by:
Blackwell Science Inc.
Commerce Place, 350 Main Street
Malden MA 02148, USA
Tel: 1-800-215-1000

Distributed in Canada by:
Login Brothers Book Company
324 Salteaux Crescent
Winnipeg, Manitoba R3J 3T2
Canada
Tel: 1-204-224-4068

Distributed in Brazil by:
Ernesto Reichmann Distribuidora de Livros, Ltda
Rua Coronel Marques 335, Tatuape 03440-000
Sao Paulo,
Brazil

Composition by Wearset, Boldon, Tyne and Wear.
Printed and bound in Great Britain by Biddles Ltd, Guildford and King's Lynn.

CONTENTS

V Therapeutic approaches

VI Patient care

Contributors

Maria Alexianu MD PhD
MDA/ALS Research Center
Department of Neurology
Baylor College of Medicine
Houston
TX 77030
USA

Peter M Andersen MD DMSc
Cecil B Day Laboratory for Neuromuscular
Research
Department of Neurology
Massachusetts General Hospital East
Harvard Medical School
Charlestown
MA 02129
USA

Stanley H Appel MD
Professor and Chairman
Director, MDA/ALS Research Center
Department of Neurology
Baylor College of Medicine
Houston
TX 77030
USA

Shahram Attarian MD
Assistant Professor
Department of Neurology and Neuromuscular
Diseases
University Hospital La Timone
Marseille 13385
France

Mark W Becher MD
Department of Pathology
University of New Mexico
School of Medicine
Albuquerque NM
USA

Daryn Belden
Statistical Coordinator
ALS Clinical Research Center
Department of Neurology
University of Wisconsin Hospital and Clinics
Madison
WI 53792-5132
USA

Benjamin R Brooks MD
Professor and Director
ALS Clinical Research Center
Department of Neurology
University of Wisconsin Hospital and Clinics
Madison
WI 53792-5132
USA
and
Staff Physician
Neurology Service
William S Middleton Memorial
VA Medical Center
Great Lakes Integrated Service Network (VISN
12)
Madison
WI 53705–2286
USA

William F Brown MD FRCPC
Professor of Neurology
Chairman, Department of Neurology
New England Medical Center
Neurology Department
Boston
MA 02111
USA

Robert H Brown Jr MD DPhil
Professor of Neurology
Harvard Medical School
Director
Cecil B. Day Laboratory for Neuromuscular
Research
Massachusetts General Hospital East
Charlestown
MA 02129
USA

Lucie I Bruijn PhD
Bristol-Myers Squibb Company
Pharmaceutical Research Institute
Neuroscience Drug Discovery
CT 06492-7660
USA

K Ming Chan MD FRCPC
Division of Physical Medicine and
Rehabilitation/Division of Neuroscience
University of Alberta
Edmonton
Canada

Don W Cleveland PhD
Professor
Ludwig Institute for Cancer Research and
Departments of Medicine and Neuroscience
University of California at San Diego
La Jolla
CA 92093
USA

Roxanne DePaul PhD
Professor
Department of Communications Disorders
University of Wisconsin-Whitewater
Whitewater
WI 53190
USA
and
ALS Clinical Research Center
Department of Neurology
University of Wisconsin Hospital and Clinics
Madison
WI 53792-5132
USA

Selmi Dogan PhD
Staff Scientist
Motor Performance Laboratory
Department of Neurology
University of Wisconsin Hospital and Clinics
Madison
WI 53792-5132
USA

Len Doyal BA, MSc
Professor of Medical Ethics
Department of Human Science and Medical
Ethics
St Bartholomew's & The Royal London
School of Medicine and Dentistry
Queen Mary and Westfield College
University of London
London
UK

Daniel B Drachman MD
Professor of Neurology and Neuroscience
John Hopkins School of Medicine
Baltimore
MD 21287–7519
USA

Andrew A Eisen MD FRCPC
Professor of Neurology
Head, Neuromuscular Diseases Unit
(Electromyography)
University of British Columbia
Head, Neuromuscular Diseases Unit
Vancouver General Hospital
Vancouver
BC V5Z 1M9
Canada

József I Engelhardt MD PhD
MDA/ALS Research Center
Department of Neurology
Baylor College of Medicine
Houston
TX 77030
USA
and
Department of Neurology and Psychiatry
Albert Szent-Györgyi Medical University
Szeged
Hungary

Deborah F Gelinas MD
Director, ALS Clinical Service
Department of Neurology
California Pacific Medical Center
Forbes H Norris MDA/ALS Center
San Francisco
CA 94115
USA

Mark E Gurney PhD
CNS Research
Pharmacia Upjohn Inc
Kalamazoo
MI 49001
USA

Mohamed Habib PhD
MDA/ALS Research Center
Department of Neurology
Baylor College of Medicine
Houston
TX 77030
USA

Mongi Ben Hamida MD
Professor of Neurology
Institut National de Neurologie
La Rabta 1007
Tunis
Tunisia

Fayçal Hentati MD
Professor of Neurology
Head of the Department of Neurology
Institut National de Neurologie
La Rabta 1007
Tunis
Tunisia

Paul G Ince MD FRCPath
MRC Clinical Scientist, Hon Senior Lecturer and
Consultant Neuropathologist
Institute for the Health of the Elderly
MRC Unit
Newcastle General Hospital
Newcastle upon Tyne
UK

Mandy Jackson MD
Department of Neurology and Neuroscience
John Hopkins University
Baltimore
MD 21287
USA

Crispin Jenkinson DPhil HonMFPHM
Deputy Director
Health Services Research Unit
University of Oxford
Institute of Health Sciences
Headington
Oxford
UK

JMB Vianney de Jong MD PhD
Department of Neurology
Academic Medical Centre
Amsterdam
The Netherlands

Katalin Juhasz-Poscine MD
Clinical Instructor
ALS Clinical Research Center
Department of Neurology
University of Wisconsin Hospital and Clinics
Madison
WI 53792-5132
USA
and
Staff Physician
Neurology Service
William S Middleton Memorial VA Medical
Center
Great Lakes Veterans Integrated Service
Network (VISN 12)
Madison
WI 53705-2286
USA

Michael Laird
Database Coordinator
ALS Clinical Research Center
Department of Neurology
University of Wisconsin Hospital and Clinics
Madison
WI 53792-5132
USA

George Levvy
Chief Executive
Motor Neurone Disease Association
Northampton
UK

Laurel Malinowski
Database Coordinator
ALS Clinical Research Center
Department of Neurology
University of Wisconsin Hospital and Clinics
Madison
WI 53792-5132
USA

Andrea Maser MS
Swallowing Clinic
Department of Rehabilitation Medicine
University of Wisconsin Hospital and Clinics
Madison
WI 53792-5132
USA

Vincent Meininger MD
Professor of Neurology
Féderation de Neurologic Mazarin
Hôpital de la Salpêtrière
Paris
France

Robert G Miller MD
Chairman, Department of Neurology
& Director, The Forbes Norris MDA/ALS
Center
California Pacific Medical Center
San Francisco
CA 94115
USA

Mitsuya Morita MD, PhD
Cecil B Day Laboratory for Neuromuscular
Research
Massachusetts General Hospital East
Charlestown
MA 02129
USA

Dennis Mosier MD PhD
MDA/ALS Research Center
Department of Neurology
Baylor College of Medicine
Houston
TX 77030
USA

Piera Pasinelli PhD
Cecil B Day Laboratory for Neuromuscular
Research
Massachusetts General Hospital-East
Charlestown
MA 02129
USA

Erik P Pioro MD DPhil
Director, ALS Center
Department of Neurology
Cleveland Clinic Foundation
Cleveland
OH 44195
USA

Jean Pouget MD
Professor of Neurology
Department of Neurology and Neuromuscular
Diseases
University Hospital La Timone
Marseille 13385
France

Donald L Price MD
Neuropathology Laboratory
Laboratory of Neuropathology
Johns Hopkins University School of Medicine
Baltimore
MD 21205
USA

Isabelle Richard MD PhD
Professor of Physical Medicine and
Rehabilitation
Medical Faculty of the University of Angers
Centre régional de rééducation et réadaptation
fonctionelle
Angers 49024
France

Wim L Robberecht MD PhD
Department of Neurology
University Hospital Gasthuisberg
Leuven 3000
Belgium

Craig Roelke
Database Coordinator
ALS Clinical Research Center
Department of Neurology
University of Wisconsin Hospital and Clinics
Madison
WI 53792-5132
USA

Kathryn Roelke RN
Research Coordinator
ALS Clinical Research Center
Department of Neurology
University of Wisconsin Hospital and Clinics
Madison
WI 53792-5132
USA

Joanna Rome MD
Assistant
Medical Faculty of the University of Nantes
Service de rééducation fonctionelle
Hopital Saint Jacques
Nantes 44093
France

Jeffrey D Rothstein MD PhD
Associate Professor of Neurology and
Neuroscience
Johns Hopkins University
Department of Neurology and Neuroscience
Baltimore
MD 21287
USA

François Salachas MD
Neurology Service
Hôpital de la Salpêtrière
Paris
France

Mohammed Sanjak PhD
Director
Motor Performance Laboratory
Department of Neurology
University of Wisconsin Hospital and Clinics
Madison
WI 53792-5132
USA
and
ALS Clinical Research Center
Department of Neurology
University of Wisconsin Hospital and Clinics
Madison
WI 53792-5132
USA

Michael Sendtner MD
Professor of Clinical Neurobiology
Clinical Research Unit of Neuroregeneration
Department of Neurology
University of Würzburg
Würzburg 97080
Germany

Jane Shannon
Database Coordinator
ALS Clinical Research Center
Department of Neurology
University of Wisconsin Hospital and Clinics
Madison
WI 53792-5132
USA

Pamela J Shaw MB BS MD FRCP
Wellcome Senior Fellow in Clinical Science and
Professor of Neurological Medicine
Department of Clinical Neurology
Royal Victoria Infirmary
Newcastle upon Tyne
UK

Láctzlós Siklós PhD
MDA/ALS Research Center
Department of Neurology
Baylor College of Medicine
Houston
TX 77030
USA
and
Institute of Biophysics
Biological Research Center of the Hungarian
Academy of Sciences
Szeged
Hungary

R Glenn Smith MD PhD
MDA/ALS Research Center
Department of Neurology
Baylor College of Medicine
Houston
TX 77030
USA

Michael J Strong MD FRCP
Motor Neuron Diseases & General Neurology
Department of Clinical Neurological Sciences
London Health Sciences Centre
University Campus
London, ON
Canada

Michael Swash MD FRCP FRCPath
Professor of Neurology
St Bartholomew's and the
Royal London School of
Medicine and Dentistry
(Queen Mary and Westfield College)
The Royal London Hospital
London
UK

Sylvie Trefouret MD
Assistant Professor
Department of Neurology
University Hospital La Timone
Marseille 13385
France

Andrew Waclawik MD
Assistant Professor
ALS Clinical Research Center
Department of Neurology
University of Wisconsin Hospital and Clinics
Madison
WI 53792-5132
USA
and
Director, EMG Laboratory
Neurology Service
William S Middleton Memorial VA Medical
Center
Great Lakes Veterans Integrated Service
Network (VISN 12)
Madison
WI 53705-2286
USA

Rustom S Wadia MD FICP FIAN
Consultant in Neurology
Ruby Hall Clinic
Poona Medical Research Foundation
Pune
India
and
Honorary Professor of Neurology
BJ Medical College
Pune
India

Toni L Williamson PhD
Trophos
Marseille 13288
Cedex 9
France

We wish to dedicate this book to our wives:
Elaine V Beilin, Nathalie Rothkoff Meininger and Caroline Swash.

Preface

Amyotrophic lateral sclerosis (ALS) is a disease that has come into the limelight after a century of neglect. Advances in understanding this fatal and neurodegenerative disease have been slow but the pace of research has recently rapidly accelerated, and there are now many ideas concerning the basic biology of the motor neuron, the key to understanding this disease. Ideas are precious in neuroscience, and often derived from observation. Much of the recent interest and progress in the disease reflects important, parallel lines of research: epidemiology and genetics, neurotrophic factors, excitotoxicity and its integral relation to energy metabolism, free radical homeostasis and its relation to apoptotic cell death, calcium metabolism and cytoskeletal proteins within the motor neuron. For example, epidemiological and clinical studies led to the realisation that ALS is not the result of any obvious environmental factor, and that a small proportion of cases are familial. The phenotypic variability within some familial cases has become of intense interest since it has been established that this variablility in expression of the disease can occur in the context of a single mutation in the SOD1 gene. Another line of research has been the unfolding of knowledge of the neurotrophic factors, a complex series of proteins that have effects of varying specificity within neuronal systems during development, and also in maintaining normal structure and function. Trials of systemically administered neurotrophic factors in people with ALS have so far had disappointing results, but these trials in themselves have led to greater understanding of the issues and problems that underlie clinical trials in ALS, a slowly progressive disease of variable presentation and rate of progress. Following these seminal observations, reclassification of the ALS and motor neuron disease syndromes is beginning, and the process of diagnosis, accordingly, has become of more importance. The introduction of an anti-excitotoxic drug, with an effect in slowing progression of ALS, has itself led to a surge in understanding and interest in the problems of sustaining quality of life in the disease, and in the ethical issues that develop during the inexorable and inevitable progression that currently characterizes ALS. Many older ideas concerning pathogenesis have been put aside for the present in the rush to understand the biology of the motor system, but these will themselves come to the fore when there is improved therapy. As in cancer therapy, cure may be a long time in coming, but each advance gives cause for hope for those afflicted with this dread disease. This hope is presently underscored by the development of powerful new tools in biomedical research that promise to accelerate the quest for a cure, including the generation of good animal models for motor neuron disease, full decoding of the human genome and all human genes, the development of micro-assay methods that allow simultaneous analysis of expression of literally scores of thousands of these genes, micro-miniaturization of a variety of protein assays, and – predicated on these advances – the development of powerful new tools for high through-put drug testing.

Readers of this book will notice that the subject matter of the individual chapters, and the editors and contributors themselves, represent many nations. The community of ALS researchers is truly worldwide, and brought together within the WFN Research Group on ALS and other motor neuron diseases. New members are welcome (www.wfnals.org).

Michael Swash
Robert H Brown Jr
Vincent Meininger

SECTION I

CLINICAL FEATURES

1

Clinical features and diagnosis of amyotrophic lateral sclerosis

Michael Swash

Terminology

The nomenclature of disorders of the motor system can be confusing (*Table 1.1*). This confusion reflects our ignorance of the underlying causes of these syndromes. Currently, terminology is based on clinical or pathological descriptions of the syndromes themselves rather than on basic underlying mechanisms. This terminological difficulty can be resolved by consideration of the historical development of the concept of anterior horn cell disease as a cause of muscle wasting.

Progressive muscular wasting was a clinical syndrome well known to physicians in the early 19th century. The term progressive muscular atrophy (PMA) was used by Aran[1] in 1850, who believed that this syndrome was a muscular disorder. Duchenne[2] gave a description of this disorder in 1849. Bell, supported by Cruveilhier,[3] who noted the thinness of the anterior spinal roots in 1853, regarded PMA as a myelopathic disorder, whereas Aran and Duchenne favoured a muscular cause. Degeneration of the anterior cells in the grey matter of the spinal cord was recognized independently by Luys[4] in Paris in 1860 and by Lockhart Clarke in London. Charcot and Joffroy[5] brought together these observations in 1869 by studying the clinical and pathological features of the disease. He described the characteristic involvement of the corticospinal tract

and proposed the term amyotrophic lateral sclerosis (ALS). The myogenic origin of other causes of progressive muscular wasting (e.g. limb-girdle muscular dystrophy) was defined by von Leyden, Landouzy, and Dejerine, and by Erb.[6] Progressive bulbar palsy was described by Duchenne.[7] Charcot and Joffroy[5] recognized its relationship to ALS when loss of motor neurones was noted in the bulbar motor nuclei in pathological studies at l'hôpital Salpétrière in Paris. Pure syndromes of

---

Idiopathic motor neurone diseases
Amyotrophic lateral sclerosis (ALS)
Progressive bulbar palsy (PBP)
Progressive muscular atrophy (PMA)
Primary lateral sclerosis (PLS)
Familial amyotrophic lateral sclerosis
Juvenile amyotrophic lateral sclerosis
Madras motor neuron disease
Monomelic motor neuron disease
(amyotrophy)

Toxin-related motor neurone diseases
Lathyrism
Konzo
Guamanian ALS

Table 1.1
The motor neurone diseases.

myelopathic weakness without muscular atrophy (e.g. primary lateral sclerosis (PLS) as described by Spiller[8]) are rare and until recently have been regarded as being related to the core syndrome of ALS.

The term motor neurone disease (MND) was introduced by Brain[9] in recognition of the relation between the syndromes of PMA, ALS, and progressive bulbar palsy (PBP), as shown by the spectrum of involvement of upper and lower motor neurones and by the topography of the muscular wasting. This term has become commonly used in the UK although Charcot's designation of ALS is preferred in other European countries and in the USA and the francophone world. Rowland[10] recognized the utility of the term MND in describing the whole clinical syndrome but stressed the importance of retaining the general usage of the plural term (motor neurone diseases) to describe all the diseases of the anterior horn cells and motor system, including the inherited spinal muscular atrophies, which are clinically and pathologically distinct from MND itself.

In this chapter, the inclusive, general term MND is used to describe the disorders described in *Table 1.1*, including all the primary degenerative lower motor neurone (LMN) and upper motor neurone (UMN) disorders, but not the spinal muscular atrophies, which are inherited disorders of the LMN; these are classified separately. Thus, the term MND is not used synonymously with the term ALS. ALS is the disorder that was recognized by Charcot (see below); it is classified here as one of the motor neurone diseases. This usage differs slightly from current US and UK practice in restricting the term ALS to the core syndrome of Charcot ALS, while using the term MND to describe, inclusively, all the motor neurone disease syndromes. However, this usage accords both with Charcot's original description and with Brain's attempt to unify thinking within the group of motor neurone diseases. In clarifying the terminology of the motor neurone diseases, including ALS, it is important to recognize previous usage, and to relate terminology to clinical syndromes.

Clinical features of motor neurone diseases

The clinical features of ALS, and other motor neurone diseases, depend on the severity of the disorder and, particularly, on the variable permutations of combined UMN and LMN dysfunction affecting the susceptible parts of the neuraxis (*Tables 1.2* and *1.3*). Depending on the site of onset, the extent of involvement of the neuraxis in the disease process, and the stage of the disease, these symptoms and signs are present in varying combinations in different anatomical regions of the body (i.e. the cranial, cervical, thoracic, and lumbosacral regions).

Charcot ALS

Charcot ALS is the core syndrome of ALS and is the most common and, by far, the most

Symptoms
Fatigue
Weakness
Cramps
Twitching of muscles
Inco-ordination

Signs
Weakness
Atrophy
Fasciculations
Suppression of reflexes
Hypotonia

Table 1.2
Lower motor neurone dysfunction.

Symptoms
Weakness
Inco-ordination
Stiffness
Slowing of distal movement

Signs
Spasticity
Brisk reflexes
Babinski and Hoffman signs
Weakness
Pseudobulbar affect

Table 1.3
Upper motor neurone dysfunction.

important of the motor neurone disorders, accounting for perhaps 85% of cases of MND. It is a relentlessly progressive, fatal disorder of the nervous system that results from the degeneration of UMNs and LMNs. The pathophysiological process is typically restricted to the UMNs and the LMNs, although more widespread changes are present in many cases at autopsy.[11] Criteria for clinical and pathological diagnosis have been defined at consensus conferences held in El Escorial, Spain in 1994[12] and at Airlie House, Virginia, USA[13] in 1998 (see http://www.wfnals.org/). In these criteria, the clinical diagnosis is based on the clinical, electrophysiological, and neuroradiological features. Currently there is no surrogate marker for the diagnosis of ALS. In considering the diagnosis of ALS, it must be recognized that a number of other conditions may mimic the ALS syndrome (*Table 1.4*). These must be excluded by careful clinical evaluation and appropriate investigation.

Diagnosis

The clinical features of MND depend on whether the presentation is with focal or generalized involvement of the motor system, as well as on the stage of the disease at which the

Spinal muscular atrophy (e.g. adult-onset proximal SMA, Kennedy's syndrome)
Radiation myelopathy
Post-traumatic syringomyelia
Endocrine diseases (e.g. thyrotoxicosis and hyperparathyroidism)
Immune mediated
   Paraproteinemic and Multifocal motor neuropathies
   Sjögren's syndrome
Exogenous toxins
   Lead
   Mercury
Tumours
   Lymphoma
   Cancer-associated neuromuscular syndromes
Inherited enzyme defects
   Hexosaminidase deficiency
Post-polio amyotrophy
Infection, such as Lyme disease

Table 1.4
Disorders that may resemble ALS and so cause diagnostic difficulty.

clinical assessment is performed. The Airlie House criteria for the diagnosis of ALS require:

1. The presence of:
   (a) evidence of LMN degeneration by clinical, electrophysiological, or neuropathological examination;
   (b) evidence of UMN degeneration by clinical examination; and
   (c) progression of the motor syndrome within a region or to other regions, as determined by history or examination; and
2. The absence of:
   (a) electrophysiological and pathological evidence of other disease processes that might explain the signs of LMN or UMN degeneration; and
   (b) neuroimaging evidence of other disease processes that might explain the observed clinical and electrophysiological signs.

Four categories of diagnostic certainty are recognized by these clinical diagnostic criteria:

(a) clinical definite ALS;
(b) clinically probable ALS;
(c) probable, laboratory-supported ALS
(d) possible ALS.

Clinically definite ALS:
Clinically definite ALS is defined by evidence on clinical grounds alone of:

(a) the presence of UMN signs as well as LMN signs in the bulbar region and at least two spinal regions; or
(b) the presence of UMN signs in two spinal regions and LMN signs in three spinal regions.

Clinically probable ALS
Clinically probable ALS is defined by evidence on clinical grounds alone of UMN and LMN signs in at least two regions with some signs rostral to the LMN signs.

Probable, laboratory-supported ALS
Probable, laboratory-supported ALS is defined, after proper application of neuroimaging and clinical laboratory protocols has excluded other causes, as:

(a) clinical evidence of UMN and LMN signs in only one region; or
(b) UMN signs alone in one region and LMN signs defined by EMG criteria in at least two limbs.

Possible ALS
Possible ALS is defined, once other diagnoses have been excluded, as:

(a) UMN and LMN signs in only one region;
(b) UMN signs alone in two or more regions; or
(c) LMN signs found rostral to UMN signs.

These diagnostic criteria are concerned with diagnostic certainty. They do not address the issue of early diagnosis nor do they attempt to provide guidance in staging the disease, either according to severity or duration. The degree of certainty of the diagnosis of ALS is necessarily related both to the severity and to the duration of disease. Although clinically definite disease is more likely to show widespread manifestations and to be of longer duration than possible or probable disease, this is not inevitable. Furthermore, these diagnostic criteria are concerned with the diagnosis of ALS for the purpose of clinical trials and other areas of ALS research; they were not devised with the intention that they be used in everyday clinical practice. However, they are clearly useful in establishing uniformity of clinical diagnosis in different centres across the world, and they represent the best available consensus of opinion concerning diagnosis. They are a standard against which diagnosis can be assessed.

The revised Airlie House criteria no longer exclude syndromes that are atypical of the core syndrome of Charcot ALS. Thus, they allow the inclusion of patients with ALS who have, or who develop, extrapyramidal features or dementia, although they do exclude patients with recognized causes of these syndromes other than ALS. These are termed ALS-plus syndromes, and are accepted as heterogeneous syndromes. However, for the purpose of entry into trials of putative new therapies, the occurrence of these additional, atypical features at presentation, rather than developing later in the course of a disease that presented with typical features of ALS itself, would be regarded as sufficiently unusual to preclude a diagnosis of Charcot ALS. Nonetheless, these features might be considered acceptable for a diagnosis of 'atypical ALS' in clinical practice.

Related syndromes

A number of other syndromes have been described that resemble Charcot ALS (see *Table 1.4*). These syndromes are also characterized by a combination of UMN and LMN features without overt sensory or other system involvement. These syndromes are uncommon, and controversial.

MND syndromes in geographic clusters

Some characteristic syndromes occur in geographic clusters or as isolates (*Table 1.5*). It is uncertain whether these are sporadic disorders; it is likely that some have a genetic origin.

Juvenile ALS — especially Tunisian families
Madras motor neurone disease
Monomelic motor neurone disease (amyotrophy)
Wasted leg syndrome
Lathyrism
Konzo
ALS–parkinsonism–dementia complex of Guam

Table 1.5
Geographic variants of ALS.

Madras motor neurone disease
In southern India, a sporadic, progressive, asymmetric disorder characterized by onset in the second or third decade is recognized.[14] Weakness, wasting, fasciculations, and pyramidal signs in the limbs are the main features,[15] and cranial nerve dysfunction — including sensorineural deafness — occurs in a proportion.[16] In a series of 40 cases, cranial nerve dysfunction occurred in 70%, and an extensor plantar response in 65%.[17] Progression is slow, and survival over a few decades is common. This syndrome does not conform to the clinical criteria for the diagnosis of Charcot ALS.

Monomelic amyotrophy
This syndrome is common in Japan[18] and India[19] and has also been reported from other countries. Characteristics include:

(a) male preponderance;
(b) insidious onset of weakness and wasting that is restricted to muscles within circumscribed cervical or lumbar spinal myotomes;
(c) absence of bulbar symptoms; and
(d) slow progression.

There may be EMG evidence of involvement of clinically unaffected muscles, and abnormally brisk reflexes have been reported;[20] these features suggest more widespread motor system involvement. Although probably a motor neurone disease, on the available evidence this syndrome does not usually progress to Charcot ALS.

Guam ALS

ALS syndromes in Guam have been studied for over 40 years.[20–24] Although the clinical phenotype of MND in Guam is usually indistinguishable from sporadic ALS of the Charcot type, a proportion of patients exhibit features of parkinsonism, and the neuropathology of this syndrome is distinct.[25] McGeer and colleagues[26] emphasized the familial nature of Guam ALS in the 15 patients they studied: a positive family history was found in 25% of cases. Infectious, genetic, and toxic theories of causation have also been proposed. Similar ALS syndromes have been reported among the indigenous people of the Kii peninsula of Japan[27] and the southern lowlands of western New Guinea.[28] Currently, it is uncertain whether all these cases are genetic in origin or whether there is a contributing environmental cause.

Paraneoplastic ALS

ALS has been associated with various tumours. A patient with clinical features of a motor neurone disease and small-cell carcinoma of the lung, tested positive for anti-Hu antibodies.[29] Three other patients with anti-Hu antibodies and small-cell tumour of the lung had an ALS-like syndrome in addition to dizziness, focal seizures, and sensory signs.[30] The ALS-like features predominated. Of five women with PLS associated with breast cancer reported by Forsyth and colleagues,[30] three later developed LMN signs, implying a diagnosis of ALS rather than PLS. A 67-year-old woman with ovarian carcinoma presented with a progressive clinical syndrome identical to ALS.[31] Anti-Purkinje cell antibodies were detected by indirect immunofluorescence and in a Western blot assay, the antibody bound to a 52 kDa neuronal protein. These reports suggest that, in an appropriate clinical setting, ALS can be considered as a paraneoplastic disorder,[32] as suggested by Brain and Norris[33] in 1965. However, precise epidemiological and clinicopathological proof of this suggested association is currently lacking.

ALS associated with other disorders

Although there is doubt as to the causative relationship in these reports, the possibility remains that the ALS syndrome may occur with increased frequency in association with cancer and gammaglobulinaemias.

ALS and lymphoproliferative diseases

There are 62 reported cases that suggest that ALS in all its phenotypic variations may be linked to lymphoproliferative disorders like Waldenstrom's macroglobulinaemia, chronic lymphocytic leukaemia, Hodgkin's and other lymphomas, and paraproteinaemia.[34,35] In more than half the reported cases, a combination of UMN and LMN signs have been noted in life and confirmed on autopsy.[35] ALS and the lymphoproliferative disorder may either present simultaneously or one may precede the other. In one case, lymphoma was detected only at autopsy. According to some authors, an elevated level of protein in the cerebrospinal fluid may signal the presence of underlying lymphoproliferative disease in ALS.[36] Immunosuppressive therapy ameliorates the neurological disorder in less than 10% of cases. The nature of the relationship between the two conditions is unknown.

Multifocal motor neuropathy

Multifocal motor neuropathy (MMN) is a motor syndrome that can closely mimic ALS. Indeed, MMN is described as an ALS-mimic in the Airlie House description of Charcot ALS (type 1a MND). MMN is therefore usually regarded as a condition that is separate from ALS. There is a suspicion, nonetheless, that there may be a relationship between the two conditions.

The clinical features of MMN consist of slowly progressive asymmetric weakness and wasting presenting between the third and fifth decade. EMG studies show conduction block away from sites of potential nerve entrapment.[37] Weakness is often confined to the territory of individual nerves. When there is multiple nerve involvement this may mimic global limb weakness. The upper limbs are first and often more severely affected.[37] Marked weakness in muscles without significant wasting, and depression of tendon reflexes are clinical clues to the diagnosis. However, in some cases, the separation of MMN from classical ALS may be blurred owing to the presence of brisk reflexes, muscle cramps, and diffuse fasciculations. Involvement of the tongue has been reported,[38] and then similarity to ALS is complete. A study of the long-term effects of intravenous immunoglobulin on MMN suggests that the clinical response is variable, and not always well sustained.[39] There is electrophysiological evidence of progression of conduction block and ongoing axonal degeneration in some cases.[39] Electrophysiologically, MMN must be distinguished from chronic inflammatory demyelinating polyradiculoneuropathy, in which sensory nerve action potentials are reduced or absent, and from Charcot ALS in which there is prominent proximal LMN involvement, including bulbar muscles, together with corticobulbar tract involvement.

Are motor neurones involved in MMN? There have been three pathological studies of MMN at autopsy.[40–42] In two of these there was axonal loss and demyelination in the anterior spinal roots with loss of anterior horn cells.[40,41] The third autopsy revealed patchy areas of demyelination in peripheral nerves at sites of conduction block.[42] However, in this third case, there was also loss of anterior horn cells and loss of axons in the corticospinal tracts — features that are consistent with a diagnosis of ALS. Therefore, clinically and pathologically, MMN appears to be a syndrome that overlaps with ALS. In noting this problem, Rowland[43] has suggested that MMN may represent focal involvement of peripheral nerves in ALS rather than a separate syndrome. This pathological evidence could also be interpreted as indicating that the diagnosis of MMN is not always secure. Nonetheless, although there remains diagnostic confusion regarding this syndrome, the diagnostic neurophysiological feature of conduction block in MMN, and the response to treatment with intravenous immunoglobulin, makes it most unlikely that all MMN is really ALS.

Familial ALS

Copper–zinc superoxide dismutase mutations and familial amyotrophic lateral sclerosis

Most families with known mutations of the copper–zinc superoxide dismutase (SOD1) gene have been identified by finding an index case with the core 'Charcot' ALS syndrome. The phenotype of familial ALS is sometimes variable. The term familial ALS has been used to describe these families.

Recognition of the role of SOD1 mutations in the pathogenesis of familial ALS has fundamentally altered clinical understanding of the ALS syndrome. SOD1-associated familial ALS is a clinical disorder in which phenotypic heterogeneity is only partially correlated with the underlying mutation. In 41 patients with SOD1 mutations from a group of 451 ALS patients screened in Scandinavia, the phenotype varied from cramps and myalgia without weakness or wasting to generalized wasting with tetraparesis and areflexia.[44] Some patients had focal limb weakness with generalized hyperreflexia. There was no phenotypic correlation with the five different SOD1 mutations found in these 41 patients, apart from a more rapidly progressive course in patients with the A4V mutation. In older studies of familial ALS, there is striking phenotypic heterogeneity including patients with features of ALS, PLS, and PMA, even within a family.[45] It is not known whether this variability reflects variable penetrance,[46] or gene–gene or gene–environment interaction, or both.[47] Cudkowicz and colleagues[48] reported absence of clinical and pathological involvement of the corticospinal tracts in 11 familial ALS patients with the A4V mutation. They proposed that the El Escorial criteria, which stress the requirement of UMN dysfunction for the diagnosis of ALS, should be modified to take cognizance of this aspect of familial ALS. Andersen and colleagues[44] have reviewed phenotypic heterogeneity in Scandinavian MND associated with SOD1 mutations. The striking heterogeneity reported in these patients with SOD1 mutations supports the view that ALS, PMA, PBP, and PLS form components of a neurological spectrum that reflects diseased motor neurones in the cortex and spinal cord,[49] a concept foreshadowed by Brain's inclusive preference for the term MND rather than ALS.

Kennedy's syndrome (X-linked spinobulbar neuronopathy)

Kennedy's syndrome is a distinct, familial, X-linked disorder characterized by progressive weakness and wasting in the proximal muscles of upper limbs and by bulbar palsy.[50] There is often a long-standing history of muscle cramps preceding the onset of weakness in the fifth decade. The presence of gynaecomastia, postural tremor of the upper limbs, perioral fasciculations, invariable involvement of the tongue, and sensory impairment in the lower limbs are clues to the diagnosis. However, in some patients these features may be subtle. In many cases there is no family history of this disorder.

A mutation in the coding region of the androgen-receptor gene results in variable increase in the number of cytosine–adenine–guanine (CAG) tandem repeats at this site.[51] This can be detected by a polymerase chain reaction test performed on peripheral blood leukocyte DNA.

Isolated patients with DNA-proven Kennedy's syndrome have had UMN signs.[52] One reported case with Kennedy's syndrome had cognitive impairment; another had corticospinal tract degeneration at autopsy, respectively.[53] In one study, 2% of patients diagnosed with MND were found to carry the characteristic Kennedy trinucleotide repeat expansion.[54] Therefore, at times Kennedy's syndrome can closely mimic ALS, and it probably deserves classification, at least in overlap, with the motor neurone diseases.

Juvenile ALS

Juvenile ALS is a hereditary disorder that presents in the second or third decade with a combination of UMN and LMN features.[55] Bulbar involvement is frequent. The disorder is slowly progressive, and survival over a few decades is usual. In Tunisia, recessively inherited juvenile ALS has been mapped to chromosome 2q33–35 in some families[56] and to chromosome 15q12–21 in others.[57] A dominantly inherited 11-generation pedigree of juvenile ALS in the USA, with an ancestry traced back to 17th-century England, has been mapped to chromosome 9q34.[58] The clinical features of this pedigree are similar to those of the Tunisian families. The three recognized syndromes may be classified as juvenile ALS 1, 2, and 3.

Transgenic mouse studies and ALS

Transgenic mice with the A4V, G93A, G37R, G85R, and G86R SOD1 mutations develop motor neurone degeneration.[59,60] In the G93A SOD1 transgenic mouse, as in the human disease, there is a prominent accumulation of neurofilaments, accompanied by slowed axonal transport of neurofilaments and other cytoskeletal proteins in the ventral root axons.[61] In human ALS, abnormalities of anterograde and retrograde fast axonal transport were described by Breuer and colleagues.[62] This is consistent with the accumulation of axonal spheroids in motor axons in the spinal cord and ventral roots in ALS.[63,64]

Transgenic mice that overexpress either the murine neurofilament light subunit[65] or the human neurofilament heavy subunit[66] develop a phenotype similar to human MND. In another model, codon 394 of the mouse neurofilament gene was mutated, introducing a leucine-to-proline substitution that disrupts neurofilament assembly. The mice developed PMA.[67] While these transgenic mouse models confirm the suspicion that disruption of neurofilament assembly and transport plays an important role in the pathogenesis of ALS, the exact role is unknown.

Classification of ALS and related syndromes

A classification of ALS has been proposed (*Table 1.6*) that recognizes phenotypic variability but gives primacy to the several underlying acquired or genetic pathogenic processes. As these pathogenic processes become better understood, this classification of ALS syndromes can evolve. Similarly, current understanding of spinocerebellar ataxias,[68,69] limb girdle muscular dystrophies,[70] and hereditary motor–sensory neuropathies[71] has led to a classification based on gene mutation and other causative mechanisms. This approach to classification[72] recognizes clinical heterogeneity within particular causations, whether genetic or acquired. Charcot ALS itself is a syndrome with varying combinations of UMN and LMN dysfunction. Phenotypic heterogeneity is a recognized feature of both sporadic and familial MND syndromes.

For the present, specific disorders from geographically distinct parts of the world are separately designated (see *Table 1.6*). When their pathogenesis is elucidated they can be reclassified. Grouping these different clinical disorders under the overall heading of MND, while retaining the individual nomenclature, emphasizes the insight that one disorder may provide for others. This is exemplified by advances in understanding of pathogenic mechanisms and phenotypic variability in familial ALS through the study of SOD1 mutations and neurofilament abnormalities. Genetic factors may modulate or predispose to a particular phenotypic expression of these various disorders of the motor neurone. This has implications for therapies and clinical trials. The classification serves to unify the nomenclature of distinct disorders of the motor neurone described in different regions of the world.

Sporadic ALS syndromes
Sporadic ALS syndrome 1 (a) — Charcot ALS
Sporadic ALS syndrome 1 (b) — Progressive muscular atrophy*
Sporadic ALS syndrome 1 (c) — Progressive bulbar palsy
Sporadic ALS syndrome 1 (d) — Primary lateral sclerosis
Sporadic ALS syndrome 1 (e) — Sporadic ALS with dementia and/or extrapyramidal signs
Sporadic ALS syndrome 2 — Paraneoplastic ALS
Sporadic ALS syndrome 3 — Madras ALS
Sporadic ALS syndrome 4 — Monomelic amyotrophy
Sporadic ALS syndrome 5 — Sporadic ALS with NF gene mutations or deletions
Sporadic ALS syndrome 6 — Sporadic Guam ALS

Familial ALS syndromes
Familial ALS syndrome 1 — ALS linked to chromosome 21 (SOD1): heterogeneous phenotype
Familial ALS syndrome 2 — ALS linked to chromosome 2 (Tunisian, recessive)
Familial ALS syndrome 3 — Autosomal dominant adult ALS not linked to chromosome 21
Familial ALS syndrome 4 — Juvenile ALS linked to chromosome 9
Familial ALS syndrome 5 — ALS linked to chromosome 15 (Tunisian recessive)
Familial ALS syndrome 6 — Familial Guam ALS

---

* PMA associated with SOD1 mutation is classified as FALS 1.
SOD1, copper–zinc super oxide dismutase; NF, neurofilament.

Table 1.6
Classification of ALS syndromes.

The rate of progression of Charcot ALS is quite variable, ranging from a few weeks to many years. This variability of progression is also a feature of the familial motor neurone syndromes, including those associated with SOD1 and neurofilament mutations. The atypical ALS syndromes, however, are generally only slowly progressive. In some, arrest of the disease has been reported, as in Madras MND. The factors modulating progression are unknown, but may be important in understanding Charcot ALS. It appears probable that these syndromes result from the interaction of several different factors, some causative or predisposing to the disease, and others related to phenotypic expression and rate of progression.

The phenotype of sporadic Charcot ALS

ALS is a relentlessly progressive, invariably fatal disease of the nervous system. It is characterized by degeneration of the UMNs and LMNs in the brain and spinal cord. There is neurogenic atrophy of muscle. The disorder is often asymmetrical at its onset, and it may be quite focal. Death results from ventilatory failure. The varying extent and localization of involvement of the motor system results in differing clinical features, but ultimately, as the disorder progresses, the clinical expression of the disease is rather uniform, with extreme muscular wasting and spasticity. In the later stages of the disease there may be evidence of involvement of extrapyramidal pathways, with parkinsonian features.[73] Dementia may develop in about 10% of cases, with a characteristic frontal affect.[74] Pathological studies have revealed far more widespread degeneration of pathways in the brain than expected clinically, including spinocerebellar tract involvement and degeneration of subcortical white matter. There may be degeneration of cortical cells in the frontal lobes, the temporal lobes, and even parts of the sensory cortex.[75]

The clinical features depend on the variable permutations of the combination of LMN and UMN involvement, and these vary not only according to the pattern of onset in any particular patient but also in relation to the stage of the disease. LMN involvement causes weakness and fatigue, with progressive muscular atrophy, fasciculation and fibrillation, reduced muscle tone, and absence of tendon reflexes. UMN involvement causes weakness, inco-ordination, stiffness and slowing of movement, with spasticity, increased tendon reflexes, clonus, and extensor plantar responses. These features are present in varying combinations in the different body segments or regions.

Asymmetric weakness and atrophy

The commonest presentation of ALS is with asymmetric distal weakness and atrophy. The patient presents with a history of unexpected tripping, difficulty negotiating curbs, dragging of a foot, and ultimately more diffuse weakness of the leg. Difficulty with buttoning clothes, turning keys in doors, picking up objects, twisting off jar caps, or simply poor co-ordination while performing fine move-

ments are the symptoms of involvement of the upper limbs. Occasionally, proximal arm muscles may be involved early in the illness, leading to difficulty with sustaining a heavy workload, with walking or running, or with climbing stairs.

Overt symptomatic weakness, and the objective demonstration of loss of strength requires considerable loss of functioning motor neurones, since compensatory reinnervation results in the maintenance of available innervated muscle fibres in the partially denervated muscle, although with enlargement of the surviving motor units. Weakness may not be detected by manual muscle testing until 50% of motor neurones have been lost.[76] However, in muscle strength testing, several additional variables are important. Of these, mood, affect, patient motivation, and general level of fatigue are especially important.[77] Despite weakness and atrophy there is usually relatively good preservation of repetitive co-ordinated movements, probably because sensory feedback is normal. However, the co-existence of spasticity, often a more severe problem than at first appreciated in ALS, results in slowness and inco-ordination of fine movement and in abnormal postures.

Some patients note otherwise asymptomatic wasting of the muscles of the dorsum of the hand. Many complain of twitching of muscles or muscle shaking (especially on direct questioning). These symptoms reflect the presence of fasciculations, a sign almost invariably noted in ALS though not specific to the disorder. Cramps or spasms are frequent, as in other denervating diseases. Myoclonus is very rare in ALS.

Bulbar onset

Bulbar features develop during the course of the disease, but may be a presenting feature, especially in middle-aged women with ALS; in

Study	Rosati et al. 1977[82]	Gubbay et al. 1985[80]	Caroscio et al. 1984[79]	Li et al. 1990[92]	Brooks et al. 1994[83]
Patients (n)	668	318	269	560	702
Bulbar onset (%)	19	22	25	19	22
Limb onset (%)	81	63	68	81	78
One arm (%)	41	11	27	44	30
Two arms (%)		9	5		9
One leg (%)	40	12	23	37	25
Two legs (%)		20	13		6
Arm and leg (%)		4			4

Table 1.7
Early symptoms in ALS.

older women, as in men, limb or axial involvement is more common. Bulbar involvement leads to difficulty speaking and swallowing, and is often closely correlated with weakened respiratory muscles and a reduced forced vital capacity. Thus, bulbar involvement carries a poor prognosis, and life expectancy in patients with bulbar ALS is less than in those who present with limb onset. The cough is weakened and the ability to sniff vigorously, a sensitive bedside test of diaphragmatic function, is reduced. Fasciculation of the tongue is a clinical sign with high diagnostic probability for ALS.[78]

Patients with predominant upper limb or bulbar involvement often have weak respiratory muscles. This results in breathlessness on minimal exertion, and especially when there is diaphragmatic weakness on lying supine. Poor nocturnal sleep, excessive daytime sleepiness, headaches on awakening, and excessive nocturnal sweating are features of early respiratory failure. Involvement of the respiratory musculature is often accompanied by activation of the accessory muscles of respiration

during normal breathing, poor cough, and an abnormal sniff test on neurological assessment. This may progress to frank respiratory failure requiring ventilatory assistance. Most patients with ALS suffer from painful muscle cramps and fatigue during the course of the illness.

Progression

The recognition of progression during the natural history of the disorder is a major component of current diagnostic criteria. In the absence of a surrogate marker for ALS this is an essential feature of the disease.[13] The pattern of onset has been much studied (*Table 1.7*). Limb onset is found in 65–80% of cases, and bulbar onset is found in 20–25%. From the onset the disease spreads to other regions.[79-83] There is evidence from EMG, from clinical assessment, and from measurement of muscle strength that this spread occurs to contiguous muscle segments, so that those nearest to the site of presentation with weakness and wasting are the next to be involved. In clinical terms, the demonstration of progression requires the development of increasing weakness and wasting.[84] These features develop only when the pace of loss of functional motor units (denervation) exceeds the reinnervative capacity of remaining functional motor units.[85] Reinnervation in ALS is not as effective or as vigorous as in more chronic neurogenic disorders (e.g. Charcot–Marie–Tooth disease). The spread of the disease can be recognized subclinically by quantitative EMG studies, which show not only that some spinal segments are more severely affected but also that the disease is invariably generalized from the time of diagnosis, and that it does not present with restricted involvement of one region with consequent spread to other regions, but is a more generalized process.[86]

UMN *features*

Since the diagnosis of ALS requires the presence of both LMN and UMN features, upper motor involvement will be present in all definite cases. However, in some patients the disorder presents with predominantly LMN features. In its extreme form, this is PMA, a disorder that may not always evolve to the Charcot ALS syndrome. Similarly, patients with relatively restricted bulbar features, or with virtually pure UMN disorder — PLS — may be encountered. These syndromes are related to Charcot ALS but are best regarded as differing in their clinical features and also in their prognosis.[72] The outcome in these syndromes is less gloomy than in Charcot ALS.

Recognition of UMN involvement in a patient with predominant wasting is not easy. There may be so little muscle mass that the tendon reflexes are difficult to elicit. However, an elicitable tendon reflex in a very wasted muscle probably signifies the co-existence of an UMN lesion, since in a pure LMN lesion the tendon reflexes would be expected to be absent. In addition, the plantar response can usually be assessed, except when there is complete paralysis of flexor or extensor muscles acting around the foot and ankle, in which case the test is inevitably unreliable. Spasticity of the tongue is often very difficult to demonstrate satisfactorily.

Other features of Charcot ALS

Other important observations on the clinical features that have been much remarked over the years include the striking relative resistance of external ocular muscles to denervation during the course of the disease. However, in unusually long survivals, as in patients kept alive beyond the onset of ventilatory failure by positive pressure ventilation, slowing of eye movements, with eventual paralysis of gaze,[87] develops relatively frequently. In some patients with bulbar onset disease, slowing of ocular movements becomes obvious before there is striking involvement of spinal regions. Nuclear involvement of external ocular muscle function is less frequent. The external ocular muscles are normally hyperneurotized, with multiple end-plate zones and, as such, are quite unlike ordinary striated skeletal muscle fibres.

The striated urinary and anal sphincter muscles are also relatively spared until the late stages of the disease. These muscles are innervated by the Onuf nucleus, in the third sacral spinal segment.[88] This nucleus has a unique neuropil structure and an unusual synaptic arrangement that indicates a differing functional specialization;[89] this may be related to the continuous tonic contraction required of these muscles during life, not only in the waking state, but also during sleep. Similarly, the abductor muscle of the larynx and the cricopharyngeal sphincter muscles, which are also in a state of continuous tonic contraction, are also resistant to denervation in ALS. These muscles, in contrast, are differentially susceptible to denervation in progressive autonomic failure, causing incontinence and ventilatory stridor.

It is generally thought that the cervical segments are the most vulnerable in ALS,[85] a clinical opinion based on the obvious and disabling weakness of the distal hand and forearm and upper arm muscles so often found in the disease.[90] This opinion is not fully supported by careful quantitative studies in large series of cases, however, which suggest that involvement of the leg musculature is just as frequent and severe, although not so immediately evident to the patient as weakness and wasting in a hand.

Epidemiology

ALS occurs in about 1–3 people per 100,000 population per year. It has a prevalence of about 5–9 per 100,000, a figure directly dependent on the survival of those affected. There are thus about 20,000 people with ALS at any one time in the USA, and 28,000 in the European Union, about 5000 of whom are in the UK. These incidence figures are probably low estimates, but the prevalence figures are likely to be more accurate estimates. No significant variations in incidence or prevalence have been reported in the developed countries, apart from foci of related syndromes in the Kii peninsula of Japan and in Guam. There is controversy as to whether the disease is increasing in incidence or whether it is more readily diagnosed than in former years.[91,92] There is consensus that, in the past, the diagnosis was often not made in the elderly, but even so the disease appears to be less frequent in very aged cohorts than in the middle-aged population.[91] Clearly, diagnostic behaviour is important in assessing changes in incidence of a disease.[93]

Until recently, in the absence of any effective treatment for ALS, there was no imperative to achieve diagnosis at any stage of its progressive course. The advent of modern imaging and of improved clinical neurophysiological assessment has enabled other conditions, such as foramen magnum neoplasms, Chiari malformation, multiple sclerosis, and motor neuropathies, to be recognized with certainty, thus ensuring that the diagnosis of ALS is itself more reliable than in the past. Most epidemiological studies of the disease have relied on coded hospital diagnostic data or on death certificates. There are well-known sources of error in both these data sets that are likely to lead to under-ascertainment. The diagnostic accuracy of death certificates in relation to ALS has been estimated at 90%, with a 6% risk of false-positive diagnosis.[94] These figures refer to cases submitted to a Scottish ALS case register. In a study in New York it was found that an incorrect diagnosis was made initially in 27% of cases during the process of diagnostic work-up.[95] These figures seem surprising to neurologists in clinical practice, but they illustrate the difficulty in establishing a firm diagnosis in a condition for which there is no absolute diagnostic test available.[96] In the early stages of the disease diagnosis may be particularly difficult to establish with certainty, but it is at this early stage that therapeutic intervention is most likely to be effective.

The work of Neilson and colleagues,[97] which involved a mathematical analysis of the epidemiological data from a number of different countries, is important in understanding the significance of these data. Neilson used a statistical technique derived form life insurance analysis (the Gompertzian analysis), which allows cohorts of data to be followed in a life model. The analysis seems to establish that, in each generation, there is a cohort of people who are susceptible to develop ALS. As other causes of death, such as myocardial

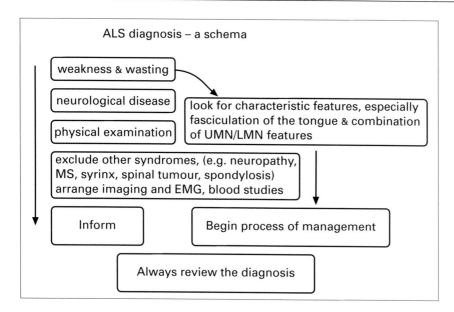

ALS diagnosis – a schema

weakness & wasting

neurological disease

physical examination

look for characteristic features, especially fasciculation of the tongue & combination of UMN/LMN features

exclude other syndromes, (e.g. neuropathy, MS, syrinx, spinal tumour, spondylosis) arrange imaging and EMG, blood studies

Inform

Begin process of management

Always review the diagnosis

Figure 1.1
Investigative approach to a patient with suspected motor neuron disease.

infarction and cancer, decrease in frequency in a population, therefore, so deaths from ALS will become more frequent among this susceptible cohort, since more of the cohort will have survived to the appropriate age to develop the disease. ALS will, therefore, become more common in developed countries as other fatal diseases come under better control. An increasing incidence of ALS does not, therefore, necessarily imply that an exposure, for example, to an exogenous toxin, is causing more mortality from this disease in the population at risk.

Features at onset of Charcot ALS

Recognition of the earliest features of ALS is dependent on the ability to make an early diagnosis (*Fig. 1.1*). In making an earlier diagnosis of ALS, the absence of overt sensory dysfunction, of sphincter dysfunction and of oculomotor dysfunction is frequently used to distinguish ALS from other disorders of the lower motor neurone and, conversely, to raise

suspicion of this diagnosis. Imaging and electrophysiology are important tools in the search for alternative diagnoses at this stage of the disease.[98]

ALS begins (*Table 1.7*) with limb involvement in 65–80% of patients, while bulbar onset is noted in 20–25%.[99–101] The disease invariably progresses with time, and symptoms and signs spread to involve contiguous body parts. EMG changes may antedate clinical weakness and atrophy, suggesting that symptom accrual is a function of the balance between denervation and reinnervation in a region after initiation of the disease process.[102]

The spread of the disease process to contiguous spinal segments within the spinal cord results in clinical and electrophysiological evidence of involvement of muscles within the corresponding spinal regions. This may sometimes cause diagnostic confusion with other diseases, particularly when root involvement is suspected. This pattern of presentation must be explicable by the pathophysiological mechanism of the disease process, and it could be consistent with an excitotoxic mechanism.

Within individual spinal segments, anterior horn cell loss is random.[90] The progressive loss of anterior horn cells results in increasing disability, ultimately leading to a bed-bound state. In contrast to other paralysing neurological conditions, bedsores are rare in ALS, in spite of the patient being bed-bound. Perhaps this is because sensation is spared in ALS; it has also been ascribed to a characteristic of the collagen in the skin of people with ALS. The usual course of ALS is relentlessly progressive, with death by 3 years in 50% of patients.[103]

Unusual or atypical features in Charcot ALS

A small proportion of patients with otherwise typical ALS may develop personality and behavioural changes. Cognitive assessment reveals impairment in planning ability, execution of strategies and ability to perform complex sequential tasks, occasionally associated with frontal lobe release signs.[74,75] Although dementia is not a primary feature of ALS, these features reflect the involvement of the frontal lobes in the disease process,[104,105] and this cortical involvement is almost invariable in autopsy series even when there is no overt clinical manifestation (see Chapter 5). These features are more common in patients with bulbar involvement.[104]

Rarely, some patients exhibit parkinsonian features in addition to the characteristic motor signs of ALS.[106] A variant of this feature is the occurrence of other extrapyramidal manifestations (e.g. a propensity for backward falls, even in the early stages of the disease, implying impairment of postural reflexes from basal ganglia involvement).[73]

Progressive bulbar palsy

PBP is a progressive disorder that presents with bulbar dysfunction caused by destruction of motor neurones in the brainstem. Usually this syndrome includes evidence of upper motor neurone dysfunction. Historically, it has been considered a bulbar form of ALS–MND, since it usually progresses to a clinical disorder that in all respects resembles the ALS syndrome. Clinically, PBP has to be differentiated from conditions with a similar initial presentation (e.g. subcortical arteriosclerotic leukoencephalopathy (Binswanger's disease, leukoariosis), Steele–Richardson–Olszewski syndrome (progressive supranuclear palsy), foramen magnum tumours, clivus chordomas, and polyneuritis cranialis.

Progressive muscular atrophy

PMA refers to MND presenting with weakness and wasting of muscles of the limbs and of trunk muscles, without evidence of UMN dysfunction. This condition may mimic adult-onset, proximal spinal muscular atrophy (SMA). The more rapid progression, and the later development of brisk reflexes may assist in differentiating PMA from SMA, since in SMA the tendon reflexes are usually reduced and the plantar responses are always flexor. The genetic background and variable phenotype of many cases of PMA is discussed above.

Primary lateral sclerosis

PLS typically presents with a slowly progressive spastic gait disorder. Over months or years, the upper limbs are involved and in some a pseudobulbar syndrome develops. Hyperreflexia and Babinski and Hoffman

Clinical
1. Insidious onset of spastic paraparesis, usually beginning in lower extremities but occasionally bulbar or the upper extremities
2. Adult onset, usually fifth decade or later
3. Absence of family history
4. Gradually progressive course (i.e. not step-like)
5. Duration >3 years
6. Clinical findings limited to those associated with corticospinal dysfunction
7. Symmetrical distribution, ultimately developing severe spastic spinobulbar paresis

Laboratory
1. Normal serum chemistry, including normal vitamin B12 levels
2. Negative serologic tests for syphilis (in endemic areas, negative Lyme and human T-cell leukaemia virus-1 serology)
3. Normal cerebrospinal fluid parameters, including absence of oligoclonal bands
4. Absent denervation potentials on EMG or, at most, occasional fibrillation and increased insertional activity in a few muscles (late and minor)
5. Absence of compressive lesions of cervical spine or foramen magnum
6. Absence of high T2 signal lesions on magnetic resonance imaging as seen in multiple sclerosis

Additionally suggestive of primary lateral sclerosis
1. Preserved bladder function
2. Absent or very prolonged latency on cortical motor-evoked response in the presence of normal peripheral stimulus-evoked compound muscle action potentials
3. Focal atrophy of the precentral gyrus on magnetic resonance imaging
4. Decreased glucose consumption in pericentral region on positron emission tomography scanning

Adapted from Pringle et al., 1992.[107]

Table 1.8
Proposed diagnostic criteria for primary lateral sclerosis.

signs are characteristic features, while LMN dysfunction and sphincter dysfunction are absent in the initial stages, although they may develop later.[107] The clinical course and survival are much longer than ALS of Charcot type. Diagnostic criteria have been suggested (*Table 1.8*); these are based on clinical, radiological, and pathological features.[36,107] PLS may be a paraneoplastic manifestation of breast carcinoma.[30]

PLS is a very rare disorder; Pringle and colleagues[107] were able to review only 23 published cases in 1992. Part of the nosological problem with PLS as a diagnosis is that, if LMN features develop, the diagnosis would be changed to ALS. The nosology of this syndrome and its relation to other pure, progressive corticospinal disorders has been reviewed by Swash and colleagues.[34,108]

Diagnosis in clinical practice

Traditionally, the diagnosis of ALS has been substantiated by electrophysiological studies utilizing Lambert's criteria.[109] These criteria were subsequently modified by the exclusion of patients with motor conduction block[110] and recently confirmed in the consensus criteria arising from the conference at Airlie House (see above). These EMG signs of LMN dysfunction should be found in at least two of the four body regions: bulbar or cranial, cervical, thoracic, and lumbosacral.

Disorders that could be mistaken for ALS

Before making a diagnosis of ALS, it is vital to ensure that syndromes that may mimic ALS have been ruled out since these have different prognoses, and some are treatable. The following conditions should be considered in the differential diagnosis of ALS (see *Table 1.4*).

Spinal muscular atrophy

Adult-onset proximal SMA may mimic progressive muscular atrophy in its presentation, with an asymmetric, limb-restricted weakness and wasting, without UMN signs.[111] Bulbar muscles are rarely affected. SMA is usually proximal, but distal-onset SMA syndromes are recognized.[112] Late-onset SMA progresses only slowly, and survival is much longer than classical MND. Autosomal-recessive inheritance may be observed in familial cases, although sporadic cases are more common. It is often difficult to distinguish sporadic adult-onset proximal SMA from PMA. The clinical features of the two can be identical, except for a more rapid rate of progress in PMA. Most SMA syndromes are linked to a mutation on chromosome 5q.13.[113]

Kennedy's syndrome

Bulbospinal neuronopathy is an X-linked recessive disorder that is characterized by the onset of weakness and wasting in the girdle muscles in men aged 40–50 years.[50] The tongue is almost always involved. Onset is preceded by the presence of arm tremors, muscle cramps, and generalized fasciculations in the previous 10–15 years. Perioral fasciculations, wasting of the tongue, and bulbar dysfunction develop. Gynaecomastia, testicular atrophy with azoospermia and diabetes mellitus are noted in some patients. The progress of the disease is slow, and again disability is not severe. Neurophysiological evaluation reveals reduced or absent sensory nerve action potentials besides widespread chronic partial denervation with evidence of reinnervation on EMG. A mutation in the coding region of the androgen-receptor gene results in variable increase in the number of cytosine–adenine–guanine tandem repeats at this site.[51] This can be detected by a polymerase chain reaction test performed on peripheral blood leukocyte DNA.

Radiation myelopathy

An LMN syndrome has been reported 3 months to 13 years after radiation to the para-aortic spinal region for malignant testicular and lymphomatous tumours.[114] The syndrome occurred when the radiation dosage exceeded 4000 rads. Asymmetric weakness, atrophy, fasciculations, cramps, and areflexia were cardinal features. Sensory, sphincter, and pyramidal tract involvement was not observed. The clinical abnormalities progressed over 1–2 years before stabilizing. Magnetic resonance imaging studies of the spinal cord were normal. Sensory, and motor nerve conduction studies were normal, as were somatosensory evoked responses. Needle EMG showed evidence of chronic partial denervation with reinnervation in affected muscles and some clinically unaffected muscles. This syndrome resulted from an endothelial vasculopathy of the spinal cord leading to anterior horn cell degeneration. There is an extensive older literature related to radiation therapy for lung, breast, oral, and maxillo-facial cancer, but the syndrome is rare in modern oncologic practice.

Thyroid disorders

ALS-like syndromes have been described in patients with thyrotoxicosis. Separating these syndromes from classical ALS may be difficult since both exhibit diffuse fasciculations, bulbar dysfunction, UMN as well as LMN dysfunction, and weight loss. The syndrome may result from a combination of myelopathy, myopathy, and motor neuropathy caused by thyrotoxicosis as resolution of the symptoms and signs follows treatment of the thyroid disorder.[115] The presence of exophthalmos and postural tremor of the outstretched hands are useful clinical clues to the underlying condition. The diagnosis is established by performing thyroid function tests.

Parathyroid disorders and osteomalacia

Up to 80% of patients with primary hyperparathyroidism, 60% of patients with secondary hyperparathyroidism, and most patients with hypophosphataemic osteomalacia develop pelvifemoral weakness and wasting. Bone pain is characteristically present but the presence of fasciculations, hyperreflexia, and Babinski signs may cause confusion with ALS.[116] The EMG may show predominantly neurogenic features but myopathic features may also be present, especially in osteomalacia.[116–118] Experimental osteomalacia causes a myopathy.[119] Treatment of hypophosphataemia with oral phosphate replacement and removal of adenomatous parathyroids results in reversal of this ALS-like disorder.

Multifocal motor neuropathy

In MMN, there is a slowly progressive asymmetric weakness and wasting, usually presenting between the third and fifth decades. Progression is very slow. Weakness is found in the territory of individual nerves but, with multiple nerve involvement, this may mimic global limb weakness. The upper limbs are more frequently and more severely affected.[37] Weakness may be marked, without significant wasting; depression of tendon reflexes is a clinical clue to the diagnosis. Sometimes, brisk reflexes, muscle cramps, and diffuse fasciculations may occur.[120] The tongue is only exceptionally involved.[38] MMN differs from chronic inflammatory demyelinating polyradiculopathy, with which there are many similarities, by the absence of abnormalities in sensory nerve conduction parameters.

The diagnosis depends on the finding of conduction block at sites away from potential entrapment sites. The value of GM_1 IgM antibodies in the diagnosis is doubtful. A favourable response to intravenous cyclophosphamide[121] or immunoglobulin therapy[122] is important in establishing the diagnosis, but the long-term response is unknown.

Toxic exposures

Lead

Acute intoxication from lead produces an encephalopathy in children and adults, while chronic exposure leads to behavioural disturbances and a motor neuropathy. Heavy and prolonged exposure to lead has also been associated with a motor disorder characterized by marked weakness and atrophy beginning in the arms, with, fasciculations, bulbar dysfunction, hyperreflexia, spasticity, and Babinski signs.[123,124] Only a history of exposure to lead, rather slow progression of events, and a response to chelation therapy can differentiate this disorder from classical ALS. Anorexia, abdominal pain, constipation, and a blue lead-line in the gums may be clues to the diagnosis. Laboratory features include anaemia, basophilic stippling of erythrocytes, and increased blood and urinary lead levels.

Mercury

Workers involved in the manufacture of electrical equipment, paint, paper, pulp, cosmetics, and nuclear devices may occasionally suffer from accidental mercury intoxication. This produces myalgia, weight loss, irritability, photophobia, abdominal pain, tremors, behavioural changes, and ataxia.[125] Rarely, brief but significant exposure to mercury may produce a rapid development of an ALS-like disorder with muscle atrophy, fasciculations, and hyperreflexia.[126] The rapid evolution and the presence of other systemic symptoms with swollen gums and blue lines are indicative of the disorder.

Organophosphates and Gulf War syndrome

An alleged increased risk of ALS among Gulf War veterans, or in people surviving exposure to organophosphorus insecticides, either in self-poisoning or lower dose exposure in agricultural work, has not been substantiated in epidemiological studies.[127,128] Some of these patients have a sensorimotor neuropathy related to the exposure.

Post-poliomyelitis syndrome

Post-poliomyelitis syndrome (post-polio amyotrophy) is the term applied to new onset of muscle weakness or to fatigue decades after recovery from acute poliomyelitis. Progressive weakness, atrophy, and fasciculation simulates MND.[129] The previous history of poliomyelitis, absence of UMN signs, slow rate of progression, the presence of pain without demonstrable cause, and the occurrence of new amyotrophy at the border zone of prior

paralysis where regeneration might predominate should all raise the suspicion of post-polio amyotrophy.

Hexosaminidase deficiency

An ALS-like syndrome may be inherited in an autosomal-recessive manner in patients of Ashkenazi Jewish descent. Onset of clinical features of a combination of UMN and LMN dysfunction in the third to fifth decade is associated with the variable presence of ataxia, stuttering, dementia, psychosis, or polyneuropathy. In some instances, a family history of Tay–Sachs disease is obtained. The disorder is caused by absence of the lysosomal hydrolase enzyme N-acetyl-hexosaminidase A, the activity of which can be measured in the serum, leukocytes, and cultured fibroblasts.[130] The finding of low activity of this enzyme in patients and in asymptomatic relatives is of relevance for establishing the diagnosis and for genetic counselling.

Autoimmune disorders

An ALS- and PLS-like syndrome has been described in patients with primary Sjögren's syndrome.[131] Some of these patients stabilize or improve after institution of corticosteroid therapy. The mechanisms underlying the neurological manifestations are unknown, but it is likely this syndrome is an autoimmune neuropathy rather than ALS.

Investigations when ALS is suspected

A detailed history and meticulous neurological assessment lay the foundation for relevant investigations in a patient with suspected ALS. Vigilance for the presence of atypical features (e.g. mode of onset, age, rate of progression, presence of associated systemic or other neurological features, and the presence of pure syndromes) assists the recognition of ALS-mimic syndromes. Every patient with suspected ALS should undergo baseline liver function tests since these may be altered by riluzole, currently the standard therapy for ALS. Haematological studies, including an erythrocyte sedimentation rate, are mandatory, since lymphoproliferative disorders masquerading as MND may be unmasked by abnormal results of these investigations. Elevated proteins or an abnormal cell count in the cerebrospinal fluid suggests causes other than ALS.

Imaging is an essential investigation to rule out other conditions. Magnetic resonance imaging of the brain and spinal cord is usually normal in ALS–MND except for the detection of occasional T2-weighted hyperintensities in the course of the corticospinal tracts and atrophy of the precentral gyrus on use of high-strength magnetic coils. Abnormal results on magnetic resonance imaging help in excluding conditions mimicking ALS in the early stages.

Clinical neurophysiological assessment is required in all cases. The investigation should not be restricted to body parts in which there is obvious abnormality clinically (*Table 1.9*). Sensory and motor nerve conduction studies are usually normal in ALS, except for occasional decrease in amplitudes of distal CMAPs. Concentric needle EMG reveals changes of chronic partial denervation with reinnervation in a widespread distribution, accompanied by diffuse fasciculations. The motor unit potentials are reduced in number and increased in amplitude and duration. On maximal voluntary activation the recruitment pattern is reduced. The distribution of these changes must be beyond the anatomical territories of peripheral nerves and nerve roots for the diagnosis of ALS to be corroborated. At least two proximal and two distal muscles in all four limbs should be sampled on concentric needle EMG. The presence of fasciculations in the tongue, either clinically or on EMG, has a high specificity for the diagnosis of ALS, especially when other clinical features are consistent.

The presence of prolonged F-wave responses, dispersion of CMAPs, conduction block, and slowing of motor conduction velocities are hallmarks of MMN. The presence of marked sensory dysfunction on sensory nerve conduction studies differentiates Kennedy's syndrome from MND.

Additional investigations may be performed on the basis of a diagnostic algorithm (see *Fig. 1.1*).

Early diagnosis

The revised Airlie House–El Escorial criteria[13] are useful in the diagnosis of the classical Charcot ALS syndrome. However, by definition, using these criteria a patient would probably have fairly advanced biological disease at the time of diagnosis. Early in the illness, focal weakness or atrophy and non-specific symptoms such as fatigue, weight loss, and fasciculations may occur. At this stage, a diagnosis of lumbar or cervical radiculopathy, compression palsy of a peripheral nerve, or brachial or lumbosacral plexus lesion is often considered. At this early stage, no specific biological test or investigation is available to establish the diagnosis of ALS. There is an imperative need to develop a test or criteria for the early diagnosis of ALS. The measurement of threshold electrotonus failed to sustain the initial promise as one such investigative technique.[132] Early diagnosis is increasingly important in the current era of emerging treatments. A schema to facilitate the diagnostic process is shown in *Fig. 1.1*.

Signs of active denervation
Fibrillation potentials and positive sharp waves

Fasciculations

Signs of chronic partial denervation
Motor unit potentials of increased duration and amplitude with high proportion of polyphasic potentials
Reduced interference pattern, usually with high firing rates (e.g. higher than 10 Hz)
Unstable motor unit potentials
Chronic partial denervation could also be demonstrated by other techniques (e.g. single-fibre EMG, macro-EMG, turns-amplitude analysis, quantitative motor unit potential analysis, and MUNE)

Features compatible with UMN involvement
Up to 30% increase in central motor conduction time
Low firing rates of motor unit potentials on effort

Features suggesting other disease processes
Evidence of motor conduction block
Motor conduction velocity lower than 70% of lower limit of normal
Distal motor latency greater than 30% of upper limit of normal
Abnormal sensory nerve conduction studies, except in the presence of co-existing entrapment syndromes or other peripheral nerve disease
F-wave or H-reflex latencies more than 30% greater than normal
Motor unit potential decrement greater than 20% on repetitive stimulation
Somatosensory-evoked potential latency greater than 20% normal
Abnormalities in autonomic function or electronystagmography
Full motor unit potential interference pattern in a clinically weak muscle

---

MUNE, motor unit number estimate.

Table 1.9
Electrophysiological evidence in the diagnosis of ALS (Airlie House Criteria, 1999).

Principles of clinical management

ALS is a progressive disorder that invariably results in death. Having made the diagnosis, the treating physician must convey the news truthfully to the patient and then help him or her cope with disability, the prospect of death, and the accompanying human fears and frustrations. Good communication skills, honesty, and empathy for the patient's plight pave the way for a balanced relationship between patient and physician. Symptomatic management includes the use of antispasticity agents, anticramping agents, antidepressants, drying agents for sialorrhoea, respiratory agents, and vaccines against influenza and pneumococcus. A multidisciplinary approach has to be formulated to plan nutritional management and physical rehabilitation (see later chapters in this volume). Though numerous potential therapies have been tested in extensive and expensive trials, none has been found to have a curative effect.

In two large, randomized, double-blind, placebo-controlled trials, the antiglutamate agent riluzole has been shown to improve tracheostomy-free survival when compared with placebo.[133,134] A Cox proportional hazards analysis was used to adjust for bad prognostic features such as bulbar onset, reduced vital capacity, rapid progression, and advanced disease.[135] This result has generated enthusiasm and support in pursuing research in quest of a cure for this disorder. However, conducting clinical trials for putative treatments for ALS is fraught with numerous difficulties and dilemmas that require further consideration. A major current clinical problem is early diagnosis.

References

1. Aran FA. Récherches sur une maladie non encore décrite du système musculaire (atrophie musculaire progressive). *Arch Gen Med* 1850; **24**: 5–35, 172–214.
2. Duchenne de Boulogne GBA. Recherches faites à l'orde des galvanisine sur l'état de la contractilité et de la sensibilité électromusculaires dans les paralysies des membres supérieurs. *C R Acad Sci (Paris)* 1849; **29**: 667.
3. Cruveilhier J. Sur la paralysie musculaire, progressive, atrophique. *Bull Acad Med (Paris)* 1852–1853; **18**: 490–546.
4. Luys JB. Atrophie musculaire progressive. Lésions histologiques de la substance grise de la moelle épinière. *Gaz Med (Paris)* 1860; **15**: 505.
5. Charcot JM, Joffroy A. Deux cas d'atrophie musculaire progressive avec lésions de la substance grise et des faisceaux antéro-latéraux de la moelle épinière. *Arch Physiol Neurol Path* 1869; **2**: 744.
6. Erb WH. Dystrophia muscularis progressiva: klinische und pathologisch-anatomische Studien. *Dtsch Nervenheil* 1891; **1**: 13–94.
7. Duchenne de Boulogne GBA. Paralysie musculaire progressive de la langue, du voile du palais et des lèvres: affection non encore décrite comme espèce morbide distincte. *Arch Gen Med* 1860; **16**: 283, 431.
8. Spiller WG. Primary degeneration of the pyramidal tracts: a study of eight cases with necropsy. *Univ Penn Med Bull* 1904; **17**: 390–395.
9. Brain WR. *Diseases of the Nervous System* 6th edn. Oxford: Oxford University Press, 1962.
10. Rowland LP. Diverse forms of motor neuron disease. In: Rowland LP, ed. *Human Motor Neuron Diseases*. New York: Raven Press, 1982, 1–13.
11. Swash M, Scholtz CL, Vowles G et al. Selective and asymmetric vulnerability of corticospinal and spinocerebellar tracts in motor neuron disease. *J Neurol Neurosurg Psychiatry* 1988; **42**: 179–183.
12. World Federation of Neurology Research Committee on Neuromuscular Diseases and SubCommittee on Motor Neuron Diseases/Amyotrophic Lateral Sclerosis. El Escorial criteria for the diagnosis of amyotrophic lateral sclerosis. *J Neurol Sci* 1994; **124 (suppl)**: 96–107.
13. Brooks BR, Miller RG, Swash M, Munsat TL. Airlie House. Revised criteria for the diagnosis of ALS. *J Neurol Sci* 1999; in press.
14. Meenakshisundaram E, Jagannathan K, Ramamurthi B. Clinical pattern of motor neuron disease seen in younger age groups in Madras. *Neurol India* 1970; **18**: 109.
15. Gourie-Devi M, Suresh TG. Madras pattern of motor neuron disease in South India. *J Neurol Neurosurg Psychiatry* 1988; **51**: 773–777.
16. Wadia PN, Bhatt MH, Misra VP. Clinical neurophysiological examination of deafness associated with juvenile motor neurone disease. *J Neurol Sci* 1987; **78**: 29–33.
17. Jagannathan K, Kumaresan G. Madras pattern of motor neuron disease. In: Gourie-Devi M, ed. *Motor Neurone Disease*. New Delhi, Oxford: IBH, 1987, 191–194.
18. Hirayama K, Tomonaga M, Kitano K et al. Focal cervical poliopathy causing juvenile muscular atrophy of distal upper extremity: a pathological study. *J Neurol Neurosurg Psychiatry* 1987; **50**: 285–290.
19. Singh N, Sachdev KK, Susheela AK. Juvenile muscular atrophy localized to arms. *Arch Neurol* 1980; **37**: 297–299.

20. Gourie-Devi M, Suresh TG, Shankar SK. Monomelic amyotrophy. *Arch Neurol* 1984; **41**: 388–394.

21. Arnold A, Edgren DC, Palladino VS. Amyotrophic lateral sclerosis: fifty cases observed on Guam. *J Nerv Ment Dis* 1953; **117**: 135–139.

22. Koerner DB. Amyotrophic lateral sclerosis on Guam: a clinical study and review of the literature. *Ann Intern Med* 1952; **37**: 1204–1220.

23. Mulder DW, Kurland LT, Iriarte LLG. Neurologic diseases on the island of Guam. *US Armed Forces Med J* 1954; **5**: 1724–1739.

24. Rogers-Johnson P, Garruto R, Yanagihara R et al. Amyotrophic lateral sclerosis and parkinsonism–dementia on Guam: a 30-year evaluation of clinical and neuropathological trends. *Neurology* 1986; **36**: 7–13.

25. Hirano A, Malamud N, Kurland LT. Parkinsonism-dementia complex, an endemic disease on the island of Guam: II. Pathological features. *Brain* 1961; **84**: 662–679.

26. McGeer PL, Schwab C, McGeer EG et al. Familial nature and continuing morbidity of the amyotrophic lateral sclerosis-parkinsonism dementia complex of Guam. *Neurology* 1997; **49**: 400–409.

27. Shiraki H, Yase Y. Amyotrophic lateral sclerosis in Japan. In: Vinken PJ, Bruyn GW, eds. *Handbook of Clinical Neurology* vol 16. New York: Elsevier, 1975, 353–418.

28. Gajdusek DC, Salazar A. Amyotrophic lateral sclerosis and parkinsonian syndromes among the Auyu and Jakai people of West New Guinea. *Neurology* 1982; **32**: 107–126.

29. Verma A, Berger JR, Snodgrass S, Petito C. Motor neuron disease: a paraneoplastic process associated with anti-Hu antibody and small cell lung carcinoma. *Ann Neurol* 1996; **40**: 112–116.

30. Forsyth PA, Dalmau J, Graus F et al. Motor neuron syndromes in cancer patients. *Ann Neurol* 1997; **41**: 722–730.

31. Khawaja S, Sripathi N, Ahmad BK, Lennon VA. Paraneoplastic motor neuron disease with type1 Purkinje cell antibodies. *Muscle Nerve* 1998; **21**: 943–945.

32. Rowland LP. Paraneoplastic primary lateral sclerosis and amyotrophic lateral sclerosis. *Ann Neurol* 1997; **41**: 703–705.

33. Brain WR, Norris FH Jr, eds. *The Remote Effects of Cancer on the Nervous System.* New York: Grune and Stratton, 1965.

34. Desai J, Swash M. IgM paraproteinaemia in a patient with primary lateral sclerosis. *Neuromusc Dis* 1999; **9**: 38–40.

35. Gordon PH, Rowland LP, Younger DS et al. Lymphoproliferative disorders and motor neuron disease: an update. *Neurology* 1997; **48**: 1671–1678.

36. Younger DS, Rowland LP, Latov N et al. Motor neuron disease and amyotrophic lateral sclerosis: relation of high CSF protein content to paraproteinemia and clinical syndromes. *Neurology* 1990; **40**: 595–599.

37. Bouche P, Moulonguet A, Younes-Chennoufi AB et al. Multifocal motor neuropathy with conduction block: a study of 24 patients. *J Neurol Neurosurg Psychiatry* 1995; **59**: 38–44.

38. Kaji R, Shibasaki H, Kimura J. Multifocal motor neuropathy: cranial nerve involvement and immunoglobulin therapy. *Neurology* 1992; **42**: 506–509.

39. Van den Berg LH, Franssen H, Wokke JHJ. The long-term effect of intravenous immunoglobulin treatment in multifocal motor neuropathy. *Brain* 1998; **121**: 421–428.

40. Adams D, Kuntzer T, Steck AJ et al. Motor conduction block and high titres of anti-GM1 ganglioside antibodies: pathological evidence of a motor neuropathy in a patient with lower motor neuron syndrome. *J Neurol Neurosurg Psychiatry* 1993; **56**: 982–987.

41. Oh SJ, Claussen GC, Odabasi Z, Palmer CP. Multifocal demyelinating motor neuropathy: pathologic evidence of 'inflammatory demyelinating polyradiculoneuropathy'. *Neurology* 1995; **45**: 1828–1832.

42. Veugelers B, Theys P, Lammens M et al. Pathological findings in a patient with amyotrophic lateral sclerosis and multifocal motor neuropathy with conduction block. *J Neurol Sci* 1996; **136**: 64–70.

43. Rowland LP. Controversies about amyotrophic lateral sclerosis. *Neurologia* 1996; **11 (suppl 5)**: 72–74.

44. Andersen PM, Nilsson P, Kernen ML et al. Phenotypic heterogeneity in motor neuron

disease patients with Cu/Zn-superoxide dismutase mutations in Scandinavia. *Brain* 1997; **120**: 1723–1737.

45. Appelbaum JS, Roos RP, Salazar-Grueso EF et al. Intrafamilial heterogeneity in hereditary motor neuron disease. *Neurology* 1992; **42**: 1488–1492.

46. Williams DB, Floate DA, Leicester J. Familial motor neuron disease: differing penetrance in large pedigrees. *J Neurol Sci* 1988; **86**: 215–230.

47. Radunovic A, Leigh PN on behalf of the European Familial ALS Group. Cu/Zn superoxide dismutase gene mutations in amyotrophic lateral sclerosis: correlation between genotype and clinical features. *J Neurol Neurosurg Psychiatry* 1996; **61**: 565–572.

48. Cudkowicz ME, McKenna-Yasek D, Chen C et al. Limited corticospinal tract involvement in amyotrophic lateral sclerosis subjects with the A4V mutation in the Cu/Zn superoxide dismutase gene. *Ann Neurol* 1998; **43**: 703–710.

49. Rowland LP. What's in a name? Amyotrophic lateral sclerosis, motor neuron disease, and alleleic heterogeneity. *Ann Neurol* 1998; **43**: 691–694.

50. Kennedy WR, Alter M, Sung JH. Progressive proximal spinal and bulbar muscular atrophy of late onset; a sex-linked recessive trait. *Neurology* 1968; **18**: 671–680.

51. LaSpada AR, Wilson EM, Lubahn DB et al. Androgen receptor gene mutations in X-linked spinal and bulbar muscular atrophy. *Narure* 1991; **352**: 77–79.

52. Ferlini A, Patrosso MC, Guidetti D et al. Androgen receptor gene (CAG)n repeat analysis on the differential diagnosis between Kennedy disease and other motor neuron disorders. *Am J Med Genet* 1995; **55**: 105–111.

53. Shaw PJ, Thagesen H, Tomkins J et al. Kennedy's disease: unusual molecular pathologic and clinical features. *Neurology* 1998; **51**: 252–255.

54. Parboosingh JS, Figlewicz DA, Krizus A et al. Spinobulbar muscular atrophy can mimic ALS; the importance of genetic testing in male patients with atypical ALS. *Neurology* 1997; **49**: 568–572.

55. Ben Hamida M, Hentati F, Ben Hamida C. Hereditary motor system diseases (chronic juvenile amyotrophic lateral sclerosis). *Brain* 1990; **113**: 347–363.

56. Hentati A, Bejaoui K, Pericak-Vance MA et al. Linkage of recessive familial amyotrophic lateral sclerosis to chromosome 2q33–35. *Nat Genet* 1994; **7**: 425–428.

57. Hentati A, Ouahchi K, Pericak-Vance MA et al. Linkage of a common locus for recessive amyotrophic lateral sclerosis. *Am J Hum Genet* 1997; **(suppl 61)**: A279.

58. Chance PF, Rabin BA, Ryan SG et al. Linkage of the gene for an autosomal dominant form of juvenile amyotrophic lateral sclerosis to chromosome 9q34. *Am J Hum Genet* 1998; **62**: 633–640.

59. Bruijn LI, Becher MW, Lee MK et al. ALS-linked SOD1 mutant G85R mediates damage to astrocytes and promotes rapidly progressive disease with SOD1 containing inclusions. *Neuron* 1997; **18**: 327–328.

60. Gurney ME, Pu H, Chiu AY et al. Motor neuron degeneration in mice that express a human Cu/Zn superoxide dismutase mutation. *Science* 1994; **264**: 1772–1775.

61. Zhang B, Tu PH, Abtahian F et al. Neurofilaments and orthograde transport are reduced in ventral root axons of transgenic mice that express human SOD1 with a G93A mutation. *J Cell Biol* 1997; **139**: 1307–1315.

62. Breuer AC, Lynn MP, Atkinson MB et al. Fast axonal transport in amyotrophic lateral sclerosis: an intra-axonal organelle traffic analysis. *Neurology* 1987; **37**: 738–748.

63. Carpenter S. Proximal axonal enlargement in motor neuron diseases. *Neurology* 1968; **18**: 841–851.

64. Hirano A. The cytopathology of amyotrophic lateral sclerosis. *Adv Neurol* 1991; **56**: 91–101.

65. Xu Z, Cork LC, Griffin JW et al. Increased expression of neurofilament subunit NF-L produces morphological alterations that resemble the pathology of human motor neuron disease. *Cell* 1993; **73**: 23–33.

66. Cote F, Collard JF, Julien JP. Progressive neuronopathy in transgenic mice expressing the human neurofilament heavy gene: a mouse model of amyotrophic lateral sclerosis. *Cell* 1993; **73**: 35–46.

67. Lee MK, Marszalek JR, Cleveland DW. A mutant neurofilament subunit causes massive selective motor neuron death: implications for the pathogenesis of human motor neuron disease. *Neuron* 1994; **13**: 975–988.

68. Rosenberg RN. Autosomal dominant cerebellar phenotypes: the genotype will settle the issue. *Neurology* 1990; **40**: 1329–1331.

69. Rosenberg RN. Autosomal dominant cerebellar phenotypes: the genotype has settled the issue. *Neurology* 1995; **45**: 1–5.

70. Ozawa E, Noguchi S, Mizuno Y et al. From dystrophinopathy to sarcoglycanopathy: evolution of a concept of muscular dystrophy. *Muscle Nerve* 1998; **21**: 421–438.

71. Mendell JR. Charcot–Marie–Tooth neuropathies and related disorders. *Semin Neurol* 1998; **18**: 41–47.

72. Swash M, Desai J. Classification of ALS. *Amyotrophic Lateral Sclerosis* 1999; **1**: in press.

73. Desai J, Swash M. Extrapyramidal involvement in ALS; backward falls and retropulsion. *J Neurol Neurosurg Psychiatry* 1999; **67**: 214–216.

74. Neary D, Snowden JS, Mann DMA et al. Frontal lobe dementia and motor neuron disease. *J Neurol Neurosurg Psychiatry* 1990; **53**: 23–32.

75. Kew J, Leigh PN. Dementia with motor neuron disease. In: Rossor MN, ed. *Unusual Dementias. Baillieres Clin Neurol* 1992: 611–626.

76. Wohlfart G. Collateral regeneration from residual motor nerve fibres in amyotrophic lateral sclerosis. *Neurology* 1957; **7**: 124–134.

77. Beasley WC. Quantitative muscle strength testing: principles and application to research and clinical services. *Arch Phys Med Rehabil* 1961; **42**: 398–425.

78. Li TM, Alberman E, Swash M. A suggested approach to the differential diagnosis of motor neurone disease from other neurological diseases. *Lancet* 1986; **ii**: 731–732.

79. Caroscio JT, Calhoun WF, Yahr MD. Prognostic factors in motor neuron disease: a prospective study of longevity. In: Rose FC, ed. *Research Progress in Motor Neurone Disease*. London: Pitman, 1984, 34–43.

80. Gubbay SS, Kahana E, Zilber N et al. Amyotrophic lateral sclerosis: a study of its presentation and prognosis. *J Neurol* 1985; **232**: 295–300.

81. Norris FH, Shepherd R, Denys E et al. Onset, natural history and outcome in idiopathic adult motor neuron disease. *J Neurol Sci* 1993; **118**: 48–95.

82. Rosati G, Pinna L, Granieri E et al. Studies on epidemiological, clinical and etiological aspects of ALS disease in Sardinia, Southern Italy. *Acta Neurol Scand* 1977; **55**: 231–244.

83. Brooks BR, Lewis D, Rawling J et al. The natural history of amyotrophic lateral sclerosis. In: Williams AC, ed. *Motor Neurone Disease*. London: Chapman and Hall, 1994, 121–169.

84. Tan YD, Dolan P, Brooks BR. Symptom progression in amyotrophic lateral sclerosis. *Ann Neurol* 1988; **24**: 14A.

85. Swash M, Schwartz MS. A longitudinal study of changes in motor units in motor neurone disease. *J Neurol Sci* 1982; **56**: 185–197.

86. Swash M. Vulnerability of lower brachial myotomes in motor neurone disease: a single fibre EMG study. *J Neurol Sci* 1980; **47**: 59–68.

87. Mizutani T, Sakamaki S, Tsuchiya N et al. Amyotrophic lateral sclerosis with ophthalmoplegia and multisystem degeneration in patients on long-term use of respirators. *Acta Neuropathol* 1992; **84**: 372–377.

88. Mannen T, Iwata M, Toyokura Y et al. Preservation of a certain motor neurone group of the sacral cord in amyotrophic lateral sclerosis; its clinical significance. *J Neurol Neurosurg Psychiatry* 1977; **40**: 464–469.

89. Carvalho M, Schwartz M S, Swash M. Involvement of the external anal sphincter in amyotrophic lateral sclerosis. *Muscle Nerve* 1995; **18**: 848–853.

90. Swash M, Leader M, Brown A et al. Focal loss of anterior horn cells in the cervical cord in motor neuron disease. *Brain* 1986; **109**: 939–952.

91. Swash M, Schwartz MS. *Neuromuscular Diseases* 3rd edn. London: Springer Verlag, 1997.

92. Li TM, Alberman E, Swash M. 560 cases of motor neuron disease: comparisons and associations. *J Neurol Neurosurg Psychiatry*

1990; **53**: 1043–1045.

93. Li TM, Swash M, Alberman E, Day SJ. Diagnosis of motor neurone disease by neurologists: a study in three countries. *J Neurol Neurosurg Psychiatry* 1991; **154**: 980–983.

94. Chancellor AM, Swingler RJ, Fraser H et al. Utility of Scottish morbidity and mortality data for epidemiological studies of motor neuron disease. *J Epidemiol Comm Health* 1993; **47**: 116–120.

95. Belsh JM, Schiffman PL. Misdiagnosis in patients with amyotrophic lateral sclerosis. *Ann Intern Med* 1990; **150**: 2301–2305.

96. Swash M. Early diagnosis of ALS. *J Neurol Sci* 1998; **160**: S33–S36.

97. Neilson S, Robinson I, Alperovitch A. Rising amyotrophic lateral sclerosis mortality in France 1968–1990: increased life expectancy and interdisease competition as an explanation. *J Neurol* 1994; **241**: 448–455.

98. Ross MA, Miller RG, Berchert RN et al. Toward earlier diagnosis of amyotrophic lateral sclerosis; revised criteria. *Neurology* 1998; **50**: 768–772.

99. Lawyer T, Netsky MG. Amyotrophic lateral sclerosis: a clinico-anatomic study of fifty three cases. *Arch Neurol Psychiatry* 1953; **69**: 171–192.

100. Vejjajiva A, Foster JB, Miller H. Motor neurone disease; a clinical study. *J Neurol Sci* 1967; **4**: 299–314.

101. Jablecki CK, Berry C, Leach KJ. Survival prediction in amyotrophic lateral sclerosis. *Muscle Nerve* 1989; **12**: 833–841.

102. Swash M, Ingram DA. Preclinical and subclinical events in motor neuron disease. *J Neurol Neurosurg Psychiatry* 1988; **51**: 165–168.

103. Mulder DW, Howard FM. Patient resistance and prognosis in amyotrophic lateral sclerosis. *Mayo Clin Proc* 1976; **51**: 537–541.

104. Abrahams S, Goldstein LH, Kew JJM et al. Frontal lobe dysfunction in amyotrophic lateral sclerosis. *Brain* 1996; **119**: 2105–2120.

105. Jackson M, Lennox G, Lowe J. Motor neuron disease-inclusion dementia. *Neurodegeneration* 1990; **5**: 339–350.

106. Qureshi AI, Wilmo G, Dihenia B et al. Motor neuron disease with parkinsonism. *Arch Neurol* 1996; **53**: 987–991.

107. Pringle CE, Hudson AJ, Munoz DG et al. Oprimary lateral sclerosis: clinical features, neuropathology and diagnostic criteria. *Brain* 1992; **115**: 495–520.

108. Swash M, Desai J, Misra P. What is primary lateral sclerosis? *J Neurol Sci* 1999; in press.

109. Lambert EH, Mulder DW. Electromyographic studies in amyotrophic lateral sclerosis. *Staff Meet Mayo Clin* 1957; **32**: 441–446.

110. Cornblath DR, Kuncl RW, Mellits D et al. Nerve conduction studies in amyotrophic lateral sclerosis. *Muscle Nerve* 1992; **15**: 1111–1115.

111. Serratrice G. Classification of adult onset chronic spinal muscular atrophies. *Cardiomyology* 1983; **2**: 255–276.

112. Pearn J, Hudgson P. Distal spinal muscular atrophy. A clinical and genetic study of 8 kindreds. *J Neurol Sci* 1979; **43**: 183–191.

113. Melki J. Spinal muscular atrophy. *Curr Opin Neurol* 1997; **10**: 381–385.

114. Bradley WG, Robison SH, Tandan R et al. Post-irradiation motor neuron syndrome. *Adv Neurol* 1991; **56**: 341–353.

115. Fisher M, Mateer JE, Ullrich I, Gutrecht JA. Pyramidal tact deficits and polyneuropathy in hyperthyroidism: combination clinically mimicking amyotrophic lateral sclerosis. *Am J Med* 1985; **78**: 1041–1044.

116. Patten BM, Engel WK. Phosphate and parathyroid disorders associated with the syndrome of amyotrophic lateral sclerosis. *Adv Neurol* 1982; **36**: 181.

117. Trebini F, Appioti A, Bacci R et al. Neurological complications in hyperparathyroidism. *Minerva Med* 1993; **84**: 73–75.

118. Dubas F, Bertrand P, Emile J. Progressive spinal muscular atrophy and parathyroid adenoma. Clinico-pathological study of a case. *Rev Neurol* 1989; **145**: 65–68.

119. Swash M, Schwartz, MS Sargeant MK. Osteomalacic myopathy: an experimental approach. *Neuropath Appl Neurobiol* 1979; **5**: 295–302.

120. Pestronk A, Chaudhry V, Feldman EL et al. Lower motor neuron syndromes defined by patterns of weakness, nerve conduction abnormalities, and high titres of antiglycolipid antibodies. *Ann Neurol* 1990; **27**: 316–326.

121. Feldman EL, Bromberg MB, Albers JW et al. Immunosuppressive treatment in multifocal motor neuropathy. *Ann Neurol* 1991; **30:** 397–401.

122. Chaudhry V, Corse AM, Cornblath DR et al. Multifocal motor neuropathy: response to human immune globulin. *Ann Neurol* 1993; **33:** 237–242.

123. Conradi S, Ronnevi LO, Norris FH. Motor neuron disease and toxic metals. *Adv Neurol* 1982; **36:** 201–231.

124. Adams CR, Zeigler DK, Lin JT. Mercury intoxication simulating amyotrophic lateral sclerosis. *JAMA* 1983; **250:** 642–643.

125. Mitchell JD. Heavy metals and trace elements in amyotrophic lateral sclerosis. *Neurol Clin* 1987; **5:** 43–60.

126. Barber TE . Inorganic mercury poisoning reminiscent of amyotrophic lateral sclerosis. *J Occup Med* 1978; **20:** 667–669.

127. Fukuda K, Nisenhaum R, Stewart G et al. Chronic multisystem illness affecting Air Force veterans of the Gulf War. *JAMA* 1998; **280:** 981–988.

128. Strauss SE. Bridging the Gulf War syndromes. *Lancet* 1999; **353:** 162–163.

129. Dalakas MC, Elder G, Hallet M. A long-term follow-up study of patients with post-poliomyelitis neuromuscular symptoms. *N Engl J Med* 1986; **314:** 959–963.

130. Mitsumoto H, Sliman RJ, Schafer IA et al. Motor neuron disease and adult hexosaminidase deficiency in two families: evidence for multisystem degeneration. *Ann Neurol* 1985; **17:** 378–385.

131. Salachas F, Lafitte C, Chassande B et al. Motor neuron disease mimicking amyotrophic lateral sclerosis and primary lateral sclerosis in primary Sjögren's syndrome (abstract). *Neurology 50* (**suppl 4**): A31.

132. Bostock H, Sharief MK, Reid MG, Murray NMF. Axonal ion channel dysfunction in amyotrophic lateral sclerosis. *Brain* 1995; **118:** 217–225.

133. Bensimon G, Lacomblez L, Meininger V et al. A controlled trial of riluzole in amyotrophic lateral sclerosis. *N Engl J Med* 1994; **330:** 585–591.

134. Lacomblez L, Bensimon G, Leigh PN et al. A dose ranging study of riluzole in amyotropic lateral sclerosis. *Lancet* 1996; **347:** 1425–1431.

135. Wagner ML, Landis BE. Riluzole; a new agent for amyotrophic lateral sclerosis. *Ann Pharmacother* 1997; **31:** 738–744.

2

Natural history of amyotrophic lateral sclerosis— impairment, disability, handicap

Benjamin Rix Brooks, Mohammed Sanjak, Daryn Belden, Katalin Juhasz-Poscine, Andrew Waclawik

Introduction

The natural history of amyotrophic lateral sclerosis (ALS) – motor neuron disease may be changing.[1-5] Although population-based studies based on data from over 5 years ago have shown no significant change in survival from time of diagnosis compared with earlier surveys,[6-9] studies of disease prognosis involving national registries[10-12] or large referral populations[13-22] give insight to differences between population-based observational studies and opt-in patient databases that are based on referral populations. Such biases[23,24] may have affected the outcome of recent clinical trials.[25-29] Furthermore, the introduction of novel drug therapies[30] may be altering the natural history of ALS.

In the past quarter of a century, the natural history of ALS has been studied with standard[21,31,32] and innovative[19,20,33,34] clinimetrics of disease outcome. Standard clinical descriptions have been the hallmark of natural history studies in the past.[21,35-37] The newer disease measures required the development of clinimetrics of:

(a) impairment — measures of impairment quantify changes in strength and function (e.g. manual muscle testing, computerized isometric strength testing, pulmonary function tests, speech and swallowing tests, and timed functional tests);

(b) disability — measures of disability identify states of dysfunction that are specific for ALS (e.g. the ALS Functional Rating Scale, the ALS Severity Scale).

(c) handicap — measures of handicap identify the impact of this disability on personal (quality of life) outcomes and societal (life role) outcomes.[38]

Some scales are hybrids of measures of impairment and disability and have unusual properties (Appel ALS Scale, Norris ALS Scale).[39,40]

This chapter reviews earlier studies of the development and progression of symptom changes in ALS and gives details of newer methods in order to present changes in physical signs specific to ALS that allow measurement of impairment (loss of strength and loss of physiological function). This is useful because these impairments develop in different physiological domains (brainstem—speech, swallowing, spinal cord—arms, breathing, legs) at different times. The chapter introduces measures that are enriched to represent changes in upper and lower motor neurons. Further, we introduce new analytical methods to define the natural history of ALS in the years to come.

Natural history of symptom development

During the symptomatic phase of the clinical period of disease, patients have a pattern of disease spread, as has been previously described, that is dependent on age, sex, site of onset, and whether the disease is sporadic or familial.[17,19] The onset of symptoms seen in ALS patients is assumed to occur when approximately an 80% loss of motor neurons has been achieved, as is the case with poliomyelitis.[41] Symptoms caused by lower motor neuron loss accrue according to a function that is dependent on the time it takes for motor neuron groups to lose neurons down to the 20% threshold at which symptoms are obvious to the patient. Patients who have symptomatic disease that begins in the arm, leg or bulbar regions may show progression of symptomatic involvement to other regions on topographically-based patterns that are consistent with more rapid progression of the disease to anatomically contiguous areas (e.g. cervical segments to cervical segments, lumbar segments to lumbar segments) before developing rostral or caudal symptoms throughout the neuraxis. The evolution of symptoms through spinal cord levels occurs faster than the accrual of symptoms in the brainstem of patients with either unilateral arm or leg onset. Patients with arm onset seem to develop bulbar symptoms more rapidly than those patients with leg onset. Surprisingly, caudal-to-rostral spread within the spinal cord and from the cervical regions to the bulbar region appears to be faster than rostral-to-caudal spread within the spinal cord.

This symptom development in ALS patients clearly demonstrates a temporal pattern of initial limb onset followed by later development of bulbar signs. Clinically, however, patients with early bulbar onset are sometimes encountered and in these patients the disease behaves in a different pattern from that seen in patients with limb onset disease.

Age and sex effects are apparent as well. The spread of disease as captured by the symptomatic self-report of the patient suggests a mechanism for staging ALS. The authors have tested this hypothesis prospectively with the use of a newly developed ALS Functional Rating Scale that clearly defines (using a disability measure) potential stages of this disease (spinal involvement followed by bulbar involvement).

Effects of the site of onset on the development of symptoms

Limb onset

The development of contralateral arm symptoms in patients with unilateral leg onset has been found to be significantly slower than symptom accumulation both in the opposite leg for 3 years of disease ($p < 0.01$) and the ipsilateral arm for 2 years of disease ($p < 0.03$). The development of ipsilateral arm symptoms in patients with unilateral leg onset was significantly faster ($p < 0.03$) than the development of contralateral arm symptoms. The development of symptoms in the opposite arm compared with the contralateral or ipsilateral leg in patients with arm onset was significantly faster ($p < 0.001$) than the development of bulbar symptoms during the first 5 years of disease. In comparison with the development of bulbar symptoms, the development of symptoms in other limbs (i.e. the opposite leg, the ipsilateral arm, and the contralateral arm) of ALS patients following unilateral leg onset was significantly faster ($p < 0.04$) for the first 5 years of disease.[42,43]

Bulbar onset

The development of cranial motor neuron symptoms by patients with unilateral arm onset was significantly faster ($p < 0.4$) than the appearance of bulbar symptoms in patients with unilateral leg onset at 2, 3, and 4 years of disease. In bulbar ALS patients with speech onset, accretion of swallowing symptoms was significantly faster ($p < 0.001$) than the accretion of both arm and leg symptoms for the first 4 years of disease. There was no significant difference between rate of development of arm symptoms and leg symptoms in patients with bulbar onset. However, the accretion of limb symptoms (arm plus leg) in patients with bulbar onset was significantly faster ($p < 0.01$) than the accretion of bulbar symptoms in patients with unilateral limb onset (arm or leg) for 6 years of follow-up.

Effects of sex on the development of symptoms

Females
Female ALS patients with leg onset demonstrated from the 3rd year onwards a larger proportion of symptom accretion in other regions than male ALS patients with leg onset. Compared with male ALS patients with unilateral leg onset, female patients were significantly more likely to develop opposite leg symptoms, ipsilateral arm symptoms, contralateral arm symptoms, and bulbar symptoms ($p < 0.02$).[43]

Males
Male ALS patients with bulbar onset demonstrated significantly more symptom accretion in arms during the first 3 years of disease than female ALS patients ($p < 0.01$).[43,44]

Effects of age on the development of symptoms

Young ALS
In the authors' study population, the proportion (25%) of young ALS patients with right arm onset was significantly higher ($p < 0.05$) than in older sporadic ALS patients (14%), but other sites are not disproportionately represented. Progression of symptoms in the bulbar region following arm or leg onset is identical in young ALS patients and older sporadic ALS patients. However, symptom progression from the bulbar region or legs to involve the arms or from the arms to involve the legs is significantly faster ($p < 0.005$) in young ALS patients than in older sporadic ALS patients.[17]

The development of symptoms in familial ALS

Autosomal dominant familial ALS
The proportions of patients with bulbar, arm or leg onset were similar in both familial ALS (57 patients) and sporadic ALS (609 patients). Symptom development in familial ALS patients who had bulbar or arm onset is identical to that seen in sporadic ALS patients. Familial ALS patients with leg onset, however, had a slower accretion of symptoms in the opposite leg, the ipsilateral arm or in either arm than sporadic ALS patients.[42]

Mechanisms and neural substrates of symptom accretion

The dependence of the evolution of symptoms in ALS patients on site of onset suggests that neuronal degeneration may occur within contiguous areas, which are more quickly involved than non-contiguous areas. The local spread to contiguous areas of motor neuron dysfunction is faster in the brainstem and the cervical and lumbar regions. The more rapid rostral-to-caudal involvement (compared with caudal-to-rostral involvement) suggests axonal transport as a possible mechanism; however, rostral-to-caudal spread via the central canal might be implicated in spread of bulbar onset disease to the spinal cord.[43]

Natural history of impairment

Muscle strength—manual muscle testing and maximum voluntary isometric contraction

In other neuromuscular diseases, such as Duchenne muscular dystrophy and facio-scapulohumeral muscular dystrophy, manual muscle testing (MMT) and maximum voluntary isometric contraction (MVIC) provide similar and adequate information for discerning clinical change over time in long-term clinical studies.[45–53] To determine the relationship between MVIC and MMT strength in ALS, MVIC and MMT assessments were performed in muscles measured independently cross-sectionally and longitudinally in 132 ALS patients by two raters. There were 93 male and 37 female patients 26 had bulbar onset, 59 had arm onset, and 47 had leg onset. MMT ratings were determined according to the Medical Research Council protocol[54] by one examiner, and MVIC in the same muscles was measured by three examiners according to established protocol.[55–57] MVIC raw data were transformed into a muscle-specific percentage predicted value determined by the age, sex, height, and weight of each patient according to regression equations developed by the National Isometric Muscle Strength Database Consortium.[49–52,56] MMTs and MVICs of shoulder extensors, shoulder flexors, elbow extensors, elbow flexors, wrist extensors, wrist flexors, hip extensors, hip flexors, leg extensors, leg flexors, and ankle dorsiflexors were studied individually (right and left) and were either analysed separately or with both right and left muscles pooled. Results for individual muscles are presented on the Internet on the University of Wisconsin ALS Clinical Research Center website

(http://www.neurology.wisc.edu/alscrc/clintrialdata1).

The MVIC strength value, expressed as percent and predicted with regard to age and sex matched normal subjects, was compared with the MMT strength rating in each muscle. Correlation analysis provided a linear relationship between MVIC and MMT for all muscles averaged per patient and was correlated with the mean muscle strength presented as mean MMT rating average per patient.

Employing a composite of all limb muscles measured cross-sectionally, the comparison of MVIC with MMT indicates that the mean MVIC is proportionate at each MMT ordinal rating (MMT-5: 94% predicted, MMT-4: 75% predicted; MMT-3: 55% predicted).[58] The mean difference in MVIC between MMT-5 and MMT-4 or MMT-4 and MMT-3 at first visit is 20 ± 4 (standard deviation) percentage predicted. Thus, between MMT5-4 and MMT4-5, approximately 20% predicted strength is lost per MMT unit decrease. This relationship does not exist below MMT-3. Similar results have been noted by other groups.[59–61] MVIC is more sensitive to change but it does parallel changes in the total ALS Functional Rating Scale score.[59]

This cross-sectional study was extended prospectively and longitudinally to look at the sensitivity of muscle strength change over time in ALS patients as measured by repeated measures (mean MMT (ordinal units); mean MVIC (% predicted)) and by a sustained fall in the muscle strength below a specific threshold (i.e. MMT $\leqslant 4$, $\leqslant 3$; MVIC $\leqslant 80\%$ predicted, $\leqslant 60\%$ predicted, $\leqslant 40\%$ predicted) or by a sustained specific drop from baseline (i.e. MMT $\geqslant 1$ ordinal unit; MVIC $\geqslant 1$ Z-unit, $\geqslant 10\%$ predicted, $\geqslant 20\%$ predicted). The findings are similar for all muscles individually and can be reviewed on the Internet.

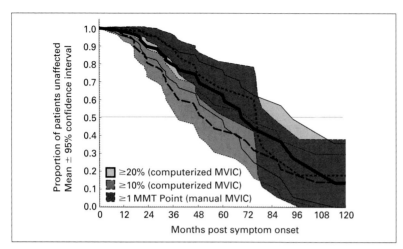

Figure 2.1a
*Arm muscles: sustained drop
from baseline.*

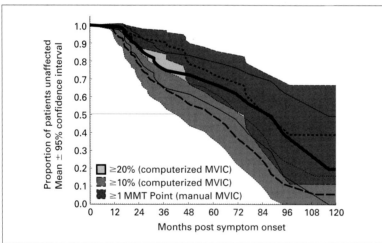

Figure 2.1b
*Leg muscles: sustained drop
from baseline.*

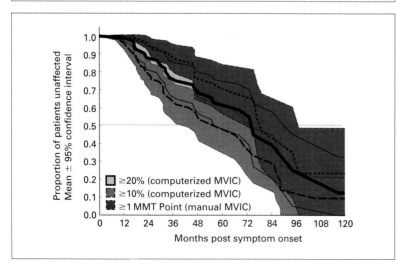

Figure 2.1c
*All muscles: sustained drop
from baseline.*

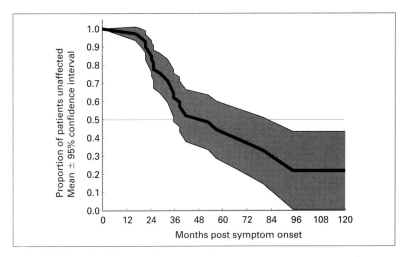

Figure 2.2a
Neck extension: sustained (≥1 MMT point) drop from baseline.

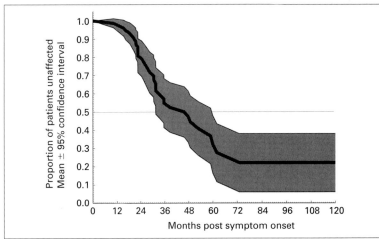

Figure 2.2b
Neck flexion: sustained (≥1 MMT point) drop from baseline.

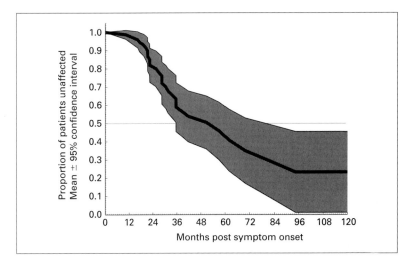

Figure 2.2c
Neck rotation: sustained (≥1 MMT point) drop from baseline.

The sustained specific drop from baseline as percentage predicted data[56] or the sustained specific 1 unit MMT drop from baseline can be shown prospectively with event history analysis (*Fig. 2.1*). The 20% predicted sustained drop from baseline overlaps the 1 unit MMT drop from baseline for arms (see *Fig. 2.1a*), legs (see *Fig. 2.1b*), and arms with legs together (see *Fig. 2.1c*). In each situation, a 10% predicted sustained drop in strength occurs significantly faster than a 20% predicted sustained drop in strength. Arm muscles demonstrate less variation over time, with half the patients declining by 1 MMT unit in 60–80 months (95% CI — confidence limit) after onset, while the 20% predicted sustained drop occurs between 60 and 96 months (95% CI) after onset. Leg muscles and the arm and leg muscle composite show wider variation, with half the patients achieving the end-point in 72–120 months (95% CI). Some muscles appear to weaken faster than the limb muscles. In particular, neck extension drops by 1 MMT unit in half the patients between 36 and 80 months (95% CI) (*Fig. 2.2a*), neck flexion drops similarly between 36 and 60 months (95% CI) (see *Fig. 2.2b*), and neck rotators drop between 36 and 66 months (95% CI) (see *Fig. 2.2c*). Bulbar isometric strength is more resistant than limb strength. While half the patients may have a 10% predicted sustained drop from baseline of tongue protrusion strength with onset as early as 30 months extending up to 96 months (95% CI) after onset, jaw clenching (masseter) strength does not change significantly in half the patients until after 120 months (*Fig. 2.3a*). The difference in the time to a 10% predicted drop in tongue muscle strength compared with jaw muscle strength is statistically significant ($p = 0.0316$). The more clinically significant 20% predicted sustained drop in tongue strength occurs in half the patients with an onset after 40 months but with an upper limit of more than 120 months (95% CI). The clinically significant 20% predicted sustained drop in jaw strength occurs in half the patients with an onset after 76 months with an indeterminate upper limit of more than 120 months (95% CI) (see *Fig. 2.3b*). These differences are not statistically significant.

Event history analysis of isometric strength measured by MMT or computerized MVIC may allow a new means of defining the natural history of strength loss in ALS patients. This may enable the performance of trials that compare the effects of different therapies on isometric muscle strength in ALS patients who have been matched for age, sex, site of onset, and time since onset.

Analysis of the properties of $\geq 10\%$ predicted drops, $\geq 20\%$ predicted drops, and 1 MMT unit sustained drops shows no statistically significant difference either among ALS patients with bulbar, arm, or leg onset or between males and females. There is no statistically significant difference for ALS patients above or below the age of 45 years.

Event history analysis of single muscles or muscle groups is presented by the University of Wisconsin ALS Clinic on its website (see URL above). In previous analyses of the change in limb muscle strength over time in ALS patients, repeated measures techniques, rate of change by mean slope techniques, and change from baseline have been presented for smaller groups of ALS patients. Changes in index finger pinch strength, wrist extension strength, jaw (masseter) strength, and tongue (protrusion) strength that have previously been studied only in limited groups of patients are presented on the website by the new event history analysis of sustained drop by $\geq 10\%$ predicted and $\geq 20\%$ predicted strength change for a large longitudinal study of the University of Wisconsin ALS Clinic patients.

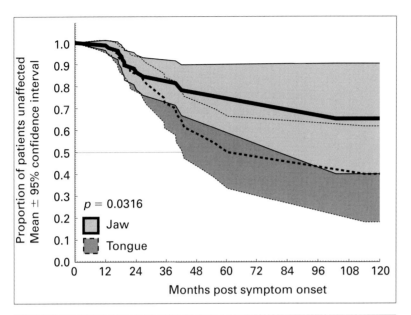

Figure 2.3a
*Bulbar strength: sustained
(≥10% predicted) drop from
baseline.*

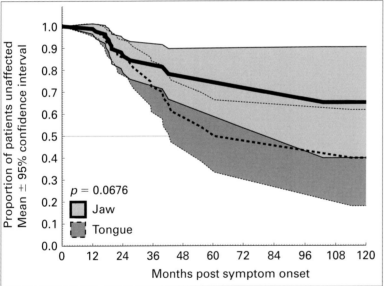

Figure 2.3b
*Bulbar strength: sustained
(≥20% predicted) drop from
baseline.*

Both MMT and MVIC strength measurements have been used in a large number of phase 1 and phase 2 clinical trials and in large multicenter phase 3 clinical trials. Intra- and inter-rater reliability have been assessed in a number of such clinical trials. Test–test reproducibility of MVIC across many centers was audited and quantified in two large phase 3 clinical trials that used MVIC as the primary clinical endpoint.[62,63] Test–retest, two weeks or more apart, across centers demonstrated a systematic decline in strength across centers in this short time period but, in addition, there was a significant ($P<0.05$) systematic inter-

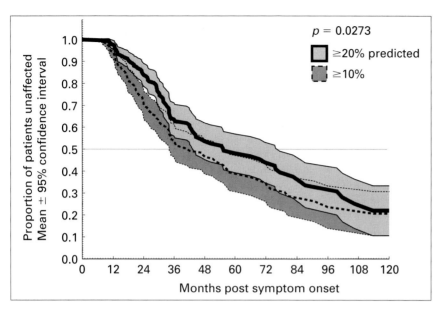

Figure 2.4a
Rapid alternating movement: sustained drop from baseline.

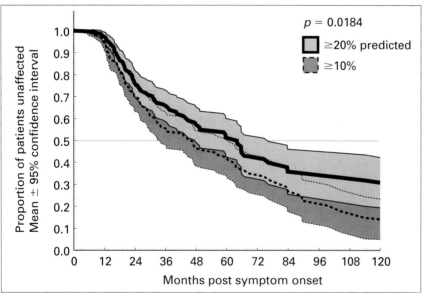

Figure 2.4b
Foot tap: sustained drop from baseline.

center difference in variance across centers.[63,64] Inter-center variance, though significant, did not affect the change in MVIC over time by center. Similar results were obtained in other studies.[65–70]

Timed functional tests — limb, axial, and bulbar tests

Newer measures of limb function indicate earlier impairments than those in isometric strength for a population of ALS patients. Rapid alternating movements of supination–

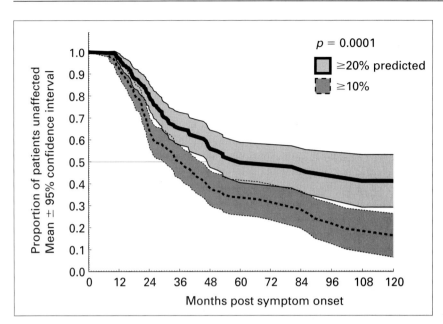

Figure 2.5a
360° turn: sustained drop from baseline.

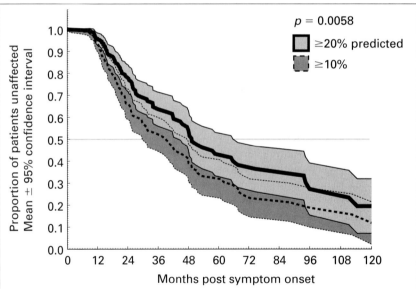

Figure 2.5b
Sit-to-stand: sustained drop from baseline.

pronation in the arms show a sustained drop by ⩾10% predicted in 50% of patients between 34 and 54 months (95% CI) after onset while a sustained drop by ⩾20% predicted occurs between 42 and 72 months (95% CI) after onset (*Fig. 2.4a*). Foot tapping shows comparable 95% CI for sustained drops of ⩾10% predicted and ⩾20% predicted (see *Fig. 2.4b*). Axial functional tests include standing velocity and 360° rotation turning velocity. Standing velocity changes by a sustained drop of ⩾10% predicted relative to normal in 50% of ALS patients between 30 and 48 months (95% CI) after onset

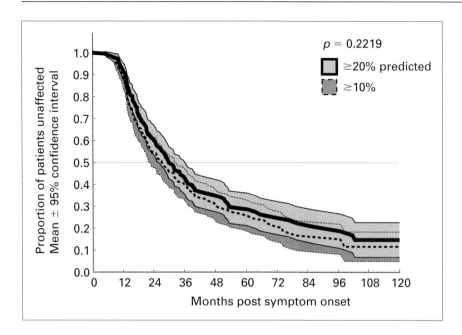

$p = 0.2219$

☐ ≥20% predicted

▨ ≥10%

Figure 2.6
30-foot walk: sustained drop from baseline.

(*Fig. 2.5a*). The comparable time for 50% of patients to show a 20% predicted drop is between 42 and 66 months (95% CI) after onset. Turning velocity in ALS patients is affected in the same time frame of 30–42 months (95% CI) for a ≥10% predicted sustained drop, but there is a wider interval (48–120 months (95% CI)) for the drop by ≥20% predicted (see *Fig. 2.5b*). Surprisingly, walking velocity decrease by ≥10% predicted occurs earlier — between 18 and 30 months (95% CI) — than changes in standing and turning velocity (*Fig. 2.6*). The sustained drop in walking velocity by ≥20% predicted occurs between 30 and 38 months (95% CI) after disease onset, which is also sooner than a similar ≥20% predicted drop in limb alternating movement tests, axial standing tests, and turning tests. Speech alternating movement rates change later than limb or axial function tests. Delayed bulbar strength, function and intelligibility changes are a hallmark of limb-onset ALS[71-84]

Alternating movement tests for the facial muscles (e.g. repetition of the word 'pepper') and for tongue muscles (e.g. repetition of the word 'ticker') change later than test of tongue strength (see *Fig. 2.3a*). A decrease in the rate of alternating movements for the facial muscles by ≥10% predicted occurs between 54 and 72 months (95% CI) after onset in 50% of ALS patients (*Fig. 2.7a*). A similar decrease in rates of alternating movements for the tongue muscles occurs between 60 and 84 months (95% CI) after onset (see *Fig. 2.7b*). The time intervals for a sustained drop by ≥20% predicted is much larger for facial muscles and tongue muscles (72–120 months; 95% CI).

Respiratory function tests

Respiratory function, measured by vital capacity, decreases significantly faster than measures of muscle strength, at a similar rate to timed functional movements of the limbs, but not as quickly as changes in walking velocity. The

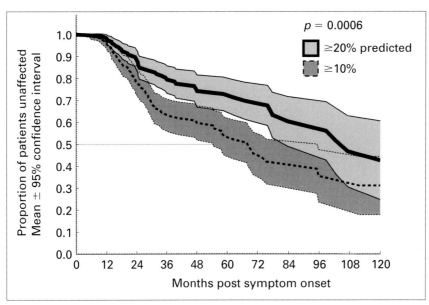

Figure 2.7a
'Pepper': sustained drop from baseline.

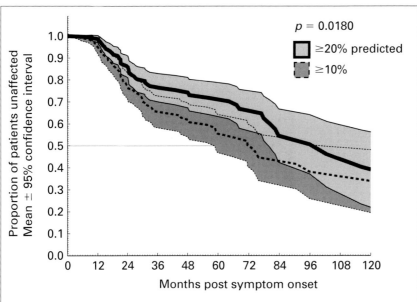

Figure 2.7b
'Ticker': sustained drop from baseline.

drop in vital capacity by ≥10% predicted occurs in 50% of ALS patients between 30 and 48 months (95% CI) after onset.[85-99] The drop in vital capacity by ≥20% predicted is significantly delayed ($p = 0.003$) in ALS patients, to 48–60 months (95% CI) after onset (*Fig. 2.8*).

Natural history of disability
Lower extremity disability

Walking velocity is one of the first functional measures to change in ALS.[59,66,100] It is not surprising, therefore, that milestones in lower extremity disability are reached earlier than

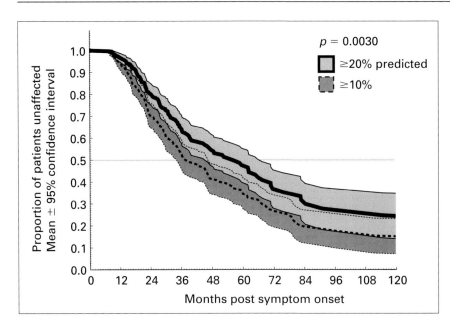

Figure 2.8
*Forced vital capacity:
sustained drop from
baseline.*

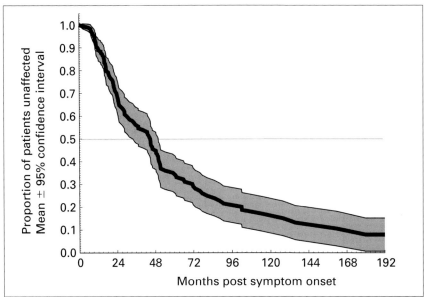

Figure 2.9
Falling in ALS patients.

milestones in other domains.[19,62,80,101–106]

Falling, measured as the time to the first fall followed by one or more successive falls, occurs in 50% of ALS patients between 30 and 48 months (95% CI) after onset (*Fig. 2.9*).

Surprisingly, the first sustained use of a cane occurs in 50% of ALS patients between 42 and 72 months (95% CI) after onset (*Fig. 2.10*), which is a slightly wider interval than the first sustained use of a walker, at

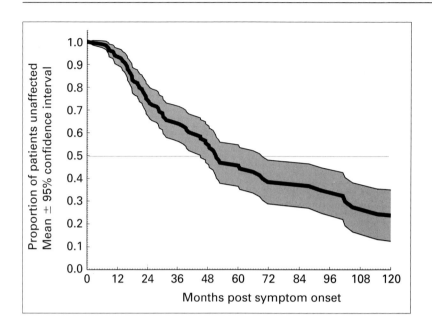

Figure 2.10
Sustained use of the cane by ALS patients.

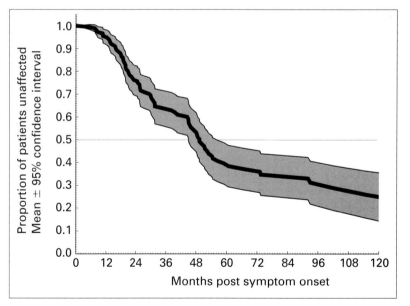

Figure 2.11
Sustained use of a walker by ALS patients.

46–58 months (95% CI) after onset (*Fig. 2.11*). However, the first sustained use of a wheelchair by 50% of ALS patients overlaps the appearance of the first sustained occurrence of falls, at 30–48 months (95% CI) after onset (*Fig. 2.12*).

Upper-extremity disability

Arm function was less likely to cause disability early in the course of ALS in the authors' patient population. The development of dressing disability to the point that help was

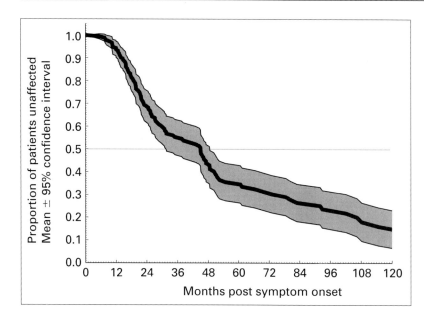

Figure 2.12
Sustained use of a wheelchair by ALS patients.

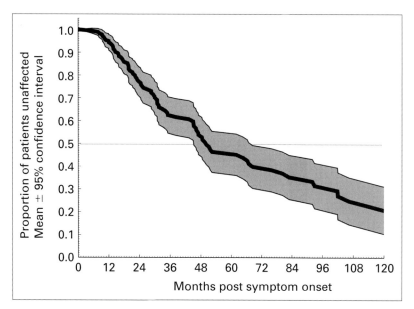

Figure 2.13
Sustained need for assisted dressing.

required from a caregiver in 50% of ALS patients did not occur until 46–66 months (95% CI) after onset (*Fig. 2.13*). It was unexpected that the development of eating disability to the point that a caregiver was required to assist in feeding the patient, did not occur until 90–120 months or later (95% CI) after onset in the authors' ALS population, and the 95% CI was rather wide (*Fig. 2.14*).

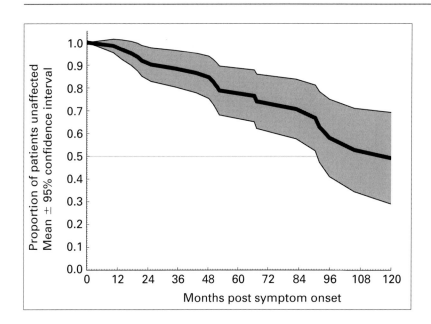

Figure 2.14
Sustained need for assisted eating.

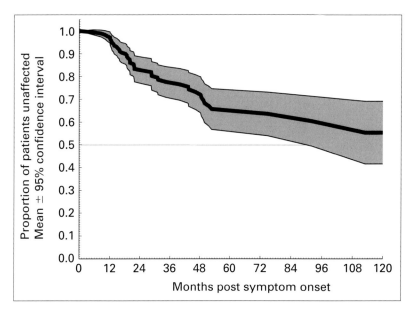

Figure 2.15
Sustained need for speech therapy.

Bulbar disability

The need for speech assistive devices, such as writing notes, letter boards, or computer-assisted speech, occurred rather late in the authors' population.[108–116] It was between 90 and more than 120 months (95% CI) after onset before these devices were used by 50% of the ALS population (*Fig. 2.15*). Another measure of bulbar function concerning swallowing involved the introduction of nutritional supplements to maintain weight. In 50% of

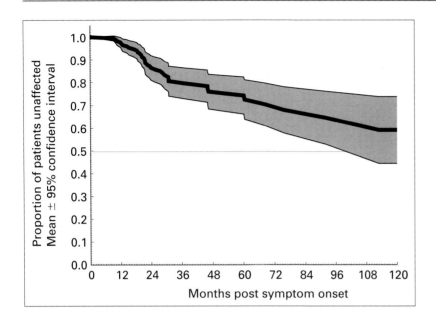

Figure 2.16
Sustained need for nutritional intervention.

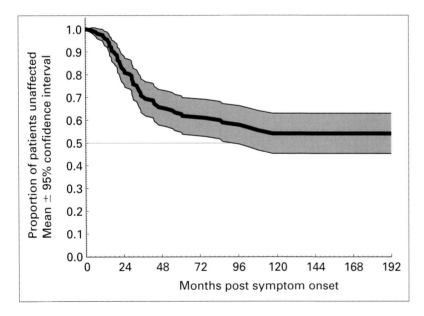

Figure 2.17
Sustained need for gastrostomy tubes.

ALS patients, such supplements were introduced between 102 and more than 120 months (95% CI) after onset (*Fig. 2.16*). The development of disability such that gastrostomy tube feeding was required follows a similar time line.[117–123] The 95% CI for 50% of

ALS patients achieving this milestone was indeterminate because only 45% of patients had gastrostomy tubes placed. An estimate is 96 to more than 120 months (95% CI) after onset (*Fig. 2.17*).

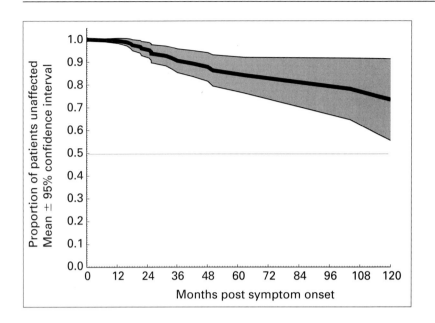

Figure 2.18
Sustained need for bi-directional positive airway pressure ventilation or permanent assisted ventilation.

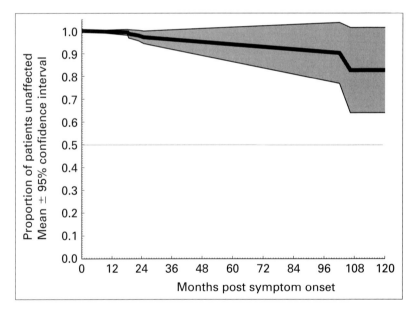

Figure 2.19
Need for permanent assisted ventilation.

Respiratory disability

Progressive loss of vital capacity leads to a decision regarding assisted ventilation in the form of non-invasive intermittent assisted ventilation (either bi-directional positive airway pressure ventilation or constant positive airway pressure ventilation) or invasive permanent assisted ventilation (either tracheotomy or permanent assisted ventilation). The 95%

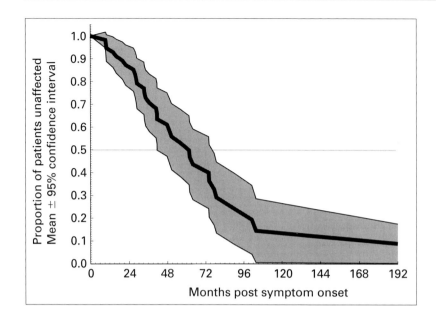

Figure 2.20
*Levels of economic
dependence due to
physical health.*

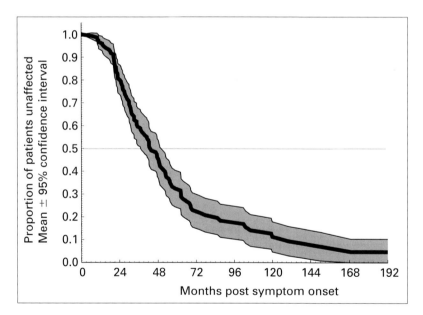

Figure 2.21
*Survival levels of ALS
patients.*

confidence limits for 50% of ALS patients achieving the milestones of either bi-directional positive airway pressure ventilation or permanent assisted ventilation were indeterminate because only 25% of patients had bi-directional positive airway pressure ventilation (*Fig. 2.18*) and only 20% of patients had tracheotomy with ventilator or permanent assisted ventilation (*Fig. 2.19*).

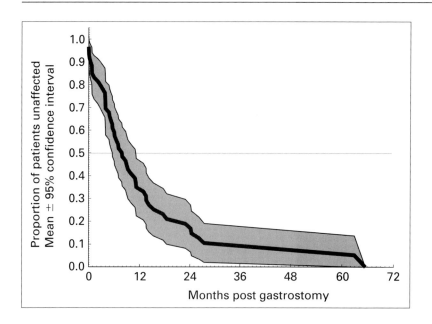

Figure 2.22
Survival levels of ALS patients after gastrostomy.

Natural history of handicap

Quality of life measures

Several quality of life (QoL) measures have been adopted or modified for use in ALS patients.[124–129] Several measures have been validated against impairment, disability, or mixed measures of the ALS process. Many studies are in the process of analysis or submission for publication. A major effort to develop a modified version of a standard QoL measure for ALS is currently ongoing.

Multiple social domains may be analysed in ALS patients. One critical domain relates to maintaining employment. In the University of Wisconsin Hospital and Clinics ALS Clinical Research Center database, 50% of ALS patients stop working between 30 and 72 months (95% CI) after onset of the disease (*Fig. 2.20*). Losing the ability to work overlaps functional decreases in vital capacity (see *Fig. 2.8*) and in hand and leg time functional tests (see *Figs 2.4–2.6*) and the development

of falling (see *Fig. 2.9*), as well as the use of proximal upper extremity assistive devices (see *Fig. 2.13*) and lower extremity assistive devices (see *Figs 2.10–2.12*).

Survival

Surprisingly, the ultimate handicap — death — is not a consequence of all the impairments and disabilities that result from ALS. The 50% survival rate in this population ranges from 36 to 48 months (95% CI) after onset (*Fig. 2.21*). Survival appears surprisingly independent of measures of limb strength (see *Figs 2.1–2.3*) and the use of gastrostomy, tracheostomy, or ventilators (see *Figs 2.17–2.19*), but it overlaps population changes in vital capacity (see *Fig. 2.8*), limb and axial functional tests (see *Figs 2.4–2.6*) as well as falling (see *Fig. 2.9*) and use of some lower extremity assistive devices (see *Fig. 2.12*).

Future studies of the natural history of ALS will require assessment of handicap measures after the introduction of specific interventions such as gastrostomy feeding. There are not yet enough data in large groups of patients to assess bi-directional positive airway pressure ventilation or other ventilator interventions. However, in a large group of patients who received gastrostomy tube feeding, 50% of ALS patients survived for 6–12 months (95% CI) after percutaneous endoscopic gastrostomy tube (*Fig. 2.22*).

Conclusion

The natural history ALS has classically been presented in terms of symptom development and impairment changes over time as measured by MMT or, recently, computerized MVIC. Changes in disability as measured by the ALS Functional Rating Scale and composite disability–impairment clinimetrics such as the Appel ALS Scale, the Norris ALS Scale, or the Charing Cross ALS Scale have looked at before–after end-point analysis, time series averages, or slope changes. Handicap may be captured by QoL measures, which attempt to provide insight to the effect of ALS on the individual's role in home, workplace, and society.

This chapter has introduced a new event history analysis of the impairment, disability, and handicap measures that may be used to describe the natural history of ALS. This novel technique of event history analysis has permitted description of the 95% CI for the time that a 50% proportion of a population of ALS patients will meet identified milestones with minimal effects of the loss to follow-up of patients who cannot return for evaluation.

The authors have used this novel, analytical technique to describe impairments, MMT and MVIC limb muscles, neck muscle strength that changes earlier than limb muscle and bulbar muscle stength that has delayed changes compared with limb muscles in ALS patients.

Timed functional tests indicate earlier functional impairment than that explained by loss of strength. Walking velocity in particular is lost more quickly by a population of ALS patients than axial functions of standing and turning or limb measures of rapid alternating movements in the hands or foot tapping. Rapid alternating movements of the tongue or facial muscles are lost later than walking and than axial and limb functional movements. Respiratory function, as measured by vital capacity, decreases significantly more quickly than measures of muscle strength, at a similar rate to limb timed functional movements, but not as quickly as walking velocity.

Measures of disability indicate that leg functional changes lead to falling and wheelchair use earlier than cane or walker use. These changes occur earlier than the need for help in dressing, which precedes the need for help in eating. Use of speech assistive devices, nutritional supplements, and gastrostomy feeding occur later in the course of the disease, at the time that non-invasive intermittent assisted ventilation (e.g. bi-directional positive airway pressure ventilation) and permanent assisted ventilation (e.g. tracheostomy) are required.

Measures of handicap derived from QoL clinimetrics and survival analysis provide startling contrasts to the impairment and disability measures.

Losing the ability to work overlaps functional decreases in vital capacity, hand and leg time functional tests, the development of falling, and the use of proximal upper extremity and lower extremity assistive devices. The 50% survival in this population ranges from 36 to 48 months (95% CI) and appears surprisingly independent of measures of limb strength and the use of gastrostomy, tracheostomy, or ventilators, but it overlaps population changes in vital capacity, limb and axial functional tests, falling, and the use of lower extremity assistive devices.

In this chapter, new relationships have been identified among the various measures of impairment, disability, and handicap in ALS. These new approaches to the natural history of ALS will allow adequate evaluation of impairment, disability, and handicap to determine whether the introduction of new therapeutic approaches will substantially improve outcomes for patients with this disease.[25]

Acknowledgments

Additional co-authors to this chapter are Roxanne DePaul, Selmi Dogan, Andrea Maser, Kathryn Roelke, Michael Laird, Laurel Malinowski, Jane Shannon and Craig Roelke.

The Clinical Studies reported were supported in part by the Muscular Dystrophy Association, the ALS Association and the Department of Veterans Affairs, Great Lakes Veterans Integrated Services Network (VISN 12). The crucial organizational support for the ALS Clinical Research Centre provided by Jennifer Parnell, Christy Weasler and Janine Diana is greatly appreciated.

References

1. Brooks BR. Diagnostic dilemmas in amyotrophic lateral sclerosis. *J Neurol Sci* 1999; **165 (suppl 1)**: S1–S9.
2. Rowland LP. Diagnosis of amyotrophic lateral sclerosis. *J Neurol Sci* 1998; **160 (suppl 1)**: S6–S24.
3. Ross MA, Miller RG, Berchert L et al. Toward earlier diagnosis of amyotrophic lateral sclerosis: revised criteria. rhCNTF ALS Study Group. *Neurology* 1998; **50**: 768–772.
4. Li TM, Swash M, Alberman E, Day SJ. Diagnosis of motor neuron disease by neurologists: a study in three countries. *J Neurol Neurosurg Psychiatry* 1991; **54**: 980–983.
5. Belsh JM, Schiffman PL. Misdiagnosis in patients with amyotrophic lateral sclerosis. *Arch Intern Med* 1990; **150**: 2301–2305.
6. McGuire V, Longstreth WT Jr, Kopesell TD, van Belle G. Incidence of amyotrophic lateral sclerosis in three counties in western Washington state. *Neurology* 1996; **47**: 571–573.
7. Annegers JF, Appel SH, Perkins P, Lee J. Amyotrophic lateral sclerosis mortality rates in Harris County, Texas. *Adv Neurol* 1991; **56**: 239–243.
8. Annegers JF, Appel S, Lee JR, Perkins P. Incidence and prevalence of amyotrophic lateral sclerosis in Harris County, Texas, 1985–1988. *Arch Neurol* 1991; **48**: 589–593.
9. Yoshida S, Mulder DW, Kurland LT, Chu CP, Okazaki H. Follow-up study on amyotrophic lateral sclerosis in Rochester, Minn., 1925 through 1984. *Neuroepidemiology* 1986; **5**: 61–70.
10. Traynor BJ, Codd MB, Corr B et al. Incidence and prevalence of ALS in Ireland, 1995–1997: a population-based study. *Neurology* 1999; **52**: 504–509.
11. Chancellor AM, Slattery JM, Fraser H et al. The prognosis of adult-onset motor neuron disease: a prospective study based on the Scottish Motor Neuron Disease Register. *J Neurol* 1993; **240**: 339–346.
12. Chio A, Magnani C, Schiffer D. Gompertzian analysis of amyotrophic lateral sclerosis mortality in Italy, 1957–1987; application to birth cohorts. *Neuroepidemiology* 1995; **14**: 269–277.
13. Jenkinson C, Swash M, Fitzpatrick R. The European Amyotrophic Lateral Sclerosis Health Profile Study. ALS-HPS Steering Group. *J Neurol Sci* 1998; **160 (suppl 1)**: S122–S126.
14. Cudkowicz ME, McKenna-Yasek D, Sapp PE et al. Epidemiology of mutations in superoxide dismutase in amyotrophic lateral sclerosis. *Ann Neurol* 1997; **41**: 210–221.
15. Brooks BR. Natural history of ALS: symptoms, strength, pulmonary function, and disability. *Neurology* 1996; **47 (suppl 2)**: S71–S82.
16. Anderson FA Jr, Miller RG. ALS CARE: a resource for measuring and improving ALS outcomes. *Neurology* 1996; **47 (suppl 2)**: S113–S116.

17. Brooks BR, Shodis KA, Lewis DH et al. Natural history of amyotrophic lateral sclerosis: quantification of symptoms, signs, strength and function. In: Serratrice G, Munsat TL, eds. *Advances in Neurology 68. Pathogenesis and Therapy of Amyotrophic Lateral Sclerosis.* Philadelphia: Lippincott–Raven, 1995, 163–184.

18. Haverkamp LJ, Appel V, Appel SH. Natural history of amyotrophic lateral sclerosis in a database population. Validation of a scoring system and a model for survival prediction. *Brain* 1995; **118**: 707–719.

19. Brooks BR, Lewis D, Rawling J et al. The natural history of ALS. In: Williams AC, ed. *Motor Neuron Disease.* London: Chapman and Hall, 1994, 131–170.

20. Ringel SP, Murphy JR, Alderson MK et al. The natural history of amyotrophic lateral sclerosis. *Neurology* 1993; **43**: 1316–1322.

21. Norris F, Shepherd R, Denys E et al. Onset, natural history and outcome in idiopathic adult motor neuron disease. *J Neurol Sci* 1993; **118**: 48–55.

22. Strong MJ, Hudson AJ, Alvord WG. Familial amyotrophic lateral sclerosis, 1850–1989: a statistical analysis of the world literature. *Can J Neurol Sci* 1991; **18**: 45–58.

23. Meininger V, Bensimon G, Lacomblez L, Salachas F. Natural history of amyotrophic lateral sclerosis. A discussion. In: Serratrice G, Munsat T, eds. *Advances in Neurology 68. Pathogenesis and Therapy of Amyotrophic Lateral Sclerosis.* Philadelphia: Lippincott– Raven, 1995, 199–207.

24. Lee JR, Annegers J, Appel SH. Prognosis of amyotrophic lateral sclerosis and the effect of referral selection. *J Neurol Sci* 1995; **132**: 207–215.

25. Miller RG, Rosenberg JA, Gelinas DF et al. Practice parameter: the care of the patient with amyotrophic lateral sclerosis (an evidence-based review): report of the Quality Standards Subcommittee of the American Academy of Neurology: ALS Practice Parameters Task Force. *Neurology* 1999; **52**: 1311–1323.

26. BDNF Study Group (Phase III). A controlled trial of recombinant methionyl human BDNF in ALS: the BDNF Study Group (Phase III). *Neurology* 1999; **52**: 1427–1433.

27. Borasio GD, Linke R, Schwarz J et al. Dopaminergic deficit in amyotrophic lateral sclerosis assessed with [I-123] IPT single photon emission computed tomography. *J Neurol Neurosurg Psychiatry* 1998; **65**: 263–265.

28. Lai EC, Felice KJ, Festoff BW et al. Effect of recombinant human insulin-like growth factor-I on progression of ALS. A placebo-controlled study. The North American ALS/IGF-I Study Group. *Neurology* 1997; **49**: 1621–1630.

29. Borasio GD. Amyotrophic lateral sclerosis: lessons in trial design from recent trials. *J Neurol Sci* 1997; **152 (suppl 1)**: S23–S28.

30. Meininger V, Dib M, Aubin F et al. The Riluzole Early Access Programme: descriptive analysis of 844 patients in France. ALS/Riluzole Study Group III. *J Neurol* 1997; **244 (suppl 2)**: S22–S25.

31. Gubbay SS, Kahana E, Zilber N et al. Amyotrophic lateral sclerosis. A study of its presentation and prognosis. *J Neurol* 1985; **232**: 295–300.

32. Bonduelle M. Amyotrophic lateral sclerosis. *Rev Neurol* 1982; **138**: 1027–1039.

33. Armon C, Moses D. Linear estimates of rates of disease progression as predictors of survival in patients with ALS entering clinical trials. *J Neurol Sci* 1998; **160 (suppl 1)**: S37–S41.

34. Ksarskis EJ, Winslow M. When did Lou Gehrig's personal illness begin? *Neurology* 1989; **39**: 1243–1245.

35. Li TM, Alberman E, Swash M. Clinical features and associations of 560 cases of motor neuron disease. *J Neurol Neurosurg Psychiatry* 1990; **53**: 1043–1045.

36. Li TM, Alberman E, Swash M. Comparison of sporadic and familial disease amongst 580 cases of motor neuron disease. *J Neurol Neurosurg Psychiatry* 1988; **51**: 778–784.

37. Li TM, Day SJ, Alberman E, Swash M. Differential diagnosis of motoneurone disease from other neurological conditions. *Lancet* 1986; **2**: 731–733.

38. Cardol M, Brandsma JW, de Groot IJ et al. Handicap questionnaires: what do they assess? *Disabil Rehabil* 1999; **21**: 97–105.

39. Brooks BR. The Norris ALS score: insight

into the natural history of ALS provided by Forbes Norris. In: Rose FC, ed. *The Forbes H Norris Memorial Volume. ALS: from Charcot to the Present and into the Future.* London: Smith–Gordon, 1994.

40. Brooks BR. Amyotrophic lateral sclerosis clinimetric scales: guidelines for administration and scoring. In: Herndon RM, ed. *Handbook of Clinical Neurological Scales.* New York: Demos Vermande, 1997, 27–79.

41. Sobue G, Sahashi K, Takahashi A et al. Degenerating compartment and functioning compartment of motor neurons in ALS: possible process of motor neuron loss. *Neurology* 1983; **33**: 654–657.

42. Brooks BR, DePaul R, Tan YD et al. Motor Neuron Disease. In: Schoenberg BS, Porter R, eds. *Controlled Clinical Trials in Neurology.* Harwood: Marcel Dekker, 1990, 249–281.

43. Brooks BR, Sufit RL, DePaul R et al. Design of clinical therapeutic trials in amyotrophic lateral sclerosis. In: Rowland LP, ed. *Advances in Neurology 58. Amyotrophic Lateral Sclerosis and Other Motor Neuron Diseases.* New York: Raven, 1991, 521–546.

44. Brooks BR. The role of axonal transport in neurodegenerative disease spread: a meta-analysis of experimental and clinical poliomyelitis compares with amyotrophic lateral sclerosis. *Can J Neurol Sci* 1991; **18** (suppl): 435–438.

45. Brooke MH, Fenichel GM, Griggs RC et al. Clinical investigation in Duchenne dystrophy: 2. Determination of the 'power' of therapeutic trials based on the natural history. *Muscle Nerve* 1983; **6**: 91–103.

46. Brooke MH, Griggs RC, Mendell JR et al. Clinical trial in Duchenne dystrophy. I. The design of the protocol. *Muscle Nerve* 1981; **4**: 186–197.

47. Brooke MH, Florence JM, Heller SL et al. Controlled trial of thyrotropin releasing hormone in amyotrophic lateral sclerosis. *Neurology* 1986; **36**: 146–151.

48. Florence JM, Pandya S, King WM et al. Intrarater reliability of manual muscle test (Medical Research Council scale) grades in Duchenne's muscular dystrophy. *Phys Ther* 1992; **72**: 115–126.

49. Tawil R, Griggs RC, McDermott MP et al. A prospective quantitative study of the natural history of facioscapulohumeral muscular dystrophy (FSHD). Implications for therapeutic trials. *Neurology* 1997; **48**: 38–46.

50. Mendell JR, Moxley RT, Griggs RC et al. Randomized, double-blind six-month trial of prednisone in Duchenne's muscular dystrophy. *N Engl J Med* 1989; **320**: 1592–1597.

51. Tawil R, McDermott MP, Mendell JR et al. Facioscapulohumeral muscular dystrophy (FSHD): design of natural history study and results of baseline testing. *Neurology* 1994; **44**: 442–446.

52. Personius KE, Pandya S, King WM et al. Facioscapulohumeral dystrophy natural history study: standardization of testing procedures and reliability of measurements. *Phys Ther* 1994; **74**: 253–263.

53. Kilmer DD, Abresch RT, McCrory MA et al. Profiles of neuromuscular diseases: facioscapulohumeral dystrophy. *Am J Phys Med Rehabil* 1995; **74**: 131–139.

54. Medical Research Council. *Aids to the Investigation of Peripheral Nerve Injury. War Memorandum* 2nd edn. London: His Majesty's Stationery Medical Office (HSMO), 1943, 11–46.

55. Sanjak M, Bleden D, Cook T, Brooks B. Muscle strength measurement. In: Lane R, ed. *Handbook of Muscle Disease.* New York: Marcel Dekker, 1996, 19–31.

56. National Isometric Muscle Strength (NIMS) Database Consortium. Muscular weakness assessment: use of normal isometric strength data. *Arch Phys Med Rehabil* 1996; **77**: 1251–1125.

57. Brinkmann JR, Andres P, Mendoza M, Sanjak M. Guidelines for the use and performance of quantitative outcome measures in ALS clinical trials. *J Neurol Sci* 1997; **147**: 97–111.

58. Brooks BR, Sanjak M, Belden D, Walclawik A. Motor neurone disease: basic designs, sample sizes and pitfalls. In: Guiloff R, ed. *Clinical Trials in Neurology.* London: Springer-Verlag, in press.

59. Andres PL, Skerry LM, Thornell B et al. A comparison of three measures of disease progression in ALS. *J Neurol Sci* 1996; **139** (suppl): 64–70.

60. Armon C, Ponraj E. Comparing composite scores based on maximal voluntary isometric contraction and on semiquantitative manual motor testing in measuring limb strength in patients with ALS. *Neurology* 1996; **47**: 1586–1587.

61. Goonetilleke A, Guiloff RJ, Nikhar N et al. The clinical assessment of muscle force (abstract). *J Neurol Sci* 1997; **150 (suppl)**: S4.

62. ALS CNTF Treatment Study (ACTS) Phase I–II Group. The Amyotrophic Lateral Sclerosis Functional Rating Scale. Assessment of activities of daily living in patients with amyotrophic lateral sclerosis. The ALS CNTF treatment study (ACTS) Phase I–II Study Group. *Arch Neurol* 1996; **53**: 141–147.

63. ALS CNTF Treatment Study (ACTS) Phase III Group. A double-blind placebo-controlled clinical trial of subcutaneous recombinant human ciliary neurotrophic factor (rHCNTF) in amyotrophic lateral sclerosis. ALS CNTF Treatment Study Group. *Neurology* 1996; **46**: 1244–1249.

64. Hoagland RJ, Mendoza M, Armon C et al. Reliability of maximal voluntary isometric contraction testing in a multicenter study of patients with amyotrophic lateral sclerosis. Syntex/Synergen Neuroscience Joint Venture rhCNTF ALS Study Group. *Muscle Nerve* 1997; **20**: 691–695.

65. Aitkens S, Lord J, Bernauer E et al. Relationship of manual muscle testing to objective strength measurements. *Muscle Nerve* 1998; **12**: 173–177.

66. Munsat TL. Issues in clinical trial design I: Use of natural history controls. A protagonist view. *Neurology* 1996; **47 (suppl 2)**: S96–S97.

67. Munsat TL, Andres PL, Finison L et al. The natural history of motoneuron loss in amyotrophic lateral sclerosis. *Neurology* 1988; **38**: 409–413.

68. Munsat TL, Andres PL, Skerry LM. The use of quantitative techniques to define amyotrophic lateral sclerosis. In: Munsat TL, ed. *Quantification of Neurologic Deficit*. Boston: Butterworths, 1989, 129–142.

69. Munsat TL, Hollander D, Andres P, Finison L. Clinical trials in ALS: measurement and natural history. In: Rowland LP, ed. *Advances in Neurology 56. Amyotrophic Lateral Sclerosis and Other Motor Neuron Diseases*. New York: Raven, 1991, 515–520.

70. Andres PL, Hedlund W, Finison L et al. Quantitative motor assessment in amyotrophic lateral sclerosis. *Neurology* 1986; **36**: 937–941.

71. De Paul R, Abbs JH. Manifestations of ALS in the cranial motor nerves: dynametric, neuropathologic and speech motor data. *Neurol Clin North Am* 1987; **5**: 231–250.

72. De Paul R, Brooks BR. Multiple orofacial indices in amyotrophic lateral sclerosis. *J Speech Hearing Res* 1993; **36**: 1158–1167.

73. De Paul R, Abbs JH, Caliguiri MP, Gracco VL. Differential involvement of hypoglossal, trigeminal and facial motoneurons in ALS. *Neurology* 1998; **38**: 281–283.

74. Dworkin JP. Tongue strength measurement in patients with amyotrophic lateral sclerosis: qualitative vs quantitative procedures. *Arch Phys Med Rehabil* 1980; **61**: 422–424.

75. Dworkin JP, Aronson AE. Tongue strength and alternate motion rates in normal and dysarthric subjects. *J Commun Disord* 1986; **19**: 115–132.

76. Dworkin JP, Culatta RA. Tongue strength: its relationship to tongue thrusting, open-bite, and articulatory proficiency. *J Speech Hearing Disorders* 1980; **45**: 277–282.

77. Dworkin JP, Hartman DE. Progressive speech deterioration and dysphagia in amyotrophic lateral sclerosis: case report. *Arch Phys Med Rehabil* 1979; **60**: 423–425.

78. Dworkin JP, Aronson AE, Mulder DW. Tongue force in normals and in dysarthric patients with amyotrophic lateral sclerosis. *J Speech Hearing Res* 1980; **23**: 828–837.

79. Hillel AD, Yorkston K, Miller RM. Using phonation time to estimate vital capacity in amyotrophic lateral sclerosis. *Arch Phys Med Rehabil* 1989; **70**: 618–620.

80. Kent JF, Kent RD, Rosenbek JC et al. Quantitative description of the dysarthria in women with amyotrophic lateral sclerosis. *J Speech Hearing Res* 1992; **35**: 723–733.

81. Kent RD, Sufit RL, Rosenbek JC et al. Speech deterioration in amyotrophic lateral sclerosis: a case study. *J Speech Hearing Res* 1991; **34**: 1269–1275.

82. Ramig LO, Scherer RC, Klasner ER et al. Acoustic analysis of voice in amyotrophic lateral sclerosis: a longitudinal case study. *J Speech Hearing Dis* 1990; **55**: 2–14.

83. Turner GS, Tjaden K, Weismer G. The influence of speaking rate on vowel space and speech intelligibility for individuals with amyotrophic lateral sclerosis. *J Speech Hearing Res* 1995; **38**: 1001–1013.

84. Weismer G, Martin R, Kent RD, Kent JF. Formant trajectory characteristics of males with amyotrophic lateral sclerosis. *J Acoust Soc Am* 1992; **91**: 1085–1098.

85. Aboussouan LS, Khan SU, Meeker DP et al. Effect of noninvasive positive-pressure ventilation on survival in amyotrophic lateral sclerosis. *Ann Intern Med* 1997; **127**: 450–453.

86. Braun SR. Respiratory system in amyotrophic lateral sclerosis. *Neurol Clin* 1987; **5**: 9–31.

87. Bach JR. Amyotrophic lateral sclerosis. Communication status and survival with ventilatory support [published erratum appears in *Am J Phys Med Rehabil* 1994; **73**: 218]. *Am J Phys Med Rehabil* 1993; **72**: 343–349.

88. Bach JR. Amyotrophic lateral sclerosis: predictors for prolongation of life by noninvasive respiratory aids. *Arch Phys Med Rehabil* 1995; **76**: 828–832.

89. Bach JR, Rajaraman R, Ballanger F et al. Neuromuscular ventilatory insufficiency: effect of home mechanical ventilator use v oxygen therapy on pneumonia and hospitalization rates. *Am J Phys Med Rehabil* 1998; **77**: 8–19.

90. Bio M, Bach JR. Positive-pressure ventilation in amyotrophic lateral sclerosis. *Ann Intern Med* 1998; **128**: 601–602.

91. Cazzolli PA, Oppenheimer EA. Home mechanical ventilation for amyotrophic lateral sclerosis: nasal compared to tracheostomy–intermittent positive pressure ventilation. *J Neurol Sci* 1996; **139** (**suppl**): 123–128.

92. Dean S, Bach JR. The use of noninvasive respiratory muscle aids in the management of patients with progressive neuromuscular diseases. *Respir Care Clin North Am* 1996; **2**: 223–240.

93. Gay PC, Westbrook PR, Daube JR et al. Effects of alterations in pulmonary function and sleep variables on survival in patients with amyotrophic lateral sclerosis. *Mayo Clin Proc* 1991; **66**: 686–694.

94. Gelinas DF, O'Connor P, Miller RG. Quality of life for ventilator-dependent ALS patients and their caregivers. *J Neurol Sci* 1998; **160** (**suppl 1**): S134–S136.

95. Hanayama K, Ishikawa Y, Bach JR. Amyotrophic lateral sclerosis. Successful treatment of mucous plugging by mechanical insufflation–exsufflation. *Am J Phys Med Rehabil* 1997; **76**: 338–339.

96. Moss AH, Casey P, Stocking CB et al. Home ventilation for amyotrophic lateral sclerosis patients: outcomes, costs, and patient, family, and physician attitudes. *Neurology* 1993; **43**: 438–443.

97. Moss AH, Oppenheimer EA, Casey P et al. Patients with amyotrophic lateral sclerosis receiving long-term mechanical ventilation. Advance care planning and outcomes. *Chest* 1996; **110**: 249–255.

98. Polkey MI, Lyall RA, Moxham J, Leigh PN. Respiratory aspects of neurological disease. *J Neurol Neurosurg Psychiatry* 1999; **66**: 5–15.

99. Schiffman PL, Belsh JM. Pulmonary function at diagnosis of amyotrophic lateral sclerosis. Rate of deterioration. *Chest* 1993; **103**: 508–513.

100. Slavin MD, Jette DU, Andres PL, Munsat TL. Lower extremity muscle force measures and functional ambulation in patients with amyotrophic lateral sclerosis. *Arch Phys Med Rehabil* 1998; **79**: 950–954.

101. Cedarbaum JM, Stambler N. Performance of the Amyotrophic Lateral Sclerosis Functional Rating Scale (ALSFRS) in multicenter clinical trials. *J Neurol Sci* 1997; **152** (**suppl 1**): S1–S9.

102. Riviere M, Meininger V, Zeisser P, Munsat T. An analysis of extended survival in patients with amyotrophic lateral sclerosis treated with riluzole. *Arch Neurol* 1998; **55**: 526–528.

103. Guiloff RJ, Goonetilleke A. Natural history of amyotrophic lateral sclerosis: observations with Charing Cross Amyotrophic Lateral Sclerosis Rating Scales. In: Serratrice G, Munsat T, eds. *Advances in Neurology 68. Patho-*

genesis and Therapy of Amyotrophic Lateral Sclerosis. Philadelphia: Lippincott–Raven, 1995, 185–198.

104. Hillel AD, Miller RM, Yorkston K et al. Amyotrophic lateral sclerosis severity scale. Neuroepidemiology 1989; 8: 142–150.

105. Appel V, Stewart SS, Smith G, Appel SH. A rating scale for amyotrophic lateral sclerosis: description and preliminary experience. Ann Neurol 1987; 22: 328–333.

106. Louwerse ES, de Jong JMBV, Kuether G. Critique of assessment methodology in amyotrophic lateral sclerosis. In: Rose FC, ed. Amyotrophic Lateral Sclerosis. Progress in Clinical Neurologic Trials. New York: Demos, 1990, 151–180.

107. Louwerse ES, Visser CE, Bossuyt PMM et al. Amyotrophic lateral sclerosis: mortality risk during the course of the disease and prognostic factors. J Neurol Sci 1997; 152 (suppl): S10–S17.

108. Anonymous. Nutritional status of patients with amyotrophic lateral sclerosis: relation to the proximity of death. Dysphagia 1997; 12: 174–175.

109. Dray TG, Hillel AD, Miller RM. Dysphagia caused by neurologic deficits. Otolaryngol Clin North Am 1998; 31: 507–524.

110. Hillel AD, Miller R. Bulbar amyotrophic lateral sclerosis: patterns of progression and clinical management. Head Neck 1989; 11: 51–59.

111. Leighton SE, Burton MJ, Lund WS, Cochrane GM. Swallowing in motor neurone disease. J R Soc Med 1994; 87: 801–805.

112. Robbins J. Swallowing in ALS and motor neuron disease. Neurol Clin 1987; 5: 213–229.

113. Strand EA, Miller RM, Yorkston KM, Hillel AD. Management of oral–pharyngeal dysphagia symptoms in amyotrophic lateral sclerosis. Dysphagia 1996; 11: 129–139.

114. Moore SR, Gresham LS, Bromberg MB et al. A self-report measure of affective lability. J Neurol Neurosurg Psychiatry 1997; 63: 89–93.

115. Eisen A, Schulzer M, MacNeil M et al. Duration of amyotrophic lateral sclerosis is age-dependent. Muscle Nerve 1993; 16: 27–32.

116. Stambler N, Charatan M, Cedarbaum JM. Prognostic indicators of survival in ALS. ALS CNTF Treatment Study Group. Neurology 1998; 50: 66–72.

117. Mazzini L, Corra T, Zaccala M et al. Percutaneous endoscopic gastrostomy and enteral nutrition in amyotrophic lateral sclerosis. J Neurol 1995; 242: 695–698.

118. Mathus-Vliegen LM, Louwerse LS, Merkus MP et al. Percutaneous endoscopic gastrostomy in patients with amyotrophic lateral sclerosis and impaired pulmonary function. Gastrointest Endosc 1994; 40: 463–469.

119. Rozier A, Ruskone Fourmestraux A, Rosenbaum A et al. Role of percutaneous endoscopic gastrostomy in amyotrophic lateral sclerosis. Rev Neurol 1991; 147: 174–176.

120. Silani V, Kasarskis EJ, Yanagisawa N. Nutritional management in amyotrophic lateral sclerosis: a worldwide perspective. J Neurol 1998; 245 (suppl 2): S13–S19; discussion S29.

121. Worwood AM, Leigh PN. Indicators and prevalence of malnutrition in motor neurone disease. Eur Neurol 1998; 40: 159–163.

122. Kasarskis EJ, Berryman S, English T et al. The use of upper extremity anthropometrics in the clinical assessment of patients with amyotrophic lateral sclerosis. Muscle Nerve 1997; 20: 330–335.

123. Kasarskis EJ, Berryman S, Vanderleest JG et al. Nutritional status of patients with amyotrophic lateral sclerosis: relation to the proximity of death. Am J Clin Nutr 1996; 63: 130–137.

124. Gray AM. ALS/MND and the perspective of health economics. J Neurol Sci 1998; 160 (suppl 1): S2–S5.

125. Swash M. Health outcome and quality-of-life measurements in amyotrophic lateral sclerosis. J Neurol 1997; 244 (suppl 2): S26–S29.

126. Fowler WM Jr, Abresch RT, Aitkens S et al. Profiles of neuromuscular diseases: design of the protocol. Am J Phys Med Rehabil 1995; 74: 62–69.

127. Fowler WM, Abresch RT, Koch TR et al. Employment profiles in neuromuscular diseases. Am J Phys Med Rehabil 1997; 76: 26–37.

128. McGuire D, Garrison L, Armon C et al. A brief quality-of-life measure for ALS clinical

trials based on a subset of items from the sickness impact profile. The Syntex–Synergen ALS/CNTF Study Group. *J Neurol Sci* 1997; **152 (suppl 1):** S18–S22.

129. McGuire D, Garrison L, Armon C et al. Relationship of the Tufts Quantitative Neuromuscular Exam (TQNE) and the Sickness Impact Profile (SIP) in measuring progression of ALS. SSNJV/CNTF ALS Study Group. *Neurology* 1996; **46:** 1442–1444.

3

Juvenile amyotrophic lateral sclerosis

Mongi Ben Hamida and Fayçal Hentati

Introduction

One hundred and thirty years after Charcot's description[1] of a disease of later life that involved the cortical motor neurons and anterior horn cells (motor neuron disease), the cause of amyotrophic lateral sclerosis (ALS) remains unknown. The familial occurrence of ALS was often denied for a long period until the description of an autosomal dominant disorder in Chamorros (the indigenous population of Guam and other Mariana Islands) by Kurland and Mulder[2] and Hirano.[3] Young patients were included in these descriptions. There are, however, few reports in old literature of juvenile ALS.[4] In many circumstances the diagnosis was questionable because of the unusual clinical associations (ophthalmoplegia, hypoacusis, choreiform movements) the extreme rarity of pathological data, and the frequent familial occurrence. In the authors' first study on ALS in Tunisia,[5] there were two distinct groups of ALS: a juvenile group with onset before 25 years of age and an adult group with onset after 35 years. Early-onset cases (between 30 and 35 years) were very rare (*Fig. 3.1*).

Juvenile or infantile ALS usually shows typical clinical features of bilateral pyramidal signs, amyotrophy of the small muscles of the hands, and fasciculations, with or without a bulbar or pseudobulbar syndrome in infancy, adolescence or early adulthood.[6,7]

Juvenile ALS, which is most often familial but may be sporadic, is generally a chronic disease with a benign long-term prognosis. A more recent and extensive report of 43 cases by Ben Hamida and colleagues[8] emphasized the clinical heterogeneity and the relative high frequency in Tunisia.

Juvenile ALS appears to be a good genetic model for Charcot disease, because of the similarity of the clinical features of the two diseases. The identification of the defective gene could be of great interest for understanding the pathophysiology of the degeneration of the motor neurons.

The severe form of juvenile ALS

Severe juvenile-onset ALS is a very rare disorder with a prognosis similar to that of classical ALS. Very rare observations of severe rapidly progressive juvenile-onset ALS have been reported.[4,9-11] In the first case reported by van Bogaert,[4] the onset was characterized by bulbar signs, and death occurred in 12 months. The history of this patient's brother, reported by the same author, had a chronic evolution over 15 years, and the neuropathological study showed a severe loss of bulbospinal motor neurons loss and disappearance of the

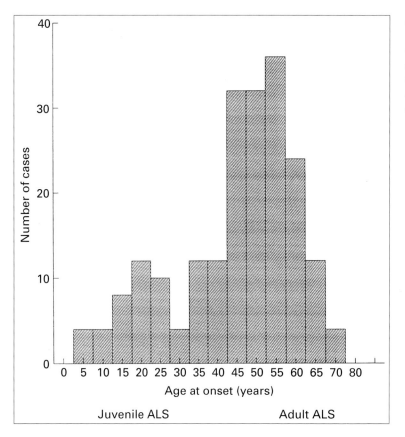

Figure 3.1
The first peak in the age of onset corresponds to juvenile ALS, with the mean age of onset around 20 years. The second peak corresponds to the adult classical form of ALS.[5]

motor neurons in anterior horns of the spinal cord with diffuse demyelination of the posterior and pyramidal tracts.

In the report by Berry and colleagues,[9] the patient was 15 years old when his illness began. He died at 16.5 years of age. The autopsy showed similar neuropathological changes to those encountered in classical ALS. The case reported by Cognazzo and Martin[12] was a girl aged 20 years who suffered from progressive amyotrophy and who died 10 months later with a bulbar syndrome. The clinical features were characteristic of ALS and the diagnosis was confirmed at autopsy. The case reported by Nelson and Prensky[11] was a

12-year-old girl who had progressively flaccid paralysis of the right upper extremity and no family history. Seven months after the onset of the illness, the weakness and a flaccid quadriparesis progressed, with increased deep tendon reflexes and ankle clonus. There were, on examination, slurred speech and numerous tongue fasciculations, and marked atrophy of the proximal and distal muscles of all extremities. The plantar response was extensor bilaterally. No sensory loss was noted. The disease progressed rapidly and the patient died approximately 1 year after the onset of the disease.

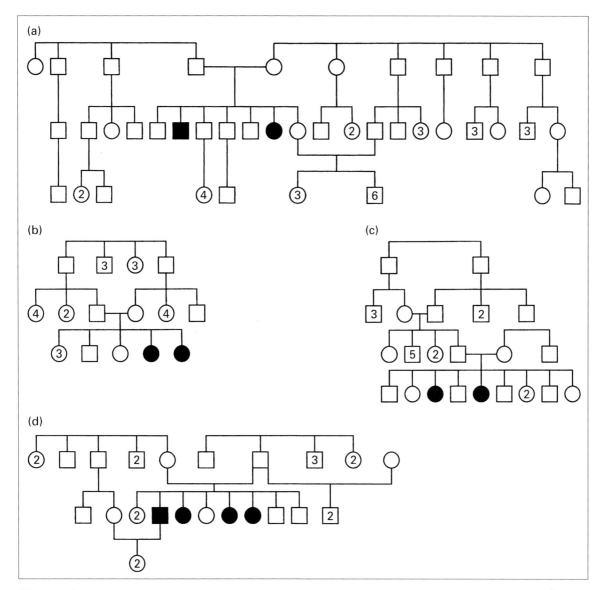

Figure 3.2
Pedigree of four families showing autosomal recessive inheritance.

The chronic form of juvenile ALS

Chronic juvenile ALS is more common than the severe form and is most often familial. The idea that ALS could occur in several members in the same family has been accepted since the Guam Island study in 1954[13] demonstrated that ALS has clinical features similar to those of Charcot disease. Several cases had been reported in the Western literature.

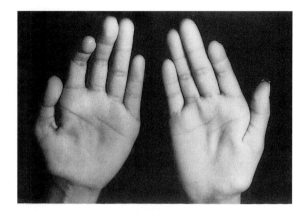

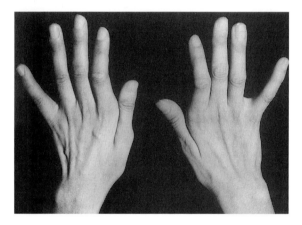

Figure 3.3
Atrophy of the small muscles of the hands.

Clinical presentation of juvenile ALS

Chronic juvenile ALS is a heterogeneous disease, characterized by autosomal recessive inheritance (*Fig. 3.2*), age of onset before 25 years, a progressive and benign course, upper and lower motor neuron involvement, and the absence of other features (sensory, cerebellar, optic vestibular, or extrapyramidal). The first

two cases (a brother and sister) were reported in Finland.[14] Careful examination of the whole family showed clear signs of motor neuron involvement. According to the large study by Ben Hamida and colleagues,[8] three clinical phenotype groups can be defined.

(a) Group 1 (the common form) is characterized by muscular atrophy of the small muscles of the hands, a pyramidal syndrome in all four limbs, and late development of a bulbar syndrome.
(b) Group 2 is characterized by spastic paraplegia with peroneal atrophy, a pyramidal syndrome of the lower limbs, and atrophy of the legs. There are no sensory disturbances.[15]
(c) Group 3 is characterized by a spastic pseudobulbar syndrome with spastic paraplegia, pseudobulbar syndrome, pyramidal syndrome of all four limbs, and mild wasting of the hands or legs, or both.

Group 1 (the common form)

This group is characterized by upper limb amyotrophy and pyramidal signs with or without a bulbar syndrome. Muscle atrophy begins in the small muscles of the hands (*Fig. 3.3*), and rarely extends progressively to the shoulders. Fasciculations appear mainly in the atrophic muscles and sometimes in the tongue. These fasciculations are arrhythmic and painless and are provoked by exposure to cold. Muscle cramps are noted in some cases. Pyramidal hypertonia is accompanied by brisk stretch reflexes. The Babinski sign is inconstant. Gait is spastic. The bulbar syndrome appears gradually with labioglossopharyngeal paralysis, dysarthria, dysphagia, tongue atrophy and paralysis of the soft palate. The masseteric reflex is brisk. There is spasmodic laughing and crying. There are no sensory disturbances.

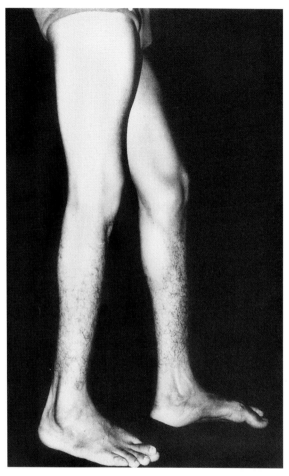

Figure 3.4
Marked atrophy of the legs. Note the atrophy of the lower part of thigh and the presence of pes cavus.

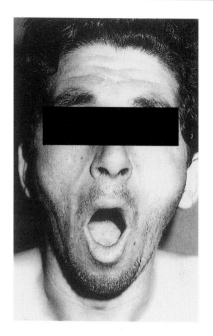

Figure 3.5
Pseudobulbar syndrome. The patient is unable to move the tongue.

Group 2 (spastic paraplegia with peroneal atrophy)

This group is characterized by spastic paraplegia, spastic gait, and atrophy of the lower limbs (*Fig 3.4*), with frequent loss of one or both ankle jerks. There are no bulbar signs. Atrophy of the hands with fasciculations can be seen. A Babinski sign is usually present. There is no bladder dysfunction or sensory disturbance.

Group 3 (spastic pseudobulbar syndrome with spastic paraplegia)

In two large families analysed by Ben Hamida and colleagues,[8] pseudobulbar syndrome and spastic paraplegia were the dominant clinical features in all cases. There were severe hypertonia of the facial muscles, with (*Fig 3.5*), spastic laughing and weeping, spastic dysarthria, atrophy of the legs more commonly than atrophy of the hands, and spastic gait. There were no fasciculations, lingual atrophy, bladder dysfunction, or sensory disturbances.

Diagnosis

In the absence of autopsy documentation, the diagnosis of chronic juvenile ALS is usually based on clinical neurophysiological and histopathological criteria.

Pathology and nerve biopsy study

In many respects, the sporadic adult disease and the juvenile disease are similar. However, in the four juvenile cases reported,[4,9–11] the changes in the brain and spinal cord involved both gray and white matter. In the gray matter, there was neuron cell loss and fibrillary astrocytosis. The most frequent neuronal abnormality was the occurrence of single or multiple inclusions within neuronal cell bodies. All inclusions showed uniform, intense argyrophilia in Bodian preparations. Neurons with inclusions were numerous in the third and fifth layers of motor cortex. Frank loss of nerve cells and fibrillary astrocytosis were most extensive in anterior horns and in the hypoglossal nucleus; these changes were seen to a moderate degree in the Vth motor nucleus and the facial nucleus and to a slight degree in the dentate nucleus.

In the white matter of the spinal cord and the medulla, moderate to marked symmetrical loss of myelin and axons, formation of lipids phagocytosis, and fibrillary astrocytosis were evident. Spinal cord lesions were located in the anterior and lateral columns, affecting mainly the crossed and uncrossed corticospinal tracts. There was moderate to marked loss of axons and myelin in the anterior nerve roots. Bilateral corticospinal tract degeneration with evidence of active demyelination was present in all cases.

Nevertheless, numerous studies based on autopsy cases have shown involvement of the non-motor pathways in Charcot disease. In this regard, mention should be made of the autopsy observation of demyelination of the posterior (Goll–Burdach) tracts by Charcot and Marie.[16] The same finding has been reported by other authors,[17–21] but they have been unable to give a satisfactory explanation. In addition, Bertrand and van Bogaert[17] stated in their neuropathological report of Charcot disease that in the peripheral nerve trunks 'the sensory fibres are as poor in myelin as are the motor fibres'. This question came out in more recent studies on peripheral sensory nerves in this disease. Dyck and colleagues[22] looked at the superficial sensory branch of the peroneal nerves of seven patients with ALS and found that one patient had a reduced density of myelinated fibers and two patients had an increased extent of axonal degeneration in single teased nerve fibers. They concluded that there was some degeneration of sensory nerves in ALS. Tohgi and colleagues[23] found a significant reduction in the number of large-diameter fibers and, to a lesser extent, small-diameter fibers in a proportion of ALS sural nerves. Kawamura and colleagues[24] found a 54% reduction in the number of large neurons in the fifth lumbar dorsal root ganglia and a 27% reduction in the number of large myelinated fibers in the fifth dorsal root in ALS patients.

In a morphometric study,[25] the sural nerves of 21 patients with ALS had more acute axonal degeneration and 30% fewer myelinated fibers ($p < 0.05$) than controls. Evidence of degeneration also extended to unmyelinated fibers. Ben Hamida and colleagues[26] reported a morphometric study of the sensory nerve in classical adult ALS (Charcot disease) and juvenile ALS. Superficial peroneal nerve was analysed in nine cases of adult ALS and compared to eight age-matched controls. There was a very significant reduction in all myelinated fibers ($p < 0.001$). Similar analysis was performed in seven patients with juvenile ALS and, compared to four age-matched controls, showed a significant reduction ($p < 0.05$) in myelinated fibers. The large unmyelinated fibers were increased later ($p < 0.01$) in adult and juvenile ALS. This later study[26] showed that the lesions of the sensory nerve are of the same type but are more obvious in adult ALS than juvenile ALS.

Skeletal muscle showed neurogenic atrophy. In addition, muscle biopsy taken in 29 cases showed neurogenic atrophy in the peroneous brevis muscle.

Electrophysiology

Electromyography is usually sufficient to establish the diagnosis of juvenile ALS. The pattern of these abnormalities is the same as in the adult forms[27] and includes:

(a) fibrillations and fasciculations in muscles of the lower and upper extremities, and sometimes also in the head and the tongue;
(b) an increase in the number, amplitude, and duration of motor unit action potentials;
(c) normal electrical excitability of the remaining fibers of motor nerves, with motor fiber conduction velocity within the normal range in nerves of relatively unaffected muscles and not less than 70% of the average normal value, according to age, in nerves of more severely affected muscles;
(d) normal excitability and conduction velocity of afferent nerve fibers, even in severely affected extremities.

This pattern of abnormalities serves to distinguish juvenile ALS from myopathies, localized lesions of the spinal cord, and disease affecting only upper motor neurons.

Discussion

In the common form of juvenile ALS, amyotrophy affects mainly the small muscles of the hand, which corresponds to degeneration of motor neurons mainly in the cervical anterior horn. There may be bulbar or pseudobulbar signs. Comparable clinical observations[28,29] have rarely been mentioned in the literature.[14,30]

These clinical features are different from the classical description of pure spastic paraplegia, in which there are normal deep tendon reflexes in the arms and no dysarthria or fasciculations. In 1966, Silver[29] reported two families characterized by autosomal-dominant inheritance and similar clinical features 'spastic paraplegia with amyotrophy of the hands'. There was no mention of fasciculations. Van Gent and colleagues[31] described a family with autosomal-dominant inheritance in which most patients had associated distal muscular atrophy of the upper limbs and upper motor neuron signs. The authors concluded that this was a type of motor neuron disorder that is slightly different from the disease described by Silver. Clinical evidence of sensory disturbances were only seen in the oldest patient, who had a mild peroneal atrophy. A few years later, Myllyla and colleagues[14] described two familial cases of juvenile ALS.

In familial spastic paraplegia there is usually no distal atrophy, except in the late evolution of the chronic form, in which atrophy of hand muscles sometimes occurs.[15] No peroneal atrophy was observed during the evolution of spastic paraplegia. The muscle atrophy of the hands had already been noted by Refsum and Skillicorn[28] and Silver.[29]

An autosomal-recessive form of spastic paraplegia, the Troyer syndrome, which produces distal muscle wasting, was described by Cross and McKusick[32] and could be considered in the frame of juvenile ALS reported by

Van Bogaert[4] and Emery and Holloway.[7] This form of spastic paraplegia is different from what Dyck[33] called hereditary sensory motor neuropathy (HSMN) type 5, which was characterized by the presence of clinical and electrophysiological sensory disturbances. In Troyer syndrome there are no sensory disturbances. The mild reduction in myelinated fibers in the superficial peroneal nerve is not significant compared to that seen in HSMN.

In Group 2 juvenile ALS, with spastic paraplegia and a pure motor peroneal atrophy, the lesion of the anterior horn is supposed to be located in the dorsolumbar cord. The abolition of ankle reflexes and the absence of a Babinski sign could be explained by the severity of motor neuron lesions in the dorsolumbar cord and the marked atrophy of the pyramidal tract at the spinal level.

In Group 3 juvenile ALS, the clinical features are close to those of primary lateral sclerosis, with undetectable anterior horn involvement. Similar clinical aspects have been reported as 'chronic progressive bilateral spinobulbar spasticity' or 'chronic progressive spastic bulbar paralysis',[35] involving only middle-aged or elderly patients. In the authors' experience, this chronic progressive spastic pseudobulbar paralysis occurs in infants and children with a possible association with peroneal atrophy and, more rarely, atrophy of the hands, indicating a possible involvement of the anterior horn.

Atypical ALS and associated forms

As classically defined, ALS is a disease purely of the motor neurons, with no involvement of the sensory nerve fibers. Nevertheless, since the observations by Charcot[34] and the neuropathology report by Bertrand and van Bogaert[17] in 1925, autopsy data in Charcot disease have confirmed the involvement of the non-motor pathways. This question has been discussed by several authors.[3,18–20] Tohgi and colleagues[23] and Bradley and colleagues[25] have shown some changes in the peripheral sensory nerves. In fact, the ALS syndrome could be associated with many other disorders.[36]

Brown–Vialetto–van Laere syndrome

This group of ALS syndromes is characterized by a progressive bulbopontine paralysis, associated with deafness and a pyramidal syndrome. There is a cranial nerve involvement (progressive bulbopontine paralysis), progressive neural deafness, spastic paraplegia, and atrophy of the hands. The progressive bulbopontine paralysis associated with deafness and pyramidal signs is closely related to the previous group and should be considered within the same category as juvenile ALS. In van Laere's opinion,[37] this syndrome is a distinct entity and it is currently accepted as Brown–Vialetto–van Laere syndrome.[38] The onset of the disease occurs early, with progressive deafness, facial diplegia, bulbar paralysis, tongue atrophy, difficulty in swallowing, and dysarthria. Pyramidal signs (brisk reflexes, a Babinski sign) are present. There may be slight abnormalities of motor nerve conduction velocity and there are no sensory disturbances.

Madras syndrome

In India, Meenakshisundaram and colleagues[39] reported a group of 11 young patients with very slowly progressive motor neuron disease. There was bilateral Bell's palsy in six cases, bulbar paralysis in seven cases, distal weakness and wasting in eight patients, with typical fasciculations. Tendon reflexes were brisk in three patients, sluggish in one, and normal in three, with bilateral extensor plantar response.

The fasciculations were noted in just the eight patients with wasted muscles. Bilateral extensor plantar response was present in all patients, except in one who had marked foot drop with brisk knee and upper tendon reflexes. Five patients showed perceptive deafness. There was no familial history and no autopsy examination was performed. The presence of deafness, bulbopontine paralysis, and pyramidal signs are exactly the same as in Brown–Vialetto–van-Laere syndrome. The six patients with normal hearing could be considered as showing infantile progressive bulbar paralysis, or Fazio–Londe syndrome.

ALS-like syndrome associated with giant axonal neuropathy

A slowly progressive autosomal-recessive form of giant axonal neuropathy (GAN) with an ALS-like syndrome (distal amyotrophy brisk reflexes, diffuse fasciculations, and bulbar signs) and deep sensory loss in the lower limbs, representing a complex multisystem degeneration, has been reported.[40] In this large kindred of six cases, the patients presented with a progressive infantile onset of distal amyotrophy, brisk reflexes, diffuse fasciculations, bulbar signs, and deep sensory loss in both lower limbs. In four patients there were giant axons filled with neurofilaments, with normal conduction velocity. This familial disorder was found to be linked to the same chromosome locus as the other GAN disorders.

Genetics

In 20% of the families with autosomal dominant ALS, the gene has been mapped on chromosome 21q.[41] The defective gene has been identified as the gene encoding for copper–zinc superoxyde dismutase.[42] Cases of recessive familial ALS are genetically heterogenous. Two genes of recessive juvenile ALS have been mapped: the gene of Group 3 juvenile ALS on chromosome 2q[43] and the gene of Group 1 juvenile ALS on chromosome 15q.[44] The gene of Group 2 juvenile ALS has not yet been identified. The three phonotypic groups of juvenile ALS are clinically and genetically different from hereditary spastic paraplegia. The pure autosomal-dominant forms have been mapped on chromosome 14q, chromosome 2q, and chromosome 15q. The Tunisian autosomal-recessive form has been mapped on chromosome 8q.[45] This locus is excluded in other autosomal-recessive Tunisian families.

References

1. Charcot JM, Joffroy A. Deux cas d'atrophie musculaire progressive avec lésions de la substance grise et des faisceaux antéro-latéraux de la moelle épinière. *Arch Physiol Norm Pathol* 1869; **2**: 354–367, 629–649, 744–760.
2. Kurland LT, Mulder DW. Epidemiology, investigations of amyotrophic lateral sclerosis, 2 familial aggregations indicative of dominant inheritance, Part II. *Neurology* (Minneapolis) 1955; **5**: 240–268.
3. Hirano A, Arumu Gasamy N, Zimmerman HM. Amyotrophic lateral sclerosis. A comparison of Guam and classical cases. *Arch Neurol* 1967; **4**: 357–363.
4. van Bogaert L. La sclérose latérale amyotrophique et la paralysie bulbaire progressive chez l'enfant. *Rev Neurol* 1925; **2**: 180–192.
5. Ben Hamida M, Hentati F. Maladie de Charcot et sclérose latérale amyotrophique juvénile. *Rev Neurol* 1984; **140**: 202–206.
6. Bonduelle M. Amyotrophic lateral sclerosis. In: Vinkin PJ, Bruyun G, eds. *Handbook of Clinical neurology: System Disorders and Atrophies* vol 22, part II. Amsterdam, Oxford: North Holland Publishing Company; New York: American Elsevier Publishing Company, 1975, 281–337.
7. Emery AEH, Holloway LP. *Familial Motor Neuron Disease. Human Motor Neuron Diseases.* New York: Raven Press, 1982, 139–147.

8. Ben Hamida M, Hentati F, Ben Hamida C. Hereditary motor system diseases (chronic juvenile amyotrophic lateral sclerosis). *Brain* 1990; **113**: 347–363.

9. Berry RG, Chambers RA, Duckett S, Torrero R. Clinico-pathological study of juvenile amyotrophic lateral sclerosis. *Neurology* (Minneapolis) 1969; **19**: 312.

10. Nishigaki S. Takahaski A, Matsuoka A. An autopsy case of sporadic amyotrophic lateral sclerosis. *Clin Neurol* 1971; **11**: 500–506.

11. Nelson JS, Prensky AL. Sporadic juvenile amyotrophic lateral sclerosis. *Arch Neurol* 1972; **27**: 300–306.

12. Cognazzo A, Martin L. A sporadic case of juvenile amyotrophic lateral sclerosis. Semiquantitative and histo-enzymological study of the denervated muscles. *Euro Neurol* 1970; **3**: 211–230.

13. Mulder DW, Kurland LT. Amyotrophic lateral sclerosis in Micronesia. *Proc Mayo Clin* 1954; **29**: 666.

14. Myllyla VV, Toivakka E, Ala-Hurula V et al. Juvenile amyotrophic lateral sclerosis. *Acta Neurol Scand* 1979; **60**: 170–177.

15. Ben Hamida M, Hentati F, Ben Hamida C, Attia-Romdhane N. Paraplégie spasmodique et atrophie distale des familles à début infantile et juvénile. Une forme clinique de sclérose latérale amyotrophique juvénile. In: Serratrice G, Pellissier JF, Desnuelle C, Pouget J, eds. *Advances in Neuromuscular diseases. Myelopathies, Neuropathies and Myopathies*. Paris: Expansion Scientifique Française, 1988, 97–105.

16. Charcot JM, Marie P. Deux nouveaux cas de sclérose latérale amyotrophique suivis d'auptosie. *Arch Neurol* 1885; 28–29.

17. Bertrand I, Van Bogaert L. La Sclérose latérale amyotrophique (anatomie pathologique). *Rev Neurol* 1925; **1**: 779–806.

18. Lawyer T, Netsky MG. Amyotrophic lateral sclerosis. A clinico-anatomic study of 53 cases. *Arch Neurol Psychiatr* 1953; **69**: 171–192.

19. Engel WK, Kurland LT, Klazo I. An inherited disease similar to amyotrophic lateral sclerosis with a pattern of posterior column involvement. An inherited form. *Brain* 1959; **82**: 203.

20. Castaigne P, Lhermitte F, Cambier J et al. Etude neuro-pathologique de 61 observations de sclérose latérale amyotrophique. Discussion nosologique. *Rev Neurol* 1972; **127**: 401–414.

21. Bradley WG, Taudan R. Amyotrophic lateral sclerosis. Part 2 (etiopathogenesis). *Ann Neurol* 1985; **4**: 419–431.

22. Dyck PJ. Inherited neuronal degeneration and atrophy affecting peripheral motor sensory and autonomic neurons. In: Dyck PJ, Thomas PK, Lambert EH, eds. *Peripheral Neuropathy* vol 2. Philadelphia, London: WB Saunders, 1975, 825–867.

23. Tohgi H, Tsukagoshi H, Toyokura Y. Quantitative changes in sural nerves in various neurological diseases. *Acta Neuropath* 1977; **38**: 95–101.

24. Kawamura Y, Dyck PJ, Shimono M et al. Morphometric comparison of the vulnerability of peripheral motor and sensory nervous in amyotrophic lateral sclerosis. *J Neuropath Exp Neurol* 1981; **40**: 667–675.

25. Bradley WG, Good P, Rascol CG, Andelman LS. Morphometric and biochemical studies of peripheral nerves in amyotrophic lateral sclerosis. *Am Neurol* 1983; **14**: 267–277.

26. Ben Hamida M, Letaief F, Hentati F, Ben Hamida C. Morphometric study of the sensory nerve in classical (or Charcot disease) and juvenile amyotrophic lateral sclerosis. *J Neurol Sci* 1987; **78**: 313–329.

27. Lambert EH. Electromyography in amyotrophic lateral sclerosis. Motor neuron disease. *Adv Neurol* 1982; **13**: 135–154.

28. Refsum S, Skillicorn SA. Amyotrophic familial spastic paraplegia. *Neurology* (Minneapolis) 1954; **4**: 40–47.

29. Silver JR. Familial spastic paraplegia with amyotrophy of the hands. *Ann Hum Genet* 1966; **30**: 69–75.

30. Gragg GW, Fogelson MH, Zwirecki RJ. Juvenile amyotrophic lateral sclerosis in two brothers from an inbred community. *Birth Defects* 1977; **7** (**original article series**): 222–225.

31. Van Gent EM, Hoogland RA, Jennekens FGI. Distal amyotrophy of predominantly the upper limbs with pyramidal features in a large kinship. *J Neurol Neurosurg Psychiatry* 1985; **48**: 266–269.

32. Cross HE, McKusick VA. The Troyer syndrome: a recessive form of spastic paraplegia with distal muscle wasting. *Arch Neurol* 1967; **16**: 473–485.

33. Dyck PJ. Inherited neuronal degeneration and atrophy affecting peripheral motor, sensory and autonomic neurons. In: Dyck PJ, Thomas PK, Lambert EH, eds. *Peripheral Neuropathy* vol 2. Philadelphia: WB Saunders, 1984, 1600–1655.

34. Charcot JM. Sclérose des cordons latéraux de la moelle épinière chez une femme hystérique, atteinte de contracture permanente des quatre membres. *Bull Soc Med* 1865; **2** (**suppl 2**): 24–42.

35. Gastaut JC, Michel B, Frigarella-Branger D, Sanma-Mauvars H. Chronic progressive spinobulbar spasticity. *Arch Neurol* 1988; **45**: 509–513.

36. Ben Hamida M, Hentati F. Juvenile amyotrophic lateral sclerosis and related syndromes. In: Rowland LP, ed. *Advances in Neurology* vol 56. *Amyotrophic Lateral Sclerosis*. New York: Raven Press, 1991, 175–179.

37. Van Laere JE. Paralysie bulbo-pontine chronique progressive familiale avec surdité: un cas de syndrome de Klippel–Trenaunay dans la même fratrie, Problèmes diagnostiques et génétiques. *Rev Neurol* 1966; **115**: 289–295.

38. Sanna G, Orefice G. Paralysi bulbare progressiva infanto-giovanile. *Acta Neurol (Napoli)* 1976; **XXXI**: 706–715.

39. Meenakshisundaram E, Jagannathan K, Ram-murthi B. Clinical pattern of motor neuron disease seen in younger age groups in Madras. *Neurol India* 1970; **XVII** (**suppl 1**): 109–112.

40. Ben Hamida M, Hentati F, Ben Hamida C. Giant axonal neuropathy with inherited multisystem degeneration in a Tunisian kindred. *Neurology* 1990; **40**: 245–250.

41. Siddique T, Figlewicz DA, Pericak-Vance MA et al. Linkage of a gene causing familial amyotrophic lateral sclerosis to chromosome 21 and evidence of genetic-locus heterogeneity. *N Engl J Med* 1991; **324**: 1381–1384.

42. Rosen DR, Siddique T, Patterson D et al. Mutations in Cu/Zn superoxide dismutase gene are associated with familial amyotrophic lateral sclerosis. *Nature* 1993; **3662**: 59–62.

43. Hentati A, Bejaoui K, Pericak-Vance MA et al. Linkage of recessive familial amyotrophic lateral sclerosis to chromosome 2q33–q35. *Nature Genet* 1994; **7**: 425–428.

44. Hentati A, Ahmed A, Yung Y et al Linkage of a commoner form of recessive amyotrophic lateral sclerosis to chromosome 15q15-q22 markers. *Neurogenetics* 1998; **2**: 55–60.

45. Hentati A, Pericak-Vance MA, Hung WY et al. Linkage of 'pure' autosomal recessive familial spastic paraplegia to chromosome 8 markers and evidence of genetic locus heterogeneity. *Hum Molec Genet* 1994; **8**: 1263–1267.

4

Atypical forms of motor neurone disease in India
Rustom S Wadia

Introduction

Atypical forms of motor neurone disease (MND) have been described in India for over 25 years. An atypical form with principal involvement of one limb occurring predominantly in males was first described by Wadia and colleagues in 1972[1] and is seen fairly commonly all over India. A second form, best labelled as Madras pattern of MND, was first described just before this.[2] In 1980, Prabhakar and colleagues[3] described a syndrome that they called 'wasted leg syndrome'. It appears similar to the first form above except that Wadia and colleagues stressed a unilateral upper limb involvement while the wasted leg syndrome is a similar disorder of the lower limb.

The atypical form of MND appears to be more common in Asia than elsewhere. The condition was first reported in Japan by Hirayama and colleagues as 'juvenile muscular atrophy of unilateral upper extremity' in 1959,[4] and by 1972 this group had collected 38 cases.[5] There are several other reports from Japan giving a total of more than 150 cases.[6,7] Peiris and colleagues[8] from Sri Lanka reported 102 cases collected over 18 years, and cases have been reported from Malaysia[9] and Hong Kong.[10] The condition has been seen in the Western world (e.g. by Harding and colleagues[11] (18 cases), Biondi and colleagues[12] (seven cases), Chaine and colleagues,[13] and O'Sullivan and McLeod.[14]

Incidence of atypical forms

There are no population-based studies of the atypical forms of MND and it is best to describe the frequency in relation to the typical forms of MND and to spinal muscular atrophy.

In our experience over the past 20 years we have had 188 typical cases of MND, with 70 of the atypical Indian variant, two of Madras MND, and 64 cases of spinal muscular atrophy. From Bangalore, Gouri Devi and colleagues[15] have reported that from 1973 to 1982 they saw 172 cases of MND, 27 cases of atypical Indian forms, and 12 cases of Madras MND. There appears to be some artefact in this comparison because in their report between 1977 and 1981[16] they saw 110 cases of MND and 23 cases (20.9%) of the atypical form. Thus, in the five additional years added in their latest report they had 62 MND and 4 atypical cases (6.4%). This probably represents underdiagnosis of the atypical form before 1977. Virmani and Vijayan[17] from Delhi had perhaps 10 atypical cases in 96 of MND and Shukla[18] from Lucknow eight atypical forms in 37 cases of MND. Chopra et al from Chandigarh have stressed the lower limb

	Number (%)
Males	67 (95.7)
Females	3 (4.3)
Mean age	23.07*
Chance finding of wasting	19 (27.14)
Upper limb only affected	54 (77.14)
Distal seventh and eighth cervical and first thoracic level affected	35 (64.8)†
Distal and proximal	6 (11.1)†
Proximal alone	13 (24.0)†
Lower limb only affected	16 (22.85)
Fasciculation	42 (60)
Minipolymyoclonus	32 (45.7)‡
Reflexes all present	34 (48.7)
Second limb affected	15 (21.42)

* Age in years
†/Percentage of upper limb cases
‡ 78% of cases with distal upper limb involvement

Table 4.1
Characteristics of benign asymmetric focal amyotrophy of young males (70 cases).

presentation and collected 62 cases of what they called the wasted leg syndrome in 14 years (1970–1983) (i.e. rougly four or five cases a year).[19] In a 5-year report on typical MND they described 62 cases (12.5 cases a year). They have not reported separately an asymmetric upper limb disorder. The author has found asymetric upper limb wasting more common than the similar syndrome affecting the lower limbs which is called wasted leg syndrome.

Benign asymmetrical focal amyotrophy of young males (atypical form of MND)

The basic features of this syndrome were described in the author's original article[1] and remain the hallmark of the condition:

(a) it affects people aged less than 30 years, predominantly males;
(b) there is focal wasting and weakness in one limb, usually the upper limb;
(c) there is no family history;
(d) it is a relatively benign disorder; and
(e) it is a neurogenic disease with normal sensation, normal sensory conduction, and no slowing of nerve conduction velocity.

The author's experience of this syndrome in Pune to date is shown in *Table 4.1*.

The findings in the rest of the country is for the most part similar. In the series by Gouri Devi and colleagues,[15] the mean age at onset was 21.9 years in the upper limb group and 24.5 years in the lower limb group. The male-to-female ratio was 24:3. In Chopra and colleagues[16] wasted leg series, the mean age was

24 years and the male-to-female ratio was 59.3. In Singh and colleagues'[20] study, 20 of 26 cases started between 16 years and 25 years and only one was aged over 27 years. Only one of their cases was in a female. A relatively lower male preponderance is seen in a study from Malaysia with 19 cases only of which 14 were in males.[9] This very high male predominance is intriguing and probably higher than any other disorder that is not X-linked. In the four large Indian series, males form 95.13% of all cases. Thirty-five of our 54 upper limb cases were distal, involving the hand and the flexors of the fingers and wrist. On several occasions the extensors were minimally affected while wrist flexors and flexors of fingers were involved, indicating that the eighth cervical and first thoracic levels were affected. In some patients the wrist extensor and finger extensors were involved in addition and the brachioradials were spared, indicating that the seventh and eighth cervical and first thoracic levels were affected. In several of these patients the triceps was also affected. The author has seen the triceps quite markedly affected with sparing of the brachioradialis. In six cases the proximal and distal group were all involved, indicating that the fifth cervical to the first thoracic levels were affected (11.1% of over 54 upper limb cases).

The author has seen another 13 cases in which the involvement was mostly proximal, indicating that the fifth and sixth cervical levels were affected. Gouri Devi and colleagues,[15] in 27 upper limb cases mentioned that all cases with proximal involvement also had distal involvement. This predominantly proximal distribution, indicating that the fifth and sixth cervical levels were affected, is very uncommon in other series. *Fig. 4.1* shows one such case.

These 13 cases appeared identical to the distal form in age and sex distribution, clinical

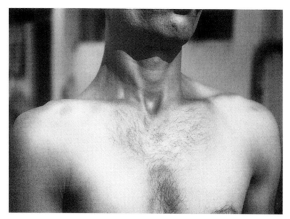

(a)

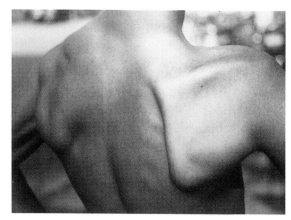

(b)

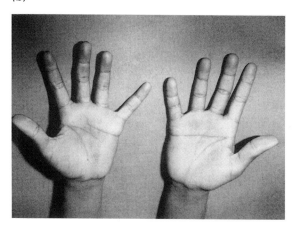

(c)

Figure 4.1
(a) and (b) Asymmetric proximal wasting upper limb. (c) Unilateral distal wasting.

onset and features and electrophysiologic findings. Thus we are inclined to believe that unilateral upper limb amytrophy may affect distal muscles only (64.8% of cases), proximal only (11.1% of cases) or both distal and proximal muscles (24% of cases). Similarly of the eight cases reported by Shukla and colleagues,[18] three were proximal.

Fasciculations were seen frequently in the wasted muscles in a total of 60% of all atypical cases, but this figure is much lower than in the author's typical MND group, where fasciculation is virtually universal. In 78% of the distal cases the author has noted minipolymyoclonus of the fingers. This finding is also noted in hereditary spinal muscular atrophy.

Hirayama and colleagues[5] stress cold paresis as a feature of this syndrome, but the author has rarely been impressed with the finding. Gouri Devi and colleagues mention that some patients feel worse when they dip their hand in cold water.[15] This is believed to be due to sensitivity of atrophic muscles to cold and it is understandable that it is more frequently seen in Japan than in India. Singh and colleagues[20] from Delhi (climate colder than Pune) mention stiffness and cramp with cold occurring in the affected hands.

The question of bilateral disease is important. One commonly used terminology is 'monomelic' atrophy. The author found that 21.42% of his cases showed bilateral involvement. Clinically, Singh and colleagues[20] saw this in 13.3% and Hirayama and colleagues[5] in 37.5% of cases. Peiris and colleagues,[8] reporting a very similar disorder from Sri Lanka apparently had 63 bilateral cases of 102. In 44 cases, the right side was more affected than the left and in 19 cases the left was more affected than the right. In this series, only five of 102 cases were both proximal and distal; the rest were distal only. Tan and colleagues[9] from Malaysia had five bilateral but

asymmetrical cases in a series of 19 cases. In Gouri Devi and colleagues'[18] series, two of 27 cases showed EMG evidence of disease in the other limb, but it is not clear if they excluded any cases with clinical bilateral disease to start with.

The author believes that such exclusion would remove 20% of cases that appear similar in all other ways. Whenever there was bilateral disease, it was more marked on one side than the other and it started in one limb before the other. Needless to say these cases were also benign with no or minimal progression over a minimum of 2–3 years. It is for this reason that the author prefers the term 'asymmetric' rather than 'monomelic' atrophy. In general there is no evidence of pyramidal affection in these cases. Virmani and colleagues'[17] study of young-age MND in Delhi is an exception: 26 of 96 cases were aged below 40 years and 13 cases had pyramidal signs. The author has rarely seen brisk reflexes in the affected limb.

Wasted leg syndrome

The question arises as to whether or not the wasted leg syndrome is the same disease as, or a similar disease to the upper limb syndrome. Both conditions occur in young males and both are markedly asymmetrical (*Fig. 4.2*).

Chopra and colleagues[19] found weakness in only 18 of their 62 cases, Gouri Devi and colleagues in five of 11 lower limb cases[15]; the author found power to be virtually normal in 61.1% of his lower limb cases. The whole of the lower limb was affected in 39 of 62 cases (62.9%) in the Chandigarh series.[19] Gouri Devi et al[15] probably had 37% affecting proximal and distal muscles in the lower limb and in our series half had proximal and distal lower limb involvement. From Chandigargh, Singh and colleagues[21] have described a similar

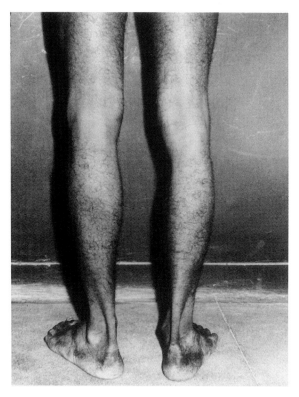

Figure 4.2
Unilateral leg wasting — 'wasted leg syndrome'.

wasted leg syndrome in which evidence of neuropathy with demyelination of nerves and slowed conduction was seen. This is, by definition, a separate condition.

Course

In the author's experience, the disease progresses for 6 months to 3 years and then becomes relatively static. The longest case on follow-up was affected in the right lower limb, mainly in the thighs and progressed for 6 months to 1 year, during which time EMG suggested that the trunk and arm muscle were affected. (This was done in Bombay.) Subsequently, this patient has stabilized and is virtu-

ally static with only one lower limb clinically affected over the past 25 years. Chopra and colleagues[18] speak of non-progressive weakness, but the wasted limb may reach half the size of the other and this must take time. An acute onset and then static disease may mean polio, a polio-like illness, or brachial neuritis and in the author's view, are all excluded from this review. There must be progress for months (at least 3 months; frequently longer). One of the features of onset, however, is that in one-quarter of the author's cases, the wasting was first brought to the attention of the patient by an observer at a swimming pool or gymnasium or by a tailor. This is a common finding in all Indian series, more so in lower limb disease; in the author's experience it is also common in the proximal upper limb group.

Radiological findings

Though the clinical picture is quite distinctive, the author believes that other focal lesions of the cervical cord must be excluded by appropriate imaging studies: myelography to start with and then magnetic resonance imaging (MRI). Though focal atrophy of the cervical cord is described, the usual finding is a normal cord. *Fig. 4.3* shows T2- and T1-weighted images of a patient which shows cord atrophy that is more marked on the left side. The author has even recently seen one such case that was thought clinically to be a clear case of benign asymmetrical focal amyotrophy of young males but that showed a syrinx on MRI.

Absence of abnormal signals on MRI in benign asymmetrical focal amyotrophy of young males probably excludes infarction or demyelination as aetiology. Biondi and colleagues[12] reported an MRI study of seven cases and was able to show asymmetric atrophy in three.

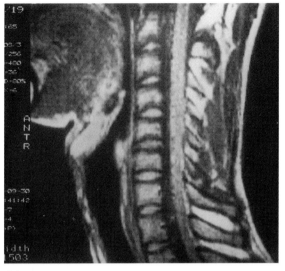

(a)

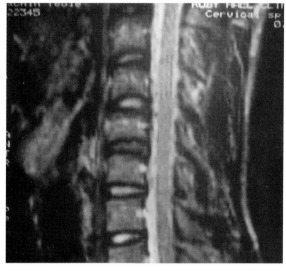

(b)

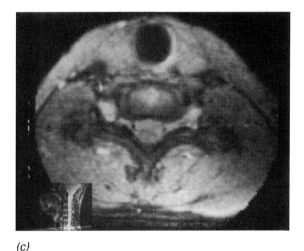

(c)

Figure 4.3
(a)–(c) T1 and T2 images of cervical cord to show focal atrophy of cord more on one side.

EMG *and nerve conduction studies*

Normal sensory conduction is a requirement for diagnosis and the author also requires motor conduction velocity, F wave latency, and distal latency to be normal. The amplitude of the compound action potential is low. EMG shows fall-out of units, and fasciculation in the majority of patients, and fibrillation are seen in up to 80%. Giant motor units are uncommon, in the author's experience, though Gouri Devi and colleagues found these in 11 of 15 upper limb cases and five of seven lower limb cases examined (total 72.7%). (The criteria they used for the term 'giant unit' is not mentioned.)

Pathology

Apparently only one case of this syndrome has been studied at post mortem. Hirayama and colleagues[22] described one patient. This patient had a lesion of the anterior horn cells of the fifth to eighth cervical level, most marked at the seventh and eighth level, with degeneration, necrosis, and mild gliosis. There was no evidence of inflammation. The muscle biopsy shows group atrophy and, in a small proportion of cases, a pseudomyopathic pattern with rounding of fibres and myophagocytosis is seen.

Aetiology

Nothing is known about the aetiology. A suggestion is made that hard muscular effort at work and occasionally in sport may predispose the segment to atrophy. This is poorly documented and no case control studies are available. Kondo and Tsubaki's study[23] has shown trauma to be a risk factor for MND in general but no special study of these cases was included. The very marked male preponderance (over 90% in most series) is most unusual. Such a high male preponderance, outside X-linked disorders, is seen very rarely in the author's experience, with perhaps ankylosing spondylitis and nasopharyngeal angiofibroma being the only similar disorders in this respect. The presence of demyelination lesions, vascular infarcts, or syrinx or other compression would exclude a case from this syndrome.

Gucuyenerk and colleagues[24] have reported two siblings in one family with monomelic atrophy but to the author's knowledge no familial cases have been reported in India.

Madras pattern of motor neurone disease

Whereas the syndrome of benign asymmetrical focal amyotrophy of young males is seen all over India, the Madras pattern of MND is seen principally in southern India and mostly from one state Tamil Nadu.[25] There is one more report from south India of 12 cases,[26] all of which came from Tamil Nadu or two adjoining states. The author has seen two cases, and three have been reported from Bombay. The Madras group[25] has described 40 cases. It is seen again in the young, all cases being below 30 years of age, but females are affected more than in benign asymmetrical focal amyotrophy of young males, with a male-to-female ratio of 4:1 in Madras and 1:1 in Bangalore. In the author's two cases, one was a female. The classic feature is bulbar palsy with the seventh to 12th cranial nerves being affected. According to the Madras group,[25] 30% have deafness but this was found in 11 of 12 cases in Bangalore.[26] In the Madras series,[25] the 12th nerve was affected in 44% of cases, the 10th nerve in 32%, and bilateral 7th nerve in 23%. The limbs are affected asymmetrically in 20–50% of cases but in this disorder UMN finding are much more common, being present is 65–75% cases. The disease is slowly progressive but benign. In the Bangalore series[26] of 12 cases, deafness preceded other signs by 9 months to 12 years in four cases.

Electrophysiology shows chronic partial denervation with normal nerve conduction and normal sensory conduction. In the Madras series,[25] some advanced cases showed slowing of motor velocity ascribed to loss of faster conducting axons. In the brain stem auditory evoked response (BAER), all waveforms are absent whereas the electrocochleogram shows normal cochlear microphonics, which suggests

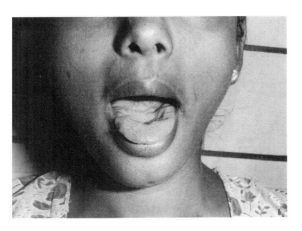

Figure 4.4
Tongue in Madras pattern motor neurone disease.

that the lesion is in the distal acoustic nerve or sensory cells of the spiral ganglion.[27]

From Madras, 10 of the cases were studied biochemically.[28] All had low blood citrate levels and high blood pyruvate levels. In contrast, in typical MND the citrate levels were always normal. This finding was reported nearly 25 years ago but is still unexplained.

The condition clinically resembles the Violetta Van Laere form of juvenile bulbar palsy. This condition has autosomal-recessive inheritances and causes deafness with juvenile bulbar palsy. When a single case is seen in a family it would be very difficult to tell one from the other. *Fig. 4.4* is one of the author's cases with bulbar palsy and deafness.

Unilateral calf hypertrophy

In 1974, Patel and colleagues[29] described unilateral calf hypertrophy as a manifestation of neurogenic anterior horn cell disease. These patients were also young and complained of pain in the leg and an enlarging calf. The creatine phosphokinase level was normal and

biopsy showed neurogenic disease. The nerve conduction was normal. The implication was that the disorder called 'neurogenic meganomelia' was a chronic anterior horn cell disorder. The author has seen three cases of the same type in the period under review and this has been described from other centres in India. These cases are sporadic. Autosomal-dominant distal spinal muscular atrophy with hypertrophied calves and benign evolution has been described outside India.[30]

References

1. Wadia RS, Karandikar R, Pallod S et al. Diseases of the anterior horn cell. *J Assoc Phys India* 1972; **200**: 415–423.
2. Meenakshi Sunderam E, Jagannath K, Ramamurthi B. Clinical pattern of motor neuron disease in younger age groups. *Neurology (India)* 1970; **suppl 1**: 104.
3. Prabhakar S, Chopra JS, Banerjee AK, Rana PVS. Wasted leg syndrome. A clinical electrophysiological and histopathological study. *Clin Neurol Neurosurg* 1981; **83**: 19–28.
4. Hirayama K, Toyokura Y, Tsubaki T. Juvenile muscular atrophy of upper extremity. A new clinical entity. *Psychiatry Neurol* (Japan) 1959; **61**: 2190–2197.
5. Hirayama K. Juvenile nonprogressive muscular atrophy localised in the hand and forearm. Observations in 38 cases. *Clin Neurol* 1972; **12**: 313–324.
6. Hashimoto O, Asada M, Ohta M, Kuroiwa Y. Clinical observations of juvenile nonprogressive muscular atrophy localised in hand and forearm. *J Neurol* 1976; **211**: 105.
7. Sobue I, Saito N, Iida M, Ando K. Juvenile type of distal and segmental muscular atrophy of upper extremities. *Ann Neurol* 1978; **3**: 429–432.
8. Peiris SB, Seneviratne KN, Wickremasinghe HR et al. Non familial juvenile distal spinal muscular atrophy of upper extremity. *J Neurol Neurosurg Psychiatry* 1989; **52**: 314–319.
9. Tan CT. Juvenile muscular atrophy of upper extremity. *J Neurol Neurosurg Psychiatry* 1985; **48**: 285–286.

10. Clan TW, Kay R, Schwartz MS. Juvenile distal spinal muscular atrophy of upper extremity in Chinese males; a single fibre electromyographic study of arms and legs. *J Neurol Neurosurg Psychiatry* 1991; **54**: 165–166.

11. Harding AE, Bradbury PG, Murray MNF. Chronic asymmetrical spinal muscularatrophy. *J Neurol Science* 1983; **59**: 69–83.

12. Biondi A, Dormont D, Weitzner I et al. MR imaging of the cervical cord in juvenile amyotrophy of distal upper extremity *AINR* 1989; **10**: 263–268.

13. Chainc P, Bouche P, Legar JM et al. Progressive muscular atrophy localized to one hand. A monomelic form of motor neuron disease. *Rev Neurol* 1988; **144**: 759–763.

14. O'Sullivan DJ, McLeod JG. Distal chronic spinal muscular atrophy involving the hands. *J Neurol Neurosurg Psychiatry* 1978; **41**: 653–658.

15. Gouri Devi M, Suresh TG, Shankar SK. Pattern of motor neurone disease in South India and monomelic atrophy. In: Gouri Devi M, ed. *Motor Neurone Disease*. New Delhi: Oxford and IBH, 1987, 171–190.

16. Gouri Devi M, Suresh TG, Shankar SK. Monomelic amyotrophy. *Arch Neurol* 1984; **41**: 388–394.

17. Virmani V, Vijayan G. Pattern of motor neurone disease in the young in North India. *J Assoc Physicians India* 1975; **23**: 695–701.

18. Shukla R, Nag D, Kar AM. Motor neurone disease at Lucknow, U.P. *Indian Med Gaz* 1979; **113**: 75–77.

19. Chopra JS, Prabhakar S, Singh AP, Banerjee AK. Pattern of motor neurone disease in North India and wasted leg syndrome. In: Gouri Devi M, ed. *Motor Neurone Disease*. New Delhi: Oxford and IBH, 1987, 147–163.

20. Singh N, Sachdev KK, Susheela AK. Juvenile muscular atrophy localized to arms. *Arch Neurol* 1980; **37**: 297–299.

21. Singh A, Jolly SS. Wasted leg syndrome. A compressive neuropathy of lower limbs. *J Assoc Physicians India* 1963; **11**: 1031–1033.

22. Hirayama K, Tomonaga M, Kitano K et al. Focal cervical poliopathy causing juvenile muscular atrophy of distal upper extremity: a pathological study. *J Neurol Neurosurg Psychiatry* 1987; **50**: 285–290.

23. Kondo K, Tsubaki T. Case control studies of motor neuron disease, association with mechanical injuries. *Arch Neurol* 1981; **38**: 220–224.

24. Gncuyenerk K, Aysun S, Topaloglu H et al. Monomelic atrophy in siblings. *Pediatr Neurol* 1991; **7**: 220–222.

25. Jagannathan K, Kumaresan G. Madras pattern of motor neurone disease. In: Gouri Devi M, ed. *Motor Neurone Disease*. New Delhi: Oxford and IBH, 1987, 191–193.

26. Gouri Devi M and Suresh TG. Madras pattern of motor neuron disease in south India. *J Neurol Neurosurg Psychiatry* 1988; **51**: 773–777.

27. Wadi PN, Bhatt MH, Misra VP. Clinical neurophysiological examination of deafness associated with juvenile motor neurone disease. *J Neurol Sci* 1897; **78**: 29–33.

28. Valmikananthan K, Mascreen M, Meenakshisunderam E, Snehalata C. Biochemical aspects of motor neurone disease. Madras pattern. *J Neurol Neurosurg Psychiatry* 1973; **36**: 753–756.

29. Patel AN, Pandya SS, Razaak ZA. Juvenile neurogenic megamonomelia (hypertrophia musculorum neuropathia). *Neurology (India)*, 1974; **22**: 15–22.

30. Groen RJ, Sie DG, van Waerden TW. Dominant inherited distal spinal muscular atrophy with atrophic and hypertrophied calves *J Neurol Sci* 1993; **114**: 81–84.

SECTION II

PATHOLOGY

5

Neuropathology
Paul G Ince

Introduction

This chapter gives an account of the classical pathology of amyotrophic lateral sclerosis (ALS) together with a review of the current consensus on molecular pathology that is typically present at autopsy. A group of related motor system disorders (ALS dementia, progressive muscular atrophy, primary lateral sclerosis, and 'motor neurone disease (MND) inclusion dementia') are then considered in relation to these pathological appearances in ALS. These can all be fitted into the conceptual framework of a common molecular pathology, which presents with considerable phenotypic diversity, on the basis of anatomical variations in individual susceptibility to, and resulting burden of, pathology. The relationship between these pathological features at autopsy and current views of the pathogenesis of the disorder are considered by addressing a number of related questions:

(a) Does a single molecular pathology characterize ALS, analogous to senile plaques and neurofibrillary tangles in Alzheimer's disease, or the Lewy body of Parkinson's disease?

(b) What is the pathological relationship between familial and sporadic ALS?

(c) Do similar molecular pathologies characterize ALS related to mutations in the gene that encodes copper–zinc superoxide dismutase (SOD1) and other forms of sporadic and familial ALS?

(d) Is there a difference between other genetically determined motor neurone degenerations (e.g. Kennedy's X-linked bulbospinal muscular atrophy, spinal muscular atrophy) and the various forms of ALS?

The absence of in vivo methods of monitoring pathological changes in motor neurones and their axons has resulted in a view of the disease process that is based on cross-sectional data, rather than on longitudinal data. Thus, key issues around the mode of cell loss, and the kinetics of the process, remain controversial in the human disease, although additional data is available from studies of in vivo morphological changes in motor nerves. Similar problems surround interpretation of upper motor neurone (UMN) changes in ALS. Two clinical approaches that will help to refine our view of motor system degeneration in ALS are various in vivo imaging modalities (structural and functional magnetic resonance imaging and magnetic resonance spectroscopy) and newer electrophysiological approaches (e.g. transcranial magnetic stimulation of the motor pathway). Concepts of pathogenesis in ALS will continue to be modified by insights from molecular pathology, clinicopathological studies, and studies of transgenic models of motor system degeneration, together with these in vivo human methods.

Neuropathological approaches to neurodegenerative diseases have been criticized on the basis that they only represent 'end-stage' pathology. This view is misguided for two reasons. First, patients with neurodegenerative diseases, including ALS, die of accidental causes or intercurrent diseases (e.g. ischaemic heart disease) in the same way as the general population. Any large collection of autopsy tissue from ALS patients will include those who have died unexpectedly at an early stage of the disease. Secondly, the distribution of ALS pathology in the central nervous system (CNS) varies from case to case. Many patients have severe bulbar–cervicothoracic disease at the time of death with relative preservation of the lumbar cord. In such cases there is an opportunity to compare severely affected and mildly affected regions of the motor system within the same patient. Observations based on patients who die unexpectedly at an early stage of the disease and on a comparison of severely diseased with relatively spared lower limb motor neurone groups in some patients have not yielded any consistent 'early' pathology that is not seen in more advanced cases.

Classical ALS

The typical clinical picture of combined UMN and lower motor neurone (LMN) signs predominates in classical ALS and is reflected in the anatomical distribution of degenerative changes in the motor system. These changes have been documented since the studies of Charcot in the mid-19th century.[1] The major pathological features, which correlate with the principal clinical manifestations, are:

(a) a reduction in both the number and size of lower motor neurones (anterior horn cells) in the spinal ventral horns and bulbar motor nuclei; and

(b) myelin pallor in the corticospinal projection pathway, a secondary consequence of axonal loss in this region.

UMN (Betz cell) soma abnormalities are much more variable, and many additional pathological features have been described using conventional and immunocytochemical stains.

Anatomical pathology

Motor system

UMNs in the motor cortex

The extent to which pathological changes can be demonstrated at autopsy in the motor cortex is highly variable even in cases with clinically typical upper motor neurone signs on examination. The most severely affected cases show an obvious absence of giant Betz cells in cortical layer 5[2] accompanied by reactive gliosis, which is demonstrable as astrocytosis (e.g. by glial fibrillary acidic protein (GFAP) immunocytochemistry) and as a diffuse microgliosis (e.g. using immunocytochemistry against antigens such as CD68 and HLA-DR). Unfortunately such findings are not direct evidence that the Betz cells have actually disappeared because there is no molecular marker that exclusively labels UMNs. Phenotypically, these large glutamatergic neurones have molecular characteristics that are similar to other pyramidal cells in the cortex. The extent to which the apparent loss of Betz cells by conventional methods (e.g. Nissl staining) is due in part to neuronal shrinkage, so that the Betz cells become indistinguishable by size criteria alone from neighbouring pyramidal cells, is unknown and probably varies from case to case. An additional factor to consider when examining individual cases is the duration and severity of UMN signs. It is the author's expe-

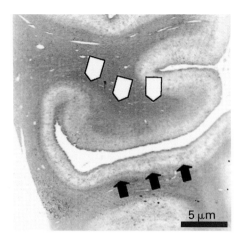

Figure 5.1
Motor cortex gliosis. The sensory cortex (black arrows) and white matter are unaffected. There is an area of diffuse brown glial staining in the subcortical white matter beneath the motor cortex (white arrows), which extends into the lower part of the cortex.

intense subcortical gliosis (*Fig. 5.1*). Other descriptions of a more patchy gliosis[3] may reflect an exaggeration of the normal discontinuous pattern of cortical astrocytic staining for GFAP.

UMNs in the pyramidal tract
Most cases of ALS show evidence of corticospinal tract myelin pallor at some level of the pathway (*Fig. 5.2*). Interpretation of such changes should be made in the light of known anatomical features of the pathway in humans. First the size of the projection, in terms of the number of projecting axons, indicates that Betz cells must contribute only a minor proportion of the total. This implies that many large pyramidal cells in the motor area and probably in the premotor area (Brodmann areas 4 and 6) contribute to the direct corticospinal projection into the brainstem and spinal cord.[4] Secondly, the density of the terminal innervation of the pathway is variable in the spinal cord. Studies in higher primates suggest that the majority of motor fibres project on to LMNs and interneurones in the cervical enlargement around the periphery of the ventral horn. These anatomical data reflect a major functional role of the pathway in fine motor control of upper limb. Consequently the size of the corticospinal tracts below the first thoracic spinal level is much reduced compared with the medullary and cervical regions. The extent of decussation in the medulla is variable, both in terms of proportion of crossed axons and the symmetry of decussation.

rience that some cases of ALS with clear UMN signs for several years can have remarkably normal morphological appearances in the motor cortex.

The intracellular lesions described in the section on molecular pathology (see below) are extremely rare in surviving Betz cells of typical sporadic ALS patients unless accompanied by dementia (see below), or in association with a mutation in the SOD1 gene (see below). The literature contains conflicting accounts of the astrocytic gliosis that is present in some ALS cases. In the author's experience, the most common form is a confluent diffuse gliosis extending variably upwards from the grey–white matter junction and merging with

Brownell and colleagues[2] emphasized the frequent finding that corticospinal tract pallor in myelin stains is most prominent in the cervical cord and medullary pyramids, which is borne out, in the author's experience, of more than 90 cases examined. In some cases this finding is apparent at all levels examined, so

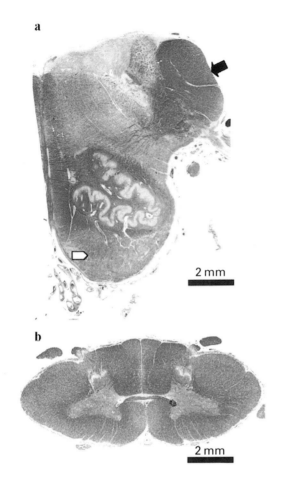

2 mm

2 mm

Figure 5.2
Corticospinal tract pallor in a specimen stained with luxol fast blue. (a) Hemi-medulla showing pallor of the pyramid (white arrowhead) compared with the unaffected inferior cerebellar peduncle (black arrow). (b) Cervical spinal cord showing more subtle pallor diffusely affecting the lateral and ventral corticospinal tracts, all the lateral and ventral white matter, and the fasiculi gracilis.

affected. The predominance of cases in which myelin pallor is not demonstrable above the level of the medulla, including cases with no discernible motor cortex pathology, leads the author to the conclusion that UMN changes in ALS most commonly arise from an axonopathy with peripheral 'dying back'.

Recent experience with macrophage markers[5,6] suggests that immunostaining with CD68 (or other markers) may offer a more sensitive method of detecting corticospinal tract changes in the absence of clear evidence of myelin pallor *(Fig. 5.3)*. Such observations must be made cautiously given the extent to which numerous brain insults, including hypoxia, are associated with increased macrophage and microglial activity. Evidence of subtle corticospinal pathology should only be interpreted in cases with otherwise typical molecular pathological evidence of ALS or MND (e.g. LMN ubiquitinated inclusions; see below) when the pattern of microglial staining is confined to white matter regions that are known to be affected in ALS and in the absence of evidence for a cause of diffuse 'non-specific' microglial activation. Inclusion of such cases probably improves the clinicopathological correlation between UMN signs and 'UMN pathology'.

LMNs
LMN loss in ALS is often subjectively more prominent than can be verified by neuronal counting. Two main reasons probably account for this. First, the mode of neuronal degeneration in ALS appears to be predominantly by shrinkage, so that careful examination reveals a proportion of surviving small dark motor neurones.[7] These neurones have recently been shown to display many biochemical features of 'programmed cell death', or apoptosis.[8] Secondly, observations made in a single section at any spinal level are unreliable because of the

that the anterior limb of the internal capsule, the central cerebral peduncle, and the lateral and ventral spinal white matter funiculi are all

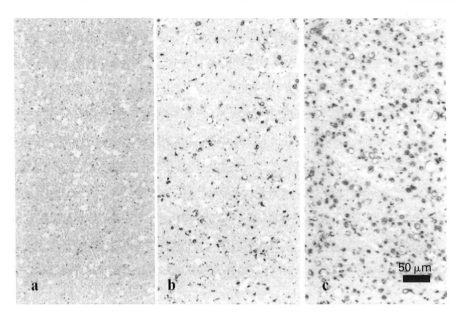

Figure 5.3
Macrophage permeation of corticospinal tract in ALS demonstrated by CD68 immunoreactivity. (a) Normal spinal white matter. (b) Mild increase in macrophages. (c) Marked macrophage permeation.

wide variation in the number of motor neurone somata that are present between one section and the next.[9] For these reasons the presence of characteristic spinal (or bulbar) motor neurone inclusion bodies is a very reassuring part of the overall pathological picture (see below). However aspects of this motor neurone loss are of interest in answering questions about the mechanisms and dynamics of motor neurone degeneration.

There is widespread interest in the possibility that neuronal loss in neurodegenerative diseases may be brought about through a mechanism of 'programmed cell death'.[8] This concept is usually encapsulated within the term 'apoptosis'. It is covered in Chapter 20, and only a few comments are included here.

First, the whole concept of cell death is often presented as a 'one-or-the-other' choice between necrosis and apoptosis, but such a concept may not be applicable in the adult CNS. It has been demonstrated that glutamatergic neurotoxicity can exhibit morphological features along a necrosis–apoptosis continuum, including 'intermediate forms' with features of both modes of cell death.[10,11] Secondly, it is the general experience of neuropathologists who have examined ALS cases that classical apoptotic bodies (such as they routinely encounter in brain tumour specimens) are not seen. In contrast, the presence of small shrunken motor neurones is widely described in pathological accounts of ALS, and this is a much more plausible candidate

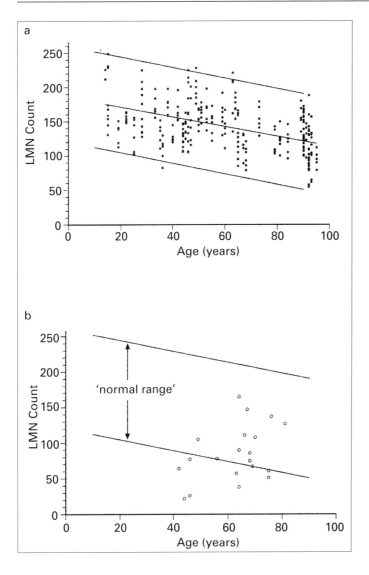

Figure 5.4
LMN counts in normal controls and ALS patients. (a) Counts from the fourth lumbar ventral horn of 50 normal individuals showing counts from six 20 μm sections spaced 100 μm apart. There is a gradual age-related fall in LMN numbers. The 95% confidence intervals for these data are indicated by the parallel lines. (b) LMN counts from the fourth lumbar ventral horn in 20 ALS patients, with the 'normal age-related range' from (a) superimposed. At least half these patients had lumbar LMN counts within the normal range despite lethal cervicobulbar neuronal depletion. (From Tomlinson et al. 1977[14] and previously unpublished data.)

for the morphological 'prequel' of eventual neuronal loss. Further evidence for the occurrence of neuronal shrinkage prior to neuronal loss comes from studies of peripheral nerves: quantitative analysis has shown a systematic reduction of axonal diameters from large to medium calibre, which is more prominent than the overall fall in absolute numbers of axons in ALS motor nerve neurones.[12] This observation correlates well with the ventral horn changes and imply that, as the neuronal somata shrink, the diameter of their axons decreases proportionately ('axodendritic pruning').[8]

Most studies that have attempted to quantify the loss of LMNs in the spinal limb enlargements show an average loss of 50% compared with age-matched controls.[13] The most comprehensive data were accumulated on 11 cases of Tomlinson BE and colleagues (unpublished data). These cases were sampled throughout the lumbosacral enlargement using 20 μm sections which were counted every 100 μm (i.e. one section in five). The results are shown in *Fig. 5.4* as estimated total LMN number for spinal level L4 in comparison with counts from 65 control cases, between the ages of 25 and 95 years, obtained using the same method.

Two observations are important. First, the controls were originally published with an analysis indicating that neuronal fallout in normal ageing did not commence before the age of 65 years.[14] A recent re-analysis of this data-set with computerized mathematical modelling shows that the data are insufficiently powerful to allow discrimination between any function used to fit to the data. Thus the original biphasic interpretation has no greater validity than, for example, a simple linear model with neuronal loss beginning in the third decade of life (Ince P and Appleton DR, unpublished observations). For this reason, the control data set is shown with 95% confidence intervals using a simple linear fit to the data. Secondly, the ALS data show an apparent inverse relationship with age. This does not reach significance at the 95% level but may indicate a trend such that younger patients are more likely to survive longer, with proportionately greater neuronal loss, owing to an higher overall level of 'fitness' at the outset of the illness. The finding that some patients have neuronal counts that are in the normal range also illustrates the extent to which the regional involvement of the spinal cord is very variable. Patients may die of respiratory failure, as a result of bulbar and cer-

vicothoracic disease, at a stage when they are ambulant with minimal lumbosacral weakness. Conversely, some patients present with lower limb signs and develop a centripetal pattern of spinal involvement whereby lower limb paralysis is an early feature. At autopsy the regional intensity of neuronal loss correlates with the pattern of clinical disease very closely, but there are no distinctions in terms of the cellular or molecular pathology of patients within this spectrum.

There appears to be no difference in the susceptibility of limb motor neurones compared with the more medially placed axial motor neurones in the ventral horns. However, two groups of otherwise typical motor neurones are characteristically spared in most cases:

(a) the sacral motor nucleus of Onufrowitz (Onuf's nucleus), which innervates muscles of the pelvic floor and associated sphincters;[15] this pathological sparing correlates with retention of urinary and faecal continence as a typical clinical feature throughout the illness; and

(b) the motor neurones of the third, fourth, and sixth cranial nerves, which innervate the external ocular muscles, are also characteristically spared so that retention of normal eye movements is a typical feature of the disease.

The basis of this selective sparing is likely to involve complex interactions of the physiological and biological properties of these neuronal groups, which relate to some of the probable disease mechanisms described in subsequent chapters. Of particular importance may be:[16–19]

(a) the expression of cytoplasmic calcium buffering proteins in spared motor nuclei;

(b) the lack of direct monosynaptic corticospinal innervation;

(c) differences in glutamatergic neurotransmission; and

(d) nitric oxide metabolism.

Non-motor CNS pathology in ALS

Involvement of extra-motor regions of the CNS is increasingly recognized as being a consistent feature of many ALS patients at autopsy. Clinical correlates of sensory, cerebellar, and extrapyramidal features are seldom described in the clinical notes of these patients, but more sensitive objective measures (e.g. evoked potentials, formal psychometry, functional brain imaging) usually show mild deficits in related modalities.

Sensory system

Pallor of the dorsal funiculi of the spinal cord is not uncommon in ALS although it has been especially emphasized in familial cases, where it is present in up to 70% of patients.[20–23] This is seen in myelin-stained sections and is usually predominant in the 'dorsal root entry zone' in the funiculus cuneatus. In addition there is also often pallor in funiculus gracilis.[22] Although these changes have been particularly associated with familial disease, they also seem to occur in sporadic cases.[21] No detailed studies have reported the relative frequency of this pathology between familial and sporadic disease. Such studies are especially difficult in this late-onset, rapidly lethal disorder, in which the lack of a known family history of ALS is not a reliable indication of sporadic disease. Involvement of neurons in the spinal posterior horns has not been reported in large 'modern' autopsy series of ALS cases.[2,20,23] However, it is certainly present in some familial cases associated with mutations in the gene that encodes SOD1.[6] Similarly, changes of neuronal atrophy in the posterior root ganglia,[24] peripheral sensory nerve,[12,25] and thalamic gliosis[2] are well documented.

Cerebellar pathways

Several papers have confirmed the frequent finding of variable myelin pallor in the ascending spinocerebellar tracts and in the thoracic nucleus of Clarke, which gives rise to the dorsal spinocerebellar pathway.[26,27] In typical cases of ALS there is a diffuse pallor of all the lateral and ventral white matter, including these cerebellar projections.[4] These changes have been interpreted as evidence of involvement of 'indirect' descending corticospinal motor pathways in addition to ascending spinocerebellar involvement.[4] The inferior olivary nuclei may show a degree of transneuronal degeneration, but cerebellar neurones have not been shown to be vulnerable in ALS. Similarly the cerebellar output projection areas (e.g. ventral pontine nuclei) are unaffected in ALS.

Substantia nigra

There are very few reports of combined ALS and 'idiopathic Lewy body Parkinson's disease'.[28] In the author's series of 90 autopsy verified cases of ALS there are two patients in whom nigral degeneration was associated with Lewy bodies, although a clinical diagnosis of Parkinson's disease was made in only one.[29] To establish this combined diagnosis it is necessary to demonstrate both the typical anatomical features and the molecular pathological features (see below) of both disorders. However, less severe nigral degeneration, so-called sub-clinical parkinsonism, is present in many patients with ALS. This takes the form of a non-Lewy body degeneration of the dopaminergic neurones of the substantia nigra in the absence of the classical inclusion bodies of either ALS or Parkinson's disease. Where such changes have been quantified at autopsy there is an association of prominent nigral degeneration with patients whose ALS is combined with a frontal lobe dementia syndrome.[30,31] Additional data from ALS patients in support of a reduction in the size of the dopaminergic projection to the basal ganglia come from in vivo scanning using 6-fluorodopa[32] that shows severe changes in about one-quarter of the patients examined. The mechanism of nigral cell loss in the absence of specific molecular pathological changes has not been determined.

Non-CNS pathology
Muscle
The typical changes of skeletal muscle atrophy were described in the earliest pathological accounts of ALS.[33–36] These comprise features of denervation atrophy with clusters of angular atrophic fibres. This clustering, together with the observation of fibre-type grouping[37] in the atrophic clusters, is a non-specific consequence of serial denervation–reinnervation–denervation. In ALS the reinnervation arises from collateral sprouting of intramuscular axons.[38]

Other tissues
Non-specific pathological changes have been reported outside the CNS in ALS. In the skin there is reported to be a change in collagen cross-linking or in the proportion of immature collagen[39] together with a more rapid degeneration in the elastin component.[40] Whether these changes have any clinical correlates (e.g. with the relative infrequency of stasis ulcers in ALS) is debatable. More recently, collagen abnormalities have been reported from the spinal cord in ALS patients at autopsy when compared with both normal and neurodegenerative disease control groups.[41]

The significance of reports of swollen mitochondria and intracellular inclusions in the liver in ALS is uncertain.[42]

Molecular pathology

The differential diagnosis of neurodegenerative disorders in later life is increasingly dominated by molecular pathological abnormalities of the neuronal (and glial) cytoskeleton. These pathological changes include both the morphological characteristics of the intraneuronal inclusion bodies that result from cytoskeletal dysfunction and also the specific molecular characteristics of the protein abnormalities involved. In Alzheimer's disease, neurofibrillary tangles and neuropil threads are composed of a triplet of tau isoforms (in contrast to the six tau isoforms found in normal mature neurones) aggregated into the 'paired helical filament' configuration that is characteristic of the disease. In contrast, there are several other 'tauopathies' with particular phenotypic spectra (e.g. corticobasal degeneration, Pick's disease, progressive supranuclear palsy, multiple system atrophy, argyrophilic grain disease), in which different combinations of lesion morphology, anatomical distribution of pathology, and specific molecular pathology are used to define each condition. A second group of disorders is characterized by lesions based on the abnormal metabolism of neurofilaments and α-synuclein; this group includes Parkinson's disease and dementia with Lewy bodies.[43]

In comparison, the molecular pathology of ALS is less well defined. Older reports have described a range of inclusion bodies in anterior horn cells and other neuronal populations using a variety of conventional tinctorial staining methods. Some of these inclusion bodies are now more fully characterized by molecular pathology and are regarded as relatively 'specific' for ALS and its variants. Other inclusion bodies can be shown to represent a different, 'non-ALS', pathological process involving motor system degeneration. The latter include the presence of neurofibrillary tangles in motor neurones in patients with the ALS–Parkinson's disease–dementia complex (ALS–PDC) of Guam. The pathology of

Guamanian ALS is that of a tau disorder, which is quite distinct from the findings in typical cases of ALS where tau pathology is absent. For this reason, ALS in Guam is best regarded as an unusual phenotype related to other taupathies, and resulting from particular environmental exposures and genetic predispositions among affected individuals. The contribution of molecular pathology is thus profound because it alters fundamental concepts of these diseases.

In relation to ALS–PDC, much writing and research on ALS during the 1980s and 1990s concerned the extent to which Guamanian ALS was a naturally occurring, high-incidence model that might provide insights into the origin of typical, sporadic ALS. The reclassification of ALS–PDC as a tau disorder alters its relevance to sporadic ALS such that it can only contribute insights as to why a pathological process (neurofibrillary degeneration) that is normally manifested as a cerebral condition is sometimes present in an atypical distribution affecting the spinal cord. This is an interesting inversion of one of the emerging features of ALS-type pathology, which most often presents as motor system degeneration, but which is now recognized as causing dementia in some individuals through cerebral involvement (see below).

Currently, the most important aspects of molecular pathology in ALS concern the ubiquitin–proteasome pathway and neurofilament metabolism.

Ubiquitinated inclusions
Ubiquitin metabolism
Ubiquitin is a 76 amino acid polypeptide that is found in all eukaryotic cells. It is a prominent feature of the neuropathology of neurodegenerative diseases because it is frequently found as a component of various inclusion bodies.[44,45] It has thus become a useful tool in the neuropathological diagnosis of neurodegenerative disease and has contributed significantly to progress in the understanding of pathogenesis.

The normal role of ubiquitin is increasingly well characterized. It is a cytosolic component with multiple functions. It binds covalently to nuclear histones and may participate in the regulation of nuclear gene expression. It is also a major pathway for extralysosomal protein degradation,[46] and it is this role that appears most relevant to neurodegeneration. It is also a heat shock protein with a potentially protective effect in cells experiencing a variety of toxic insults.[47] Protein degradation via the ubiquitin–proteasome pathway is an energy-dependent, multi-step cascade that involves several enzymes. Ubiquitin monomers are cleaved from polyubiquitin chains and then covalently attached to thiol residues of target peptides, a step that requires the activity of an ATP-dependent enzyme. The resulting covalently tagged peptide is then degraded in the proteolytic channel of the 26S proteasome. Finally, there is an enzyme pathway involved; this cleaves ubiquitin from the target peptide to enable recycling.

Although many of the inclusion bodies of neurodegenerative diseases, including ALS, are heavily ubiquitinated there is no evidence for any primary abnormality of the ubiquitin–proteasome pathway in these diseases. Rather it appears that ubiquitination is a consequence of the accumulation of abnormal proteins despite the availability of multiple lysosomal and non-lysosomal pathways for protein degradation.

Ubiquitinated inclusions in ALS
Given the common association of ubiquitination with the inclusion bodies of many neurodegenerative diseases it was logical to apply antiubiquitin immunocytochemistry to ALS.

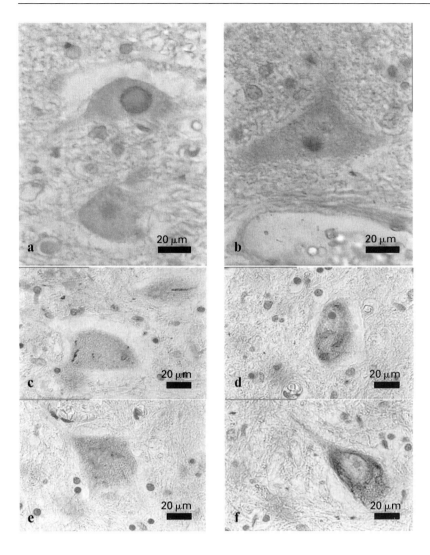

Figure 5.5
Ubiquitinated inclusions in spinal motor neurons in ALS. (a,b) Compact 'Lewy-like' inclusions. (c,d,e,f) 'Skein' type inclusions.

This revealed the very frequent finding of either 'skein-like', or 'Lewy body-like' accumulations of ubiquitinated material in the LMNs of most cases.[48,49] These filamentous bodies (*Fig. 5.5*) probably represent a continuous range of morphologies across a spectrum ranging from more compact and dense masses of filamentous protein to skein-like multi-stranded filaments.[50] In some neurones these lesions may exist only as a single small strand or fleck of ubiquitinated material. The dense compact bodies seem to correspond to many of the rounded, 'Lewy body-like' inclusion bodies, which were previously described, in conventional stains, as either 'eosinophilic' or 'basophilic'. The existence of the filamentous skeins was not appreciated before ubiquitin immunocytochemistry. Ubiquinated inclusions

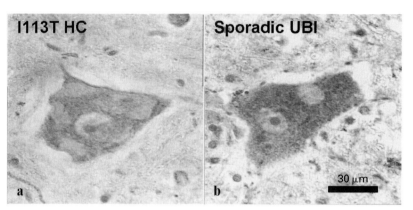

Figure 5.6
Absence of α-synuclein staining in neuronal inclusions in ALS (a) Hyaline inclusions (pale cytoplasmic areas) in an ALS case with SOD1 mutation I113T. (b) Ubiquitinated ALS inclusion (rounded pale area of cytoplasm) in sporadic ALS.

(UBIs) are found in otherwise normal-appearing neurones, in the lipofuscin cap of motor neurones, and in some dark shrunken neurones. There is therefore no clear correlation between the presence of an inclusion body and degeneration of the affected neurone. Taken with the role of ubiquitin in the elimination of abnormal peptides and its involvement in cell stress responses, it is possible that the UBI functions as a cytoprotective mechanism for sequestering an abnormal harmful protein. The absence of up-regulation of other cell stress genes in ALS, such as HSP72,[52] suggests that the role of ubiquitin in UBIs is primarily concerned with the non-lysosomal proteolysis pathway.

Both types of UBI contain filaments and tubules of 15–25 nm diameter by electron microscopy,[49,52–55] together with smaller filaments (10–15 nm in diameter), which may represent neurofilaments. The nature of the larger filaments is not known, and no specific protein targets for ubiquitination have been discovered in ALS. In particular the ubiquitinated inclusion bodies of ALS do not show co-localization with tau, neurofilaments,[56] or α-synuclein (*Fig. 5.6*), features that character-

ize many other late-onset neurodegenerative disorders. In this respect, our understanding of the molecular pathology of ALS is less advanced than our understanding of Alzheimer's disease, the various 'taupathies' (e.g. Pick's disease, progressive supranuclear palsy, corticobasal degeneration, multiple system atrophy), or the spectrum of Lewy body disorders, including Parkinson's disease and dementia with Lewy bodies.

Clinical pathology of UBIs in ALS
The discovery of UBIs has had a major impact on the clinicopathological understanding of ALS, and they provide a useful diagnostic marker. Despite their importance, there are no systematic prospective studies of the specificity and sensitivity of the lesions in ALS and its variants. Their abundance varies between cases and there are no data correlating this variation with any other aspect of phenotype. In cases with severe neuronal loss they may be very infrequent and yet still be present in a high percentage of surviving motor neurones. In these cases, and in cases in which pathology is minimal in the area under examination, they may be found only after examination of multi-

ple serial sections. Consensus protocols for sampling have not been agreed, and it remains uncertain how thoroughly a case should be sampled, in terms of multiple sites and numbers of sections examined, before excluding the presence of UBIs. In the author's series, of more than 90 cases, very few of the cases did not contain UBIs if serial strips of 10×10 µm sections, from multiple levels of the motor system, were stained for ubiquitin. The cases that did not show UBIs were usually atypical LMN syndromes with prolonged survival, or unusual familial cases of progressive muscular atrophy type. Thus it is likely that these lesions characterize at least 80–100% of sporadic cases of ALS,[57] as well as many of its variants (see below). Even at the lower end of this range they correlate as closely with the clinical diagnosis of ALS as Lewy bodies do with clinically diagnosed Parkinson's disease and as Alzheimer-type pathology in demented patients does with Alzheimer's disease. Morphologically, the skein-type inclusion predominates. Many cases show a mixture of skeins and 'Lewy body-like' UBIs, but some cases have almost exclusively one type or the other.[48,57]

Data on both normal controls and other neurological conditions are also limited. UBIs are not described in normal subjects but they have been very infrequently described in patients with other multisystem-type degenerative disorders.[57,58] Future studies will need to examine the latter cases carefully and extensively, using panels of antisera, to distinguish atypically generalized ALS-type degeneration from patients with genuinely mixed pathologies. Other motor disorders, including poliomyelitis[59] and the post-poliomyelitis syndrome (Ince P, unpublished observations), or spinal muscular atrophy[60] (Ince P, unpublished observations) do not show UBIs.

UBIs are mainly found in susceptible LMN groups of the spinal cord and brainstem. They are also found in the cerebrum in some cases, especially in the presence of dementia,[57,61] and such demented cases are discussed below (see below). LMN groups that are usually spared in ALS (i.e. the oculomotor nuclei of the midbrain and pons[57] and Onuf's nucleus of the sacral spinal cord[62]) do not usually show UBIs.

Bunina bodies

In 1962, Bunina[63] described the presence of small eosinophilic bodies in anterior horn cells in ALS.[64] These Bunina bodies comprise short refractile linear bodies in the soma of motor neurones and are clearly distinguishable from other kinds of inclusions that are visible in haematoxylin and eosin sections of ALS spinal cord (*Fig. 5.7*). Ultrastructure suggests lysosomal derivation.[65,66] These inclusions have been described in both sporadic and familial disease and are reported to be present in 30–50% of cases. This is possibly a smaller proportion of all ALS–MND cases than for UBIs, although there is a similar lack of detailed quantitative studies from which to advise on optimal sampling strategies. Bunina bodies are not described in other disorders and may be specific for ALS, although with lower sensitivity than UBIs. More recently they have been shown to be immunoreactive for cystatin C.[67] Others have postulated that they may be a precursor of the UBI. Given the lack of staining of UBIs for cystatin C, and of quantitative data, there is little evidence to support this hypothesis. The pathogenesis of these structures and their relationship to neurodegeneration and neurone loss is not characterized.

Hyaline conglomerate inclusions

A second type of intraneuronal inclusion body is found in some patients with ALS — hyaline

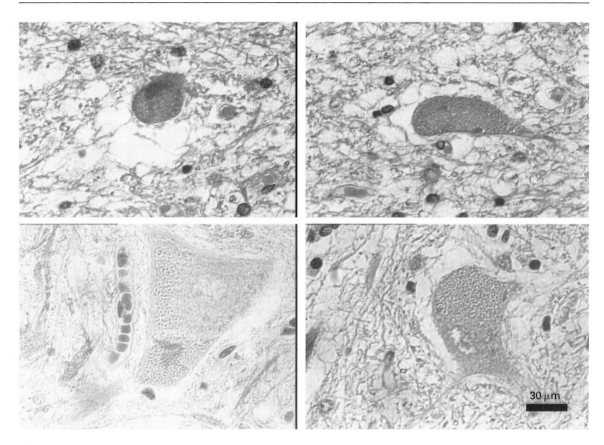

Figure 5.7
Bunina bodies stained with haematoxylin and eosin.

conglomorate inclusions (HCIs) (*Fig. 5.8*). These have been termed variously as hyaline bodies and hyaline conglomerates.[68,69] They consist of large aggregates of 10–15 nm-diameter neurofilaments associated with other 'entrapped' cytoplasmic proteins and organelles.[64,69–71] They are strongly immunoreactive for both phosphorylation-dependent and phosphorylation-independent neurofilament epitopes.[6,72] They have also been described in a few neurologically normal control subjects and in patients with other neurological diseases,[72,73] so that they are probably

less specific for ALS compared with UBIs. The pathogenesis of these lesions is no more clearly understood than that of UBIs, although they must be regarded as the result of a separate process. This conclusion can be drawn on the basis that:

(a) they undoubtedly have a major component of neurofilament protein, which is not a significant feature of UBIs;[56]
(b) in the author's experience of more than 90 autopsy-proven cases of ALS they were much less common than UBIs and were

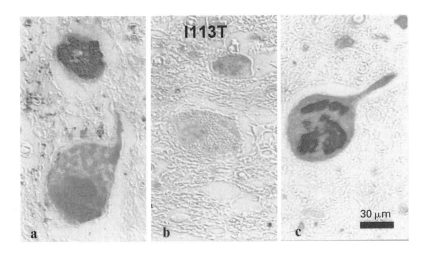

Figure 5.8
Hyaline inclusions in LMNs from a case with SOD1 mutation I113T. (a) SMI 31. (b) Ubiquitin. (c) SMI 32.

restricted to two cases, both of which had the SOD1-gene mutation I113T;[6]

(c) although one of these two cases also had UBIs, these were infrequent and were restricted to the hypoglossal nucleus, whereas HCIs were frequent in both motor and non-motor neurones in many CNS regions;

(d) there are no reports of intermediate forms of inclusions with characteristics of both UBIs and HCIs in the literature; and

(e) neurofilament immunoreactivity in UBIs has only rarely been reported in the Lewy-like bodies and is usually associated with the periphery of the inclusion.[53,74] However, both of these familial cases[53,74] predate the introduction of screening for SOD1-gene mutations and it is not certain if these lesions really represent UBIs or HCIs. In confocal microscopy studies using a range of neurofilament antisera, the author found only a few examples of compact UBIs (Lewy body-like inclusions), which showed slight peripheral immunore-

activity to neurofilament but only to a polyclonal antibody to phosphorylated neurofilament heavy chain.[6]

This comparison of UBIs and HCIs highlights two main issues. First, if UBIs contain neurofilaments as a primary component of their structure, then these proteins must be so highly altered that they have lost all antigenic epitopes that can be recognized by the very wide array of monoclonal and polyclonal neurofilament antisera that have been employed in ALS research across the world. Secondly, much of the nomenclature in the literature is confusing. HCIs are composed of neurofilaments but UBIs do not appear to be so. Since Lewy bodies contain neurofilaments (in addition to α-synuclein[75,76]), it is not logical to describe any sub-group of UBIs as 'Lewy-body like'. As described above, UBIs form a continuous spectrum from fine filamentous skeins to increasing compact aggregates of filaments, thus the 'Lewy-body like UBI' is better termed a 'compact UBI'.

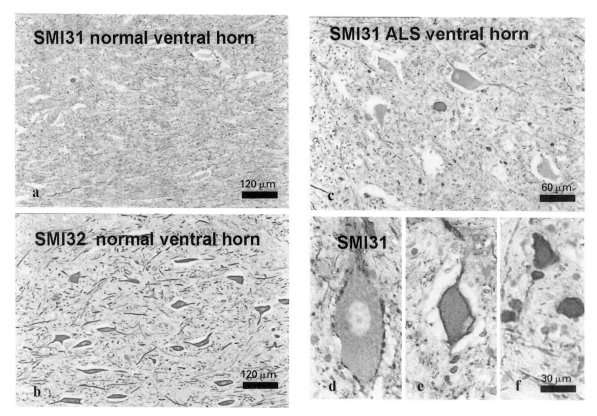

Figure 5.9
Neurofilament staining of ventral horn. (a) Normal phosphorylated neurofilament staining (SMI 31). (b) Normal non-phosphorylated neurofilament staining (SMI 32). (c) Phosphorylated neurofilament staining in ALS. (d) Normal LMN (SMI 31). (e) Darkly staining LMN stained for SMI 31 in ALS. (f) LMN and spheroids in ALS (SMI 31).

Other neurofilament alterations

Neurofilaments are the major class of cytoskeletal intermediate filaments that characterize neurons (*Fig. 5.9*). There are three isoforms (low, medium, and high molecular weight), which have some differential expression in development. Medium and heavy chain neurofilament proteins particularly characterize large projection neurones, such as motor neurones, and are associated with the slow component of axonal transport. Details of neurofilament biology have been extensively reviewed.[77] A key feature of this biology is the extensive array of phosphorylation sites expressed by the larger isoforms, and the extent of phosphorylation has important functional correlates. In normal neurones the somatic neurofilaments are predominantly non-phosphorylated (NF-P$^-$) whereas axonal neurofilaments have much higher levels of phosphorylation (NF-P[+]). These differences are readily demonstrable in tissue sections using antibodies that specifically recognize epitopes in either the P[-] or P[+] states. Cytoskeletal abnormalities in ALS have been linked to abnormalities in the normal metabolism of neurofilament transport.

Globules and spheroids
Axonal swellings in the anterior horn have been described in ALS. These 'spheroids' and 'globules'[70,77,78] are composed of abnormally orientated conglomerations of neurofilaments and are usually rich in phosphorylated epitopes. They generally resemble fusiform swellings in serial sections and are presumed to represent focal abnormalities of axonal cytoskeletal regulation with a failure of axonal transport. To that extent they are rather similar to the 'axonal spheroids' of diffuse non-missile head trauma. Both the larger spheroids and the smaller globules are present in normal subjects and have no disease specificity. Spheroids tend to be in proximal axons close to the motor neurone somata whereas globules tend to be more peripheral in the ventral horn.[73] Some spheroids may be in dendrites.[79] There has been speculation as to whether spheroids are transported in an anterograde or retrograde fashion[80] but it seems most likely that they simply accumulate at a point where the axonal cytoskeleton fails by accumulation of slow anterograde transport of neurofilaments.

The numbers of spheroids is almost certainly increased in ALS,[72,73,81] in contrast to globules, but this is not reliably demonstrable in a single tissue section. Sometimes they have been described in the soma of spinal motor neurones,[64,69,78] which raises the issue of their relationship to the HCIs described above. Spheroids are composed exclusively of NF-P[+] epitopes whereas HCIs contain both NF-P[-] and NF-P[+] epitopes. However this may simply

reflect the fact that the axon contains very little non-phosphorylated neurofilament protein so that only neurofilament containing NF-P[+] is added to the spheroid. In contrast the soma normally has very little NF-P[+] so that neurofilament aggregation at that site would be expected to initially contain only NF-P[-]. It is possible that, in the soma, this disorganized conglomerate of neurofilament is acted on inappropriately by somatic protein kinases so that there is progressive phosphorylation of the aggregated neurofilament, leading to the mixed pattern detected by immunocytochemistry.

Another feature of neurones that contain HCIs is the absence of staining, in that part of the soma that is unoccupied by the conglomerate, of either NF-P[-] or NF-P[+], suggesting that the whole neurofilament cytoskeleton has collapsed into the conglomerate. These observations raise the possibility that both spheroids and HCIs arise from a similar underlying failure of cytoskeletal regulation, which results in slightly different molecular and morphological features because of the neuronal compartment (soma or axon) that is involved.

Diffuse somatic phosphorylation of neurofilaments
Some authors have reported a diffuse increase in neurofilament phosphorylation affecting the soma of spinal motor neurones in ALS.[73,81–83] In normal ageing, a proportion of motor neurones show strong neurofilament immunoreactivity using antibodies to detect phosphorylated epitopes.[58] In the author's series of 20 sporadic ALS cases and 10 controls, in which lumbar spinal cord sections were stained with the antibodies SMI 31 and SMI 32 (detecting phosphorylated and non-phosphorylated neurofilament medium (NF-M) and neurofilament heavy (NF-H) epitopes respectively), the total number of motor

neurones was reduced by 54% in ALS. Controls and ALS cases both showed SMI 31 immunoreactivity in the somata of some motor neurones in the ventral horn. However, there was a marked difference in that the proportion of strongly immunoreactive neurons in ALS was 25.8% (range 0–85%) of the SMI 31 staining neurons, compared with 4.5% (range 0–14.6%; $p < 0.01$) in controls.

Other studies have reported no differences in somatic neurofilament phosphorylation in ALS,[72] which may reflect differences in tissue preparation and antibody specificity. There are no data regarding the implications of this finding of abnormal cytoskeletal function: it would, for example, be valuable to know whether neurones that are affected show other pathological abnormalities related to oxidative stress or apoptosis.

ALS dementia

It is now generally accepted that up to 5% of patients with typical motor features of ALS develop a frontotemporal dementia syndrome, either shortly before or soon after their motor disorder.[21,84–92] The cerebral pathology of this syndrome includes several non-specific features. There is diffuse atrophy of the cerebral hemispheres with frontotemporal accentuation,[93] together with microvacuolation of cortical layer 2 in the worst affected areas.[94] Another non-specific feature is the presence of variable, but usually intense, subcortical gliosis of white matter in the frontotemporal regions; this may extend into the caudate nucleus.[93] Recent stereological work has indicated that diffuse cortical neuronal loss can be widespread even in non-demented patients with ALS.[95] Substantia nigra degeneration in the absence of Lewy body formation is another common finding.

The most specific feature of the pathology of these patients is the presence of ubiquiti-nated neuronal inclusion bodies in a more widespread distribution than is seen in typical ALS.[61,89,90,96,97] These are characteristically present in the hippocampal dentate granule cells (*Fig. 5.10*) and more variably in the neurones of cortical layers 2 and 3 in the frontotemporal regions. Molecular pathology studies indicate that they share the features of the motor neurone UBIs of ALS. However, since the major protein constitution of UBIs has not yet been demonstrated, this interpretation is to some extent speculative. Conceptually it is proposed that, in some patients, susceptibility to the disease process that characterizes ALS extends to cerebral regions that are not normally affected. This cerebral degeneration is manifested pathologically by the presence of UBIs in cerebral cortical regions, and the distribution of the pathology provides an adequate anatomical substrate for the neuropsychological features of ALS dementia. Further support for this concept of an extended regional involvement in ALS to non-motor areas comes from observations in non-demented ALS patients. Studies of cerebral function by positron emission tomography scanning[98–100] as well as detailed neuropsychological testing in non-demented ALS patients[101] show that many patients have evidence of sub-clinical cerebral involvement of non-motor regions. In addition, pathological examination of the hippocampus in ALS patients at autopsy shows hippocampal inclusions in a greater proportion of cases than were known to show cognitive impairment in life (Lowe J, personal communication).

ALS variants

The traditional view of MND regards the three syndromes of ALS, progressive bulbar palsy, and progressive muscular atrophy as variants of the same disease process.[102] Most

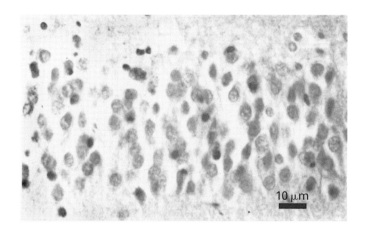

Figure 5.10
Dentate granule cell ubiquitinated inclusions in ALS dementia.

cases that present as progressive bulbar palsy go on to develop typical ALS during the course of the illness. Greater controversy has persisted over the status of primary lateral sclerosis in relation to this disease spectrum. Modern pathological studies, based on defining disease processes through molecular pathological markers, indicates that both primary lateral sclerosis and a type of frontotemporal dementia (MND inclusion dementia) should be considered as syndromes that arise via the same pathological cascade as occurs in ALS–MND,[103] but with different anatomical selectivity.

Pathological observations that link these disorders are summarized below. The key to firmly establishing these syndromes within an overall spectrum of neurodegeneration is the UBI. At present, morphological (light and electron microscopy) pathological findings and molecular pathological findings suggest that the UBI is a characteristic lesion for ALS, despite an imperfect understanding of the basis of the lesion. Thus, UBIs are sufficiently distinct from neurofibrillary tangles, Lewy bodies, glial cell inclusions (of multiple system

atrophy), cortical balloon cells, and various lesions that characterize the other late-onset neurodegenerative disorders, so that they can be considered to define a particular pathway of degeneration. ALS is the most familiar syndrome that arises from this pathway, but it has been proposed that the other syndromes discussed in this section represent the continuation of a spectrum that arises from the specific anatomical vulnerability of each individual patient.[43,50] This spectrum of clinicopathological syndromes is summarized in *Table 5.1*.

Anatomopathological correlates of clinical phenotypes

Progressive muscular atrophy

This phenotype denotes a pure LMN degeneration in the absence of UMN signs. The differential diagnosis includes Kennedy's syndrome (X-linked spinobulbar muscular atrophy) and adult forms of spinal muscular atrophy, both of which are characterized by genetic abnormalities. Kennedy's syndrome patients have an enlarged cytosine–adenine–guanine repeat region in the gene that encodes the androgen receptor (coded on chromosome X), and cases of spinal motor atrophy are increasingly linked to deletions in the *smn* and *naip* genes (coded on chromosome 5). On this basis diagnostic confusion can be overcome directly by genetic means. The author has performed post mortem studies of two patients with Kennedy's syndrome[104] and four patients with Werdnig–Hoffman disease (infantile spinal motor atrophy). None of these cases showed any evidence of UBIs in multiple sections examined throughout the motor system and elsewhere in the brain. In the author's series of 90 autopsied ALS–MND cases there were 14 in whom UMN signs had not been detected clinically at any stage. Of these, 12 showed UBIs at some level of the spinal cord or bulbar motor neurone groups. There were two exceptions: one patient with an unusual family history[105] and an elderly patient with an indolent 10-year history of progressive weakness. It is likely that these two patients did not have true ALS–MND.

An important issue in such patients with progressive muscular atrophy is the reliability of clinical methods in detecting UMN signs at a late stage of the disease, when there is severe global weakness and amyotrophy. The possibility that corticospinal tract degeneration can be detected in such circumstances is currently under investigation. A variety of methods has been used to show long tract degeneration in autopsy tissues. In the author's experience neither conventional myelin stains nor the Marchi impregnation technique are as sensitive as an immunocytochemical stain for active microglia and macrophages.[5,6] Of the 12 cases mentioned above, these various techniques showed sub-clinical corticospinal tract involvement in seven patients. This type of observation underlines the difficulty of classifying cases of ALS–MND on the basis of clinical signs alone. Many cases of progressive

muscular atrophy, but not all, show some progression towards ALS when examined at autopsy, and the molecular pathology of motor neurone degeneration in most cases of progressive muscular atrophy is indistinguishable from that of ALS.

Primary lateral sclerosis

Primary lateral sclerosis is a slowly progressive spastic paraparesis; it has been less securely linked to ALS from clinical and pathological studies. The differential diagnosis includes hereditary spastic paraparesis, multiple sclerosis, human T-cell leukaemia virus-1-associated tropical paraparesis, and human immunodeficiency virus myelopathy. Pathological reports are few and have recently been reviewed.[106] Ten cases of primary lateral sclerosis have been reported in the literature since 1977,[106–112] and in addition the author has studied one further case (Lowe J, unpublished observations, study of the brain). In all but three of these there was significant atrophy of the prefrontal gyrus and an associated loss of Betz cell somata. Most of the cases (seven of 11) pre-date the use of ubiquitin immunocytochemistry to detect UBI and Bunina bodies, but three showed eosinophilic inclusions within anterior horn cells or the hypoglossal nucleus. Among the more recent cases,[106,112] there were two in whom typical UBI were identified in a few LMNs at autopsy.

In the case examined by the author (Lowe J, Ince P, unpublished observations, study of the spinal cord), there was no evidence of LMN involvement either by immunocytochemical examination of multiple sections from many spinal levels or by detailed quantification of motor neurone numbers based on previously reported methods for optimum counting.[14] These observations are consistent with the hypothesis that primary lateral sclerosis cases represent a spectrum of ALS-type degeneration

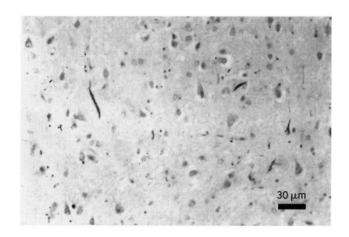

Figure 5.11
Frontal neurites in MND inclusion dementia as seen by ubiquitin immunocytochemistry.

30 μm

presenting as an UMN disorder, with possible late sub-clinical extension to involve LMNs. An additional important feature of these cases is the presence of UBI in the cerebral cortex in a distribution typical of ALS dementia cases[106] (Lowe J, unpublished observations), which suggests that cases of primary lateral sclerosis (PLS) also merge into the spectrum of ALS dementia. However, some differences have been reported in that substantia nigra degeneration may be inconspicuous in PLS.[106] Two cases of HSP studied by the author showed no evidence of either UBI or Bunina bodies in any area examined and are clearly distinct from PLS.

MND inclusion dementia

Frontotemporal dementia syndromes (e.g. dementia of frontal lobe type[113] and dementia lacking distinctive histological features[114]) have been sub-divided into several histopathological groups.[115] In a proportion of such cases the molecular pathology of the cerebral hemispheres is identical to that found in ALS dementia. This observation has resulted in the

term MND inclusion dementia for such cases.[103]

The original pathological reports were based on patients from whom only the cerebrum was retained for examination because of the absence of clinical features related to spinal disease. On the basis of these incomplete autopsies it remained speculative as to whether this disorder is truly part of the spectrum of ALS and its variants. More recently four cases of MND inclusion dementia have been studied (Lowe J, unpublished observations) in which the spinal cord was examined. These cases all showed some typical UBIs in anterior horn cells or in the hypoglossal nucleus despite the lack of clinical features of amyotrophy. Curiously there was no evidence of corticospinal tract degeneration or of involvement of the motor cortex in these cases. Among a further three cases of frontotemporal dementia with ALS-type cerebral inclusions, one showed both mild corticospinal tract pallor and anterior horn cell UBIs.[116] This combination of severe cognitive failure with sub-clinical LMN pathology appears to be yet another stereotyped pattern of selective vulnerability within a particular group of patients. Cases of MND inclusion dementia also show extension of the pathological distribution of UBIs to the basal ganglia, although similar changes have also been described in a patient with ALS dementia.[117]

In the frontotemporal cortex of patients with MND inclusion dementia there are thread-like dystrophic neurites showing immunoreactivity to ubiquitin; these are negative for tau and neurofilament staining (*Fig. 5.11*). These lesions resemble the neurites described in Huntington's disease[118] and dementia with Lewy bodies,[119] although they have a rather different distribution.

Additional support for a direct relationship between ALS and MND inclusion dementia emerges from examples of familial disease. In the kindred described by Jackson and colleagues,[103] disease was present in each of four generations of a family, involving nine out of 15 family members. Of these affected individuals, six had pure frontotemporal dementia (demonstrated pathologically to be MND inclusion dementia in the only autopsied case) while one had ALS with no dementia, one had ALS with parkinsonism, and another had ALS dementia. This clearly indicates that a single autosomal-dominant locus can variably cause one family to both develop ALS and MND inclusion dementia (together with overlap syndromes).

Spectrum of ALS and relation to ALS variants

The clinical phenotype in ALS is heavily dominated by motor system degeneration so that the pathological involvement of other CNS regions is usually undetected unless it is the subject of research studies. These extramotor features may frequently arise late in the course of the disease, which adds to the difficulty in

detecting them. This concept is supported by the finding of widespread CNS degeneration in brain regions that are classically unaffected by ALS in Japanese patients who, maintained on artificial ventilation, survived long beyond the stage when respiratory failure would normally result in death.[120] Among patients with 'classical' ALS there is a spectrum of multisystem involvement which probably merges imperceptibly into the changes associated with ALS dementia. Pathologically, ALS dementia merges with 'pure' MND inclusion dementia and with primary lateral sclerosis. Similarly, many patients with a clinical phenotype of progressive muscular atrophy show subtle UMN degeneration at autopsy. From this perspective, ALS emerges as a frequent clinico-pathological syndrome, and the best recognized one, within a continuous spectrum (ranging from pure progressive muscular atrophy at one end to primary lateral sclerosis and MND inclusion dementia at the other) arising from a common pathogenetic cascade. Molecular pathology suggests that the best markers for this degenerative process are the UBI and the Bunina body. The spectrum of pathological involvement of different CNS regions in these disorders is outlined in *Table 5.1*.

Familial ALS

Various motor system disorders show inheritance, including:

(a) autosomal-dominant inheritance (familial ALS, hereditary spastic paraparesis);
(b) autosomal-recessive inheritance (spinal motor atrophy, hereditary spastic paraparesis); and
(c) X-linked inheritance (Kennedy's syndrome).

As described above, the pathological features of hereditary spastic paraparesis, progressive muscular atrophy, and Kennedy's

Phenotype	Regions affected				
	Frontotemporal cortex	Hippocampus dentate fascia	UMN or corticospinal tract	LMN (spinal/bulbar)	Other
Progressive muscular atrophy	—	—	—	+	Some cases have sub-clinical corticospinal tract pathology
ALS	±	±	+	+	? Substantia nigra; spinocerebellar tracts; dorsal columns; thalamus (especially familial and SOD1-linked cases)
ALS dementia	+	+	+	+	As for ALS
Primary lateral sclerosis	±	±	+	—	? Substantia nigra
MND inclusion dementia	+	+	±	±	Basal ganglia, thalamus, ? substantia nigra

ALS, amyotrophic lateral sclerosis; MND, motor neurone disease; LMN, lower motor neuron; UMN, upper motor neuron. —, no regular involvement; ±, variable involvement, usually slight; +, typically involved; ?, pathology often present but not typical ALS inclusions.

Table 5.1
Proposed spectrum of clinicopathological phenotypes characterized by molecular pathological features characteristic of ALS.

disease are sufficiently distinct from ALS to indicate a different pathological mechanism for neurodegeneration. However up to 10% of ALS patients have a positive family history, which usually indicates autosomal-dominant inheritance. It is therefore difficult to draw firm conclusions from much of the previous literature because of the uncertainty of ascertainment of familial disease. The absence of a firm family history of ALS is not conclusive evidence for sporadic disease. The only groups between which definite comparisons can be made are those known to have mutations in the gene that encodes SOD1 and those shown to have a normal SOD1 genotype. For this reason the literature on the pathology of familial ALS must be regarded in two parts. The literature on the pathology of familial ALS before 1994 does not include data from SOD1-gene analysis and is therefore difficult to relate to current observations on cases with fully characterized gene defects. It would be very valuable to have retrospective genetic analysis of the many cases reported in this older literature. The most recent literature looks at the pathology in cases with defined 'causal' genetic mutations. For practical purposes, this group includes at present only cases with an SOD1-gene mutation.

Pathology of familial ALS cases with an uncharacterized genetic basis

The earlier literature suggested that degeneration of the posterior columns was more frequent in familial cases.[64] The suggestion that spinocerebellar involvement or dementia[21] are over-represented in familial ALS are not well supported by published studies. However, there are no large comparative studies of extramotor pathology in familial ALS and sporadic disease in the literature. Familial ALS cases have also

been reported to have neuropathological features that are identical to sporadic ALS.[121] It has been demonstrated that UBIs are present in both sporadic and familial cases.[57]

ALS linked to mutations in the SOD1 gene

At present at least 19 cases have been reported in which an SOD1-gene abnormality was characterized and in which neuropathology was performed.[5,6,122–129] The extent of pathological evaluation was variable and the cases do not all provide fully comparable conclusions. There is no evidence of a consistent pathological phenotype. Many examples have a typical ALS-type distribution of pathology with no significant non-motor involvement.[6,126] However, there are also a substantial number of the cases in which the disease is clearly multisystem.[6,124,126,129] Many of these cases show posterior column pallor and this may be more common in SOD1-related cases than in sporadic cases.[5,6,126,127] Hippocampal UBIs have been found in SOD1 familial ALS in cases not known to have been clinically demented.

A major feature of these reports is the prominence of neurofilamentous HCIs in SOD1 familial ALS cases. This inclusion is particularly associated with the A4V and I113T mutations[6,125,127,129] but has also been reported in the H48Q mutation.[128] The other cases reported showed typical UBIs and a few contained both types of inclusion body. Given the considerable heterogeneity of clinical and pathological phenotypes that are observed, both between different SOD1 mutations and also within a single mutation, these molecular pathological observations are unusually consistent for A4V and I113T. The other striking example of consistent phenotype in relation to a particular SOD1 mutation is the observation of limited corticospinal tract involvement in

A4V cases. This is also found at autopsy,[129] although some variation in corticospinal tract involvement is present. Such findings highlight the extent to which disease phenotype in ALS (both clinical and pathological) must be strongly modified in each individual patient by interactions with other genetic host factors, even in cases in which the disease is 'driven' by a highly penetrant autosomal dominant gene defect.

References

1. Charcot JM. De la sclérose latérale amyotrophique. *Prog Med* 1874; **2**: 325–327, 341–342, 453–455.

2. Brownell B, Oppenheimer DR, Hughes JT. The central nervous system in motor neurone disease. *J Neurol Neurosurg Psychiatry* 1970; **33**: 338–357.

3. Kamo H, Haebara H, Akiguchi I et al. A distinctive pattern of reactive gliosis in the precentral cortex in amyotrophic lateral sclerosis. *Acta Neuropathol* 1987; **74**: 33–38.

4. Chou SM. Pathology of motor system disorder. In: Leigh PN, Swash M , eds. *Motor Neuron Disease: Biology and Management.* London: Springer-Verlag, 1995, 53–92.

5. Ince PG, Shaw PJ, Slade JY et al. Familial amyotrophic lateral sclerosis with a mutation in exon 4 of the Cu/Zn superoxide dismutase gene: pathological and immunocytochemical changes. *Acta Neuropathol* 1996; **92**: 395–403.

6. Ince PG, Tomkins J, Slade JY et al. Amyotrophic lateral sclerosis associated with genetic abnormalities in the gene encoding superoxide dismutase: molecular pathology of five new cases and comparison with 73 sporadic cases and previous reports. *J Neuropathol Exp Neurol* 1998; **57**: 895–904.

7. Hirano A, Iwata M. Pathology of motor neurons with specific reference to amyotrophic lateral sclerosis. In: Tsubaki T, Toyokura Y, eds. *Amyotrophic Lateral Sclerosis.* Baltimore: University Park Press, 1978, 107–133.

8. Martin LJ. Neuronal death in amyotrophic lateral sclerosis is apoptosis: possible contribution of a programmed cell death mechanism. *J Neuropathol Exp Neurol* 1999; **58**: 459–471.

9. Tomlinson BE, Irving D, Rebeiz JJ. Total numbers of limb motor neurons in the human lumbosacral cord and an analysis of the accuracy of various sampling procedures. *J Neurol Sci* 1973; **20**: 313–327.

10. Portera-Cailliau C, Hedreen JC, Price DL, Koliatsos VE. Evidence for apoptotic cell death in Huntingdon disease and excitotoxic animal models. *J Neurosci* 1995; **15**: 3774–3787.

11. Portera-Cailliau C, Price DL, Martin IJ. Non-NMDA and NMDA receptor-mediated excitotoxic neuronal deaths in adult brain are morphologically distinct: further evidence for an apoptosis-necrosis continuum. *J Comp Neurol* 1997; **378**: 88–104.

12. Dyck PJ, Stevens JC, Mulder DW, Espinosa RE. Frequency of nerve fibre degeneration of peripheral and sensory neurons in amyotrophic lateral sclerosis. *Neurology* 1975; **25**: 781–785.

13. Ince PG, Slade J, Chinnery RM et al. Quantitative study of synaptophysin immunoreactivity of cerebral cortex and spinal cord in motor neuron disease. *J Neuropathol Exp Neurol* 1995; **54**: 673–679.

14. Tomlinson BE, Irving D, Rebeiz JJ. The number of limb motoneurons in the human lumbosacral cord throughout life. *J Neurol Sci* 1977; **34**: 213–225.

15. Iwata M, Hirano A. Sparing of the Onufrowicz nucleus in sacral anterior horn lesions. *Ann Neurol* 1978; **4**: 245–249.

16. Alexianu ME, Ho BK, Mohammed AH et al. The role of calcium-binding proteins in selective motoneuron vulnerability in amyotrophic lateral sclerosis. *Ann Neurol* 1994; **36**: 846–858.

17. Ince P, Stout N, Shaw PJ et al. Parvalbumin and calbindin D-28k in the human motor system and in motor neurone disease. *Neuropathol Appl Neurobiol* 1993; **19**: 291–299.

18. Shaw PJ, Chinnery RM, Ince PG. Non-MNDA receptors in motor neuron disease (MND): a quantitative autoradiographic study in spinal cord and motor cortex using [3H]CNQX and [3H]kainate. *Brain Res*

1994; **655**: 186–194.

19. Shaw PJ, Ince PG, Matthews JNS et al. N-methyl-D-aspartate (NMDA) receptors in the spinal cord and motor cortex in motor neurone disease: a quantitative autoradiographic study using [3H]MK-801. *Brain Res* 1994; **637**: 297–302.

20. Castaigne P, Lhermitte F, Cambier J et al. Etude neuropathologique de 61 observations de sclérose latérale amyotrophique: discussion nosologique. *Rev Neurol* 1972; **127**: 401–414.

21. Hudson AJ. Amyotrophic lateral sclerosis and its association with dementia, parkinsonism and other neurological disorders: a review. *Brain* 1981; **104**: 217–247.

22. Iwata M, Hirano A. Current problems in the pathology of amyotrophic lateral sclerosis. In: Zimmerman HM, ed. *Progress in Neuropathology* vol. 4. New York: Raven Press, 1979, 277–298.

23. Lawyer TJ, Netsky MG. Amyotrophic lateral sclerosis: a clinicopathological study of 53 cases. *Arch Neurol Psychiatry* 1953; **69**: 171–192.

24. Kawamura Y, Dyck PJ, Shimono M et al. Morphometric comparison of the vulnerability of peripheral motor and sensory neurons in amyotrophic lateral sclerosis. *J Neuropathol Exp Neurol* 1981; **40**: 667–675.

25. Bradley WG, Good P, Rasool CG, Adelman LS. Morphometric and biochemical studies of peripheral nerves in amyotrophic lateral sclerosis. *Ann Neurol* 1983; **14**: 267–277.

26. Swash M, Leader M, Brown A, Swettenham KW. Focal loss of anterior horn cells in the cervical cord in motor neuron disease. *Brain* 1986; **109**: 939–952.

27. Averback P, Crocker P. Regular involvement of Clarke's nucleus in sporadic amyotrophic lateral sclerosis. *Arch Neurol* 1982; **39**: 155–156.

28. Eisen A, Calne D. Amyotrophic lateral sclerosis, Parkinson's disease and Alzheimer's disease: phylogenetic disorders of the human neocortex sharing many characteristics. *Can J Neurol Sci* 1992; **19 (suppl 1)**: 117–120.

29. Williams TL, Shaw PJ, Lowe J et al. Parkinsonism in motor neuron disease: case report and literature review. *Acta Neuropathol* 1995; **89**: 275–283.

30. Burrow JNC, Blumbergs PC. Substantia nigra degeneration in motor neurone disease. *Aust N Z J Med* 1992; **22**: 469–472.

31. Kato S, Oda M, Tanabe H. Diminution of dopaminergic neurones in the substantia nigra of sporadic amyotrophic lateral sclerosis. *Neuropathol Appl Neurobiol* 1993; **19**: 300–304.

32. Takahashi H, Snow BJ, Bhatt M et al. Evidence for a dopaminergic deficit in sporadic amyotrophic lateral sclerosis. *Lancet* 1993; **342**: 1016–1018.

33. Aran FA. Recherches sur une maladie non encore décrite du système musculaire (atrophie musculaire progressive). *Arch Gen Med* 1850; **24**: 5–35, 172–214.

34. Charcot JM, Joffroy A. Deux cas d'atrophie musculaire progressive avec lésions de la substance grise et des fasciaeux antérolateraux de la moelle épinière. *Arch Physiol (Paris)* 1869; **2**: 354–367, 629–644, 744–760.

35. Kojewnikoff A. Cas de sclérose latérale amyotrophique, la dégénérescence des faisceaux pyramidaux se propageant à traverstout l'encéphale. *Arch Neurol* 1883; **6**: 356–376.

36. Martin JE, Swash M. The pathology of motor neuron disease. In: Leigh PN, Swash M, eds. *Motor Neuron Disease: Biology and Management.* London: Springer-Verlag, 1995, 93–118.

37. Hughes JT. Pathology of amyotrophic lateral sclerosis. In: Rowland LP, ed. *Human Motor Neuron Diseases.* New York: Raven Press, 1982, 61–74.

38. Wohlfart G. Collateral regeneration from residual motor nerve fibres in amyotrophic lateral sclerosis. *Ann Neurol* 1957; **7**: 124–134.

39. Ono S, Yamauchi M. Collagen cross-linking of skin in patients with amyotrophic lateral sclerosis. *Ann Neurol* 1992; **31**: 305–310.

40. Ono S, Yamauchi M. Elastin cross-linking in the skin from patients with amyotrophic lateral sclerosis. *J Neurol Neurosurg Psychiatry* 1994; **57**: 94–96.

41. Ono S, Imai T, Munakata S. Collagen abnormalities in the spinal cord from patients with amyotrophic lateral sclerosis. *J Neurol Sci* 1998; **160**: 140–147.

42. Nakano I, Hirayama K, Terao K. Hepatic ultrastructural changes and liver dysfunction in amyotrophic lateral sclerosis. *Arch Neurol* 1987; **44**: 103–106.

43. Ince PG, Morris CM, Perry EK. Dementia with Lewy bodies: a distinct non-Alzheimer dementia? *Brain Pathol* 1998; **8**: 299–324.

44. Love S, Saitoh T, Quijada S et al. Alz-50, ubiquitin and tau immunoreactivity of neurofibrillary tangles, Pick bodies and Lewy bodies. *J Neuropathol Exp Neurol* 1988; **47**: 393–405.

45. Lowe J, Blanchard A, Morrell K et al. Ubiquitin is a common factor in intermediate filament inclusion bodies of diverse type in man, including those of Parkinson's disease, Pick's disease and Alzheimer's disease as well as Rosenthal fibres in cerebellar astrocytomas, cytoplasmic inclusion bodies in muscle and Mallory bodies in alcoholic liver disease. *J Pathol* 1988; **155**: 9–15.

46. Hershko A, Ciechanover A, Heller H et al. Proposed role of ATP in protein breakdown: conjugation of proteins with multiple chains of the polypeptide of ATP-dependent proteolysis. *Proc Natl Acad Sci U S A* 1980; **77**: 1783–1786.

47. Bond U, Schlesinger MJ. Ubiquitin is a heat shock protein in chicken embryo fibroblasts. *Mol Cell Biol* 1985; **5**: 949–956.

48. Leigh PN, Anderton BH, Dodson A et al. Ubiquitin deposits in anterior horn cells in motor neurone disease. *Neurosci Lett* 1988; **93**: 197–203.

49. Lowe J, Lennox G, Jefferson D et al. A filamentous inclusion body within anterior horn neurons in motor neuron disease defined by immunocytochemical localisation of ubiquitin. *Neurosci Lett* 1988; **93**: 203–210.

50. Ince PG, Lowe J, Shaw PJ. Amyotrophic lateral sclerosis: current issues in classification, pathogenesis and molecular pathology. *Neuropathol Appl Neurobiol* 1998; **24**: 104–117.

51. Garofalo O, Kennedy PGE, Swash M et al. Ubiquitin and heat shock protein expression in amyotrophic lateral sclerosis. *Neuropathol Appl Neurobiol* 1991; **17**: 39–45.

52. Mizusawa H, Nakamure H, Wakayama I et al. Skein-like inclusions in the anterior horn cells in motor neuron disease. *J Neurol Sci* 1991; **105**: 14–21.

53. Murayama S, Ookawa Y, Mori H et al. Immunocytochemical and ultrastructural study of Lewy body-like inclusions in familial amyotrophic lateral sclerosis. *Acta Neuropathol* 1989; **78**: 143–152.

54. Murayama S, Mori H, Ihara Y et al. Immunocytochemical and ultrastructural studies of lower motor neurons in ALS. *Ann Neurol* 1990; **27**: 137–148.

55. Schiffer D, Autilio-Gambetti L, Chio A et al. Ubiquitin in motor neuron disease: a study at the light and electron microscopical level. *J Neuropathol Exp Neurol* 1991; **50**: 463–473.

56. Mather K, Martin JE, Swash M et al. Histochemical and immunocytochemical study of ubiquitinated neuronal inclusions in amyotrophic lateral sclerosis. *Neuropath Appl Neurobiol* 1993; **19**: 141–145.

57. Leigh PN, Whitwell H, Garofalo O et al. Ubiquitin-immunoreactive intraneuronal inclusions in amyotrophic lateral sclerosis: morphology, distribution and specificity. *Brain* 1991; **114**: 775–788.

58. Cruz-Sánchez FF, Moral A, Tolosa E et al. Evaluation of neuronal loss, astrocytosis and abnormalities of cytoskeletal components of large motor neurons in the human anterior horn in ageing. *J Neural Transm* 1998; **105**: 689–701.

59. Lowe J, Aldridge F, Lennox G et al. Inclusion bodies in motor cortex and brainstem of patients with motor neuron disease are detected by immunocytochemical localisation of ubiquitin. *Neurosci Lett* 1989; **105**: 7–13.

60. Murayama S, Bouldin TW, Suzuki K. Immunocytochemical and ultrastructural studies of Werdnig–Hoffman disease. *Acta Neuropathol* 1991; **81**: 408–417.

61. Wightman G, Anderson VER, Martin J et al. Hippocampal and neocortical ubiquitin-immunoreactive inclusions in amyotrophic lateral sclerosis. *Neurosci Lett* 1992; **139**: 269–277.

62. Kihira T, Yoshida S, Uebayashi Y et al. Involvement of Onuf's nucleus in ALS. Demonstration of intraneuronal conglomerate inclusions and Bunina bodies. *J Neurol Sci* 1991; **104**: 119–128.

63. Bunina TL. Intracellular inclusions in familial

amyotrophic lateral sclerosis. *Zh Nevropatol Psikhiatr* 1962; **62**: 1293–1299.

64. Hirano A, Kurland LT, Sayre GP. Familial amyotrophic lateral sclerosis: a subgroup characterized by posterior and spinocerebellar tract involvement and hyaline inclusions. *Arch Neurol* 1967; **16**: 232–243.

65. Sasaki S, Maruyama S. Ultrastructural study of Bunina bodies in the anterior horn neurons of patients with amyotrophic lateral sclerosis. *Neurosci Lett* 1993; **154**: 117–120.

66. Tomonaga M, Saito M, Yoshimura M et al. Ultrastructure of the Bunina bodies in anterior horn cells of amyotrophic lateral sclerosis. *Acta Neuropathol* 1978; **42**: 81–86.

67. Okamoto K, Hirai S, Amari M et al. Bunina bodies in amyotrophic lateral sclerosis immunostained with rabbit antiserum. *Neurosci Lett* 1993; **162**: 125–128.

68. Hirano A, Donnefeld H, Sasaki S, Nakano I. Fine structural observations on neurofilamentous changes in amyotrophic lateral sclerosis. *J Neuropathol Exp Neurol* 1984; **43**: 461–470.

69. Schochet JS, Hardmann JM, Ladewig PP, Earle KM. Intraneuronal conglomerates in sporadic motor neuron disease. *Arch Neurol* 1969; **20**: 548–553.

70. Chou SM. Pathognomy of intraneuronal inclusions in ALS. In: Tsubaki T, Toyokura Y, eds. *Amyotrophic Lateral Sclerosis*. Tokyo and Baltimore: Tokyo University Press and University Park Press, 1979, 135–177.

71. Kondo A, Iwaki T, Tateishi J et al. Accumulation of neurofilaments in a sporadic case of amyotrophic lateral sclerosis. *Jpn J Psychiatry Neurol* 1986; **40**: 677–684.

72. Leigh PN, Dodson A, Swash M et al. Cytoskeletal abnormalities in motor neuron disease: an immunocytochemical study. *Brain* 1989; **112**: 521–535.

73. Sobue G, Hashizume Y, Yasuda T. Phosphorylated high molecular weight neurofilament protein in lower motor neurons in ALS and other neurodegenerative diseases involving the ventral horns. *Acta Neuropathol* 1990; **79**: 402–408.

74. Mizusawa H, Matsumoto S, Yen SH et al. Focal accumulation of phosphorylated neurofilaments within the anterior horn cell in familial amyotrophic lateral sclerosis. *Acta Neuropathol* 1989; **79**: 37–43.

75. Pollanen MS, Dickson DW, Bergeron C. Pathology and biology of the Lewy body. *J Neuropathol Exp Neurol* 1993; **52**: 183–191.

76. Spillantini MG, Crowther RA, Jakes R, Hasegawa M. α-synuclein in filamentous inclusions of Lewy bodies from Parkinson's disease and Dementia with Lewy bodies. *Proc Natl Acad Sci U S A* 1998; **95**: 6469–6473.

77. Robinson PA, Anderton BH. Neurofilament probes: a review of neurofilament distribution and morphology. *Rev Neurosci* 1988; **2**: 1–40.

78. Carpenter S. Proximal axonal enlargement in motor neuron disease. *Neurology* 1968; **18**: 841–851.

79. Sasaki S, Kamei H, Yamane K, Murayama S. Swelling of neuronal processes in motor neuron disease. *Neurology* 1988; **38**: 1114–1118.

80. Leigh PN, Garofalo O. The molecular pathology of motor neuron disease. In: Leigh PN, Swash M, eds. *Motor Neuron Disease: Biology and Management*. London: Springer-Verlag, 1995, 144–150.

81. Mannetto V, Sternberger NH, Perry G et al. Phosphorylation of neurofilaments is altered in amyotrophic lateral sclerosis. *J Neuropathol Exp Neurol* 1988; **47**: 642–653.

82. Arima K, Ogawa M, Sunohara N et al. Immunohistochemical and ultrastructural characterisation of ubiquitinated eosinophilic fibrillary neuronal inclusions in sporadic amyotrophic lateral sclerosis. *Acta Neuropathol* 1998; **96**: 75–85.

83. Munoz DG, Greene C, Perl DP, Selkoe DJ. Accumulation of phosphorylated neurofilaments in anterior horn motoneurons of amyotrophic lateral sclerosis patients. *J Neuropathol Exp Neurol* 1988; **47**: 9–18.

84. Wilkstrom J, Paetau A, Palo J et al. Classic amyotrophic lateral sclerosis with dementia. *Arch Neurol* 1982; **39**: 681–683.

85. Mitsuyama Y. Presenile dementia with motor neuron disease in Japan: clinicopathological review of 26 cases. *J Neurol Neurosurg Psychiatry* 1984; **47**: 953–959.

86. Gallassi R, Montaga P, Ciardulli C et al. Cognitive impairment in motor neuron dis-

ease. *Acta Neurol Scand* 1985; **71**: 480–484.

87. Mitsuyama Y, Kogoh H, Ata K. Progressive dementia with motor neuron disease: an additional case report and neuropathological review of 20 cases in Japan. *Eur Arch Psychiatry Neurol Sci* 1985; **235**: 1–8.

88. Morita K, Kaiya H, Ikeda T, Namba M. Presenile dementia combined with amyotrophy: a review of 34 Japanese cases. *Arch Gerontol Geriatr* 1987; **6**: 263–277.

89. Neary D, Snowden JS, Mann DMA et al. Frontal lobe dementia and motor neurone disease. *J Neurol Neurosurg Psychiatry* 1990; **53**: 23–32.

90. Peavy GM, Herzog AG, Rubin NP, Mesulam MM. Neuropsychological aspects of dementia of motor neuron disease: a report of two cases. *Neurology* 1992; **42**: 1004–1008.

91. Caselli RJ, Windebank AJ, Petersen RC, Komori T. Rapidly progressive aphasic dementia and motor neuron disease. *Ann Neurol* 1993; **33**: 200–207.

92. Mitsuyama Y. Presenile dementia with motor neuron disease. *Dementia* 1993; **4**: 137–142.

93. Kew JJM, Leigh PN. Dementia with motor neurone disease. In: Rossor MN, ed. *Unusual Dementias. Bailliere's Clinical Neurology* vol. 1. London: Bailliere Tindall, 1992, 611–626.

94. Lowe J. New pathological findings in amyotrophic lateral sclerosis. *J Neurol Sci* 1994; **124 (suppl)**: 38–51.

95. Latsoudis H, Everall I, McKay D et al. Extramotor cortical lesions in MND: unbiased stereological estimation of the neuronal numerical density using the optical dissector. *Neuropathol Appl Neurobiol* 1999; **25**: 163–164.

96. Okamoto K, Hirai S, Yamazaki Y et al. New ubiquitin-positive intraneuronal inclusions in the extra-motor cortices in patients with amyotrophic lateral sclerosis. *Neurosci Lett* 1991; **129**: 233–236.

97. Brun A, Englund B, Gustafson L et al. Consensus on clinical and neuropathological criteria for frontotemporal dementia. *J Neurol Neurosurg Psychiatry* 1994; **57**: 416–418.

98. Abrahams S, Goldstein LH, Kew JJM et al. Frontal lobe dysfunction in amyotrophic lateral sclerosis. A PET study. *Brain* 1996; **119**:

2105–2120.

99. Kew JJM, Goldstein LH, Leigh PN et al. The relationship between abnormalities of cognitive function and cerebral activation in amyotrophic lateral sclerosis. A neuropsychological and positron emission tomography study. *Brain* 1993; **116**: 1399–1423.

100. Ludolph AC, Elger CE, Bottger IW et al. Frontal lobe function in amyotrophic lateral sclerosis: a neuropsychological and positron emission tomography study. *Acta Neurol Scand* 1992; **85**: 81–89.

101. Chari G, Shaw PJ, Sahgal A. Non-verbal visual attention, but not recognition memory or learning processes are impaired in motor neurone disease. *Neuropsychologica* 1996; **34**: 377–385.

102. Dejerine J. Etude anatomique et clinique sur la paralysie labio-glosso-laryngée. *Arch Physiol Norm Ser* 1883; **3**: 180–227.

103. Jackson M, Lennox G, Lowe J. Motor neurone disease-inclusion dementia. *Neurodegeneration* 1996; **5**: 339–350.

104. Shaw PJ, Thagesen H, Tomkins J et al. Kennedy's disease: new molecular pathological and clinical features. *Neurology* 1998; **51**: 252–255.

105. Shaw PJ, Ince PG, Slade J et al. Lower motor neuron degeneration and familial predisposition to colonic neoplasia in two adult siblings. *J Neurol Neurosurg Psychiatry* 1991; **54**: 993–996.

106. Konagaya M, Sakai M, Matsuoka Y et al. Upper motor neuron predominant degeneration with frontal and temporal lobe atrophy. *Acta Neuropathol* 1998; **96**: 532–536.

107. Fisher CM. Pure spastic paralysis of corticospinal origin. *Can J Neurol Sci* 1977; **4**: 251–258.

108. Beal MF, Richardson EPJ. Primary lateral sclerosis: a case report. *Arch Neurol* 1981; **38**: 630–633.

109. Kuzahara S, Natori H, Inomata F, Toyokura Y. A case of clinical and pathological manifestations of primary lateral sclerosis with remarkable atrophy of the frontal and temporal lobes mimicking Pick's disease [Japanese]. *Neuropathol* 1985; **6**: 295–296.

110. Younger DS, Chou S, Hays AP et al. Primary

lateral sclerosis: a clinical diagnosis reemerges. *Arch Neurol* 1988; **45:** 1304–1307.

111. Kato S, Hirano A, Llena JF. Primary lateral sclerosis: a case report [Japanese]. *Neurol Med Chir (Tokyo)* 1990; **32:** 501–506.

112. Watanabe R, Iino M, Honda M et al. Primary lateral sclerosis. *Neuropathology* 1997; **17:** 220–224.

113. Mann DMA, South PW, Snowden JS, Neary D. Dementia of frontal lobe type: neuropathology and immunohistochemistry. *J Neurol Neurosurg Psychiatry* 1993; **56:** 605–614.

114. Knopman DS, Mastri AR, Frey WH et al. Dementia lacking distinctive histological features: a common non-Alzheimer degenerative dementia. *Neurology* 1990; **40:** 251–266.

115. Cooper P, Jackson M, Lennox G et al. Tau, ubiquitin, and αB crystallin immunohistochemistry define the principal causes of degenerative frontotemporal dementia. *Arch Neurol* 1995; **52:** 1011–1015.

116. Holton JL, Revesz T, Crooks R, Scaravilli F. Motor neuron disease-inclusion dementia: evidence for pathological involvement of the spinal cord. *Neuropathol Appl Neurobiol* 1999; **25:** 164.

117. Kawashima T, Kikuchi H, Takita M et al. Skein-like inclusions in the neostriatum from a case of amyotrophic lateral sclerosis with dementia. *Acta Neuropathol* 1998; **96:** 541–545.

118. Cammarata S, Caponnetto C, Tabaton M. Ubiquitin-reactive neurites in the cerebral cortex of subjects with Huntington's chorea: a pathological correlate of dementia? *Neurosci Lett* 1993; **156:** 96–98.

119. Dickson DW, Ruan D, Crystal H et al. Hippocampal degeneration differentiates diffuse Lewy body disease (DLBD) from Alzheimer's disease: light and electron microscopic immunocytochemistry of CA2-3 neurites specific to DLBD. *Neurology* 1991; **41:** 1402–1409.

120. Mizutani T, Sakamaki S, Tsuchiya N. Amyotrophic lateral sclerosis with ophthalmoplegia and multisystem degeneration in patients on long-term use of respirators. *Acta Neuropathol* 1992; **84:** 372–377.

121. Williams DB. Familial amyotrophic lateral sclerosis. In: Vinken PJ, Bruyn GW, Klawans HL, de Jong JBMV, eds. *Diseases of the Motor System. Handbook of Clinical Neurology* vol. 59. Amsterdam: Elsevier, 1991, 242–251.

122. Pramatorova A, Goto J, Nanba E et al. A two base pair deletion in the SOD1 gene causes familial amyotrophic lateral sclerosis. *Hum Mol Genet* 1994; **3:** 2061–2062.

123. Takahashi H, Makifuchi T, Nakano R et al. Familial amyotrophic lateral sclerosis with a mutation in the Cu/Zn superoxide dismutase gene. *Acta Neuropathol* 1994; **88:** 185–188.

124. Orrell RW, King AW, Hilton DA et al. Familial amyotrophic lateral sclerosis with a point mutation of SOD-1: intrafamilial heterogeneity of disease duration associated with neurofibrillary tangles. *J Neurol Neurosurg Psychiatry* 1995; **59:** 266–270.

125. Chou SM, Wang HS, Taniguchi A. Role of SOD1 and nitric oxide/cyclic GMP cascade on neurofilament aggregation in ALS/MND. *J Neurol Sci* 1996; **139 (suppl):** 16–26.

126. Kato S, Shimoda M, Watanabe Y et al. Familial amyotrophic lateral sclerosis with a two base pair deletion in superoxide dismutase 1 gene: multisystem degeneration with intracytoplasmic hyaline inclusions in astrocytes. *J Neuropathol Exp Neurol* 1996; **55:** 1089–1101.

127. Rouleau GA, Clark AW, Rooke K. SOD1 mutation is associated with accumulation of neurofilaments in amyotrophic lateral sclerosis. *Ann Neurol* 1996; **39:** 128–131.

128. Shaw CE, Enayat ZE, Powell JF et al. Familial amyotrophic lateral sclerosis: molecular pathology of a patient with a SOD1 mutation. *Neurology* 1997; **49:** 1612–1616.

129. Cudkowicz ME, McKenna-Yasek D, Chen C et al. Limited corticospinal tract involvement in amyotrophic lateral sclerosis subjects with the A4V mutation in the copper/zinc superoxide dismutase gene. *Ann Neurol* 1998; **43:** 703–710.

6

Biochemical pathology
Pamela J Shaw

Introduction

Many of the neurochemical changes identified to date in amyotrophic lateral sclerosis (ALS) are likely to be a consequence, rather than an underlying cause, of motor neurone loss. Neurochemical studies on human post-mortem tissue have often produced conflicting results, which may be due in part to neurochemical changes occurring during the agonal state and after death, and in part to technical difficulties in the measurement of certain neurochemical parameters in biological samples. No neurochemical changes have been identified in ALS that are equivalent in importance to the nigrostriatal dopamine deficiency identified in Parkinson's disease. Nevertheless, some aspects of the biochemical pathology identified in ALS may provide important clues into pathogenetic mechanisms of the disease. Examples include the evidence for an imbalance between excitatory and inhibitory neurotransmission and the evidence for oxidative stress as contributory factors to motor neurone injury.

This chapter reviews the current state of knowledge in relation to the normal neurochemistry of motor neurones; alterations in the expression of ubiquitin and neurofilament proteins; changes in ALS in neurotransmitter systems, neuropeptides, neurotrophic factors, metals and trace ele-

ments; and biochemical markers of oxidative stress.

Neurochemical features of normal human motor neurones that may contribute to vulnerability to neurodegeneration

Aspects of the neurochemistry of specific neuronal groups within the human central nervous system (CNS) are likely to be important in the development of late-onset selective neurodegeneration (*Table 6.1*). In relation to certain inherited neurodegenerative disorders such as copper–zinc superoxide dismutase (SOD1)-related familial ALS or Huntington's disease, the affected gene is known to be widely expressed in many cell systems in the CNS, and yet the ensuing cell death affects only specific neuronal groups. This must result from an interaction between the mutant protein and neurone-specific molecular and neurochemical features. Before considering the neurochemical alterations that occur in the motor system in ALS, it is therefore worth considering the current state of knowledge relating to the normal neurochemistry of human motor neurones.

Human motor neurones are amongst the

Large cells with very long axonal processes

High metabolic rate

High neurofilament content

Exposure outside the CNS (at neuromuscular junction)

High cell surface expression of glutamate receptors

Cell-specific profile of glutamate receptors (low expression of GluR2 AMPA receptor subunits)

No expression of certain calcium-binding proteins

High expression of copper–zinc superoxide dismutase

Table 6.1
Factors that may contribute to selective vulnerability of human motor neurones to neurodegeneration.

largest cells in the CNS. They have very long axonal processes, which may be up to 1 m in length. Because of these morphological features, they require a robust cytoskeletal structure, with a high content of neurofilament proteins, and a high metabolic rate. Unlike most other neurones, they have external contact outside the blood–brain barrier at the neuromuscular junction. Motor neurones have a high expression of cell surface glutamate receptors. In addition, their cell specific profile of glutamate receptors appears to differ from that of many other groups of neurones. The GluR2 subunit of the α-amino-3-hydroxy-5-methyl-4-isoxazole propionic acid (AMPA) subtype of glutamate receptor appears not to be expressed at a low level in human motor neurones, whereas it is present in most other neuronal groups.[1] The presence of the GluR2 subunit normally renders activated AMPA receptors impermeable to calcium. Its low expression in motor neurones means that these cells are likely to be activated by atypical, calcium-permeable AMPA receptors. Also, motor neurones that are vulnerable to pathology in ALS do not express the major calcium-binding

proteins parvalbumin and calbindin D-28k, which are thought to have an important role in buffering intracellular calcium.[2,3] These two neurochemical features may render motor neurones more vulnerable than other cell groups in the CNS to potentially toxic, calcium-dependent biochemical processes. Finally, perhaps because of their high metabolic rate, motor neurones have a higher expression of free radical scavenging enzymes, including SOD1, than other neurons.[4,5] While this may be important as a normal physiological defence against oxidative stress, it may also render motor neurones selectively vulnerable when the neurochemical properties of SOD1 are altered by point mutations in the SOD1 gene.

Alterations in the ubiquitin–proteasome system

Ubiquitin is a 76 amino acid polypeptide whose name is derived from its ubiquitous expression in eukaryotic cells. Ubiquitin has been shown to be a component of intraneuronal inclusion bodies found in various neurodegenerative diseases. It is a member of the heat-shock family of proteins[6] and is present both free within the cytoplasm and conjugated to other proteins. At present, the best known role of ubiquitin is in the non-lysosomal degradation of short-lived and damaged proteins.[7] The biochemistry of the ubiquitin conjugation pathway and the current state of knowledge regarding ubiquitin-dependent protein degradation have been reviewed previously.[7,8] In summary, ubiquitin is joined reversibly to other proteins via linkage between the α-carboxyl group of ubiquitin and lysine ε-amino groups of the acceptor proteins (isopeptide bonds). In an energy-dependent reaction, ubiquitin is first activated by an enzyme called E1, to which it becomes linked by a high-energy thiolester bond. Ubiquitin then forms a thiolester bond with a second protein, the ubiquitin-conjugating enzyme (E2). E2, often with the activation of an additional factor, E3, catalyses isopeptide bond formation between ubiquitin and the substrate. For substrates destined for proteolytic degradation, additional ubiquitin molecules are usually added to the substrate by the same enzyme cascade, to form chains of ubiquitin molecules in isopeptide linkage to one another. Degradation of such multi-ubiquitinated proteins occurs via a large proteinase called the 26S proteasome complex.

Ubiquitin immunocytochemistry in tissue from patients with ALS has revealed the presence of several types of ubiquitin-immunoreactive inclusions within surviving motor neurones.[9,10] Filamentous or skein-like inclusions are the most abundant type (*Fig. 6.1a*). They form fine interlacing bundles in the cell bodies or dendrites, or both, of surviving motor neurones and may also be seen in several other neuronal groups. Ultrastructurally they are composed of bundles of filaments measuring 10–25 nm in diameter, arranged as tubular structures, and associated with granu-

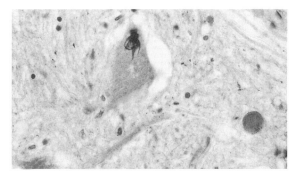

(a)

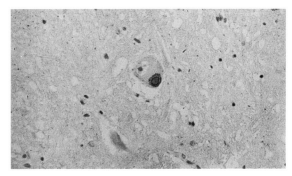

(b)

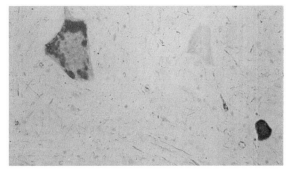

(c)

Figure 6.1
Inclusion bodies within surviving motor neurones in ALS. (a) Skein-like ubiquitinated inclusion in a lumbar motor neurone from a sporadic ALS case. (b) Lewy-like compact ubiquitinated inclusion in a lumbar motor neurone from a sporadic ALS case. (c) Hyaline conglomerate inclusions immunostained with an antibody to phophorylated neurofilament in a lumbar motor neurone from a case of familial ALS with the I113T mutation.

lar material. The second type of ubiquitinated inclusion is the dense body or Lewy body-like inclusion (see *Fig. 6.1b*). These inclusions are composed of radially arranged filaments with a granulofilamentous core that often contains lipofuscin. Some of the filaments are 10–15 nm in diameter and therefore probably represent neurofilaments, while other filaments are slightly larger, with a diameter of 15–25 nm. Double-labelling studies have shown that these compact inclusions may show immunoreactivity for neurofilament epitopes.[11,12] In some cases of SOD1-related familial ALS, large argyrophilic hyaline conglomerate inclusions have been observed in the perikarya and axons of motor neurones and in certain other neuronal groups (see *Fig. 6.1c*).[11,13] These inclusions show strong immunoreactivity for both phosphorylated and non-phosphorylated neurofilament epitopes, but only faint staining for ubiquitin.

It has been considered likely that the presence of ubiquitinated inclusions in ALS reflects the presence of ubiquitin–protein conjugates, which are resistant to degradation via the ubiquitin–proteolytic pathway, although this has not been proven. Although there is some evidence for the presence of neurofilament epitopes in some ubiquitinated inclusions in ALS, as described above, biochemical and molecular characterization of these inclusions is far from complete. Screening with a wide range of antibodies against other cytoskeletal proteins has so far produced negative results. It is possible that the proteins associated with inclusions are damaged to the extent that they are no longer recognized by conventional antibodies. Future work directed towards identification of the abnormal proteins associated with ubiquitinated inclusions in ALS is likely to yield important insights into the biochemical processes associated with cell death.

Alterations in neurofilaments

Neurofilament proteins form a major component of the neuronal cytoskeleton and serve several important functions including the maintenance of cell shape, axonal calibre, and axonal transport. Neurofilaments are particularly abundant in large neurones with long axons, such as motor neurones. They are composed of three subunit polypeptides: neurofilament light (molecular weight 68 kDa), neurofilament medium (molecular weight 150 kDa), and neurofilament heavy (molecular weight 200 kDa), which are assembled in a 6:2:1 ratio to form macromolecular filaments.[14] Each neurofilament subunit consists of conserved head and rod domains and a more variable acidic tail domain. The rod domains are principally composed of α-helices, which wrap around each other to form a superhelix of parallel coiled coils.[15] The head domains is important for lateral interactions between neurofilaments.[16] Neurofilament dimers assemble into protofilaments in a head-to-tail arrangement. Two protofilaments wrap around each other to form protofibrils, which in turn combine with three other protofibrils to form the characteristic 10 nm diameter neurofilaments seen by electron microscopy. The assembly of neurofilaments involves many complex interactions between subunits, stabilized by hydrophobic interactions that often involve tyrosine residues.[16] The neurofilament subunits are assembled in the motor neurone cell body and are transported down the axon by slow axonal transport at a rate of 1 mm per day. Some phosphorylation of neurofilaments occurs within the cell body, but phosphorylation progressively increases as the neurofilament proteins are transported down the axon. Increased phosphorylation of neurofilaments within the perikaryon can be observed after several neuronal insults. Consensus has not been reached as to whether phosphorylated neurofilaments are increased in the perikarya of surviving motor neurones in ALS. Some studies have reported an increased expression of phosphorylated neurofilaments,[17–19] but others have failed to confirm this finding.[20]

Neurofilament proteins are of interest as possible candidate targets of damage in ALS for several reasons. Neuronal spheroids, consisting of disorganised 10 nm filaments characteristic of neurofilaments, are regularly seen in the proximal axons of motor neurones in ALS.[21] While spheroids may also be seen in normal control cases, they are more numerous and often larger in size in the spinal cord of ALS patients. As described in the preceding section, compact or Lewy body-like inclusions in ALS may contain neurofilament epitopes, and the hyaline conglomerate inclusions seen in some SOD1-related familial ALS cases show strong reactivity for both phosphorylated and non-phosphorylated neurofilament proteins.

The importance of neurofilaments in the normal health of motor neurones is emphasized by the observation of occasional cases of sporadic ALS with deletions or insertions in the KSP repeat region of the neurofilament heavy gene.[22,23] In addition, motor neurone pathological changes develop in transgenic mice that overexpress the neurofilament light or heavy subunits[24,25] or in mice that express mutations in the neurofilament light gene.[26] Axonal transport is demonstrably disrupted in neurofilament heavy transgenic mice.[27] Thus, disruption of neurofilament assembly can selectively injure motor neurones, possibly by interfering with the retrograde transport of trophic support from target muscle tissue.

In neuronal cell culture models of oxidative stress, neurofilament proteins appear to show differential vulnerability to free radical damage.[28] Motor neurone cell lines transfected with mutant SOD1 show accumulations of all three neurofilament proteins, and this increase is exaggerated when the cells are subjected to oxidative stress.[29] These alterations are not seen in the presence of normal SOD1. One of the major hypotheses for the toxic gain of function associated with SOD1 mutations is that altered substrate affinity of the active site of the mutant enzyme may lead to the formation of nitronium residues from peroxynitrite with nitration of tyrosine residues of susceptible proteins.[30] Crowe and colleagues[31] showed that the tyrosine residues in the rod and tail domains of neurofilament light are more susceptible to SOD1-catalysed tyrosine nitration than other proteins in the CNS.

Alterations in neurotransmitter systems
Excitatory amino acid neurotransmission

Glutamate, and in some cases other excitatory amino acids (EAAs), is the major excitatory neurotransmitter in the mammalian nervous system. Glutamatergic excitation of human motor neurones is likely to arise from the descending corticospinal tracts,[32,33] from collaterals of the A α-fibres that innervate muscle spindles and Golgi tendon organs,[34,35] and from excitatory interneurones in the spinal cord.[36] There is great structural and functional diversity in the ionotropic glutamate receptor family, which results from combinations of 14 known gene products and their splice variants, with or without additional RNA editing.[37] Human motor neurones appear to express an unusual profile of glutamate receptors, in particular having a low or absent expression of the GluR2 AMPA receptor subunit, which may lead to increased calcium entry on glutamate receptor activation and may contribute to vulnerability to glutamate-mediated injury.[1]

Glutamate exists in the CNS in several different compartments. The large neuronal compartment contains about 80–90% of the CNS glutamate. Most of this is in a metabolic pool, but a small proportion represents the neurotransmitter fraction. Approximately 20% of CNS glutamate is located in glial cells.[38,39] None of the enzymes responsible for glutamate synthesis is known to be specific for the neurotransmitter pool, and post mortem studies do not allow differentiation between the different compartments of glutamate in the CNS.

There is a body of circumstantial evidence that disturbance of glutamatergic neurotransmission may contribute to motor neurone injury in ALS. This has been the subject of several recent reviews,[40–43] and only the major neurochemical aspects are highlighted here.

Glutamate levels in CNS tissue, CSF and plasma in ALS

A hypothesis has arisen that there may be a defect in metabolism, transport, or storage of glutamate, based on the following neurochemical studies. Significant reductions in the levels of glutamate in several CNS regions have been reported in post mortem studies of ALS patients.[44] Perry and colleagues[45] and Plaitakis and colleagues[46] identified reduced levels of glutamate in ALS tissue, both in the brain and in the spinal cord. Malessa and colleagues[47] also found decreased tissue levels of glutamate in cervical and lumbar spinal cord, involving white as well as grey matter. Reduced levels of aspartate have also been reported in the spinal cord.[46,47]

In contrast, several groups have reported that the level of glutamate in cerebrospinal fluid (CSF) is significantly raised in ALS,[48,49] although not all groups have been able to confirm this finding.[50] There are technical difficul-

ties in measuring glutamate levels in biological samples. This is reflected by the finding that different studies have reported a 15-fold variation in the levels of CSF glutamate in normal human controls. The levels of CSF glutamate measured by automated high-performance chromatography (HPLC) are 10-fold lower than when measured by ion exchange chromatography.[51] Other possible difficulties lie in the selection of patients. Levels of glutamate in CSF and plasma may vary with age and sex.[52] Moreover, ALS patients may be heterogeneous with respect to CSF glutamate. One recent study suggested that the increase in CSF glutamate may be present in only 30% of ALS patients, the remainder having levels within the normal range.[49]

Conflicting results have also arisen from different laboratories in relation to fasting plasma glutamate levels in ALS. One group reported that fasting plasma glutamate levels are elevated by approximately 100% in ALS patients compared to controls, and that oral glutamate loading produced abnormally high levels in the ALS group.[53] Other groups, however, have failed to replicate this result and have reported a normal profile of plasma amino acids in ALS.[49,50]

At present, therefore, the data on CSF and plasma glutamate are conflicting and do not provide clear evidence for or against the glutamatergic hypothesis or motor neurone injury.

During normal glutamate neurotransmission, the excitatory signal is terminated by active removal of glutamate from the synaptic cleft by several types of glutamate reuptake transporter proteins. There has been considerable interest in one of the glial glutamate transporter proteins, GLT-1 or excitatory amino acid transporter 2 (EAAT2) in relation to the pathogenesis of ALS (see Chapter 15). In summary, studies of sodium-dependent glutamate uptake, autoradiographic studies of radioligand binding to glutamate transporters, and studies of the expression of EAAT2 protein in ALS and control spinal cord have shown reduced function and expression of the glutamate transport system in ALS.[54–57] This may be a secondary rather than a primary neurochemical change, as suggested by the finding that the expression of the murine equivalent of EAAT2, GLT-1, decreases in SOD1-mutant transgenic mice.[58] Nevertheless, reduced efficiency of glutamate clearance from the vicinity of motor neurones could still contribute to the cascade of motor neurone injury. It is of interest that lower motor neurone groups that are vulnerable to pathology in ALS, such as spinal motor neurones, have a much higher perisomatic expression of the EAAT2 protein than motor neurone groups such as the oculomotor neurones, which are less vulnerable to the disease process.[59]

Experimental studies

Several experimental studies have provided evidence that glutamate receptor agonists may contribute to motor neurone injury. Thus, intrathecal injection of kainic acid in mice preferentially injures motor neurones and induces the formation of abnormally phosphorylated neurofilaments within them, a cytoskeletal abnormality that has been demonstrated in ALS.[60] The CSF of ALS patients has been shown to be toxic to cultured neurones via activation of AMPA–kainate glutamate receptors.[61] However, it has not yet been demonstrated whether such toxicity correlates with the level of CSF glutamate.

Glutamate receptor binding sites

Autoradiographic studies have shown an increased density of binding sites for N-methyl-D-aspartate (NMDA) and non-NMDA receptor ligands in ALS, particularly in the intermediate grey matter of the spinal cord and the deep layers of the motor cortex.[62,63] This may reflect an increased excitatory drive to surviving motor neurones in a failing motor system, but it may also contribute to an escalating cascade of neuronal injury. These neurochemical findings may underlie the abnormal excitability of the motor system in ALS patients in life that is demonstrated by transcranial magnetic stimulation and positron emission tomographic imaging.[64–66]

Glutamate dehydrogenase

Glutamate dehydrogenase (GDH) is an important enzyme in glutamate metabolism and in the detoxification of ammonia (NH_3). Its predominant action is thought to be the synthesis of glutamate from α-ketoglutarate, NADH, and NH_4^+. It is uncertain whether GDH has a specific role in the production of neurotransmitter glutamate, and it does not appear to be specifically co-localized to glutamatergic pathways.

Several research groups have measured leukocyte GDH activity in ALS. Plaitakis and Caroscio[53] found no change in the enzyme activity, whereas Hugon and colleagues[67] reported decreased activity in approximately 60% of ALS patients. Malessa and colleagues[47,68] measured GDH activity in spinal cord homogenates and found that the enzyme activity in the cervical cord was significantly increased in the dorsal horn and lateral and ventral white matter but was normal in the ventral horn and dorsal white matter. In the lumbar spinal cord, less marked changes were observed. Since GDH within the CNS is located primarily in astrocytes, these changes in ALS tissue may be due to reactive gliosis. It is conceivable, however, that increased GDH activity could contribute to neuronal injury by increasing neurotransmitter glutamate release.

N-acetyl-aspartyl glutamate

N-acetyl-aspartyl glutamate (NAAG) is a dipeptide that can be synthesized from glutamate and aspartate. It is converted to N-acetyl aspartate (NAA) and glutamate by the enzyme N-acetyl-α-linked acidic dipeptidase. NAAG has been localized by immunocytochemistry to a number of neuronal systems in the mammalian brain, including motor neurones in the brainstem and spinal cord.[69] The concentration of NAAG is highest in the spinal cord.[70] The physiological role of NAAG is uncertain, but it has been suggested that it may act as a precursor or store of neurotransmitter glutamate. It fulfils several criteria as a neurotransmitter or neuromodulatory compound, and it has an excitatory effect on spinal neurones mediated by NMDA receptors.[71,72] In ALS, the levels of NAAG and its metabolite NAA have been reported to be increased in CSF and decreased in spinal cord tissue.[44] The significance of these findings is uncertain, particularly given the lack of knowledge of the normal physiological functions of NAAG.

Cysteine and sulphur-containing compounds in ALS

An increase in plasma cysteine levels and a decrease in plasma inorganic sulphate have been reported in ALS patients compared to controls.[73] A defect in sulphur oxidation in ALS was reported by the same group.[74] These findings led to the proposal that neuronal degeneration in ALS might result from neurotoxicity of L-cysteine or from defective oxidation of exogenous or endogenous toxic sulphur-containing compounds. However, it is apparent that these changes are not specific for ALS, having also been found in Parkinson's disease and Alzheimer's disease. Moreover, Perry and colleagues[75] have challenged these findings and this group was unable to substan-

tiate any changes in either the plasma content of cysteine or inorganic sulphate, or brain levels of cysteine.

Inhibitory neurotransmitter systems in ALS

An imbalance between excitatory and inhibitory neurotransmission could potentially contribute to neuronal injury. Several aspects of inhibitory neurotransmission have been investigated in ALS patients and disease models. The approaches involved include:

(a) the investigation of receptor or transporter expression;
(b) the measurement of inhibitory amino acids in plasma, CSF, and CNS tissue;
(c) the quantification of the numbers of inhibitory interneurones in CNS tissue
(d) neurophysiological studies.

A loss of γ-aminobutyric acid (GABA)-ergic inhibitory interneurones has been reported in the motor cortex of ALS patients by using immunocytochemical identification of parvalbumin as a marker of these cells.[76] Physiological studies have shown that recurrent inhibition is decreased in ALS patients compared to controls.[77] Neurophysiological studies using transcranial magnetic stimulation of the motor cortex have also indicated abnormalities in local inhibitory circuitry in ALS patients.[78,79]

Glycine

Glycine is an important inhibitory neurotransmitter in the mammalian CNS. The greatest densities of glycine receptors, assessed by [³H]strychnine binding, are present in the spinal cord and brainstem.[80] Strychnine-sensitive glycine receptors are present on spinal cord motor neurones and their activation produces increased chloride conductance, which leads to hyperpolarization. In the spinal cord, glycine is thought to be released by propriospinal fibres and segmental interneurones, including Renshaw cells.[81] As well as its role in inhibitory neurotransmission, glycine acts as a co-agonist with glutamate at a strychnine-insensitive allosteric site on the excitatory NMDA glutamate receptor.[82]

In 1972, a report was published of three brothers who developed spastic paraparesis and lower limb wasting in the context of non-ketotic hyperglycinaemia.[83] Subsequently, de Belleroche and colleagues[84] reported that the level of glycine in CSF was increased in ALS patients compared to controls. Iwasaki and colleagues[85] reported increased concentrations of glycine in the plasma of ALS patients, and Lane and colleagues[86] reported reduced clearance of glycine from plasma at 4 hours after an oral glycine load. These results led to the hypothesis that the altered level of glycine might potentiate activation of spinal cord NMDA receptors with neurotoxic consequences. However, these observations in relation to plasma and CSF glycine levels have not been substantiated by other groups. Thus, the significance of altered glycine tolerance in ALS patients is at present uncertain.

No alterations in the levels of glycine have been reported in brain and spinal cord CNS tissue in ALS patients compared to controls.[46,47,87,88] Binding to strychnine-sensitive glycine receptors is reduced in the ventral horn of the spinal cord in ALS cases compared to controls.[89,90] Because inhibitory glycine receptors are normally present on motor neurones, it is assumed that, at least in part, these observed changes may simply occur as a consequence of motor neurone depletion. Glycine transporter mRNA has been shown to be decreased in the spinal ventral horn of patients with motor neurone disease.[91]

GABA

GABA is a major inhibitory neurotransmitter that acts at two pharmacologically distinct receptor types. In relation to the motor system, GABA is known to mediate presynaptic inhibition of primary afferent fibres and may also be involved in post-synaptic forms of motor neurone inhibition. The $GABA_A$ receptor is a ligand-gated chloride channel[92] and mediates fast inhibition, which relates to frequency modulation. Antagonism of the $GABA_A$ receptors in rat primary motor cortex leads to spontaneous motor activity.[93] $GABA_B$ receptors modulate calcium and potassium conduction[94,95] and are responsible for slow inhibition. Antagonism of $GABA_B$ receptors in the cat spinal cord results in increased amplitude of monosynaptic reflexes.[96] There is emerging evidence for the presence of GABA as well as glycine receptors on lower motor neurones. Thus, GABA and glycine have been shown to co-localize in terminals projecting on to motor neurones in the rat abducens nucleus,[97] and the $GABA_B$ receptor agonist baclofen has been shown to suppress activity of hypoglossal motor neurones in a dose-dependent manner.[98]

No alterations in the levels of GABA have been documented in the CSF[50] or spinal cord tissue[47] from ALS patients. Studies on the levels of GABA in CNS tissue in ALS have been inconclusive. Normal values have been reported in motor cortex,[87] frontal cortex, and cerebellar cortex; reduced levels have been reported in lumbar spinal cord.[46] In many of the 13 CNS regions analysed by Perry and colleagues,[45] GABA levels were found to be low in ALS. However, Malessa and colleagues[47] reported no significant changes in spinal cord GABA levels in ALS. Hayashi and colleagues[89] found no change in GABA-receptor binding in homogenates from the thoracic cord of ALS patients. In a later study, which examined cervical, thoracic, and lumbar spinal cord, GABA receptor binding was reduced in ventral horn tissue from ALS patients.[90] A more recent study examined benzodiazepine receptor binding sites in cortical membranes and found no difference between controls and ALS patients.[99]

Taurine

Taurine is not established as a classical inhibitory neurotransmitter, but it is known to stabilize membrane excitability and exert a depressant effect on neuronal firing, as well as interacting with several neurotransmitter systems.[100] In the spinal cord it is likely that taurine is formed from cysteine by the enzymatic activity of cysteine dioxygenase.[101] The physiological role of taurine is at present poorly understood. Taurine levels appear to remain stable in post mortem tissue.[88] In CNS tissue from ALS patients, taurine levels have been reported as normal[46,102] or increased in cervical spinal cord, cortex, and several subcortical regions.[45,47,87] The implications of these changes are uncertain.

Cholinergic neurotransmission

Choline acetyl transferase (ChAT), the acetyl choline neurotransmitter synthesizing enzyme, is an excellent marker of cholinergic cells, and its activity appears to remain stable in post mortem tissue.[103,104] In the mammalian spinal cord, ChAT has been localized to large and small motor neurones and to synaptic terminals.[105,106] ChAT activity in ALS spinal cord is reduced in the ventral horn and also the dorsal grey matter.[107,108] The majority of the observed decrease is likely to be due to loss of large motor neurones. A reduction of cholinergic receptors has also been demonstrated in the post mortem spinal cord of ALS cases. The density of muscarinic cholinergic receptor binding sites is reduced by approximately

50–60% of normal values in the ventral horn from ALS patients.[90,109,110] However, these studies also reported reductions in muscarinic binding sites in the dorsal horn of ALS patients and the pathological correlate of the cholinergic deficit in this non-motor area of the spinal cord is uncertain. No alterations in nicotinic cholinergic receptors have been reported in ALS.[109]

Monoamine neurotransmitter systems

Serotonin (5-hydroxytryptamine)

Anatomical studies in mammals have shown that the brainstem raphe nuclei, which have a high density of serotonergic neurons, project to many regions of the CNS.[111,112] In the spinal cord the dorsal and ventral horns and the region surrounding the central canal are richly innervated by serotonergic neurons,[113–116] which descend predominantly from the medullary and pontine raphe nuclei via small unmyelinated fibres within ventral and lateral white matter tracts. The ventral horn receives the densest serotonergic fibre input of all the spinal grey matter regions, and serotonin–containing varicosities have been observed to make intimate contact with motor neurone cell bodies and their processes.[113,114] In some of these terminals, substance P or thyrotropin-releasing hormone (TRH), or both, are co-localized with serotonin. Serotonin has been shown to have an excitatory action on motor neurones.[117,118] This can occur either as a direct effect[117,119] or through enhancement of the excitatory effect of glutamate.[120,121] Serotonin can also indirectly influence the activity of motor neurones by activating excitatory or inhibitory interneurones in the vicinity of motor neurones.[122]

Four studies have examined the levels of serotonin and its metabolite 5-hydroxy-indole acetic acid (5-HIAA) in the spinal cord in ALS cases and controls.[123–126] In normal spinal cord there is a rostrocaudal gradient of serotonin concentration, with higher levels in the lumbar region than in the cervical region.[124,126] These studies reported no change in the levels of serotonin itself in ALS spinal cord. Conflicting findings have been reported in relation to 5-HIAA. Different laboratories have reported unchanged,[124] decreased,[123,125] and increased[126] levels of 5-HIAA. The reason for the discrepancies between these different studies is unclear, although 5-HIAA is more susceptible to degradation in post mortem material than is serotonin itself.[127]

The density of serotonergic fibres detected by immunocytochemistry is normal in ALS spinal cord.[128] Serotonin reuptake sites, assessed in autoradiographic studies by [³H]paroxetine binding, are present at very low density in the human cortex. In the spinal cord, [³H]paroxetine binding sites are most abundant in the ventral horn, central grey matter, and the substantia gelatinosa. In ALS, a significant increase was observed in the density of [³H]paroxetine binding in the lateral ventral horn of the cervical spinal cord, but not in other spinal areas.[129]

Serotonin-1a receptor binding sites (assessed by the binding of [³H]8-hydroxy-N,N-dipropyl-2-aminotetraline) have been assessed in the normal human motor system and in ALS. In the motor cortex the highest density of receptors is observed in the superficial laminae, and no changes are observed in ALS. In the spinal cord, the density of serotonin-1a receptors is highest in the substantia gelatinosa, and an increased number of binding sites is found in the cervical compared to the lumbar spinal cord. In ALS, one study reported that the laminar pattern and rostrocaudal gradient of serotonin-1a receptors was preserved, with a significant decrease in sero-

tonin-1a binding sites in the intermediate and ventral grey matter at cervical level.[126] Manaker and colleagues,[110] however, reported an increase in serotonin-1a receptor binding sites in the ventral horn of ALS spinal cord, and a lowered binding affinity of the receptor. A significant reduction in the level of serotonin-1d receptor binding sites has been reported in the ventral and central grey matter regions of the lumbar cord in ALS.[129] No differences were observed at the cervical level. No significant differences were observed in serotonin-1e receptors in the spinal cord or motor cortex between ALS cases and controls.[129]

Serotonin-2 receptors can be assessed by [³H]ketanserin binding. In the normal human motor cortex, there is a trilaminar pattern of binding, with the highest density of binding in the middle laminae. In the spinal cord ligand, binding density is highest in the ventral horn and around the central canal. 'Hot spots' of binding are observed in relation to the cell bodies of lower motor neurones. In the motor and premotor cortex regions of ALS patients, a significant reduction in serotonin-2 receptor binding has been documented compared to controls.[126] In ALS spinal cord, there were no significant differences in the overall levels of serotonin-2 receptor binding sites. However, loss of motor neurones was reflected in a reduction in ventral horn hot spots. The preservation of overall binding density, despite the loss of these foci, may indicate some diffuse increase in serotonin-2 binding sites on surviving neurones in ALS.[126]

Several hypotheses have been put forward to explain the possible functional significance of the alterations in parameters of serotonergic neurotransmission in ALS. It has been suggested that there may be a reduced tonic excitatory drive to motor neurones in ALS owing to reduced release of serotonin in the spinal cord and that this may result in an increase in glutamatergic excitation with neurotoxic consequences. Forrest and colleagues[126] suggested a different hypothesis. Since the serotonergic projections are intact in ALS (spinal serotonin levels are preserved and there is no evidence of pathology in the raphe nuclei), it is likely that the changes observed are physiological adaptations to failing motor function. The increased 5-HIAA:serotonin ratio observed by this group may indicate an increased turnover of serotonin at remaining receptors. The localization of serotonin-2 receptors as foci of high-binding intensity around motor neurone somata and the preservation of overall serotonin-2 receptor binding, despite loss of these hot spots in ALS, is consistent with a role for this receptor in facilitating motor neurone excitability.

The serotonin-1a receptor has been identified as the receptor mediating the inhibitory action of serotonin on motor neurones.[122,130] The loss of serotonin-1a receptors in ALS spinal cord may reflect the loss of inhibitory interneurones in the disease.

The exact anatomical and cellular correlates of the observed decreases in serotonin-2 receptor binding in ALS motor and pre-motor cortex are uncertain. It is of interest, however, that detailed neuropsychological testing in ALS patients has demonstrated impairment in processes involving frontostriatal circuitry. In particular, focal attentional deficits have been shown in up to 25% of ALS patients.[131] It has recently been suggested that a major behavioural consequence of reduced cortical serotonin-2a receptor activity is an impairment of attentional function.[132] It is therefore possible that the observed changes in serotonin-2 receptors in the frontal cortex may begin to provide a neurochemical substrate for the observed subclinical deficits in frontal lobe function in ALS.

Dopamine

The dopaminergic neurotransmitter system has not been extensively studied in the human spinal cord. No alterations have been found in the levels of dopamine or its major metabolites in ALS spinal cord, but the levels measured were close to the limits of detection, using HPLC with electrochemical detection.[124] In addition, no differences in dopamine receptor binding sites have been identified in ALS.[89,110]

Norepinephrine

One report has suggested that sympathetic activity is increased in ALS and that norepinephrine (noradrenaline) levels in the CSF are elevated.[133] The results of studies reporting levels of norepinephrine in ALS spinal cord tissue have been conflicting: Ohsugi and colleagues[124] reported no alteration but Malessa and Leigh[134] reported a significant increase in lumbar and thoracic cord. No differences in β-adrenergic receptor binding sites have been observed in ALS spinal cord.[89,110]

Alterations in neuropeptides

Neuropeptides in the CNS are of potential importance as neurotransmitters and neuromodulators and as trophic factors necessary for the maintenance of neuronal integrity. Electrophysiological actions have been shown for some peptides that are present in nerve terminals synapsing on motor neurones. Thyrotropin-releasing hormone, substance P, neurotensin, and bombesin induce depolarization of ventral roots and motor neurones in vivo and in vitro.[135–138] The action of neurotensin and bombesin is thought to be indirect and mediated via interneurones.

Substance P

In the spinal cord some descending serotonergic fibres contain substance P or thyrotrophin-releasing hormone, or both. The highest density of substance P fibres has been demonstrated in lamina I of the dorsal horn and in relation to autonomic groups of neurones.[139] Substance P has an important role in the transmission of pain impulses and in modulating somatic motor reflexes.[140] There is evidence that substance P exerts a trophic influence on both sensory and motor neurones.[141-143] In ALS spinal cord, a decrease in substance P receptors has been observed in the spinal ventral horn, which probably reflects loss of motor neurones.[144] The levels of substance P have been reported to be decreased in the dorsal and ventral horn of ALS cases.[107,145] Controversy exists regarding the loss or preservation of substance P immunoreactive fibres in the ventral horn of the spinal cord in ALS. Gibson and colleagues[145] and Schoenen and colleagues[139] reported a loss of substance P-positive fibres, whereas Dietl and colleagues[144] reported no change in substance P immunoreactivity.[144]

Thyrotropin-releasing hormone

Thyrotropin-releasing hormone (TRH)-positive fibres in the spinal cord are thought to originate from the medullary raphe nuclei and are concentrated in lamina IX and the intermediolateral nuclei.[146] TRH immunoreactive fibres may also contain serotonin or substance P, or both.[147] TRH has been shown to increase motor neurone excitability, and there are several lines of evidence that it also has neurotrophic effects on this cell group.[141,147,148] Three studies have reported decreased TRH levels in the spinal cord in ALS.[149-151] Two other studies have failed to confirm alterations in TRH levels.[145,152] Manaker[110,153] reported a decrease in TRH receptors in lamina II and lamina IX of the spinal cord in ALS. In lamina IX, the decrease observed is compatible with the presence of post-synaptic TRH receptors

on motor neurones, which decrease as a result of death of the motor neurones. The decrease in TRH receptors in the dorsal horn remains unexplained.

Calcitonin gene-related peptide

Calcitonin gene-related peptide (CGRP) is a 37 amino acid neuropeptide that appears to have a role in sensory autonomic, and motor systems.[154] CGRP immunoreactivity and mRNA have been localized to brainstem and spinal motor neurones. Ultrastructurally, CGRP immunoreactivity localizes to the Golgi complex and adjacent vesicles. In the human spinal cord, lower motor neurones show strong CRGP immunoreactivity.[155,156] CGRP has a well-described action as a motor neurone derived anterograde muscle trophic factor that is released from the neuromuscular junction.[157] A number of actions have been ascribed to this peptide, including contraction of striated muscle, increasing the level of cAMP in muscle and myocytes, and regulation of acetylcholine receptor channel properties at the neuromuscular junction. The ability of motor neurones to synthesize and transport this peptide to the motor end-plates may thus have a direct trophic effect on muscle fibre function and thus in turn on the integrity of the motor neurones. Developmentally, CGRP contributes to the maintenance of high densities of acetylcholine receptors when myotubes develop, as well as effecting neuronal sprouting of motor nerves after injury.[158,159]

Early studies suggested an overall reduction in CGRP-immunoreactive neurones in the spinal cord.[145] However, Kato and colleagues,[160] using cases with relatively short postmortem delays, showed an increase in CGRP immunoreactivity in the ventral horn in ALS. Studies by the same group showed that CGRP-immunoreactivity occurs in spheroids, neurofilament-rich abnormal swellings of motor neurone axons.[161] These authors postulated that defects in axonal transport may result in proximal accumulation of CGRP and loss of the supply of this peptide to the neuromuscular junction. No studies of CGRP gene expression at mRNA level have been reported to date.

Endothelin

Endothelin is the only other major neuropeptide so far identified to be expressed in the motor neurones of human adults.[162] Low densities of endothelin receptors are present in the spinal cord, suggesting that the synthesized peptide exerts its action on receptors located on distant structures.[163] To date this neuropeptide has not been fully investigated in the spinal cord in ALS. The physiological role of endothelin in the motor neurone has not yet been identified and no action on skeletal muscle activity has so far been demonstrated.

Alterations in neurotrophic factors

Neurotrophic factors regulate neuronal proliferation, differentiation, survival, and maintenance. They act on specific neurones by binding to the extracellular domain of a transmembrane protein, thereby inducing an intracellular signal transduction cascade that results in alteration in gene expression. A large number of trophic molecules from different gene families have been shown to promote the survival of motor neurones in vitro or in vivo (Fig. 6.2, Table 6.2). However, few of these polypeptides have specific effects only on motor neurones. Adult motor neurones express trkB receptors, which mediate the effects of brain-derived neurotrophic factor and neurotrophin 4 and neurotrophin 5, and trkC receptors, which mediate the effects of neurotrophin 3.[164,165]

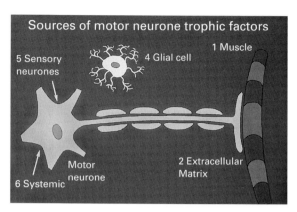

Figure 6.2
Sources of neurotrophic support for motor neurones.

The loss of trophic factor support has been regarded as an attractive hypothesis for the cell death of motor neurones in ALS.[166] Little work has yet been done on the normal levels of expression of neurotrophic factors in the human motor system, and it is not possible at present to exclude the possibility that neurotrophic factor deficiency may contribute to the pathogenesis of ALS. One study screened for non-specific trophic factor deficits in ALS and failed to show any significant abnormalities.[167] The expression of specific neurotrophic factor receptors in the post mortem CNS of ALS patients has not yet been investigated.

Metals and trace elements

Metal ions and trace elements have long been suspected to play a role in the pathogenesis of ALS.[168,169] In particular, the following elements have been suggested to play a role in motor neurone degeneration: lead, mercury, aluminium, selenium, manganese, and iron.

Brain-derived neurotrophic factor
Cardiotrophin-1
Choline acetyl transferase development factor
Ciliary neurotrophic factor
Fibroblast growth factor-1
Fibroblast growth factor-2
Fibroblast growth factor-5
Glial-derived neurotrophic factor
Insulin
Insulin-like growth factor-1
Insulin-like growth factor-2
Interleukin-6
Leukaemia inhibitor factor
Neurite promoting factor
Neurotrophin-3
Neurotrophin-4
Platelet-derived growth factor
Protease nexin-1
S-100
Transforming growth factor-β
Vasoactive intestinal peptide

Table 6.2
Neurotrophic factors and growth factors that have been shown to promote motor neurone survival in vivo or in vitro.

Lead

Lead poisoning may present clinically as a disorder that closely resembles ALS[170-172] and the possibility remains that this metal participates in the pathogenesis of the disease in a proportion of cases. It is interesting that inter-individ-ual variation in susceptibility to lead toxicity has been suggested. Possible mechanisms for the neurotoxicity of lead include:

(a) acceleration of the peroxidation of membrane lipids induced by hydrogen peroxide;[173]
(b) alteration in synaptic activity;
(c) changes in calcium homeostasis;
(d) alteration in cholinergic function; and
(e) alteration in the distribution of glutamate in the brain.[174,175]

Studies measuring the levels of lead in the plasma and CSF of ALS patients have produced conflicting results.[176-178] Examination of spinal cord tissue has shown elevated lead levels in ALS,[179] but it has been argued that this reflects non-specific uptake in disease tissues rather than primary accumulation.[180] Therapeutic trials of lead chelation therapy in ALS have not shown any definite benefit.[170-172]

Mercury

There have been several reports of ALS-like syndromes in people exposed to mercury.[181-183] Rat motor neurones have been shown to take up mercury selectively.[184] The chemical steps in mercury absorption and detoxification are not fully understood. The metabolic handling of mercury, however, involves the action of the enzyme thiol methyl transferase, the activity of which has been reported to be increased in ALS.[185] Potential mechanisms of mercury toxicity include:

(a) depletion of brain levels of the anti-oxidant ascorbate;[186]
(b) reduced activity of NADPH-specific glutathione reductase;[187]
(c) stimulation of superoxide radical production; and
(d) promotion of iron-catalysed lipid peroxidation.[188]

Muscle levels of mercury have been reported to be normal in ALS, but hair and nail levels have been reported to be increased in a Japanese population with ALS, including both classical cases and cases from the Kii peninsula.[189] Data on the measurement of tissue levels of mercury in ALS are scarce. One study showed an elevated mercury : selenium ratio in the brain but not in the spinal cord.[190] No treatment trials looking specifically at elimination of mercury overload in ALS have been reported to date.

Aluminium

The possibility that aluminium may be involved in motor system degenerative disorders has come from several sources. Firstly, one of the major hypotheses put forward to explain the high incidence of ALS in the western Pacific has been that an abnormality of mineral homoeostasis (owing to environmental deficiencies of calcium and magnesium and high levels of aluminium and manganese) may result in the deposition of toxic metal ions, including aluminium, within motor neurones.[191–193] Secondly, aluminium has been shown to be toxic to motor neurones in animal models, where it leads to an abnormality of axonal transport and the development of intracellular inclusions composed of abnormal neurofilament protein.[194] An analogy has been drawn between ALS and the chronic progressive myelopathy and motor neurone degeneration seen in the New Zealand white rabbit following intracisternal injection of low dose aluminium chloride.[195]

Increased aluminium levels have been reported in post mortem hippocampal tissue of ALS patients.[193] However, in a recent large study of the spinal cord of 31 ALS cases and 17 controls, where aluminium was measured using a graphite furnace atomic absorption analysis, no significant elevation was found in the ALS cases.[196] These authors concluded that there was no evidence to support the hypothesis of a primary role for aluminium in the pathogenesis of ALS.

Selenium

Selenium is a major trace element and a component of an important antioxidant enzyme, glutathione peroxidase. Interest in selenium in ALS arose from a cluster of cases in a region of South Dakota, USA, where the selenium content of the soil is high.[197] No definite evidence of toxic accumulation of selenium in these cases was confirmed. Mitchell and colleagues[168] demonstrated elevated levels of selenium in the spinal cord, liver, and bone of ALS patients compared to controls. More recently, in a study using instrumental neutron activation analysis, the levels of selenium in lumbar spinal cord were found to be significantly elevated in 38 ALS patients compared to controls.[198] This study also showed an increase in the activity of the selenoprotein enzyme glutathione peroxidase in ALS spinal cord. It was postulated that the increase in selenium might simply be due to the increased activity of glutathione peroxidase, an enzyme whose activity is known to be inducible in the presence of oxidative stress.

Manganese

Interest in manganese in relation to ALS arose from a report of an ALS-like syndrome in a worker exposed to this metal. The element is also abundant in Guam and in the Kii peninsula of Japan (both foci of high incidence of ALS). A motor system disorder in the aboriginal population of Groote Eyelandt has been ascribed to the mining of manganese in this area.[199] Studies using neutron activation analysis to measure manganese in the spinal cord of the cases in Guam[199] and sporadic cases of motor neurone disease[168] have shown elevated levels compared to controls.

Iron

Iron is the most abundant metal in the human body. It exists mainly in the ferric (III) oxidation state and is tightly bound into transport or storage proteins such as transferrin or ferritin. Non-protein-bound iron, particularly when reduced to the ferrous (II) state, has the capacity to catalyse the generation of highly damaging hydroxyl radicals by the Haber–Weiss reaction. Ferrous iron is present in very low concentrations except in the presence of iron overload, when iron is decompartmentalized (e.g. by rupture of cell or organelle membranes), or when iron is displaced by other metal ions. Kurlander and Patten[200] reported that the iron content of anterior horn cell tissue from seven patients with ALS was higher than the content in controls. However, Mitchell and colleagues[168] reported normal iron levels in spinal cord and liver in ALS patients. A larger and more recent study used neutron activation analysis to measure the iron content of lumbar spinal cord samples of 38 ALS patients compared to controls. The mean iron level in the spinal cord of ALS patients was 39% higher than in controls, with 25% of ALS patients having iron levels greater than 2 standard deviations above the mean control level.[198,201] The levels of iron in the lumbar spinal cord in the ALS patients did not correlate with the degree of lower limb weakness at death or with motor neurone counts from adjacent spinal segments, suggesting that the findings did not simply reflect depletion of motor neurones. The cellular distribution and oxidation state of the excess iron in ALS spinal cord are at present uncertain, and the question as to whether this neurochemical alteration may contribute to oxidative stress is also unanswered.

Oxidative stress

Oxidative stress is one of the major potential causes of age-related deterioration in neuronal function (*Table 6.3*) and cumulative damage

Fibroblasts from patients with sporadic ALS show increased sensitivity to oxidative stress
Increased levels of protein carbonyl in spinal cord and frontal cortex
Increased 3-nitrotyrosine in spinal cord
Increased 8-hydroxy 2-dioxyguanosine in motor cortex and spinal cord
Increased level of selenium and increased activity of selenoprotein enzyme glutathionine peroxidase in spinal cord
Increased SOD1 mRNA in surviving motor neurones
Increased glial expression of SOD1, MnSOD and catalase in spinal cord
Increased expression of metallothionein in spinal cord
MnSOD, manganese superoxide dismutase; SOD1, copper–zinc superoxide dismutase.

Table 6.3
Neurochemical evidence that oxidative stress may contribute to motor neurone injury in sporadic ALS.

by free radicals may contribute to the later-life onset and progressive nature of neurodegenerative diseases such as ALS. Genetically determined abnormalities in the cellular free radical defence system caused by mutations in the SOD1 enzyme underlie 20% of all cases of familial ALS or approximately 2% of ALS as a whole.[202,203] The primary role of SOD1 is to dismutate superoxide radicals to hydrogen peroxide, which is then further metabolized by the antioxidant enzymes glutathione peroxidase or catalase. Subsidiary activities of SOD1 include peroxidase activity resulting in the generation of hydroxyl radicals from hydrogen peroxide,[204] the production of nitronium species from peroxynitrite, which can nitrate the tyrosine residues of target proteins,[205] and the protection of the enzyme calcineurin from inactivation.[206] The discovery of SOD1 mutations in some cases of familial ALS has generated great interest in oxidative stress as a potential mechanism of motor neurone injury. Because of the close clinical and pathological similarity between the familial and sporadic forms of ALS, there has also been interest in the possibility that oxidative stress may be operating as a mechanism of cellular injury in sporadic ALS. Oxidative stress as a potential pathophysiological mechanism in ALS is covered in detail in Chapter 11, and only aspects of neurochemical relevance are mentioned here.

Because only a small number of cases of human ALS with defined SOD1 mutations have undergone detailed post mortem neurochemical investigation, relatively little data are available on the neurochemical pathological changes in this subgroup of patients. Ferrante and colleagues[207] found increased immunostaining for hemoxygenase-1, malondialdehyde modified protein and 8-hydroxy 2'-dioxyguanosine in the spinal cord in five cases of SOD1-linked familial ALS. It has been shown in mutant SOD1 transgenic mice that indices of lipid peroxidation are increased in spinal cord and cerebral cortex and that markers of nitrosylation of proteins by peroxynitrite derivatives are increased in the spinal cord of affected mice.[208]

In relation to sporadic ALS, several lines of evidence have emerged that suggest that oxidative stress may contribute to motor neurone injury. Fibroblasts from patients with sporadic ALS have been shown to exhibit heightened sensitivity to oxidative stress.[209]

Biochemical indices of oxidative damage

Studies from two different laboratories have shown that protein carbonyls, formed by the oxidative modification of certain amino acid residues in proteins, are present at an increased level in the spinal cord[210] and frontal cortex[211] of sporadic ALS patients compared to normal controls and also compared to disease controls with a similar agonal status to the ALS group. Beal and colleagues[212] reported an increased concentration of 3-nitrotyrosine, a marker of oxidative damage mediated by peroxynitrite, in the spinal cord of ALS patients. In addition, increased 3-nitrotyrosine immunoreactivity was observed in residual motor neurones from cases of both sporadic and familial ALS. Ferrante and colleagues[207] reported increased protein carbonyl and nuclear 8-hydroxy 2'-dioxyguanosine levels in the motor cortex of sporadic ALS cases, as well as an increase in indices of oxidative damage to protein and DNA in the spinal cord.

Biochemical indices that may indicate a compensatory response to oxidative stress

The content of selenium and the activity of the selenium-containing enzyme glutathione peroxidase are increased in the spinal cord of ALS cases compared to controls.[198] However, a decrease was reported in the activity of this free radical scavenging enzyme in the cortex of ALS patients.[213] SOD1 mRNA has been shown to be increased in individual motor neurones from sporadic ALS cases.[214] Immunohistochemical studies have shown increased glial expression of SOD1, manganese SOD (SOD2), and catalase in the spinal cord of ALS cases, especially in the vicinity of the corticospinal tracts or in the neuropil of the ventral horn, or both.[4] Increased expression of metallothionein has been demonstrated in ALS spinal cord.[215] Metallothioneins are metal binding proteins with free radical scavenging capabilities; they are also involved in the detoxification and storage of metals.

Summary and conclusions

Insights are beginning to emerge in relation to the normal neurochemistry of motor neurones, which may help explain the vulnerability of this cell group to neurodegeneration. Future work aimed at further elucidating the abnormal proteins associated with ubiquitinated inclusions in ALS will yield important insights into the biochemical processes associated with cell death. Neurofilament proteins represent an important target for injury in the cell death process in both sporadic and familial ALS.

There is a large body of circumstantial evidence that an imbalance between the excitatory or glutamatergic neurotransmission and inhibitory neurotransmission may contribute to motor neurone injury in ALS. Even if this imbalance is secondary to another primary pathogenetic process, it still represents an important target for therapeutic intervention in the cell death cascade. Less is known about other motor system neurotransmitters, but agents such as TRH and serotonin may clearly have an important modulatory effect on the excitability of motor neurons.

Heavy metal toxicity can result in a clinical disease state resembling ALS in occasional patients, but there is no firm evidence that such toxicity represents a common pathogenetic mechanism in ALS. Some of the changes in levels of metals in the spinal cord of ALS cases are of interest in relation to oxidative stress and associated compensatory mechanisms.

Compelling evidence is emerging that oxidative stress may be a contributory pathogenetic mechanism in both SOD1-related ALS and sporadic ALS. The discovery of SOD1 mutations in familial ALS has allowed the development of cellular and animal models of the human disease. These models can be expected, in coming years, to yield important insights into the sequential molecular events underlying motor neurone death, as well as the development of more effective strategies for therapeutic intervention.

Acknowledgements

Pamela J Shaw is supported by the Wellcome Trust as a Senior Fellow in Clinical Science.

References

1. Williams TL, Day NC, Ince PG et al. Calcium-permeable alpha-amino-3-hydroxy-5-methyl-4-isoxazole propionic acid receptors: a molecular determinant of selective vulnerability in amyotrophic lateral sclerosis. *Ann Neurol* 1997; **42**: 200–207.
2. Ince PG, Stout N, Shaw PJ et al. Parvalbumin and calbindin D-28k in the human motor system and in motor neuron disease. *Neuropath Appl Neurobiol* 1993; **19**: 291–299.
3. Alexianu ME, Ho BK, Mohammed AH et al. The role of calcium-binding proteins in selective motoneurone vulnerability in amyotrophic lateral sclerosis. *Ann Neurol* 1994; **36**: 846–858.

4. Shaw PJ, Chinnery RM, Thageson H et al. Immunocytochemical study of the distribution of free radical scavenging enzymes Cu/Zn superoxide dismutase (SOD1), Mn superoxide dismutase (SOD2) and catalase in the normal human spinal cord and in motor neuron disease. *J Neurol Sci* 1997; **147**: 115–125.

5. Pardo CA, Xu Z, Borchelt DR et al. Superoxide dismutase is an abundant component in cell bodies, dendrites and axons of motor neurons and in a subset of other neurons. *Proc Natl Acad Sci USA* 1995; **92**: 954–958.

6. Bond U, Schlesinger MJ. Ubiquitin is a heat shock protein in chicken embryo fibroblasts. *Mol Cell Biol* 1985; **5**: 949–956.

7. Hochstrasser M. Ubiquitin, proteasomes, and the regulation of intracellular protein degradation. *Curr Opin Cell Biol* 1995; **7**: 215–223.

8. Leigh PN, Garofalo O. The molecular pathology of motor neuron disease. In: Leigh PN, Swash M, eds. *Motor Neuron Disease. Biology and Management.* London: Springer-Verlag, 1995, 139–161.

9. Leigh PN, Anderton BH, Dodson A et al. Ubiquitin deposits in anterior horn cells in motor neuron disease. *Neurosci Lett* 1988; **93**: 197–203.

10. Lowe J, Lennox G, Jefferson D. A filamentous inclusion body within anterior horn neurons in motor neuron disease defined by immunocytochemical localisation of ubiquitin. *Neurosci Lett* 1988; **94**: 203–210.

11. Ince PG, Tomkins J, Salde JY et al. Amyotrophic lateral sclerosis associated with genetic abnormalities in Cu/Zn superoxide dismutase: molecular pathology of five new cases and comparison with previous reports. *J Neuropathol Exp Neurol* 1998; **57**: 895–904.

12. Murayama S, Ookawa Y, Mori H et al. Immunocytochemical and ultrastructural study of Lewy-body-like inclusions in familial amyotrophic lateral sclerosis. *Acta Neuropathol* 1989; **78**: 143–152.

13. Rouleau GA, Clark AW, Rooke K et al. SOD1 mutation is associated with accumulation of neurofilaments in amyotrophic lateral sclerosis. *Ann Neurol* 1996; **39**: 128–131.

14. Nixon RA, Shea TB. Dynamics of neuronal intermediate filaments: a developmental perspective. *Cell Motil Cytoskeleton* 1992; **22**: 81–91.

15. Lupas A. Coiled coils: new structures and new functions. *Trends Biol Sci* 1996; **21**: 375–382.

16. Heins S, Wong PC, Muller S et al. The rod domain of NF-L determines neurofilament architecture, whereas the end domains specify filament assembly and network formation. *J Cell Biol* 1993; **123**: 1517–1533.

17. Munoz DG, Green C, Perl D, Selkoe DJ. Accumulation of phosphorylated neurofilaments in anterior horn motoneurons of ALS patients. *J Neuropathol Exp Neurol* 1988; **47**: 9–18.

18. Manetto V, Sternberger NH, Perry G et al. Phosphorylation of neurofilaments is altered in amyotrophic lateral sclerosis. *J Neuropathol Exp Neurol* 1988; **47**: 642–653.

19. Sobue G, Hashizume Y, Yasuda T. Phosphorylated high molecular weight neurofilament protein in lower motor neurons in ALS and other neurodegenerative diseases involving ventral horn cells. *Acta Neuropathol* 1990; **79**: 402–408.

20. Leigh PN, Dodson A, Swash M et al. Cytoskeletal abnormalities in motor neuron disease: an immunocytochemical study. *Brain* 1989; **112**: 521–535.

21. Delisle MB, Carpenter S. Neurofibrillary axonal swellings and ALS. *J Neurol Sci* 1984; **63**: 241–252.

22. Figlewicz DA, Krizus A, Martinoli MG et al. Variants of the heavy neurofilament subunit are associated with the development of amyotrophic lateral sclerosis. *Hum Mol Genet* 1994; **3**: 1757–1761.

23. Tomkins J, Usher P, Slade JY et al. Novel 84bp insertion in the KSP repeat region of the heavy neurofilament subunit in amyotrophic lateral sclerosis. *NeuroReport* 1998; **9**: 3967–3970.

24. Xu Z, Cork L, Griffin J, Cleveland D. Increased expression of neurofilament subunit NF-L produces morphological alterations that resemble the pathology of human motor neuron disease. *Cell* 1993; **73**: 23–33.

25. Cote F, Collard JF, Julien JP. Progressive neuropathy in transgenic mice expressing the human neurofilament heavy gene: a mouse

model of amyotrophic lateral sclerosis. *Cell* 1993; **73**: 35–46.

26. Lee MK, Marszalek JR, Cleveland DW. A mutant neurofilament subunit causes massive, selective motor neuron death: implications for the pathogenesis of human motor neuron disease. *Neuron* 1994; **13**: 975–988.

27. Collard JF, Cote F, Julien JP. Defective axonal transport in a transgenic mouse model of amyotrophic lateral sclerosis. *Nature* 1995; **375**: 12–13.

28. Cookson MR, Thatcher NM, Ince PG, Shaw PJ. Selective loss of neurofilament proteins after exposure of differentiated IMR-32 neuroblastoma cells to oxidative stress. *Brain Res* 1996; **738**: 162–166.

29. Cookson MR, Tomkins J, Manning P et al. Cu/Zn superoxide dismutase mutations cause perikaryal accumulation of neurofilament proteins in a cell culture model of amyotrophic lateral sclerosis. *Proceedings of the 8th International Symposium on ALS/MND*, Glasgow 1997.

30. Beckman JS, Carson M, Smith CD, Koppenol WH. ALS, SOD and peroxynitrite. *Nature* 1993; **364**: 584.

31. Crowe JP, Ye YZ, Strong M et al. Superoxide dismutase catalyzes nitration of tyrosines by peroxynitrite in the rod and head domains of neurofilament-L. *J Neurochem* 1997; **69**: 1945–1953.

32. Young AB, Penney JB, Dauth GW et al. Glutamate or aspartate as a possible neurotransmitter of cerebral corticofugal fibres in the monkey. *Neurol* 1983; **33**: 1513–1516.

33. Young AB, Penney JB. Pharmacological aspects of motor dysfunction. In: Asbury AK, McKham GM, McDonald WI, eds. *Diseases of the Nervous System, Clinical Neurobiology*. Philadelphia: WB Saunders, 1992, 343–352.

34. Burke RE. Spinal cord: ventral horn. In: Shepherd GM, ed. *The Synaptic Organisation of the Brain*. New York: Oxford University Press, 1990, 88–132.

35. Molander C, Xu Q, Rivero-Mellian C, Grant G. Cytoarchitectonic organization of the spinal cord in the rat. II. The cervical and thoracic cord. *J Comp Neurol* 1989; **289**: 375–385.

36. O'Brien RJ, Fischbach GD. Characterization of excitatory amino acid receptors expressed by chick motor neurone in vitro. *J Neurosci* 1986; **6**: 3290–3296.

37. Hollmann M, Heinemann S. Cloned glutamate receptors. *Annu Rev Neurosci* 1994; **17**: 31–108.

38. Fonnum F. Glutamate: a neurotransmitter in mammalian brain. *J Neurochem* 1984; **42**: 1–11.

39. Plaitakis A. Glutamate dysfunction and selective motor neuron degeneration in ALS: an hypothesis. *Ann Neurol* 1990; **28**: 3–8.

40. Shaw PJ, Ince PG. Glutamate, excitotoxicity and amyotrophic lateral sclerosis. *J Neurol* 1997; **244 (suppl 2)**: S3–S14.

41. Ince PG, Egget C, Shaw PJ. Role of excitotoxicity in neurological disease. *Rev Contemp Pharmacol* 1997; **8**: 195–212.

42. Rothstein JD, Excitotoxic mechanisms in the pathogenesis of amyotrophic lateral sclerosis. *Adv Neurol* 1995; **68**: 7–20.

43. Zeman S, Lloyd C, Medrum B, Leigh PN. Excitatory amino acids, free radicals and the pathogenesis of motor neuron disease. *Neuropathol Appl Neurobiol* 1994; **20**: 219–231.

44. Tsai G, Stauch-Slusher B, Sim L et al. Reductions in acidic amino acids and N-acetyl-aspartyl glutamate (NAAG) in amyotrophic lateral sclerosis CNS. *Brain Res* 1991; **655**: 195–201.

45. Perry TL, Hansen S, Jones K. Brain glutamate deficiency in amyotrophic lateral sclerosis. *Neurol* 1987; **37**: 1845–1848.

46. Plaitakis A, Constantakakis E, Smith J. The neuroexcitotoxic amino acids glutamate and aspartate are altered in the spinal cord and brain in amyotrophic lateral sclerosis. *Ann Neurol* 1988; **24**: 446–449.

47. Malessa S, Leigh PN, Bertel O et al. Amyotrophic lateral sclerosis: glutamate dehydrogenase and transmitter amino acids in the spinal cord. *J Neurol Neurosurg Psychiatry* 1991; **54**: 984–988.

48. Rothstein JD, Tsai G, Kuncl RW. Abnormal excitatory amino acid metabolism in amyotrophic lateral sclerosis. *Ann Neurol* 1990; **28**: 18–25.

49. Shaw PJ, Forrest V, Ince PG et al. CSF and

plasma amino acid levels in motor neuron disease: elevation of CSF glutamate in a subset of patients. *Neurodegeneration* 1995; **4**: 209–216.

50. Perry TL, Krieger C, Hansen S, Eisen A. Amyotrophic lateral sclerosis: amino acid levels in plasma and cerebrospinal fluid. *Ann Neurol* 1990; **28**: 12–17.

51. Rothstein JD, Tsai G, Kuncl RW et al. Abnormal excitatory amino acid metabolism in amyotrophic lateral sclerosis. *Ann Neurol* 1991; **30**: 224–225.

52. Ferraro TN, Hare TA. Free and conjugated amino acids in human CSF: influence of age and sex. *Brain Res* 1985; **338**: 53–60.

53. Plaitakis A, Caroscio JT. Abnormal glutamate metabolism in amyotrophic lateral sclerosis. *Ann Neurol* 1987; **22**: 575–579.

54. Rothstein JD, Chang RR, Kuncl RW. Amyotrophic lateral sclerosis: abnormal glutamate transport and models of chronic glutamate toxicity. In: Simon RP, ed. *Excitatory Amino Acids*. New York: Thieme Medical Publishers, 1992, 223–228.

55. Shaw PJ, Chinnery RM, Ince PG. [3H]D-Aspartate binding sites in the normal human spinal cord and changes in motor neuron disease: a quantitative autoradiographic study. *Brain Res* 1994; **655**: 195–201.

56. Bristol LA, Rothstein JD. Glutamate transporter gene expression in amyotrophic lateral sclerosis motor cortex. *Ann Neurol* 1996; **39**: 676–679.

57. Fray AE, Banner SJ, Ince PG et al. The expression of the glial glutamate transporter EAAT2 in motor neurone disease: an immunohistochemical study. *Eur J Neurosci* 1998; **10**: 2481–2489.

58. Bruijn LI, Becher MW, Lee MK et al. ALS-linked SOD1 mutant G85R mediates damage to astrocytes and promotes rapidly progressive disease with SOD1 containing inclusions. *Neuron* 1997; **18**: 327–338.

59. Milton ID, Banner SJ, Ince PG et al. The immunohistochemical expression of the glial glutamate transporter EAAT2 in the human CNS. *Mol Brain Res* 1997; **52**: 17–31.

60. Hugon J, Vallat JM. Abnormal distribution of phosphorylated neurofilaments in neuronal degeneration induced by kainic acid. *Neurosci Lett* 1990; **119**: 45–48.

61. Couratier P, Hugon J, Sindou P et al. Cell culture evidence for neurone degeneration in amyotrophic lateral sclerosis being linked to AMPA/kainate receptors. *Lancet* 1993; **341**: 265–268.

62. Shaw PJ, Ince PG, Matthews JNS et al. N-methyl-D-aspartate receptors in the spinal cord and motor cortex in motor neuron disease: a quantitative autodiographic study using [³H]MK-801. *Brain Res* 1994; **637**: 297–302.

63. Shaw PJ, Chinnery RM, Ince PG. Non-NMDA receptors in motor neuron disease (MND): a quantitative autoradiographic study in spinal cord and motor cortex using [3H]CNQX and [3H]kainate. *Brain Res* 1994; **655**: 186–194.

64. Eisen A, Pant B, Stewart H. Cortical excitability in amyotrophic lateral sclerosis: a clue to pathogenesis. *Can J Neurol Sci* 1993; **20**: 11–16.

65. Mills KR. Motor neurone disease: studies of the corticospinal excitation of single motoneurons by magnetic brain stimulation. *Brain* 1995; **118**: 971–982.

66. Kew JJM, Leigh PN, Playford ED et al. Cortical function in amyotrophic lateral sclerosis: a positron emission tomography study. *Brain* 1993; **116**: 644–680.

67. Hugon J, Tabaraud F, Rigaud M et al. Glutamate dehydrogenase and aspartate aminotransferase in leukocytes of patients with motor neuron disease. *Neurology* 1989; **39**: 956–958.

68. Malessa S, Leigh PN, Hornykiewicz O. Glutamate dehydrogenase in amyotrophic lateral sclerosis. *Lancet* 1988; **ii**: 681–682.

69. Anderson KJ, Managhan DT, Cangro CB et al. Localization of N-acetylaspartylglutamate-like immunoreactivity in selected areas of the rat brain. *Neurosci Lett* 1986; **72**: 14–20.

70. Koller KJ, Coyle JT. Ontogenesis of N-acetyl-aspartate and N-acetyl-aspartyl-glutamate in rat brain. *Brain Res* 1984; **317**: 137–140.

71. Zollinger M. Amsler U, Do KQ et al. Release of N-acetylaspartylglutamate on depolarization of rat brain slices. *J Neurochem* 1988; **51**: 1919–1923.

72. Westbrook GL, Mayer ML, Namoodiri MAA, Neale JH. High concentrations of N-

acetylaspartyl-glutamate (NAAG) selectively activate NMDA receptors on mouse spinal cord neurons in cell culture. *J Neurosci* 1986; **6**: 3385–3392.

73. Heathfield MT, Fearn S, Steventon GB et al. Plasma cysteine and sulfate levels in patients with motor neuron, Parkinson's and Alzheimer's disease. *Neurosci Lett* 1990; **110**: 216–220.

74. Steventon G, Williams AC, Waring PH et al. Xenobiotic metabolism in motor neuron disease. *Lancet* 1988; **ii**: 644–647.

75. Perry TL, Krieger C, Hansen S, Tabatabaei A. Amyotrophic lateral sclerosis: fasting plasma levels of cysteine and inorganic sulfate are normal as are brain contents of cysteine. *Ann Neurol* 1991; **41**: 487–490.

76. Nihei K, McKee AC, Kowall NW. Patterns of neuronal degeneration in the motor cortex of amyotrophic lateral sclerosis patients. *Acta Neuropathol* 1993; **86**: 55–64.

77. Raynor EM, Shefner JM. Recurrent inhibition is decreased in patients with amyotrophic lateral sclerosis. *Neurology* 1994; **44**: 2148–2153.

78. Enterzari-Taher M, Eisen A, Stewart H, Nakajima M. Abnormalities of cortical inhibitory neurons in amyotrophic lateral sclerosis. *Muscle Nerve* 1997; **20**: 65–71.

79. Ziemann U, Winter M, Reimers CD et al. Impaired motor cortex inhibition in patients with amyotrophic lateral sclerosis: evidence from paired transcranial magnetic stimulation. *Neurology* 1997; **49**: 1292–1297.

80. Zarbin MA, Wamsley JK, Kuhar MJ. Glycine receptor: light microscopic autoradiographic localization with (3H)strychnine. *J Neurosci* 1981; **1**: 532–547.

81. Geyer SW, Gudden W, Betz H et al. Co-localization of choline acetyltransferase and post-synaptic glycine receptors in motor neurons of rat spinal cord demonstrated by immuno-cytochemistry. *Neurosci Lett* 1987; **82**: 11–15.

82. Bonhaus DW, Burge BC, McNamara JP. Biochemical evidence that glycine allosterically regulates an NMDA receptor-coupled ion channel. *Eur J Pharmacol* 1987; **142**: 489–490.

83. Bank WJ, Morrow G. A familial spinal cord disorder with hyperglycinemia. *Arch Neurol* 1972; **27**: 136–144.

84. de Belleroche J, Recordati A, Rose FC. Elevated levels of amino acids in the CSF of motor neuron disease patients. *Neurochem Pathol* 1984; **2**: 1–6.

85. Iwasaki Y, Ikeda K, Shiojima T, Kinoshita M. Increased plasma concentrations of aspartate, glutamate and glycine in Parkinson's disease. *Neurosci Lett* 1992; **145**: 175–177.

86. Lane RJM, Bandopadhyay R, de Belleroche J. Abnormal glycine metabolism in motor neurone disease: studies on plasma and cerebrospinal fluid. *J R Soc Med* 1993; **86**: 501–505.

87. Yoshino Y, Koike H, Akai K. Free amino acids in motor cortex of amyotrophic lateral sclerosis. *Experientia* 1979; **35**: 219–220.

88. Perry TL, Hansen S, Grandham SS. Postmortem changes of amino compounds in human and rat brain. *J Neurochem* 1981; **36**: 406–412.

89. Hayashi H, Suga M, Satake M, Tsubaki T. Reduced glycine receptor in the spinal cord in amyotrophic lateral sclerosis. *Ann Neurol* 1981; **9**: 292–294.

90. Whitehouse PJ, Wamsley JK, Zarbin MA et al. Amyotrophic lateral sclerosis: alterations in neurotransmitter receptors. *Ann Neurol* 1983; **14**: 8–16.

91. Virgo L, de Belleroche J. Induction of the immediate early gene c-jun in human spinal cord in amyotrophic lateral sclerosis with concomitant loss of NMDA receptor NF-1 and glycine transporter mRNA. *Brain Res* 1995; **676**: 196–204.

92. Enna SJ, Maggi A. Biochemical pharmacology of GABAergic agonists. *Life Sci* 1979; **24**: 1727–1728.

93. Castro-Alamancos MA, Borrell J. Motor activity induced by disinhibition of the primary cortex of the rat is blocked by a non-NMDA glutamate receptor antagonist. *Neurosci Lett* 1993; **150**: 183–186.

94. Bowery NG, Hill DR, Hudson AL et al. Baclofen decreases neurotransmitter release in the mammalian CNS by an action at a novel GABA receptor. *Nature* 1980; **283**: 92–94.

95. Gahwiler BH, Brown DA. GABA$_B$ receptor activated K$^+$ current in voltage clamped CA3

pyramidal cells in hippocampal cultures. *Proc Natl Acad Sci USA* 1985; **82**: 1558–1562.

96. Curtis DR, Lacey G. GABA_B receptor-mediated spinal inhibition. *Neuroreport* 1994; **5**: 540–542.

97. Lahjouji F, Barbe A, Chazal G, Bras H. Evidence for colocalization of GABA and glycine in afferents to retrogradely labelled rat abducens motoneurones. *Neurosci Lett* 1996; **206**: 161–164.

98. Okabe S, Woch G, Kubin L. Role of GABA_B receptors in the control of hypoglossal motoneurons in vivo. *Neuroreport* 1994; **5**: 2573–2576.

99. Gredal O, Pakkenberg B, Nielsen M. Muscarinic, N-methyl-D-aspartate (NMDA) and benzodiazepine receptor binding sites in cortical membranes from amyotrophic lateral sclerosis patients. *J Neurol Sci* 1996; **143**: 121–125.

100. Oja SS, Kontro P. Taurine. In: Lajtha A, ed. *Handbook of Neurochemistry* vol 3. New York: Plenum Press, 1983, 501–533.

101. Yamaguchi K, Hosokawa Y. Cysteine dioxygenase. *Methods Enzymol* 1987; **143**: 395–403.

102. Robinson N. Chemical changes in the spinal cord in Friedreich's ataxia and motor neuron disease. *J Neurol Neurosurg Psychiatry* 1968; **31**: 330–333.

103. Rossier J. Choline acetyltransferase: a review with special reference to its cellular and subcellular localisation. *Int Rev Neurobiol* 1977; **20**: 284–337.

104. Spokes EGS, Koch DJ. Post-mortem stability of dopamine, glutamate decarboxylase and choline acetyltransferase in the mouse brain under conditions simulating the handling of human autopsy material. *J Neurochem* 1978; **31**: 381–387.

105. Houser CR, Crawford GD, Barber RP et al. Organization and morphological characteristics of cholinergic neurons: an immunocytochemical study with a monoclonal antibody to choline acetyltransferase. *Brain Res* 1983; **266**: 97–119.

106. Kimura H, McGeer PL, Peng JH, McGeer EG. The cholinergic system studied by choline acetyltransferase immunocytochemistry in the cat. *J Comp Neurol* 1981; **200**: 151–201.

107. Gillberg PG, Aquilonius SM, Eckern SA et al. Choline acetyltransferase and substance P-like immunoreactivity in the human spinal cord: changes in amyotrophic lateral sclerosis. *Brain Res* 1982; **250**: 394–397.

108. Nagata Y, Okuya M, Watanabe R, Honda M. Regional distribution of cholinergic neurons in human spinal cord transections in patients with and without motor neuron disease. *Brain Res* 1982; **244**: 223–229.

109. Gillberg PG, Aquilonius SM. Cholinergic, opiod and glycine receptor binding sites localized in human spinal cord by in vitro autoradiography: changes in amyotrophic lateral sclerosis. *Acta Neurol Scand* 1985; **72**: 299–306.

110. Manakar S, Calne SB, Winokur A. Alterations in receptors for thyrotropin-releasing hormone, serotonin, and acetylcholine in amyotrophic lateral sclerosis. *Neurology* 1988; **38**: 1464–1474.

111. Bradley PB, Engel G, Feniuk W et al. Proposals for the classification and nomenclature of functional receptors for 5-hydroxytryptamine. *Neuropharmacology* 1986; **25**: 563–576.

112. Fuxe K. Evidence for the existence of monoamine neurons in the central nervous system. IV. The distribution of monoamine terminals in the central nervous system. *Acta Physiol* 1965; **64 (suppl 247)**: 37–85.

113. Bowker RM, Westlund KM, Sullivan MC, Coulter JD. Organization of descending serotonergic projections to the spinal cord. *Prog Brain Res* 1982; **57**: 239–265.

114. Dahlstrom A, Fuxe K. Evidence for the existence of monoamine containing neurons in the central nervous system. I. Demonstration of monoamines in the cell bodies of brain stem neurons. *Acta Physiol Scand* 1964; **62 (suppl 232)**: 1–55.

115. Kojima M, Takeuchi T, Goto M, Sano Y. Immunohistochemical study on the localisation of serotonin fibres and terminals in the spinal cord of the monkey (*Macaca fuscata*). *Cell Tissue Res* 1983; **229**: 23–36.

116. Segu L, Calas A. The topographical distribution of serotonergic terminals in the spinal cord of the cat: quantitative radioautographic studies. *Brain Res* 1978; **153**: 449–464.

117. Bedard PJ, Tremblay LE, Barbeau H et al.

Action of 5-hydroxytryptamine, substance P, thyrotropin-releasing hormone and clonidine on motor neurone excitability. *Can J Neurol Sci* 1987; **14**: 506–509.

118. Zhang L. Effects of 5-hydroxytryptamine on cat spinal motoneurons. *Can J Physiol* 1991; **69**: 154–163.

119. Takahashi T, Berger A. Direct excitation of rat spinal motoneurones by serotonin. *J Physiol* 1990; **423**: 63–76.

120. White SR. A comparison of the effects of serotonin, substance P and thyrotropin releasing hormone on excitability of rat spinal motoneurons in vivo. *Brain Res* 1985; **335**: 63–70.

121. White SR, Fung SJ. Serotonin depolarises cat spinal motoneurons in situ and decreases motoneuron after hyperpolarizing potentials. *Brain Res* 1989; **502**: 205–213.

122. Wang MY, Dun NJ. 5-hydroxytryptamine responses in neonate rat motoneurones in vitro. *J Physiol* 1990; **430**: 87–103.

123. Bertel O, Malessa S, Sluga E, Hornykiewicz O. Amyotrophic lateral sclerosis: changes of noradrenergic and serotonergic transmitter systems in the spinal cord. *Brain Res* 1991; **566**: 54–60.

124. Ohsugi K, Adachi K, Mukoyama M, Ando K. Lack of change in indoleamine metabolism in spinal cord of patients with amyotrophic lateral sclerosis. *Neurosci Lett* 1987; **79**: 351–354.

125. Sofic E, Riederer P, Gsell W et al. Biogenic amines and metabolites in spinal cord of patients with Parkinson's disease and amyotrophic lateral sclerosis. *J Neural Transm* 1991; **3**: 133–142.

126. Forrest V, Ince P, Leitch M et al. Serotonergic neurotransmission in the spinal cord and motor cortex of patients with motor neuron disease and controls: quantitative autoradiography for 5-HT$_{1a}$ and 5-HT$_2$ receptors. *J Neurol Sci* 1996; **139** (**suppl**): 83–90.

127. Lackovic Z, Jakupcevic M, Bunarevic A et al. Serotonin and norepinephrine in the spinal cord of man. *Brain Res* 1988; **443**: 199–203.

128. Schoenen J, Reznik M, Deleaide PJ, Vanderhaeghen JJ. Etude immunocytochimique de la distribution spinale de substance P, des enkephalines, de cholecystokinine et de serotonine dans la sclérose latérale amyotrophique. *C R Soc Biol* 1985; **179**: 528–534.

129. Forrest VA. *Aspects of Serotonergic and Glutamatergic Neurotransmission in the Human Motor System and in Motor Neurone Disease* (PhD Thesis). University of Newcastle upon Tyne, 1996.

130. Davies MF, Deisz RA, Prince DA, Peroutka SJ. Two distinct effects of 5-hydroxytryptamine on single cortical neurons. *Brain Res* 1987; **423**: 347–352.

131. Chari G, Shaw PJ, Saghal A. Non-verbal visual attention but not recognition memory or learning processes are impaired in motor neurone disease. *Neuropsychologica* 1996; **34**: 377–385.

132. Steckler T, Sahgal A. The role of serotonergic-cholinergic interactions in the mediation of cognitive behaviour. *Behav Brain Res* 1995; **67**: 165–169.

133. Chida K, Sakamaki S, Takasu T. Alteration in autonomic function and cardiovascular regulation in amyotrophic lateral sclerosis. *J Neurol* 1989; **236**: 127–130.

134. Malessa S, Leigh PN. Neurochemistry of motor neuron disease. In: Leigh PN, Swash M, eds. *Motor Neuron Disease. Biology and Management*. London: Springer-Verlag, 1995, 163–182.

135. Nicoll RA. The action of thyrotrophin-releasing hormone, substance P and related peptides on frog spinal motoneurones. *J Pharmacol Exp Ther* 1978; **207**: 817–824.

136. Ono H, Fukuda H. Ventral root depolarization and spinal reflex augmentation by a TRH analog in rat spinal cord. *Neuropharmacology* 1982; **21**: 39–44.

137. Nistri A, Fisher ND, Gurnell M. Block by the neuropeptide TRH of an apparently novel K$^+$ conductance of rat motoneurones. *Neurosci Lett* 1990; **120**: 25–30.

138. Strand FL, Rose KJ, Zuccarelli LA et al. Neuropeptide hormones as neurotrophic factors. *Physiol Rev* 1991; **71**: 1017–1046.

139. Schoenen J, Lotstra F, Vierendeels G et al. Substance P, enkephalins, somatostatin, cholecystokinin, oxytocin and vasopressin in human spinal cord. *Neurology* 1985; **35**: 881–890.

140. Krivoy WA, Couch JR, Steward JM, Zimmerman E. Modulation of cat monosynaptic reflexes by substance P. *Brain Res* 1980; **202:** 356–372.

141. Iwasaki Y, Kinoshita M, Ikeda K et al. Trophic effect of various neuropeptides on the cultured ventral spinal cord of rat embryo. *Neurosci Lett* 1989; **101:** 316–320.

142. Hokfelt T, Vincent S, Hellsten I et al. Immunohistochemical evidence for a 'neurotoxic' action of (D-Pro², D-Try⁷,⁹) substance P, an analogue with substance P activity. *Acta Physiol Scand* 1981; **113:** 571–573.

143. Gordh JT, Post C, Olsson Y. Evaluation of the toxicity of subarachnoid clonidine, guanfacine and a substance P-antagonist on rat spinal cord and nerve roots: light and electron microscopic observations after chronic intrathecal administration. *Anesth Analg* 1986; **65:** 1301–1311.

144. Dietl MM, Sanchez M, Probst A, Palacios JM. Substance P receptors in the human spinal cord: decrease in amyotrophic lateral sclerosis. *Brain Res* 1989; **483:** 39–49.

145. Gibson SJ, Polak JM, Katagiri T et al. A comparison of the distribution of eight peptides in spinal cord from normal controls and cases of motor neuron disease with special reference to Onuf's nucleus. *Brain Res* 1988; **474:** 255–278.

146. Johansson O, Hokfelt T, Jeffcoate SL. Immunohistochemical support of three putative transmitters in one neuron: coexistence of 5-hydroxytryptamine, substance P- and thyrotropin releasing hormone-like immunoreactivity in medullary neurons projecting to the spinal cord. *Neuroscience* 1981; **6:** 1857–1881.

147. Fone KCP, Dix P, Tomlinson DR et al. Spinal effects of chronic intrathecal administration of the thyrotropin-releasing hormone analogue (CG 3509) in rats. *Brain Res* 1988; **455:** 157–161.

148. Banda RW, Means ED. Effect of thyrotropin-releasing hormone on neural loss secondary to axotomy. *Neurology* 1989; **39 (suppl 1):** 401.

149. Banda RW, Kubek JM, Means ED. Decreased content of thyrotropin releasing hormone (TRH) in cervical ventral horns of patients with amyotrophic lateral sclerosis (ALS). *Neurology* 1986; **36 (suppl):** 139.

150. Mitsuma T, Nogimori T, Adachi K et al. Concentrations of immunoreactive thyrotropin-releasing hormone in spinal cord of patients with amyotrophic lateral sclerosis. *Am J Med Sci* 1984; **287:** 34–36.

151. Jackson IMB, Adelman LS, Munsat TL et al. Amyotrophic lateral sclerosis: thyrotropin-releasing hormone and histidyl proline diketopoperazine in the spinal cord and cerebrospinal fluid. *Neurology* 1986; **36:** 1218–1233.

152. Court JA, McDermott JR, Gibson AM et al. Raised thyrotropin-releasing hormone, proglutamylamino peptidase, and proline endopeptidase are present in the spinal cord of wobbler mice but not in human motor neuron disease. *J Neurochem* 1989; **49:** 1084–1090.

153. Manaker S, Shulman LH, Winokur A, Rainbow TC. Autoradiographic localization of thyrotropin-releasing hormone receptors in amyotrophic lateral sclerosis. *Neurology* 1985; **35:** 1650–1653.

154. Rosenfeld MG, Mermod JJ, Amara SG et al. Production of a novel neuropeptide encoded by the calcitonin gene via tissue-specific RNA processing. *Nature* 1983; **304:** 129–135.

155. Gibson SJ, Polak JM, Bloom SR et al. Calcitonin gene-related peptide immunoreactivity in the spinal cord of man and of eight other species. *J Neurosci* 1984; **4:** 3101–3111.

156. Harmann PA, Chung K, Briner RP et al. Calcitonin gene-related peptide (CGRP) in the human spinal cord: a light and electron microscopic analysis. *J Comp Neurol* 1988; **269:** 371–380.

157. New HV, Mudge AW. Calcitonin gene-related peptide regulates muscle acetylcholine receptor synthesis. *Nature* 1986; **323:** 809–811.

158. Fontaine B, Klarsfeld A, Hokfelt T, Changeux JP. Calcitonin gene-related peptide, a peptide present in spinal cord motor neurons, increases the number of acetylcholine receptors in primary cultures of chick embryo myotubes. *Neurosci Lett* 1986; **71:** 59–65.

159. White DM, Zimmerman M. Changes in the content and release of substance P and calci-

tonin gene-related peptide in rat cutaneous nerve neuroma. In: Dubner R, Gebhart GF, Bond MR, eds. *Proceedings of the Vth World Congress on Pain, Pain Research and Clinical Management.* Amsterdam: Elsevier, 1988, 109–113.

160. Kato T, Hirano A, Manaka H. Calcitonin gene-related peptide immunoreactivity in familial amyotrophic lateral sclerosis. *Neurosci Lett* 1991; **133**: 163–167.

161. Kato T, Katagiri T, Hirano A et al. Calcitonin gene-related peptide immunoreactivity in spinal spheroids in motor neuron disease. *Acta Neuropathol* 1991; **82**: 302–305.

162. Giaid A, Gibson SJ, Ibrahim NBN et al. Endothelin 1, an endothelium-derived peptide is expressed in neurones of the human spinal cord and dorsal root ganglia. *Proc Natl Acad Sci USA* 1989; **86**: 7634–7638.

163. Polak JM, Gibson SJ. Neuropeptides: occurrence in motor nerves and relevance to motor neurone disease. In: Williams AC, ed. *Motor Neuron Disease.* London: Chapman and Hall, 1994, 603–658.

164. Ip NY, Stitt TN, Tapley P et al. Similarities and differences in the way neurotrophins interact with Trk receptors in neuronal and nonneuronal cells. *Neuron* 1993; **10**: 137–149.

165. Oppenheim RW. Neurotrophic survival molecules for motoneurons: an embarrassment of riches. *Neuron* 1996; **17**: 195–197.

166. Appel SH. A unifying hypothesis for the cause of amyotrophic lateral sclerosis, parkinsonism, and Alzheimer's disease. *Ann Neurol* 1981; **10**: 499–505.

167. Ebenedal T, Askmark H, Aquilonius SM. Screening for neurotrophic disturbances in amyotrophic lateral sclerosis. *Acta Neurol Scand* 1989; **79**: 188–193.

168. Mitchell JD. Heavy metals and trace elements in amyotrophic lateral sclerosis. *Neurol Clin* 1987; **5**: 43–60.

169. Conradi S, Ronnevi L-O, Vesterburg O. Increased plasma levels of lead in amyotrophic lateral sclerosis compared to controls, as determined by atomic absorption spectrophotometry. *J Neurol Neurosurg Psychiatry* 1978; **41**: 389–393.

170. Campbell AMG, Williams ER, Barltrop D. Motor neurone disease and exposure to lead. *J Neurol Neurosurg Psychiatry* 1970; **33**: 877–885.

171. Livesley B, Sessons CE. Chronic lead intoxication mimicking motor neurone disease. *Br Med J* 1968; **4**: 387–388.

172. Simpson JA, Seaton DA, Adams JF. Response to treatment with chelating agents of anemia, chronic encephalopathy and myelopathy due to lead poisoning. *J Neurol Neurosurg Psychiatry* 1964; **27**: 536–541.

173. Quinlan GJ. Action of lead (II) and aluminium (III) on iron-stimulated lipid peroxidation in liposomes, erythrocytes and rat liver microsomal fractions. *Biochim Biophys Acta* 1988; **962**: 196–200.

174. Pall H. Metals and free radicals. In: Williams AC, ed. *Motor Neuron Disease.* London: Chapman and Hall, 1994, 497–534.

175. Patel AK, Michaelson IA, Cremer JE, Balazs R. The metabolism of ^{14}C glucose by the brains of suckling rats intoxicated with inorganic lead. *J Neurochem* 1974; **22**: 581–590.

176. Conradi S, Ronnevi LO, Nise G et al. Abnormal distribution of lead in amyotrophic lateral sclerosis. Re-estimation of lead in the cerebrospinal fluid. *J Neurol Sci* 1980; **48**: 413–418.

177. Stober T, Stelte W, Kunze K. Lead concentrations in blood plasma, erythrocytes and cerebrospinal fluid in amyotrophic lateral sclerosis. *J Neurol Sci* 1983; **61**: 21–26.

178. Manton WJ, Cook JD. Lead content of CSF and other tissues in amyotrophic lateral sclerosis. *Neurology* 1979; **29**: 611–612.

179. Petkau A, Sawatzky A, Hillier CR. Lead content of neuromuscular tissue in amyotrophic lateral sclerosis: case report and other considerations. *Br J Ind Med* 1974; **31**: 275–287.

180. Mandybur TI, Cooper GP. Increased spinal cord lead content in amyotrophic lateral sclerosis. Possibly a secondary phenomenon. *Med Hypotheses* 1979; **5**: 1313–1315.

181. Brown IA. Chronic mercurialism. A cause of the clinical syndrome of amyotrophic lateral sclerosis. *Arch Neurol Psychiatry* 1954; **72**: 674–681.

182. Adams CR, Ziegler DK, Lin JT. Mercury intoxication simulating amyotrophic lateral sclerosis. *JAMA* 1983; **250**: 642–643.

183. Barber TE. Inorganic mercury intoxication reminiscent of amyotrophic lateral sclerosis. *J Occup Med* 1978; **20**: 667–669.

184. Moller-Madson B, Danscher G. Localization of mercury in CNS of the rat. I Mercuric chloride (HgCl$_2$) per os. *Environ Res* 1986; **41**: 29–43.

185. Waring RH, Sturman SG, Williams AC et al. S-methylation in motor neurone disease and Parkinson's disease. *Lancet* 1989; **ii**: 356–357.

186. Blackstone S, Hurley RJ, Hughes RE. Some interrelationships between vitamin C (absorbic acid) and mercury in the guinea pig. *Food Cosmet Toxicol* 1974; **12**: 511–516.

187. Pekkanen TJ, Sandholm M. The effect of experimental methyl mercury poisoning on the activity of NADPH-specific glutathione reductase of rat brain and liver. *Acta Vet Scand* 1972; **13**: 14–19.

188. Halliwell B, Gutteridge JM. *Free Radicals in Biology and Medicine*. Oxford: Clarendon Press, 1989.

189. Mano Y, Takayanagi T, Ishitani A, Hirota T. Mercury in hair of patients with amyotrophic lateral sclerosis. *Rinsho Shinkeigaku* 1990; **29**: 844–848.

190. Khare SS, Ehmann WD, Kasarskis EJ, Markesbery WR. Trace element imbalances in amyotrophic lateral sclerosis. *Neurotoxicology* 1990; **11**: 521–532.

191. Yase Y. The role of aluminium in CNS degeneration with interaction with calcium. *Neurotoxicology* 1980; **1**: 101–109.

192. Yoshimasu F, Yasui M, Yase Y et al. Studies on amyotrophic lateral sclerosis by neutron activation analysis. 3. Systematic analysis of metals on Guamian ALS and PD cases. *Folia Psychiatr Neurol Jpn* 1982; **36**: 173–180.

193. Piccardo P, Yanagihara R, Garruto RM et al. Histochemical and X-ray microanalytical localisation of aluminium in amyotrophic lateral sclerosis and parkinsonism–dementia of Guam. *Acta Neuropathol* 1988; **77**: 1–4.

194. Tronscoso JC, Hoffmann PN, Griffin JW et al. Aluminium intoxication: a disorder of neurofilament transport in motor neurons. *Brain Res* 1985; **342**: 172–175.

195. Strong MJ, Garruto RM. Chronic aluminium-induced motor neuron degeneration. *Can J Neurol Sci* 1991; **18 (suppl 3)**: 428–431.

196. Deibel MA, Ehmann WD, Candy JM et al. Aluminium in motor neuron disease spinal cord. *Trace Elem Electrol* 1997; **14**: 51–54.

197. Kilness AW, Hochberg FH. Amyotrophic lateral sclerosis in a high-selenium environment. *JAMA* 1977; **237**: 2843–2844.

198. Ince PG, Shaw PJ, Candy JM et al. Iron, selenium and glutathione peroxidase activity are elevated in sporadic motor neuron disease. *Neurosci Lett* 1994; **183**: 87–90.

199. Miyata S, Nakamura S, Nagata H et al. Increased manganese level in spinal cords of amyotrophic lateral sclerosis determined by radiochemical neutron activation analysis. *J Neurol Sci* 1983; **61**: 283–293.

200. Kurlander HM, Patten BM. Metals in spinal cord tissue of patients dying of motor neurone disease. *Ann Neurol* 1979; **6**: 21–24.

201. Markesbery WR, Ehmann WD, Candy JM et al. Neutron activation analysis of trace elements in motor neuron disease spinal cord. *Neurodegeneration* 1995; **4**: 383–390.

202. Rosen DR, Siddique T, Patterson D et al. Mutations in Cu/Zn superoxide dismutase are associated with familial amyotrophic lateral sclerosis. *Nature* 1993; **362**: 59–62.

203. Radunovic A, Leigh PN. Cu/Zn superoxide dismutase gene mutations in amyotrophic lateral sclerosis: correlation between genotype and clinical features. *J Neurol Neurosurg Psychiatry* 1996; **61**: 565–572.

204. Wiedau-Pazos M, Goto JJ, Rabizadeh S et al. Altered reactivity of superoxide dismutase in familial amyotrophic lateral sclerosis. *Science* 1996; **271**: 515–518.

205. Beckman JS, Carson M, Smith CD, Koppenol WH. ALS, SOD and peroxynitrite. *Nature* 1993; **364**: 584.

206. Wang X, Culotta VC, Klee CB. Superoxide dismutase protects calcineurin from inactivation. *Nature* 1996; **383**: 434–437.

207. Ferrante RJ, Browne SE, Shinobu LA et al. Evidence of increased oxidative damage in both sporadic and familial amyotrophic lateral sclerosis. *J Neurochem* 1997; **69**: 2064–2074.

208. Ferrante RJ, Shinobu LA, Schulz JB et al. Increased 3-nitrotyrosine and oxidative damage in mice with a human copper/zinc superoxide dismutase mutation. *Ann Neurol* 1997; **42**: 326–334.

209. Aguirre T, van den Bosch L, Goetschalckx P et al. Increased sensitivity of fibroblasts from ALS patients to oxidative stress. *Ann Neurol* 1998; **43**: 452–457.

210. Shaw PJ, Ince PG, Falkous G, Mantle D. Oxidative damage to protein in sporadic motor neuron disease spinal cord. *Ann Neurol* 1995; **38**: 691–695.

211. Bowling AC, Shulz JB, Brown RH, Beal MF. Superoxide dismutase activity, oxidative damage and mitochondrial energy metabolism in familial and sporadic amyotrophic lateral sclerosis. *J Neurochem* 1993; **61**: 2322–2325.

212. Beal MF, Ferrante RJ, Browne SE et al. Increased 3-nitrotyrosine in both sporadic and familial amyotrophic lateral sclerosis. *Ann Neurol* 1997; **42**: 646–654.

213. Przedborski S, Donaldson D, Jakowec M et al. Brain superoxide dismutase, catalase and glutathione peroxidase activities in amyotrophic lateral sclerosis. *Ann Neurol* 1996; **39**: 158–165.

214. Bergeron C, Muntasser S, Somerville MJ et al. Copper/zinc superoxide dismutase mRNA levels are increased in sporadic amyotrophic lateral sclerosis motoneurons. *Brain Res* 1994; **659**: 272–276.

215. Sillevis Smitt PAE, Mulder TPJ, Verspaget HW et al. Metallothionein in amyotrophic lateral sclerosis. *Biol Signals* 1994; **3**: 193–197.

SECTION III

FUNCTIONAL AND PHYSIOLOGICAL STUDIES

7

Spinal motor neurons in amyotrophic lateral sclerosis: pathophysiology and motor unit counting

William F Brown and K Ming Chan

Introduction

Amyotrophic lateral sclerosis (ALS) is a rapidly progressive disease primarily affecting upper and lower motor neurons, which have an average survival time, from the appearance of the earliest symptoms and signs, of only 3–5 years.[1–3] The clinical presentation, especially in the early stages, varies considerably from case to case depending on the mix and relative intensities with which pyramidal cells in the motor cortex and motor neurons in the brainstem and spinal cord are affected. Despite careful clinical examination, sometimes it may be difficult to differentiate early ALS from other differential diagnosis such as cervical spondylitic myelopathies, radiculopathies, various mononeuropathies, and multifocal motor neuropathies. The certainty of the diagnosis may, however, be enhanced through the appropriate application of electrophysiological studies.

The objectives in this chapter are:

(a) to provide a comprehensive review of the pathophysiological changes in spinal motor neurons in ALS;
(b) to illustrate how the latter changes may be applied to the electrophysiological diagnosis of ALS, including a review of motor unit number estimating techniques; and
(c) to discuss how electrophysiological data might be usefully incorporated into clinical studies of the natural history and response to treatment of the disease.

Overview of the patho-physiological changes in ALS

The pathophysiological changes in ALS are dictated by the rates at which motor neurons are lost at various levels of neuraxis, the severity of those losses, the extent to which surviving motor neurons adapt to the losses of motor neurons or are themselves affected by the disease, and the severity of the involvement of the cortical motor neurons. Apart from the prominent motor neuron involvement, pathological studies have shown that other neurons, such as those in the sensory tracts, Clarke's column, and other central systems, may also be affected in ALS.[4,5] However, the latter pathological changes are relatively minor and, except for occasional mild abnormalities in somatosensory evoked potentials and sensory nerve conduction late in the disease, there is little indication that these neurons are specifically targeted in ALS.[6,7]

The pathophysiological changes in motor neurons may usefully be divided into those that primarily reflect changes in:

(a) the 'central' motor drive to lower motor neurons;

(b) the numbers, sizes, and excitabilities of the motor neurons themselves;

(c) the excitabilities and impulse transmitting capacities of the motor axons;

(d) neuromuscular transmission;

(e) the post-junctional muscle fibers; and

(f) the force-generating capacities of the motor units (MUs).

However useful the foregoing subdivisions may be for the purposes of discussion, they should not cloud the fact that various combinations of these abnormalities may sometimes be found to co-exist within the same spinal segments.

Pathophysiological changes in 'central' drive to motor neurons

Although the pathophysiological changes in upper motor neurons are reviewed in Chapters 8 and 9, some of the pertinent pathophysiological indications of impaired 'central' motor drive to motor neurons are highlighted here because these changes clearly affect the patients' ability to recruit lower motor neurons. Indications of losses and dysfunction of upper motor neurons in ALS include:

(a) mild prolongations in central motor conduction times and reductions in the responses of muscles evoked by magnetic–electrical stimuli delivered to the motor cortex;[8]

(b) the sizes of the maximum corticomotor neuronal excitatory post-synaptic potentials in response to cortical magnetic–electrical stimulation were reduced in ALS;[9,10]

(c) the presence of H reflexes in muscles where H reflexes are not normally found;

(d) finding an appreciable twitch in response to delivering a supramaximal stimulus to the motor nerve during a maximum voluntary contraction;

(e) the failure of voluntary contraction to potentiate a late 'transcortical' response in response to a supramaximal stimulus delivered to the motor nerve.

Pathophysiological changes in lower motor neurons

Pathophysiological changes in lower motor neurons include:

(a) losses of motor neurons;

(b) adaptive changes in surviving motor neurons; and

(c) dysfunctional changes in surviving motor neurons as they, in turn, succumb to the disease.

Evidence for losses of motor neurons may be both indirect and direct. Indirect evidence for losses of motor neurons in ALS includes reductions in the sizes of the maximum compound muscle action potentials (CMAPs) evoked by a supramaximal stimulus delivered to motor nerves and reduced recruitment of MUs despite voluntary attempts to contract the affected muscles maximally. Reduced recruitment may of course reflect losses of lower motor neurons or reduced 'central' drive to motor neurons. The distinction rests on differences in the recruitment patterns between the two. Loss of 'central' drive is suggested by difficulties in voluntarily recruiting MUs, which can otherwise be activated by electrical stimulation of the appropriate motor nerve. Lack of 'central' drive is also suggested by the inability to drive MUs at appropriately high enough frequencies or to sustain the discharges of MUs despite maximal voluntary efforts to do so.

On the other hand, losses of lower motor neurons are suggested by difficulties in producing full interference patterns in the face of appropriately high firing frequencies in those

MUs that are recruited. Of course, impaired 'central' drive and losses of lower motor neurons often go hand in hand in ALS, and the resulting recruitment patterns of MUs reflects the two influences.

Losses of motor neurons

More direct evidence for losses of motor neurons is provided by reductions in the numbers of MUs by any of several techniques for estimating the numbers of MUs. Studies employing different techniques are in general agreement in that they all show rapid losses of MUs, which far exceeded any age-related losses. In some instances, the losses of MUs are so severe that it is possible to count the numbers of MUs. Serial motor unit number estimates (MUNEs) have shown an initially very rapid loss of lower motor neurons in most instances, with a tendency for the rate of losses to slow somewhat later in the course of the disease (*Fig. 7.1*).[11] The various approaches for estimating the numbers of MUs in humans are covered later in this chapter, after a summary of the electrophysiological diagnosis of ALS.

Expansion of the innervation field in ALS

The pathophysiological changes in ALS include of course not only the loss of motor neurons but adaptive responses on the part of surviving motor neurons. These adaptive responses include the development of sprouts from axons of surviving motor neurons and the formation of new synaptic contacts between these sprouts and muscle fibers that have lost their 'natural' innervating motor neurons. Strong indirect evidence for such an expansion of the innervation fields of MUs in ALS includes findings such as fiber grouping in muscle biopsies taken from affected muscles and pathophysiological changes such as:

(a) significant and sometimes very substantial increases in the size of motor unit action potentials (MUAPs), whether detected with surface electrodes, intramuscular

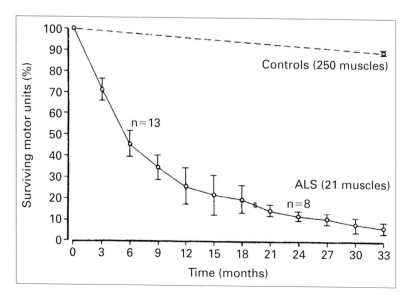

Figure 7.1
The rate of decline of the estimated number of surviving motor units in ALS patients followed from the time of initial diagnosis for up to 33 months. (From Dantes and McComas,[11] with permission.)

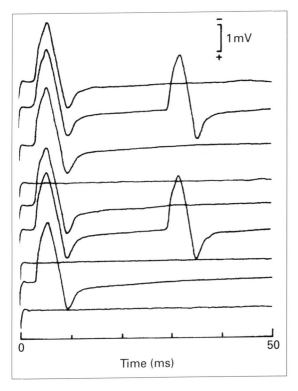

Figure 7.2
Surface recorded motor unit action potential (MUAP) of a thenar motor unit in an ALS patient. The tracings were from nine consecutive surface stimulation applied to the median nerve at the wrist at threshold stimulus intensity. The 'all-or-none' response suggests that the action potentials were from a single motor unit. The identical size and configuration of the late response, the F response, to the direct response further confirms this. The negative peak area of this MUAP was almost 10 times above the upper limit of normal obtained from the thenar muscles of a sample of healthy subjects in the same age group.[46]

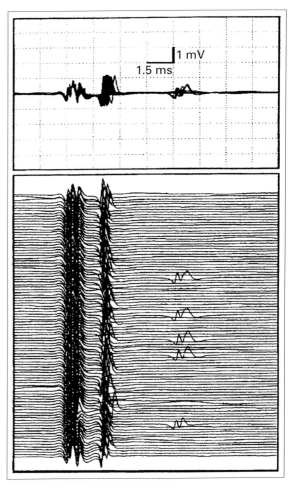

Figure 7.3
Single fiber EMG recording of a voluntarily recruited motor unit in the common extensor digitorum muscle of an ALS patient. The lower panel displays a raster of 100 consecutive firings of this motor unit, which are shown superimposed in the top panel. Note the markedly increased jitter and fiber density in this motor unit. Marked conduction block and increased jitter were present in the pair of muscle fibers on the extreme right, which only fired five out of 100 times. The appearance and disappearance of this pair of muscle fibers in unison indicate that the site of conduction block was at the terminal arbor of the motor axon.

macroelectrodes, or concentric needle electrodes (*Fig. 7.2*);[12,13]

(b) increased fiber densities (*Fig. 7.3*);[14,15]

(c) increases in the transverse territories of MUs; and

(d) increases in the twitch tensions of MUs.[12]

Dysfunctional changes in motor axons

Evidence of pathophysiological changes in motor axons include findings such as:

(a) abnormal excitability in single MUs and axons as indicated by fasciculation and repetitive firing;[14,16]
(b) axonal blocking (*Fig. 7.4*); and
(c) modest reductions in conduction velocities of motor nerves, especially in the latter stages of the disease.

Hyperexcitability in motor neurons and their axons may manifest as muscular cramping, myokymia, fasciculations, and repetitive firing. None of these is pathognomonic of ALS, but their presence in the company of other dysfunctional changes of the lower motor neurons are important clues to the diagnosis of ALS. Baldiserra and colleagues[17] showed convincing evidence that the generation sites for cramps and myokymia may lie in the soma and dendritic trees of the motor neuron, possibly as a result of changes in the conductance of calcium and potassium channels and, consequently, partial depolarization of the motor neuron. On the other hand, fasciculation and repetitive firing are phenomena that may be generated at various sites throughout the motor axon, including the terminal and pre-terminal branches of the axon.[18,19]

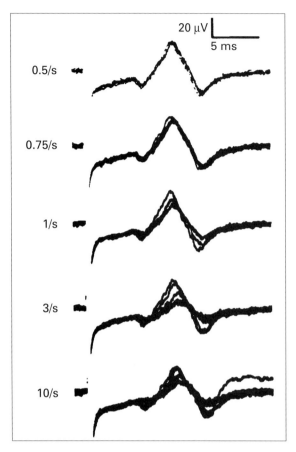

Figure 7.4
Surface recorded motor unit action potentials (MUAPs) of a thenar motor unit (MU) from an ALS patient. The MU was repetitively stimulated at frequencies of 2–10 Hz. Note that decrement of the MUAP started at 1 Hz and the maximum decrement occurred at 3 Hz.

Dysfunctional changes at the neuromuscular junction

Evidence of dysfunctional changes at the neuromuscular junction are common and include:

(a) increased variability in the shapes and sizes of voluntarily recruited MUAPs;
(b) decrements in the sizes of MUAPs and maximum CMAPs in response to repetitive stimulation of the motor nerve;[20] and

(c) increased jitter and blocking at single neuromuscular junctions.[14,15]

These findings might indicate either the breakdown of synaptic transmission in 'dysfunctional' motor neurons or failures of neuromuscular transmission at new and 'immature' neuromuscular junctions formed by relatively healthy expanding motor neurons.

Post-junctional changes in muscle fibers

Fibrillation potentials and positive sharp waves, indications of the presence of denervated muscle fibers, are common findings in ALS, especially in muscles in which there is evidence of loss of MUs.

Fiber grouping is a common finding in pathological studies in ALS. Such a finding is not surprising in any disease in which motor neurons have been lost and the surviving motor neurons develop axonal sprouts and form new synaptic contacts with denervated muscle fibers. Corollary evidence for such reinnervation are increased fiber densities and sizes of the MUAPs of MUs in ALS.

Dengler and colleagues[12] have shown that, in mildly affected cases of ALS, the areas of macro-EMG potentials of MUs in the first dorsal interosseous muscle were significantly increased compared to the controls, and that there was a corresponding increase in the twitch tensions and fiber densities of these MUs. However, in more severely affected patients, the correlations between recruitment threshold, twitch force, and macro-EMG size tended to break down and, for any given recruitment threshold and macro size, the twitch tensions were often reduced. Earlier studies by Milner-Brown and colleagues[21] also showed that the twitch tensions of some MUs in ALS were smaller than what might be expected from the size of their corresponding surface detected MUAPs.

Summary of the electrophysiological changes in MUs in ALS

Indications that as many as 50–80% of the normal pool of motor neurons may be lost before wasting or weakness become apparent in affected muscles, together with the findings of increases in the sizes of MUAP, suggest that, at least early in the course of the disease, most if not all motor neurons retain remarkable capacities to adapt to the loss of neighboring motor neurons by expanding their innervation fields.[13,22] Further progression, however, is increasingly marked by 'dysfunctional' changes in the motor axons, the neuromuscular junction, and the capacities of affected motor neurons to maintain their innervation fields and to generate the requisite force in response to pre-synaptic impulses. Evidence for such dysfunctional changes might be marked by progressive slowing of conduction of nerve impulses in affected motor axons; increasingly frequent failures in neuromuscular transmission; and reduction in the sizes of MUAPs, twitch, and tetanic tensions in affected MUs.

The electrophysiological diagnosis of ALS

The purposes of electrophysiological studies are to provide supporting evidence for the diagnosis of ALS while at the same time excluding other possible diagnostic considerations such as multifocal block neuropathy, myasthenia gravis, and other ALS 'look-alikes'. *Table 7.1* describes the principal electrophysiologic findings consistent with the diagnosis of ALS.

Motor unit number estimation

Since one of the central pathophysiological features of ALS is the loss of lower motor neurons, reliable and practical methods for estimating the numbers of motor neurons should be of value in the diagnosis of ALS, clinical

Denervation and reinnervation in the territories of two or more non-contiguous regions of the neuraxis including the brainstem (trigeminal, facial, or tongue muscles), cervical cord (cervical and various related shoulder girdle and limb muscles), thoracic cord (paraspinal, intercostal, or upper abdominal muscles), and lumbosacral cord (paraspinal, lower abdominal, and lower limb muscles)

Normal maximum motor conduction velocities and motor terminal latencies. These, however, may become mildly abnormal in the later stages of the disease and where there has been a severe loss of motor units

Evidence of abnormal motor axonal excitability such as fasciculations or repetitive firing

Normal peripheral sensory conduction in mixed peripheral nerves where there has been a clear loss of motor axons (units)

Normal somatosensory evoked potentials. Sensory conduction may become abnormal late in the disease, resulting in reduced sensory nerve action potential amplitudes and mildly prolonged cortical evoked potentials.

Evidence of upper motor neuron involvement as indicated by:
(a) reduced recruitment in the presence of normal or nearly normal numbers of motor units;
(b) the inability to voluntarily recruit a motor unit which can be activated by stimulation of its axon;
(c) the finding of H reflexes in muscles where H reflexes are not normally found;
(d) a significantly increased interpolated twitch response during a maximum voluntary contraction;
(e) the inability to potentiate an H reflex or a late M2 response; and
(f) reduced motor responses to magnetic-electrical stimulation of the motor cortex together with normal or mildly prolonged central motor conduction times

The absence of conduction block in motor nerves or other evidence of a demyelinating neuropathy

Evidence of instabilities in neuromuscular and/or axonal transmission including:
(a) variations in the shapes and sizes of motor unit action potentials generated by specific motor units;
(b) decrements in the sizes of motor unit action potentials in response to repetitive stimulation, often at frequencies as low as 1 Hz;
(c) increased 'jitter' and impulse blocking; and
(d) axonal blocking

Evidence of motor unit losses as indicated by reduced motor unit number estimates and reduced motor unit recruitment and sizes of maximum compound muscle action potentials

Table 7.1
Principal electrophysiologic findings in ALS.

studies of the natural history of motor neurons in ALS, and the assessment of the effectiveness of any new treatment. The pioneering work of McComas and co-workers[23] in the early 1970s and the later development of various modifications to their original method have produced a number of practical and attractive methods for estimating motor unit numbers. Many of these newer approaches incorporate computer-assisted automation. These advances, plus the added stimulus and attractiveness of adopting methods for estimating motor unit numbers in clinical trials, have doubtlessly driven further interest in developing robust, dependable methods for estimating the numbers of MUs in various muscles.[24] Since these methods have been recently reviewed, what follows is a brief summary of the newer approaches to MUNEs with the authors' views on their values, pitfalls, and possible applicability to the clinical diagnosis and clinical trials in ALS.

Methods for estimating the numbers of MUs in human muscles

McComas introduced the original method of estimating the MU numbers in 1971.[23] In this method, a supramaximal stimulus was applied to the motor nerve to determine the size of the maximum CMAP as detected with surface electrodes. The latter potential represents the sum of all the MUAPs generated by the constituent MUs detected with the same surface electrodes. Finely graded stimuli were then delivered to the motor nerve through a bipolar electrode applied to the surface over the motor nerve to excite the first five to 10 successively higher threshold single motor axons. From the cumulative sum of these surface-recorded (S)-MUAPs, the average S-MUAP was determined and the MUBE calculated by:

$$MUNE = \frac{\text{the size of the maximum CMAP}}{\text{the size of the average S-MUAP}}$$

Unfortunately, the thresholds of all but the lowest threshold motor axons at any given site of stimulation all too often overlap to the degree that it is impossible to avoid activating various combinations of motor axons. This phenomenon of 'alternation' is especially a problem in young healthy subjects in whom there is a full complement of motor axons with similar thresholds. 'Alternation' is probably the single most vexing problem with the manual method of estimating MUs. It causes erroneously low average S-MUAP size and, consequently, over-estimation of the number of MUs present. Other methods were subsequently derived to eliminate or minimize this source of error.

The automated incremental stimulation technique

In 1991, a fully automated method for estimating motor unit numbers was introduced by Galea and colleagues.[25] This method incorporated a program that automatically governed the intensity of successively delivered stimuli and an algorithm for template matching designed to minimize 'alternation'. In the authors' experience, although this automated method generally produces estimates well within the range of other methods, its test–retest reliability is relatively poor. Moreover, the putative MUAPs produced by the algorithm often bear little resemblance to the shapes of actual MUAPs derived using other secure means for stimulating single motor axons.

Statistical approaches to MUNEs

Shortly after this, Daube[26,27] described another fully automated approach to estimating motor unit numbers. This approach was based on the proposition that the fluctuations in the size of the M potential in response to series of stimuli of constant intensity approximates a Poisson distribution, in which case the variance observed is equal to the mean MUAP size. The mean MUAP size was derived at each of several stimulus intensity levels between threshold and supramaximal intensities. From each of the mean MUAP sizes thus derived, the overall average MUAP size was calculated and the MUNE was determined by division of the maximum CMAP by the overall average MUAP size.

Although the assumption that the CMAPs from a series of stimuli follow a Poisson distribution is true in normal motor axons, it may not be correct in diseased motor axons since their relative excitability could change as they become progressively more dysfunctional. Furthermore, the application of Poisson statistics requires large sample sizes and therefore its validity becomes increasingly problematic as the number of surviving motor neurons rapidly dwindles, which is common in ALS. However, this approach does have a number of advantages: it is relatively 'hands-off', fast, and reasonably reliable.

Multiple point stimulation

This method was designed to circumvent 'alternation' by accepting only MUAPs associated with stimulation of the lowest threshold motor axon at each of several sites along the course of a motor nerve.[28,29] The development of software to subtract the 'null' response from the 'all' response associated with the generation of the MUAP made it possible to:

(a) explore stimulus sites close to the motor point by minimizing, through template subtraction, stimulus artefact;

(b) collect, in some instances, MUAPs associated with the second and even third higher

threshold motor axons, again using template subtraction;

(c) set the latencies of MUAPs obtained by stimulation at differing distances from the motor point to zero; and

(d) sum the sample of MUAPs 'data point by data point' in a manner approximating the actual summation of MUAPs in the maximum CMAP (*Fig. 7.5*).

Multiple point stimulation is most applicable to motor nerves, such as the median, ulnar, and common peroneal nerves, that are relatively accessible to surface stimulation. Additional advantages of this approach include the fact that pathophysiological phenomena, such as decrements in response to repetitive stimulation and repetitive firing, both of which are especially common in ALS, may be readily identified. Furthermore, in some instances the approach lends itself to identification of the same motor axons and MUs in serial studies.[30] Set against these advantages, which offer important additional information about the status of individual MUs, is the fact that this approach, probably more than any other, demands vigorous training and experience in order to take full advantage of the method.

MUNEs derived using the F response

By developing software to extract single MUAPs from the F response, Doherty and colleagues[31,32] were able to obtain a sample of MUAPs from which a mean MUAP size and thereby a motor unit estimate could be determined. Recurrent discharge of single motor neurons (the F response) sometimes follows invasion of the somadentritic tree of the motor neuron by the antidromically transmitted nerve impulses originating at a peripheral site of stimulation. In healthy subjects, the chance of such a recurrent discharge in any single

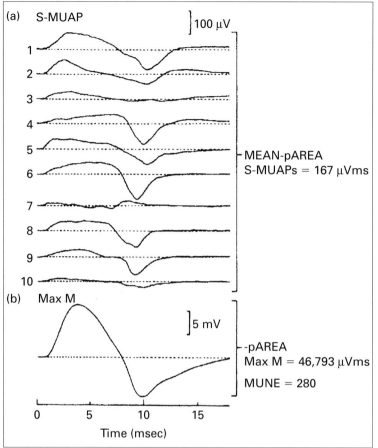

Figure 7.5
Motor unit number estimation using the multiple point stimulation technique. The surface-recorded motor unit action potentials (S-MUAPs) of 10 motor units in the thenar muscles of a healthy 27-year-old male subject is shown in (a) and the maximal 'M' potential in (b). The motor units were activated by stimulating at different sites along the accessible portion of the median nerve at the wrist, elbow, and upper arm. The dissimilarity in the sizes and shapes of the different S-MUAPs can be readily discerned on visual inspection. Before an 'average' S-MUAP was calculated, the onset of these S-MUAPs was aligned so that 'data point by data point' summation could be carried out. The average negative peak area in this case was 167 μVms (a). In comparison, the maximal M potential had a negative peak area (-PAREA) of 46,793 μVms (b), thus yielding a motor unit number estimate of 280.

motor neuron is quite low — of the order of 1–10% and usually closer to 1% of antidromically conducted impulses. Therefore, the chance that specific combination of F responses in two or more MUs will repeat a sufficient number of times in a train of 200–300 stimuli to be counted as a single MUAP is very small indeed. The method may therefore be used as a reliable means of deriving a representative sample of MUAPs from which an average MUAP can be obtained. In addition, the conduction velocities of single motor axons can also be determined.

It turns out, however, that in ALS the chance of an F response occurring in any single motor axon may change. In some instances, an F response may occur as often as 50% of the time in some MUs yet be unobtainable in other MUs. As a result, estimates derived using the F response technique in ALS, in the authors' judgement, are far less reliable than is the case with multiple point stimulation

Spike-triggered averaging

This approach is also designed to circumvent 'alternation' but, unlike other preceding methods, it uses voluntary contraction rather than electrical stimulation to activate the MUs.[33,34] The method is readily applicable to proximal muscles whose innervating nerves are usually much less accessible to surface electrical stimulation. In this method, the associated MUAPs of some of the voluntarily recruited MUs may be selectively recorded by using an intramuscular needle electrode. The tracking of specific intramuscularly detected MUAPs may be further facilitated by using a window discriminator. Once chosen, the latter may then serve as triggers with which their associated surface-detected MUAPs may be extracted using signal averaging. More recently, decomposition and template recognition have been coupled with spike-triggered averaging to increase the yield of MUAPs obtainable at any single intramuscular detection site and broaden the range of intensities of contraction over which the MUs may be selected.[24,35] Apart from providing an estimate of the MU number, this technique can also provide an additional range of useful physiological information, including the recruitment threshold, macro-EMG size, and firing rate of each MU. However, decomposition and template recognition software presents its own special problems; furthermore, as is the case with other software, it is tied to specific manufacturers' hardware, to date at least.

MUNEs derived using force

Measurements of the contractile forces associated with single human MUs have only been carried out infrequently because of the technical difficulties attendant to measuring single MU twitches. In 1990, Stein and Yang[36] employed spike-triggered averaging as well as intramuscular microstimulation to measure the twitch tensions generated by single MUs. The maximum twitch tension was then divided by the mean twitch tension of a sample of MUs to estimate the number of MUs in the thenar and EDB muscles. The values derived using this technique were somewhat lower than those derived using a variety of other techniques. The motor unit number estimates on different muscles in healthy individuals using different methods are summarized in *Table 7.2*.[23,27,28,31,34,36–39]

Requirements for any technique for estimating MU numbers

Methods for estimating MU numbers in clinical settings should meet the following requirements:

(a) there should be no systematic bias in the selection of the MUs used to derive the average MU size;

(b) the sample size used to determine the average MU size should be sufficiently large so as to be representative of the distributions of MU sizes in the muscle;

(c) the test–retest reliability of the technique should be high; and

(d) the technique should be as non-invasive and cause as little discomfort to the patient as possible.

In the authors' experience, the only two approaches that meet these requirements at present are multiple point stimulation and Daube's statistical method. Of the two, the former potentially offers more information about the pathophysiological characteristics of the surviving MUs while the latter offers the advantage of being 'more hands-off' and perhaps less demanding of operator skill.

Method		Authors	Muscle	MUNE (mean ± SD)	Subjects (n)	Age (years)
Electrical stimulation	Direct response	McComas et al, 1971[23]	Extensor digitorum brevis	199 ± 60	41	4–58
		Brown, 1972[37]	Thenar	253 ± 34	61	<40
		Ballantyne and Hansen, 1974[38]	Extensor digitorum brevis	197 ± 49	39	35 ± 14
		Stein and Yang, 1990[36]	Thenar	170 ± 62	10	26–49
		Doherty and Brown, 1993[28]	Thenar	288 ± 95	17	20–40
				139 ± 68	20	63–81
	F response	Stashuk et al, 1994[31]	Thenar	245 ± 105	18	31 ± 11
					15	68 ± 3
	Force	Stein and Yang, 1990[36]	Thenar	116 ± 45	10	26–49
Spike trigger averaging		Brown et al, 1988[34]	Biceps-brachialis	911 ± 254	40	<60
				479 ± 220		>60
	Force	Stein and Yang, 1990[36]	Thenar	135 ± 27	10	26–49
		Stein and Yang, 1990[36]	Thenar	130 ± 39	10	26–49
Statistical methods		Daube, 1995[27]	Thenar	234/95*	30	†
		Daube, 1995[27]	Hypothenar	256/115*	30	†
		Daube, 1995[27]	Extensor digitorum brevis	158/58*	30	†
		Slawnych et al, 1996[39]	Thenar	107 ± 55	23	16–57
		Slawnych et al, 1996[39]	Extensor digitorum brevis	87 ± 37	29	16–57

* means/lower limit
† age not stated

Table 7.2
Composite table of motor unit number estimates (MUNE) using different techniques.

The application of electrophysiological studies to clinical trials in ALS

Characteristically, patients with ALS suffer from progressive weakness and often wasting of affected muscles. Strength is usually assessed by asking the patient to make maximum voluntary contractions in various muscles. The natural history and responses of patients with ALS to treatment has been assessed by measuring maximum voluntary contractions in selected limb muscles and quantitatively assessing key respiratory and bulbar functions.[40,41] These measures have been incorporated in various combinations in outcome measure scales.

Although serial measurements of the force output of muscles, disability scales, and activities of daily living assessments are important measures of disease progression, they provide only a crude and indirect measure of the pathophysiological changes in ALS. For example, while it is true that maximum voluntary contractions in well-trained and motivated subjects closely approximate the maximum forces generated by tetanic stimulation of the motor nerve or direct stimulation of the muscles, the same cannot be said for untrained subjects. In untrained subjects, a supramaximal stimulus delivered to the motor nerve during a maximal effort may reveal a sizeable twitch superimposed on the voluntarily generated force, which indicates the extent to which the subject's effort falls short of a truly maximum voluntary contraction.[42,43] Assessment of maximum voluntary contractions cannot differentiate between weakness resulting from losses of lower and upper motor neurons. Furthermore, even marked lower motor neuron losses can be masked by the enormous capacities of surviving motor neurons to expand their innervation territories. This makes it imperative to include some measure of the numbers of motor neurons as well as the force output of the muscle. Apart from serving as an aid to the diagnosis of ALS, such electrophysiological studies may shed new light on the sequence of pathophysiological changes in upper and lower motor neurons accompanying the course of the disease. These studies are important if we are to learn more about:

(a) the relationships between the numbers of MUs, their functional status, and the force output of the affected muscles at various stages of the disease;
(b) the sequence of changes beginning with the initial adaptive responses of the surviving motor neurons and subsequent appearance of 'dysfunctional' changes;
(c) the capacities of surviving motor neurons to expand their innervation fields in response to losses of neighboring motor neurons; and
(d) the factors that govern survival times in motor neurons in ALS.

This information is of clinical and scientific relevance. For example, is there a 'point of no return' in motor neurons beyond which rescue is no longer possible? If so, can such a point be recognized by identifying specific pathophysiological features in the associated MU? Are the survival times of lower motor neurons influenced in any way by the extent to which the upper motor neurons are affected and vice versa? Do the physiological characteristics of lower motor neurons in any way influence their survival, as Dengler and colleagues[12] have suggested? Lastly, can physiological studies serve as sensitive markers for the progression of the disease and its response to new drugs?

The authors believe that recent developments, including reliable estimates of MU numbers and sensitive measures of the functional status in the surviving motor neurons, can provide sensitive, practical, non-invasive, and well-tolerated means for assessing the progress and response of the disease that could be adopted in clinical trials in ALS. For instance, recent studies have confirmed that MUNE is a more sensitive guide to disease progression than measures of strength or independence in daily activities since these other measure may be masked by collateral reinnervation or influenced by other extraneous factors such as motivation, depression, or pain.[44,45] The combination of physiological measures, including serial assessments of neuromuscular transmission, the MUAP sizes, and possibly the contractile properties and number of the surviving MUs with muscle strength, may provide physiologically relevant and clinically useful information. In addition, the foregoing studies might be supplemented by similar studies in specific motor neurons throughout the course of the disease. Together, they may offer a potentially sensitive and powerful means of assessing the progress of the disease and its response to new treatments in ALS.

References

1. Jablecki CK, Berry C, Leach J. Survival prediction in amyotrophic lateral sclerosis. *Muscle Nerve* 1989; **12**: 833–841.
2. Ringel SP, Murphy JR, Alderson MK et al. The natural history of amyotrophic lateral sclerosis. *Neurology* 1993; **43**: 1316–1322.
3. Mulder DW, Howard FM. Patient resistance and prognosis in amyotrophic lateral sclerosis. *Mayo Clin Proc* 1976; **51**: 537—541.
4. Averback P, Crocker P. Regular involvement of Clarke's nucleus in sporadic amyotrophic lateral sclerosis. *Arch Neurol* 1982; **39**: 155–156.
5. Brownell B, Oppenheimer DR, Hughes JT. The central nervous system in motor neurone disease. *J Neurol Neurosurg Psychiatry* 1970; **33**: 338–357.
6. Shefner JM, Tyler HR, Krarup C. Abnormalities in the sensory action potential in patients with amyotrophic lateral sclerosis. *Muscle Nerve* 1991; **14**: 1242–1246.
7. Radtke RA, Erwin A, Erwin CW. Abnormal sensory evoked potentials in amyotrophic lateral sclerosis. *Neurology* 1986; **36**: 796–780.
8. Schriefer TN, Hess CW, Mills KR, Murray NMF. Central motor conduction studies in motor neurone disease using magnetic brain stimulation. *Electroencephalogr Clin Neurophysiol* 1989; **74**: 431–437.
9. Nakajima M, Eisen A, McCarthy R et al. Reduced corticomotoneuronal excitatory postsynaptic potentials (EPSPs) with normal Ia afferent EPSPs in amyotrophic lateral sclerosis. *Neurology* 1996; **47**: 1555–1561.
10. Awiszus F, Feistner H. Abnormal EPSPs evoked by magnetic brain stimulation in hand muscle motoneurons of patients with ALS. *Electroencephalogr Clin Neurophysiol* 1993; **89**: 408–414.
11. Dantes M, McComas AJ. The extent and time course of motoneuron involvement in amyotrophic lateral sclerosis. *Muscle Nerve* 1991; **14**: 416–421.
12. Dengler R, Konstanzer A, Kuther G et al. Amyotrophic lateral sclerosis: macro-EMG and twitch forces of single motor units. *Muscle Nerve* 1990; **13**: 545–550.
13. McComas AJ, Sica RE, Campbell MJ, Upton AR. Functional compensation in partially denervated muscles. *J Neurol Neurosurg Psychiatry* 1971; **34**: 453–460.
14. Janko M, Trontelj JV, Gersak K. Fasciculations in motor neuron disease: discharge rate reflects extent and recency of collateral sprouting. *J Neurol Neurosurg Psychiatry* 1989; **52**: 1375–1381.
15. Stalberg E, Schawartz MS, Trontelj JV. Single fibre electromyography in various processes affecting the anterior horn cell. *J Neurol Sci* 1975; **24**: 403–415.
16. Bostock H, Sharief MK, Reid G, Murray NMF. Axonal ion channel dysfunction in amyotrophic lateral sclerosis. *Brain* 1995; **118**: 217–225.
17. Baldissera F, Caballari P, Dworzak F. Motor neuron 'bistability — a pathogenic mechanism for cramps and myokymia. *Brain* 1994; **117**: 929–939.

18. Conradi S, Grimby L, Lundemo G. Pathophysiology of fasciculation in ALS as studied by electromyography of single motor units. *Muscle Nerve* 1982; **5**: 202–208.

19. Roth G. The origin of fasciculations. *Ann Neurol* 1982; **12**: 542–547.

20. Killian JM, Wilfong AA, Burnett L et al. Decremental motor responses to repetitive nerve stimulation in ALS. *Muscle Nerve* 1994; **17**: 747–754.

21. Milner-Brown HS, Stein RB, Lee RG. Contractile and electrical properties of human motor units in neuropathies and motor neurone disease. *J Neurol Neurosurg Psychiatry* 1974; **37**: 670–676.

22. Hansen S, Ballantyne JP. A quantitative electrophysiological study of motor neurone disease. *J Neurol Neurosurg Psychiatry* 1978; **41**: 773–783.

23. McComas AJ, Fawcett PR, Campbell MJ, Sica RE. Electrophysiological estimation of the number of motor units within a human muscle. *J Neurol Neurosurg Psychiatry* 1971; **34**: 121–131.

24. Doherty T, Simmons Z, O'Connell B et al. Methods for estimating the numbers of motor units in human muscles. *J Clin Neurophysiol* 1995; **12**: 565–584.

25. Galea V, de Bruin H, Cavasin R, McComas AJ. The numbers and relative sizes of motor units estimated by computer. *Muscle Nerve* 1991; **14**: 1123–1130.

26. Daube JR. Statistical estimates of number of motor units in thenar and foot muscles in patients with amyotrophic lateral sclerosis or the residual of poliomyelitis. *Muscle Nerve* 1988; **11**: 957–958.

27. Daube JR. Estimating the number of motor units in a muscle. *J Clin Neurophysiol* 1995; **12**: 585–594.

28. Doherty TJ, Brown WF. The estimated numbers and relative sizes of thenar motor units as selected by multiple point stimulation in young and older adults. *Muscle Nerve* 1993; **16**: 355–366.

29. Kadrie HA, Yates SK, Milner-Brown HS, Brown WF. Multiple point electrical stimulation of ulnar and median nerves. *J Neurol Neurosurg Psychiatry* 1976; **39**: 973–985.

30. Chan KM, Doherty TJ, Andres LP et al. Longitudinal study of the contractile and electrical properties of single human thenar motor units. *Muscle Nerve* 1998; **21** (7): 839–849.

31. Stashuk DW, Doherty TJ, Kassam A, Brown WF. Motor unit number estimates based on the automated analysis of F responses. *Muscle Nerve* 1994; **17**: 881–890.

32. Doherty TJ, Komori T, Stashuk DW et al. Physiological properties of single thenar motor units in the F-response of younger and older adults. *Muscle Nerve* 1994; **17**: 860–872.

33. Strong MJ, Brown WF, Hudson AJ, Snow R. Motor unit estimates in the biceps–brachialis in amyotrophic lateral sclerosis. *Muscle Nerve* 1988; **11**: 415–422.

34. Brown WF, Strong MJ, Snow R. Methods for estimating numbers of motor units in biceps–brachialis muscles and losses of motor units with aging. *Muscle Nerve* 1988; **11**: 423–432.

35. Stashuk DW, Doherty TJ, Brown WF. EMG signal decomposition applied to motor unit estimates. *Muscle Nerve* 1992; **15**: 1191.

36. Stein RB, Yang JF. Methods for estimating the number of motor units in human muscles. *Ann Neurol* 1990; **28**: 487–495.

37. Brown WF. A method for estimating the number of motor units in thenar muscles and the changes in motor unit count with aging. *J Neurol Neurosurg Psychiatry* 1972; **35**: 845–852.

38. Ballantyne JP, Hansen S. A new method for the estimation of the number of motor units in a muscle. *J Neurol Neurosurg Psychiatry* 1974; **37**: 907–915.

39. Slawnych M, Laszlo C, Hershler C. Motor unit estimates obtained using the new 'MUESA' method. *Muscle Nerve* 1996; **19**: 626–636.

40. Andres PL, Thibodeau LM, Finison LJ, Munsat TL. Quantitative assessment of neuromuscular deficit in ALS. *Neurol Clin* 1987; **5**: 125–141.

41. Andres PL, Finison LJ, Conlon T et al. Use of composite scores (megascores) to measure deficit in amyotrophic lateral sclerosis. *Neurology* 1988; **38**: 405–408.

42. Merton PA. Voluntary strength and fatigue. *J Physiol* 1954; **123**: 553–564.

43. Allen GM, Gandevia SC, Mckenzie DK. Reliability of measurements of muscle strength and voluntary activation using twitch interpolation. *Muscle Nerve* 1995; **18**: 593–600.

44. Bromberg MB, Forshew DA, Nau KL et al. Motor unit number estimation, isometric strength, and electromyographic measures in amyotrophic lateral sclerosis. *Muscle Nerve* 1993; **16**: 1213–1219.
45. Felice KJ. A longitudinal study comparing thenar motor unit number estimates to other quantitative tests in patients with amyotrophic lateral sclerosis. *Muscle Nerve* 1997; **20**: 179–185.
46. Doherty TJ, Brown WF. Age related changes in human thenar motor unit twitch contractile properties. *J Appl Physiol* 1997; **82**: 93–101.

8

Corticospinal motor neurons: pathophysiology
Andrew A Eisen

Introduction

Upper motor neuron deficit is an essential component of the El Escorial criteria for probable and definite amyotrophic lateral sclerosis (ALS). However, until recently relatively little attention has been paid to the assessment of upper motor neuron dysfunction or to the possible mechanisms that underlie these deficits in ALS. The scarcity of information reflects the difficulty in sorting out upper versus lower motor neuron weakness when they co-exist and a lack of good clinical methods to measure upper motor neuron deficit. Initial results with functional imaging using magnetic resonance imaging (MRI) magnetic resonance spectroscopy (MRS), and positron emission tomography (PET) hold promise in evaluating upper motor neuron dysfunction in ALS. However, these techniques are presently restricted because of their expense and because of their limited ability to cone down on a circumscribed area as small as the motor cortex. The advent of transcranial magnetic stimulation (TMS) opened the door for inexpensive, in vivo evaluation of the motor pathways in awake humans. The technique has become sufficiently sophisticated to allow inferences to be made about the functioning of relatively few corticomotoneurons and the anterior horn cells that they innervate. Much of this chapter is devoted to single unit recording using TMS.

The corticomotoneuronal hypothesis

The corticomotoneuronal (CM) system in humans and, to a lesser extent, in non-human primates has greatly expanded at the expense of other descending tracts. The cells of origin of the CM system are amongst the largest in the nervous system and include the Betz cells. Their large size makes them particularly vulnerable to excitotoxic and oxidative stresses. Anatomical and physiological studies indicate that the CM neurons make monosynaptic connections with the motor neuron pools of all spinal motor neurons (SMNs) except those that innervate the external ocular muscles and Onuf's nucleus, whose cell bodies innervate the bladder wall.[1-4] These two groups of spinal motor neurons are almost invariably spared in ALS. The above observations, and the absence of an animal model that truly mimics human ALS, initiated the 'corticomotoneuronal' hypothesis of ALS. This hypothesis postulates that ALS is primarily a disorder of the corticomotoneuron or its presynaptic terminal, which secondarily affects the lower motor neurons and possibly other neurons.[5-7] The idea that ALS might originate in the motor cortex is far from new: this concept was originally proposed by Charcot.[8,9] Others, however, have proposed that ALS commences in the spinal motor neurons and spreads retrogradely to the upper motor neurons.[10] It is also possible that both the upper and lower motor neurons are involved independently of each other. For example, one hallmark of ALS is the accumulation of axonal spheroids in the lower motor neuron and conglomerates in the upper motor neurons. Chou and colleagues[11] have performed experiments suggesting that neurofilamentous accumulations result from the co-localization of peroxynitrite and superoxide, which affects neurofilament assembly. These findings support the idea that both cells are subjected to a common insult affecting them independently of each other. Kiernan and Hudson,[12] and more recently Pamphlett and colleagues,[13] have examined the pathological correlates of upper and lower motor neuron demise and concluded that both types of neuron die independently of each other. However, autopsy material reflects end-stage disease and cannot be used in a reliable way to determine the earliest structures that are involved in ALS and the events that succeed them.[6]

Other arguments countered against the CM hypothesis include the issue of the primary muscular atrophy (PMA) form of ALS and the reasons why motor stroke does not also cause lower motor neuron loss. Most cases of adult-onset PMA are hereditary and the responsible gene has been identified.[14,15] Sporadic ALS, beginning with lower motor neuron findings, is common but more than 85% of patients develop upper motor neuron findings in a few weeks or months and, if the lower motor neuron loss is severe, upper motor neuron findings may be difficult to detect. Some cases of lower motor neuron disease mimicking ALS turn out to have motor neuropathy with conduction block or hexosaminidase-B deficiency. The CM hypothesis depends on intact but impaired functioning of the corticomotoneurons that may be subjected to glutamate excitotoxicity (see Chapter 14) which may similarly excite the anterior horn cell. This would not be possible in an acutely destructive process such as stroke.

Investigating the CM system

Recent in vivo studies, using MRI, ^{1}H-MRS, and PET have given interesting information regarding dysfunction of the motor cortex early in ALS. T2-weighted MRI scans can show signal loss confined to the motor cortex. The abnormality may be bilateral and may extend from the vertex to the centrum semiovale; sometimes it is seen along the pyramidal tract, extending between the internal capsule to the cerebral peduncles.[16,17] It remains to be seen how these changes correlate with upper versus lower motor neuron changes.

Long echo time ^{1}H-MRS provides spectral information on the methyl resonances of N-acetyl acetate (NAA), choline (Cho)-containing compounds, creatine (Cr), phosphocreatine (PCr), and, when elevated, lactate. The concentration of N-acetylaspartate as measured by ^{1}H-MRS provides an index for the viability of the neuronal pool in the brain area measured. Pioro and colleagues[18] found that in ALS patients with definite upper motor neuron signs the ratio of the NAA spectrum to the Cr spectrum was significantly decreased ($p < 0.001$) in the primary motor cortex compared to normal controls (*Fig. 8.1*). In patients with probable upper motor neuron signs, the NAA-to-Cr ratio was also reduced but at a lower significance ($p < 0.05$, compared to $p < 0.001$). In patients who had only lower motor neuron signs the NAA-to-Cr ratio was not significantly different from normal. The linearity in the decline of the NAA-to-Cr ratio in patients with definite upper motor neuron signs, probable upper motor neuron signs, and without upper motor neuron signs compared

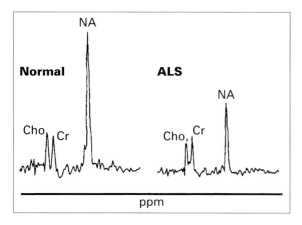

Figure 8.1
¹H-MRS spectra in a normal subject (left) and a patient with ALS (right). The size of the N-acetyl (NAA) component, which is restricted to neurons and is a good marker of neuronal integrity, is reduced in the patients with upper motor neuron signs. In order to take account of background 'noise', the neuronal loss is usually expressed as the NAA-to-creatine ratio. This ratio is also very much reduced in the patient. Cho, choline; Cr, creatine. (Modified from Pioro et al.[18])

to normal controls is impressive ($r^2 = 0.99$). More recent studies by others have confirmed these results.[19,20] The ability to analyse smaller brain volumes has allowed measurement of the NAA-to-Cr ratio in the brainstem and the medulla. Values in these regions are as reduced as they are in the motor cortex, presumably reflecting loss of neurons in the cranial motor nuclei.[21] ¹H-MRS may also prove to be a useful tool for the longitudinal evaluation of ALS patients, especially patients receiving therapies designed to alter levels of intracellular concentrations of glutamate, aspartate, or their metabolites, especially NAA and *N*-acetyl aspartyl glutamate (NAAG). Abnormalities have been reversed after treatment with riluzole, indicating that ¹H-MRS can detect neuronal dysfunction that is reversible.

PET in ALS indicates that there is a significantly lower regional cerebral blood flow (rCBF) in the primary sensorimotor cortex at rest. This is not unexpected given the neuronal loss within the motor cortex in ALS. Paradoxically, however, there is a greater increase of rCBF accompanying movement than occurs in normal subjects.[22,23] In ALS patients with upper motor neuron signs, activation — for example, movement of a joystick with the right hand — increases rCBF in the hand and arm area of the sensorimotor cortex bilaterally and the face area of the contralateral sensorimotor cortex as well as the contralateral pre-motor and supplementary motor cortices. The increased rCBF seen in ALS during movement has been interpreted as being due to the opening of new

Unusual nature of fasciculation in ALS

Double (repetitive) discharges

Reduced cortical threshold to transcranial magnetic stimulation

Shortened cortical silent period

Failure of inhibition in a conditioning-test paradigm

Table 8.1
Evidence for hyperexcitability of the motor cortex in ALS.

descending pathways.[23] However, an alternative explanation is that the changes are due to loss of local circuit inhibitory interneurons. This would result in relative overexcitation of surviving corticomotoneurons during movement.

In recent years a variety of neurophysiological methods using transcranial magnetic stimulation have been designed to investigate the integrity of the motor cortex and its descending pathways (see Chapter 9). Studies using transcranial magnetic stimulation with surface EMG recording from the target muscle have shown a range of abnormalities. These have resulted in a clearer understanding of the pathophysiological mechanisms underlying cortical dysfunction in ALS. Most of the abnormalities (*Table 8.1*) can be interpreted as implying that the motor cortex is hyperexcitable in ALS. For example, the threshold (stimulus strength of the magnetic field) required to activate the motor cortex with a magnetic coil is reduced compared to normal. This appears most prominent in early disease.[24–27] The cortical inhibitory circuitry, which is mediated through local circuit inhibitory interneurons and modulates the firing of the corticomotoneuron, is also impaired in ALS. This can be demonstrated through evoking the cortical silent period. Its duration, which is approximately 120 msec when recorded form a hand muscle, is a measure of corticospinal inhibition. However, most of the inhibition is due to cortical mechanisms.[28] The cortical silent period is produced when a fully contracting target muscle is subjected to an intervening transcranial magnetic stimulus (*Fig. 8.2*). Compared to normal subjects the cortical silent period is shortened in ALS.[28,29]

Another way of studying cortical inhibition is to use a conditioning-test paradigm. When a subthreshold conditioning magnetic stimulus shortly precedes a suprathreshold test mag-

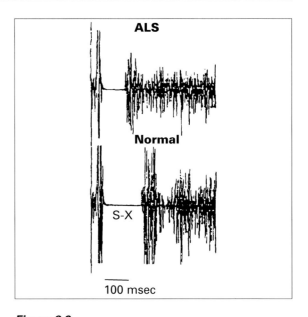

Figure 8.2
The cortical silent period is shortened in ALS (top trace). A supramaximal cortical stimulus was delivered and EMG activity was recorded from the thenar muscle, which was contracting at 80% of maximum force. The interval between the motor evoked potential and the return of EMG activity is the silent period (S–X interval). This shortening of the cortical silent period reflects loss of inhibitory control by the local circuit inhibitory interneurons. A recording in a normal subject is shown in the lower trace.

netic stimulus, there is normally complete inhibition of the test response. However, in ALS this ability of the conditioning stimulus to inhibit the test response is largely lost (*Fig. 8.3*).[30,31] It is outside the scope of this chapter to discuss fasciculation and repetitive discharges of the motor unit in the context of ALS. However, both are also probable manifestations of a hyperexcitable motor system in ALS.[32]

A more sophisticated physiological approach to investigating the CM system in

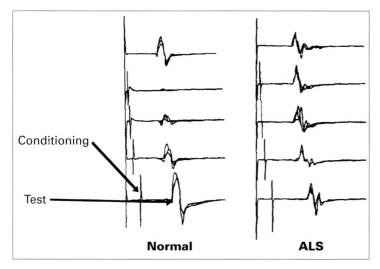

Normal   **ALS**

Figure 8.3
When transcranial double stimulation is applied to the normal motor cortex using a subthreshold conditioning stimulus followed by a threshold test stimulus 1–4 msec later, there is marked attenuation of the test response (left). The suppression is due to local circuit cortical inhibitory mechanisms because electrical brain stimulation, which stimulates post-synaptic structures, does not cause attenuation of the test response. In the patient with ALS (right), attenuation of the test response does not occur. (Modified from Yokota et al.[30])

Conditioning

Test

considerable detail is that of peristimulus time histograms (PSTHs). In humans, the CM system is the main descending motor pathway. Its transmitter is glutamate. The CM system is composed of colonies of corticomotoneurons (the CM colony), which converge upon a single spinal motoneuron.[33,34] The number of corticomotoneurons in each colony can exceed 100 in number. Those that innervate hand and forearm muscles have the greatest number of neurons per colony converging upon a single anterior horn cell. Divergence also occurs, i.e. one corticomotoneuron will synapase with many different anterior horn cells of a given motor neuron poll but also those of agonistic muscles. This remarkable arrangement underlies the large repertoire of fractionated movement that humans are able to master. Loss of fractionation is frequently an early upper motor neuron clinical deficit in ALS.

The PSTH measures changes in the firing probability of a single voluntary activated motor unit when it is subjected to a series of intervening transcranial magnetic stimuli.[35–39]

When the PSTH is recorded from a forearm or a hand muscle there is typically a large increase in firing of the motor unit that occurs at about 20–25 msec after the stimulus. This is recorded as the primary peak in the PSTH (*Fig. 8.4*). The configuration of the primary peak (namely its amplitude, dispersion, and duration) is a measure of the composite excitatory post-synaptic potential (EPSP), which is induced when the corticomotoneurons of the colony that innervate the recruited motor unit. discharge.[40,41]

Method and theory underlying PSTHs

In recording a PSTH, a needle electrode is used to record an index motor unit potential (MUP) from a target muscle. Steady recruitment of the index MUP is maintained. This can be aided by auditory visual feedback of the spike discharges. A window discriminator helps to separate the index from other conta-

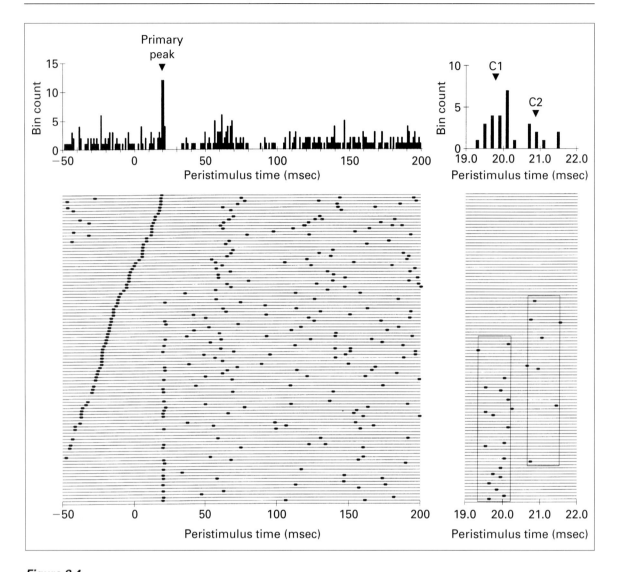

Figure 8.4
Peristimulus time histogram (PSTH) of the firing of a motor unit recorded from the common extensor digitorum muscle in a healthy 42-year-old man (top). Transcranial magnetic stimulation was delivered at time 0 msec and the total sweep duration was 250 msec. Discharges were collected into 1 msec bins. At about 20 msec after the stimulus there is a marked increase in the firing of the motor unit recognized as the primary peak. The primary peak is also shown on the right, where discharges were collected into 0.2 msec bins between 19.0 msec and 22.0 msec. This shows that the primary peak is composed of two subcomponents labeled C1 and C2 (shown in boxes in the raster display below). The raster displays of individual motor unit discharges underneath the PSTHs show that stimulus-induced firing of the motor unit could only occur when the interval between the preceding voluntary discharge of the motor unit and the stimulus-induced firing of the motor unit was at least 30 msec.

minating motor units. Only motor units whose amplitude exceeds 150 μV and who rise times is less than 50 μsec should be accepted. A magnetic stimulator randomly delivers a series of not less than 120 threshold stimuli at intervals of 1–5 seconds to the contralateral motor cortex during recruitment of the index MUP. Changes in the firing probability of the motor unit are collected into 1 msec bins of stimulus-triggered sweeps and are expressed as a peristimulus time histogram (PSTH) (see *Fig. 8.4*). A convenient analysis time for each stimulus-triggered sweep is 250 msec (50 msec before the stimulus and 200 msec after the stimulus).

In most PSTHs, an initial period of increased firing probability — the primary peak — is readily discernible at about 20–40 msec after the stimulus. In certain subjects the onset latency of the primary peaks derived from different but adjacent motor units varies. Onsets tend to cluster somewhat periodically at 2–3 msec intervals and in normal subjects the onset latency ranges from 18 to 27 msec. The rather regular 2–3 msec periodicity in occurrence of the primary peak indicates that its onset latency cannot be exclusively a function of the length and conduction velocity of the motor pathway, but reflects the time required for temporal summation of consecutively arriving descending volleys. In ALS, onset latency of the primary peak can be much longer than normal (*Fig. 8.5*). As discussed below, the prolongation seen in ALS is not due to slowing in the pyramidal pathways but to increased temporal dispersion of repetitive descending volleys.[54] In fact, central motor conduction measured using surface recorded compound motor evoked potentials is frequently normal in ALS.

The total number of bins in the primary peak that have counts exceeding the mean prestimulus background by more than 2 standard deviations is used to measure its rise time and magnitude of the composite EPSP generated in the indexed motor neuron. This in turn is a reflection of the strength of the descending volley(s). The number of descending volley(s) required for full depolarization of the anterior horn cell is determined by the strength of individual descending volleys and also by the inherent properties of the spinal motor neurons, such as the membrane resistance, which facilitates temporal summation.[39,42] Failure of the descending volley to depolarize the anterior horn cell could be the result of disease of dysfunction of the CM colony of an inability of the spinal motor neuron to react to the descending volley, or both. As described below, the evidence favours the former.[55] Firing of the index motor unit within the range of the primary peak is dependent upon the time of stimulation and its relation to the preceding voluntary discharge (see *Figs 8.4* and *8.5*). Raster plots of individual discharges show that a stimulus-induced discharge can occur within the primary peak only when the magnetic stimulus is given after the preceding voluntary motor unit discharge (i.e. when the stimulus arrives at the spinal motor neuron at least 20 msec after its voluntary firing). If the stimulus is given too shortly before or after the preceding discharge, the motor neuron cannot discharge within the primary peak and does so at its own inherent frequency (see *Figs. 8.4* and *8.5*).

Multiple peaks (subcomponents) can occur within the primary peak of the PSTH.[35,36,39,43] In humans, subcomponents can be regularly induced by high-voltage transcranial electrical stimulation. In normal subjects, subcomponents in the primary peak are less frequently induced by threshold transcranial stimulation. They can only be readily identified using 0.2 msec bin collections (see *Figs. 8.4* and *8.5*). Subcomponents tend to occur at 2 msec

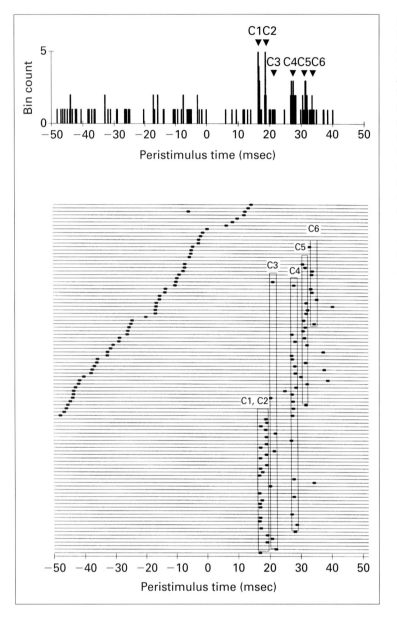

Figure 8.5
Prestimulus time histogram of the motor unit discharges in a 70-year-old woman with ALS. The arrangement is the same as shown in Fig. 8.4, except that the post-stimulus period is displayed for up to 50 msec and the discharges are collected into 0.2 msec bins. Individual motor unit discharges are shown in the raster display below. In this example, the primary peak commenced normally at about 17 msec after the stimulus but was very prolonged and consisted of six subcomponents, labeled C1–C6.

intervals. This time interval corresponds closely to that of multiple descending volleys in the pyramidal tract that are evoked by a single electrical cortical stimulation.[44–46] In the baboon, an anodal electrical stimulus delivered to the exposed motor cortex produces an initial descending volley — direct (D) wave — followed by up to five subsequent volleys — indirect (I) waves.[45] The I waves recur at characteristic intervals of 2.0–2.5 msec. Day and colleagues[36] studied PSTH peaks of single motor units after transcranial electric and

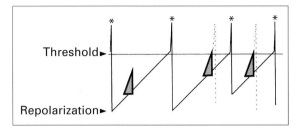

Figure 8.6
Model depicting the membrane excursions of the spinal motor neuron during voluntary, tonic contraction and how the neuron might respond to an intervening cortical stimulus. Voluntary spikes are indicated by asterisks (*). The shadowed triangle indicates a composite EPSP induced by a threshold cortical stimulation. The interrupted line indicates anticipated stimulation-induced firing of the motor unit. A stimulus-induced EPSP that arrives too soon after a preceding voluntary discharge will not be able to bring the membrane potential to threshold (depicted in the first EPSP). With stimulus-induced EPSPs arriving progressively later the membrane potential will first equal and then exceed the potential difference between the interspike trajectory and the threshold. This EPSP interacts with the voluntary excursion and brings the neuron to threshold (depicted in the second EPSP). When the interspike interval is shorter and the depth of post-spike repolarization is small, as may occur in ALS (shown on the right side), the magnitude of EPSP equals the potential difference earlier during a post-spike membrane excursion.

magnetic stimulation and concluded that multiple PSTH peaks can be explained on the D and I wave hypothesis of pyramidal neuron activation. Unlike electrical stimulation, magnetic stimulation does not easily produce a D wave in normal subjects.[47] In ALS subjects, there are more subcomponents in the PSTH than in normal subjects.

Figure 8.6 models how the shape and size of the composite EPSP can be estimated from

the primary peak;[40] a train of voluntary spikes of a discharging spinal motor neuron is shown. It is assumed that the trajectory of the membrane potential excursion during the interspike interval is linear and that the depth of repolarization is proportional to the interspike interval. A stimulus-induced EPSP of a given amplitude can arrive at any time during the interspike interval in which the membrane potential progressively returns towards its firing threshold. When the EPSP arrives shortly after the preceding voluntary spike its magnitude is insufficient to bring the membrane potential to threshold. EPSPs arriving at progressively later times will have magnitudes that equal or exceed the potential difference between the interspike trajectory and the threshold for firing, as exemplified in the second and third EPSPs in *Fig. 8.6*. When the motor unit fires more rapidly, as frequently happens in ALS (see *Fig. 8.6*, right third), the interspike interval is shorter and the magnitude of EPSP equals the potential difference earlier during a post-spike membrane excursion, since the depth of post-spike repolarization is small. This means that a composite EPSP of a given amplitude is able to bring the neuron to threshold with a greater probability. On the basis of this model, the amplitude of the composite EPSP can be estimated from the number of events collected during the primary peak (bin count), the number of stimuli delivered, and the interspike interval using the following equation:

$$\text{EPSP (mV)} = \frac{\text{bin count} \times \text{mean interspike interval} \times 10^{-1}}{\text{number of stimuli}}$$

The equation assumes a membrane potential excursion of 10 mV (-65 to -55 mV) at a firing rate of 10 Hz.[35,39]

PSTH studies in ALS

The abnormalities in the primary peak, which reflects the composite EPSP, are quite diverse in ALS (*Fig. 8.7*). The primary peak may be small (or absent) or it may be large with an increased temporal dispersion.[7,48–53] The diversity of abnormalities probably parallels functional changes in the CM colony that occur with disease progression.[54] The evidence that the abnormalities are supraspinal in origin is compelling[49,54,55] and supports the corticomotoneuronal hypothesis. The next sections describe experiments that support a supraspinal origin for the abnormalities seen in the PSTH in ALS, with explanations for the diversity of results.

Correlates of abnormal PSTH to motor function

The PSTH assesses the functional integrity of a given CM colony and its target, single, spinal motor neuron. The clinical progression of ALS is heterogeneous and different CM colonies and the spinal motor neurons that they innervate are at different stages of demise. There is even a spectrum of abnormalities in the PSTHs recorded from closely adjacent motor units in the same muscle of a given patient. This diversity of abnormalities in different motor units of the same muscle makes correlation of PSTH abnormalities with disease duration difficult (see *Fig. 8.7*). However, there is a correlation between the PSTH and clinical deficit. The number of subcomponents in the PSTH is increased even in patients who are not weak in the studied extremity, so that weakness or wasting are not prerequisites for this abnormality. This implies that the abnormality (increase in number of subcomponents) must occur early in the disease process. Increased number of subcomponents in the PSTH indicates repetitive firing of the parent CM colony, which is yet

another manifestation of hyperexcitability within the motor cortex. Hyperexcitability of the CM colony may be the earliest physiological change in the CM system of ALS. It could result in excessive excitatory drive of the target spinal motor neuron. It is unlikely that the changes simply reflect compensation for a partial loss of some corticomotoneurons because the strength of unitary descending volleys, as measured by the size of the primary peak, is often preserved in strong muscles and only modestly weak muscles.

In patients with weak limbs, the increased number of subcomponents is additionally associated with delayed onset latencies of the primary peak and attenuation of the unitary EPSP. These abnormalities are inter-related. Prolongation of the primary peak onset latency in ALS is probably due to attenuation of the unitary EPSP, a result of partial demise of the CM colony that occurs as the disease progresses. Attenuation of the EPSP could also be caused by dysfunction of the spinal motor neurons. However, there is still an increased number of subcomponents in the PSTH of patients with weakness, suggesting that the spinal motor neurons are still able to integrate repetitively arriving descending volleys (temporal summation). Further evidence for this follows.

Comparison of PSTHs obtained by peripheral versus cortical stimulation

Comparison of the size of the composite EPSP resulting from cortical stimulation with one that is generated by stimulation of peripheral Ia afferent fibers measured in the same motor unit provides an indirect assessment of the integrity of the anterior horn cell. If the anterior horn cell surface membrane is abnormal, the EPSPs resulting from both cortical and Ia

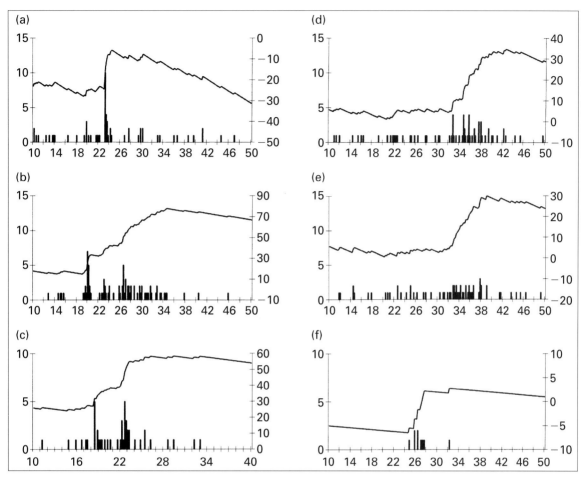

Figure 8.7
The progression of disease in different CM colonies and the spinal motor neurons that they innervate is heterogeneous. They are at different stages of demise and the spectrum of abnormalities in the PSTHs recorded from closely adjacent motor units even in the same muscle of a given patient is broad and variable. These PSTHs were recorded from six adjacent motor units in the common extensor digitorum muscle of the same patient with ALS. PSTH (a) is normal. PSTH (b) and PSTH (c) are dispersed and show an increase in the number of components of the primary peak. PSTH (d), PSTH (e), and PSTH (f) are all small, the result of reduced numbers of corticomotoneurons in the CM colony. The cumulative summation transform (CUSUM) is also shown in each trace. This allows better identification of direction change in the PSTH.

stimulation are likely to be small or unmeasure-able. If the problem lies within the motor cortex, the EPSP evoked by Ia stimulation should be normal. Using the tibialis anterior as the target muscle, Awiszus and Feistner[49] showed that in patients with ALS, the response to Ia peripheral nerve stimulation was identical to that of controls, but that about 50% of motor units had abnormally prolonged composite EPSPs with transcrancial stimulation.

Very similar results were obtained by Naka-jima and colleagues,[55] who used the first dorsal interosseus muscle (FDI) as the target muscle. In normal subjects, the cortical EPSP, recorded from the FDI, is almost always larger than the Ia EPSP, indicating that composite cortical synaptic facilitation is larger than Ia afferent facilitation to this particular motor neuron pool. The reverse is the case for soleus motor units, where normally the Ia EPSP is larger than the cortical EPSP composite events.[55] These differences probably reflect the very different function of the two muscles. The FDI is involved in a large repertoire of fractionated movements, necessitating a large cortical facilitation, whereas the soleus is essentially involved in postural maintenance and requires greater Ia afferent information. The composite CM EPSP for the FDI is 2–3 mV, compared to about 0.6 mV for the soleus.[55]

In ALS, the ratio of the cortical EPSP to the Ia afferent EPSP is significantly reduced because of a reduction in the size of the cortically evoked EPSP. These findings imply that the spinal motor neuron remains normally functional, even when the CM colony that innervates it is compromised. This supports the corticomotoneuronal hypothesis.

Macro-EMG studies and cortical PSTHs

Macro-EMG can be used to estimate the total size of the motor unit. Although there are no available anatomical data, it is reasonable to assume that spinal motor neurons that have an enlarged motor unit territory with a larger macro-EMG amplitude also have an enlarged cell body — possibly in response to increased metabolic demands. The input resistance of such motor units should be decreased and this would tend to reduce the estimated amplitude of their composite EPSPs. A composite EPSP depolarizing the spinal motor neuronal membrane alters its membrane potential at a common trigger zone, the axon hillock, raising it to threshold for firing. The amplitude of the composite EPSP depends on the total output at the spinal motor neuron and varies with the product of the CM synaptic current (input) and its own input resistance, given by Ohm's law:[56]

$$E = IR$$

where E is the estimated amplitude of the composite EPSP, I is the CM synaptic current, and R is the input resistance of the spinal motor neuron. In keeping with the Henneman size principle,[57] spinal motor neurons that generate larger twitch tensions and larger motor unit potentials at the skin surface have a larger cell body. There is an inverse relationship between the surface area of a neuron and its input resistance: the larger the neuron, the smaller its passive input resistance. Larger motor unit potentials as estimated by macro-EMG will generate smaller composite EPSPs because they have a smaller passive input resistance. This argument assumes that, in normal subjects, spinal motor neurons of different sizes, within a given motor neuron poll innervating a muscle, receive a similar total CM synaptic current input.[56]

In ALS the normal inverse relationship between the composite EPSP and the input resistance of the spinal motor neuron is lost.[58] ALS motor neurons with a large macro-EMG have larger rather than smaller composite EPSPs, and conversely, most motor neurons that have a reduced composite EPSP do not have large macro-MUPs. These findings indicate that in ALS, changes in the estimated amplitude of composite EPSPs must result from an abnormal synaptic current (input). The small composite EPSP in ALS simply reflects a reduced number of CM synapses, resulting from a loss of corticomotoneurons, a loss of their presynaptic terminals, or both.

Impaired cortical inhibitory mechanisms in ALS

It is possible that inhibitory modulation of the corticomotoneuron, which is mediated through several different classes of cortical interneurons, is impaired in ALS. This would result in overexcitation of the corticomotoneuron and consequently the anterior horn cell. Distinct types of inhibitory interneurons have been identified by their immunohistochemical reactivity to the calcium-binding proteins calbindin, parvalbumin, and calretinin.[59–61] Calcium-binding proteins are a family of proteins that have a unique distribution in the brain and are important in buffering intracellular calcium. Glutamate neurotoxicity is a process by which the overactivation of glutamate receptors can cause the influx of excessive extracellular calcium, leading to neuronal cell death (see Chapter 14). Neurons that contain calcium-binding proteins may be more resistant to glutamate neurotoxicity owing to their increased ability to buffer calcium.

The axon terminals of the local circuit inhibitory interneurons form symmetric inhibitory synapses on the dendritic shafts, somata, or proximal axonal segments of pyramidal neurons.[61] Neurons that terminate exclusively on the corticomotoneuronal cell soma are called wide arbor neurons and they react to parvalbumin. They may be responsible for synchronizing events of the cell. Neurons that terminate on the apical dendrite are referred to as double-bouquet neurons, and they demonstrate immunoreactivity to calretinin and less frequently to calbindin. They modulate the response of the pyramidal neuron to excitatory inputs. Neurons that terminate on the initial axonal segment of the pyramidal cell are called chandelier neurons, and they immunoreact to parvalbumin and influence the probability of the cell firing.[61,62] As with other local circuit inhibitory interneurons, chandelier neurons are γ-aminobutyric acid (GABA)-ergic. They are significantly depleted in ALS motor cortex[63,64] but are normal in number in the oculomotor, trochlear, and abducens nuclei, all of which are usually spared in ALS.[65]

Postnatally the inhibitory input to the axon hillock of the pyramidal neuron can be determined by the density of its parvalbumin immunoreactivity. This increases by about 50% during the first two postnatal months and gradually decreases around the time of puberty.[66] These results suggest that subpopulations of cortical neurons may be regulated by dynamic interactions between excitatory and inhibitory inputs during development. These interactions are critical in the postnatal refinement in cortical circuitry. Inappropriate or incomplete synaptogenesis might predispose aging neurons to succumb to the cascade of cellular events resulting in ALS.

Summary

It is most difficult to arrive at meaningful conclusions regarding the temporal sequence of events in ALS affecting the corticomotoneuronal system on the basis of autopsy studies. The results of the physiological studies described in this chapter point compellingly to a primary pre-synaptic, supraspinal, disturbance early in the disorder. This is most likely within the motor cortex. There is evidence that dysfunction and subsequent demise of corticomotoneuronal colonies occurs initially when spinal motor neurons function normally. PSTHs of the firing pattern of voluntarily activated motor units subjected to transcranial magnetic stimulation indicates that the descending cortical volley is inadequate in ALS. The primary peak of the PSTH, which reflects the strength of the excitatory postsynaptic potential generated at the spinal motor neuron, is dispersed and contains increased numbers of subcomponents. This is a function of increased repetitive firing of the corticomotoneuron, which is hyperexcitable. Overexcitation of the corticomotoneuron may be secondary to loss of cortical inhibitory modulation normally mediated through local circuit inhibitory interneurons. With the demise of the corticomotoneuronal colony, the PSTH becomes small and eventually unrecordable.

The sequence of events described has therapeutic implications. Both agents that inhibit glutamatergic transmission and enhance GABA-ergic inhibitory control have a role in the treatment of ALS. Delivery of these compounds would need to access the cerebral cortex readily.

References

1. Gandevia SC, Rothwell JC. Activation of the human diaphragm from the motor cortex. *J Physiol* 1980; **303**: 351–364.
2. Gandevia SC, Plassman BL. Responses in human intercostal and truncal muscles to motor cortical and spinal stimulation. *Respir Physiol* 1988; **73**: 325–338.
3. Colebatch JG, Rothwell JC, Day BL et al. Cortical outflow to proximal arm muscles in man. *Brain* 1990; **113**: 1843–1856.
4. Iwatsubo T, Kuzuhara S, Kanemitsu B et al. Corticofugal projections to the motor nuclei of the brainstem and spinal cord in humans. *Neurology* 1990; **40**: 309–312.
5. Eisen A, Kim S, Pant B. Amyotrophic lateral sclerosis (ALS): a phylogenetic disease of the corticomotoneuron? *Muscle Nerve* 1992; **15**: 219–228.
6. Eisen A. Amyotrophic lateral sclerosis is a multifactorial disease. *Muscle Nerve* 1995; **18**: 741–752.
7. Eisen A, Nakajima M, Enterzari-Taher M, Stewart H. The corticomotoneuron: aging, sporadic amyotrophic lateral sclerosis (ALS) and first degree relatives. In: Kimura J, Kaji R, eds. *Physiology of ALS and Related Diseases*. Amsterdam: Elsevier, 1997, 155–175.
8. Charcot JM. Sclérose des cordons latéraux de la moelle épinère chez femme hystérique atteinte de contracture permanente des quatre membres. *Bull Soc Med Hop Paris* 1865; **2 (suppl 2)**: 24–42.
9. Charcot JM, Joffroy A, Deux cas d'atrophie musculaire progressive avec lésions de la substance grise et des faisceaux anteriolatéraux de la moelle épinère. *Arch Physiol Norm Pathol* 1869; **2**: 354–367, 629–649, 744–760.
10. Chou SM, Norris FH. Amyotrophic lateral sclerosis: lower motor neuron disease spreading to upper motor neurons. *Muscle Nerve* 1993; **16**: 864–869.
11. Chou SM, Wang HS, Komai K. Colocalization of NOS and SODI in neurofilament accumulation within the motor neurons of amyotrophic lateral sclerosis: an immunohistochemical study. *J Chem Neuroanat* 1996; **10**: 249–258.
12. Kiernan JA, Hudson AJ. Changes in sizes of cortical and lower motor neurons in amyotrophic lateral sclerosis. *Brain* 1991; **114**: 843–853.
13. Pamphlett R, Kril J, Hng TM. Motor neuron disease: a primary disorder of corticomotoneuron? *Muscle Nerve* 1995; **18**: 314–318.
14. Melki J, Abdelhak S, Sheth P et al. Gene for chronic proximal spinal muscular atrophies maps to chromosome 5q. *Nature* 1990; **344**: 767–768.
15. Roy N, Mahadevan MS, McLean M et al. The gene for neuronal apoptosis inhibitory protein is partially deleted in individuals with spinal muscular atrophy. *Cell* 1995; **80**: 167–178.
16. Ishikawa K, Nagura H, Yokota T, Yamanouchi H. Signal loss in the motor cortex on magnetic resonance images in amyotrophic lateral sclerosis. *Ann Neurol* 1993; **33**: 218–221.
17. Iwasaki Y, Ikeda K, Shiojima T et al. Clinical significance of hypointensity in the motor cortex on T2-weighted images. *Neurology* 1994; **44**: 1181.

18. Pioro EP, Antel JP, Cashman NR, Arnold DL. Detection of cortical neuron loss in motor neuron disease by proton magnetic resonance spectroscopy imaging in vivo. *Neurology* 1994; **44**: 1933–1938.

19. Jones AP, Gunawardena WJ, Coutinho CMA et al. Preliminary results of proton magnetic resonance spectroscopy in motor neuron disease (amyotrophic lateral sclerosis). *J Neurol Sci* 1995; **129 (suppl)**: 85–89.

20. Gredal O, Rosenbaum S, Topp S et al. Quantification of brain metabolites in amyotrophic lateral sclerosis by localized proton magnetic resonance spectroscopy. *Neurology* 1997; **48**: 878–881.

21. Cwik VA, Hanstock CC, Boyd C et al. Regional neuronal dysfunction in amyotrophic lateral sclerosis (ALS): in vivo measurement with protein magnetic resonance spectroscopy (MRS). *Neurology* 1997; **48 (suppl)**: A216.

22. Kew JJM, Goldstein LH, Leigh PN et al. The relationship between abnormalities of cognitive function and cerebral activation in amyotrophic lateral sclerosis. A neuropsychological and positron emission tomography study. *Brain* 1993; **116**: 1399–1423.

23. Kew JJ, Brooks DJ, Passingham RE et al. Cortical function in progressive lower motor neuron disorders and amyotrophic lateral sclerosis: a comparative PET study. *Neurology* 1994; **44**: 1101–1110.

24. Caramia MD, Bernardi G, Zarola F, Rossini PM. Neurophysiological evaluation of the central nervous impulse propagation in patients with sensorimotor disturbances. *Electroencephalogr Clin Neurophysiol* 1988; **70**: 16–25.

25. Caramia MD, Cicinelli P, Paradiso C et al. Excitability changes of muscular responses to magnetic brain stimulation in patients with central motordisorders. *Electroencephalogr Clin Neurophysiol* 1991; **81**: 243–250.

26. Eisen A, Pant B, Stewart H. Cortical excitability in amyotrophic lateral sclerosis: a clue to pathogenesis. *Can J Neurol Sci* 1993; **20**: 11–16.

27. Mills KR, Nithi KA. Corticomotor threshold is reduced in early sporadic amyotrophic lateral sclerosis. *Muscle Nerve* 1997; **20**: 1137–1141.

28. Prout AJ, Eisen A. The cortical silent period and amyotrophic lateral sclerosis. *Muscle Nerve* 1994; **17**: 217–223.

29. Disiato MT, Caramia MD. Towards a neurophysiological marker of amyotrophic lateral sclerosis as revealed by changes in cortical excitability. *Electroencephalogr Clin Neurophysiol* 1997; **105**: 1–7.

30. Yokota T, Yoshino A, Saito Y. Double cortical stimulation in amyotrophic lateral sclerosis. *J Neurol Neurosurg Psychiatry* 1996; **61**: 596–600.

31. Ziemann U, Winter M, Reimers K et al. Impaired cortico-cortical inhibition in patients with amyotrophic lateral sclerosis. A transcranial magnetic stimulation study (abstract). *Electroencephalogr Clin Neurophysiol* 1996; **99**: 346.

32. Eisen A, Krieger C. *Amyotrophic Lateral Sclerosis: a Synthesis of Research and Clinical Practice*. Cambridge University Press, 1998.

33. Phillips CG, Porter R. *Corticospinal Neurones: Their Role in Movement*. London: Academic Press, 1977, 155.

34. Porter R, Lemon RN. *Corticospinal Function and Voluntary Movement*. Monographs of the Physiological Society No. 45. Oxford: Clarendon Press, 1993, 122–209.

35. Day BL, Rothwell JC, Thompson PD et al. Motor cortex stimulation in intact man. II. Multiple descending volleys. *Brain* 1987; **110**: 1191–1209.

36. Day BL, Dressler D, Maertens de Noordhout A et al. Electric and magnetic stimulation of human motor cortex. Surface EMG and single motor unit responses. *J Physiol (Lond)* 1989; **412**: 449–473.

37. Brouwer B, Asby P. Corticospinal projection to upper and lower limb spinal motoneurons in man. *Electroencephalogr Clin Neurophysiol* 1990; **76**: 509–519.

38. Palmar E, Ashby P. Corticospinal projections to upper limb motoneurones in humans. *J Physiol (Lond)* 1992; **448**: 387–412.

39. Bawa P, Lemon RN. Recruitment of motor units in response to transcranial magnetic stimulation in man. *J Physiol (Lond)* 1993; **471**: 445–464.

40. Ashby P, Zilm D. Relationship between EPSP shape and cross-correlation profile explored by computer simulation for studies on human motoneurons. *Exp Brain Res* 1982; **47**: 33–40.

41. Fetz EE, Gustafsson B. Relation between shapes of post-synaptic potentials and changes in firing probability of cat motoneurons. *J Physiol (Lond)* 1983; **341**: 387–410.

42. Kandel ER, Schwartz JH. Directly gated transmission at central synapses. In: Kandel ER, Schwartz JH, Jessell TM, eds. *Principles of Neural Science* 3rd edn. New York: Elsevier, 1991, 153–172.

43. Boniface SJ, Mills KR, Schubert M. Responses of single motoneurons to magnetic brain stimulation in healthy subjects and patients with multiple sclerosis. *Brain* 1991; **114**: 643–662.

44. Patton HD, Amassian VE. Single- and multiple-unit analysis of cortical stage of pyramidal tract activation. *J Neurophysiol* 1954; **17**: 345–363.

45. Kernell D, Wu Chieb-Ping. Responses of the pyramidal tract to stimulation of the baboon's motor cortex. *J Physiol (Lond)* 1967; **191**: 653–672.

46. Boyd SG, Rothwell JC, Cowan JMA et al. A method of monitoring function in corticospinal pathways during scoliosis surgery with a note on motor conduction velocities. *J Neurol Neurosurg Psychiatry* 1986; **49**: 251–257.

47. Amassian VE, Quirk GJ, Stewart M. A comparison of corticospinal activation by magnetic coil and electrical stimulation of monkey motor cortex. *Electroencephalogr Clin Neurophysiol* 1990; **77**: 390–401.

48. Awiszus F, Feistner H. Abnormal EPSPs evoked by magnetic brain stimulation in hand muscle motoneurons of patients with amyotrophic lateral sclerosis. *Electroencephalogr Clin Neurophysiol* 1993; **89**: 408–414.

49. Awiszus F, Feistner H. Comparison of single motor unit response to transcranial magnetic and peroneal nerve stimulation in the tibialis anterior muscle of patients with amyotrophic lateral sclerosis. *Electroencephalogr Clin Neurophysiol* 1995; **97**: 90–95.

50. Mills KR. Motor neuron disease. Studies of the corticospinal excitation of single motor neurons by magnetic brain stimulation. *Brain* 1995; **118**: 971–982.

51. Eisen A, Entezari-Taher M, Stewart H. Cortical projections to spinal motoneurons: changes with aging and amyotrophic lateral sclerosis.

Neurology 1996; **46**: 1396–1404.

52. Kohara N, Kaji R, Kojima Y et al. Abnormal excitability of the corticospinal pathway in patients with amyotrophic lateral sclerosis: a single motor unit study using transcranial magnetic stimulation. *Electroencephalogr Clin Neurophysiol* 1996; **101**: 32–41.

53. Mills KR, Kohara N. Magnetic brain stimulation in ALS: single motor unit studies. In Kimura J, Kaji R, eds. *Physiology of ALS and Related Diseases*. Amsterdam: Elsevier, 1997; 177–192.

54. Nakajima M, Eisen A, Stewart H. Diverse abnormalities of corticomotoneuronal projections in individual patients with amyotrophic lateral sclerosis. *Electroencephalogr Clin Neurophysiol* 1997; **105**: 451–457.

55. Nakajima M, Eisen A, McCarthy R et al. Reduced corticomotoneuronal excitatory post-synaptic potentials (EPSPs) with normal Ia afferent EPSPs in amyotrophic lateral sclerosis. *Neurology* 1996; **47**: 1555–1561.

56. Ghez C. Muscles: effectors of the motor systems. In: Kandel ER, Schwartz JH, Jessell TM, eds. *Principles of Neural Science* 3rd edn. New York: Elsevier, 1991, 548–563.

57. Henneman E, Somien G, Carpenter DO. Functional significance in cell size in spinal motoneurons. *J Neurophysiol* 1965; **28**: 560–580.

58. Nakajima M, Eisen A, Stewart H. Comparison of corticomotoneuronal EPSPs and macro-MUPs in amyotrophic lateral sclerosis. *Muscle Nerve* 1998; **21**: 18–24.

59. Celio MR. Calbindin D-28K and parvalbumin in rat nervous system. *Neuroscience* 1990; **35**: 375–475.

60. Bainbridge KG, Celio MR, Rogers JH. Calcium-binding proteons in the nervous system. *Trends Neurosci* 1992; **15**: 259–264.

61. Conde F, Lund JS, Jacobowitz DM et al. Local circuit neurons immunoreact for calretinin, calbindin D-28k or parvalbumin in monkey prefrontal cortex: distribution and morphology. *J Comp Neurol* 1994; **341**: 95–116.

62. DeFelipe J, Jones EG. High-resolution light and electron microscopic immunohistemistry of colocalized GABA and calbindin D-28k in somata and double bouquet cell axons of monkey somatosensory cortex. *Eur J Neurosci*

1992; **4**: 46–60.

63. Nihei K, McKee AC, Kowall NW. Patterns of neuronal degeneration in the motor cortex of amyotrophic lateral sclerosis patients. *Acta Neuropathol* 1993; **86**: 55–64.

64. Alexianu ME, Ho BK, Mohamed AH et al. The role of calcium-binding proteins in selective motoneuron vulnerability in amyotrophic lateral sclerosis. *Ann Neurol* 1994; **36**: 846–858.

65. Reiner A, Medina L, Figuerdo-Cardenas G et al. Brainstem motoneuron pools that are selectively resistant in amyotrophic lateral sclerosis are preferentially enriched in parvalbumin: evidence from monkey brainstem for a calcium-mediated mechanism in sporadic ALS. *Exp Neurol* 1995; **131**: 239–250.

66. Andeson SA, Classey JD, Conde F et al. Synchronous development of pyramidal neuron dendritic spines and parvalbumin-immunoreactice chandelier neuron axon terminals in layer III of monkey prefrontal cortex. *Neuroscience* 1995; **67**: 7–22.

9

Transcranial magnetic stimulation

Jean Pouget, Sylvie Trefouret and Shahram Attarian

Introduction

Investigation of the corticospinal motor pathway is essential in amyotrophic lateral sclerosis (ALS) because upper motor neuron deficit is a component of the diagnosis. However, clinical methods to explore this dysfunction are often not sensitive. The techniques of imaging or functional imaging to assess upper motor neuron deficit are scarce and restricted. In 1980, Merton and Morton[1] reported the possibility of electrically stimulating the motor cortex using surface electrodes placed on the scalp of unanesthetized humans. This approach to cortical stimulation has not become widespread primarily because of the discomfort it causes to subjects. Much of the current applied to the scalp through surface electrodes remains in the soft tissue above the skull and high current intensity excites pain receptors.

Transcranial magnetic stimulation (TMS) was first devised in 1985.[2] It allows a non-invasive, virtually pain-free evaluation of upper motor neuron function in awake subjects. The exact site of the motor cortex stimulated through magnetic stimulation is still controversial. The motor responses observed in contralateral muscles after TMS have some variability probably owing to the existence of at least one synapse between the stimulated structures and the high responding spinal motor neurons.

It was shown that there are two types of responses that occur in the pyramidal axons after motor cortex stimulation:[3] direct (D) waves make up the first descending volley and originate by depolarization of the axons of corticomotoneurons; indirect (I) waves are multiple waves that occur some milliseconds later and are thought to originate through synaptic excitation of corticomotoneurons. Usually transcranial electrical stimulation produces D waves followed by I waves whereas TMS produces mainly I waves. However, D waves may be obtained by TMS depending on the shape or the position of the coil on the scalp.

Procedure of TMS *in clinical practice*

The stimulation coil is positioned on the scalp and has to be slightly adapted in every case to achieve optimal excitation. Orientation of the coil depends upon the type of the stimulation and the current wave from going through the coil. Flat orientation typically produces more robust stimulation, whereas tangential orientation produces more focal stimulation. Clockwise stimulation current is used for target muscles on the right side and counterclockwise current for those on the left.

Voluntary contraction of the target muscle has a facilitatory effect on the motor response obtained by TMS, inducing a shortening of the latency and an increased amplitude. This facilitation can be explained either by the recruitment of faster-conducting neurons at the cortical level or by the lowering of the motor neuron threshold at the spinal level, and probably by both mechanisms. Usually, weak voluntary contraction, about 10–20% of maximal voluntary contraction force, is used. Alternative facilitation have been proposed, such as contralateral homologous muscle contraction or non-specific maneuvers such as counting aloud. Because of the influence of facilitation on latency and amplitude of motor responses, the level of voluntary contraction has to be kept constant during the recording.

Several parameters of the motor responses obtained after TMS can be evaluated and have a different significance:

(a) the motor evoked potential;
(b) central motor conduction time;
(c) the threshold for cortical activation;
(d) the silent period; and
(e) the effects of a paired TMS either on the same hemisphere or on both hemispheres.

Motor evoked potential

The motor evoked potential (MEP) is the compound muscle action potential produced by a single transcranial magnetic stimulus. It is usually recorded during a weak voluntary contraction to obtain a facilitation as previously mentioned. Several tests are carried out to define the shortest onset latency and the highest amplitude of the response. The amplitude of the MEP is usually, but not always, smaller than the compound muscle action potential evoked by electrical stimulation of the peripheral nerve.[4,5] The MEP amplitude is expressed as a percentage of the maximum amplitude M wave of the motor response obtained by motor nerve stimulation. It is never less than 20%, and a value under 10% can be regarded as abnormal.[5] Some authors prefer to use the amplitude recorded after radicular stimulation than the amplitude recorded at the peripheral sites (wrist for the upper limb, fibula head for the lower limb) to avoid the misleading result that may result from a peripheral nerve disorder.[4] The MEP latency increases with increasing height, limb length, and age, but the central motor conduction time does not.[4]

Central motor conduction time

The central motor conduction time (CMCT) is obtained by subtracting from the MEP latency the peripheral conduction time. This peripheral conduction time is calculated by stimulating, usually magnetically to avoid pain, the spinal root at the seventh cervical level for the upper limb and at the first lumbar level for the lower limb. It can also be estimated by recording F waves latency using the formula:

$$CMCT = \frac{F - M - I}{2}$$

Because motor responses are not constantly observed by the lumbar roots magnetic stimulation in normals,[4] the second technique is usually preferred.

Threshold for cortical activation

The threshold for cortical activation is established by increasing the stimulus strength, given in percentage of maximum output, in 5% steps. The threshold is defined as the lowest intensity that gives a reproducible response three times. Mills and Nithi[6] defined an upper and lower threshold. The lower threshold is the maximum intensity that does not produce a recordable MEP in response to 10 consecutive stimuli. The upper threshold is the minimal intensity that produces MEP in response to 10 consecutive stimuli. Motor threshold is an index of the excitability level of corticomotoneurons.

Cortical silent period

The cortical silent period is determined by applying TMS during a sustained voluntary contraction of the studied muscle. After the MEP there is an inhibition period of voluntary activity, which is the silent period. This inhibition is attributed to the activation of inhibitory cortical structures. The duration of the silent period is dependent on the stimulus intensity and on the studied muscle, but it is not influenced by the force level of the voluntary contraction.

Paired TMS

Paired TMS allows study of cortical inhibition by using a conditioning-test paradigm. When paired TMS is applied on the same motor cortical area, the test response is inhibited if the interstimulus interval is 1–5 msec or 30 msec whereas it is facilitated if the interstimulus interval is 8–15 msec. When TMS is applied on the motor area of each hemisphere, transcallosal inhibition is observed for interstimulus interval from 6–30 msec.

Transcranial magnetic stimulation in ALS

Motor evoked potential

The first studies[7,8] of the cortical motor conduction in ALS were performed by electrical cortical stimulation and essentially considered CMCT abnormalities. Using TMS, Schriefer and colleagues[9] observed an abnormal CMCT in 64% of 22 patients with motor neuron disease. Conversely, Eisen and colleagues[10] noted that MEP latencies were only modestly prolonged and that the essential abnormality was reduced MEP amplitude. MEPs were often absent when pseudobulbar features predominated. When all MEP abnormal parameters

were considered and three different upper limb muscles were studied, the sensitivity of TMS abnormalities in ALS increased to 92.5%. It was confirmed by Uozumi and colleagues[11] that a reduced MEP/M wave amplitude has a higher correlation with pyramidal tract involvement than a prolonged MEP onset latency. In 63 ALS patients in whom MEP were studied in two muscles (some patients being re-examined once or twice), Claus and colleagues[12] found an abnormal CMCT in 51% of patients without significant change during follow-up. They considered CMCT to be an insensitive parameter without significant prognostic value. Recently Mills and Nithy[13] noted CMCT abnormalities in only 17% of 65 ALS patients without correlation with physical signs.

In summary, although as a group CMCT patients with ALS showed MEP abnormalities, CMCT cannot be considered to be a sensitive and specific parameter to detect subclinical upper motor neuron defect in individual patients. MEP amplitude is probably more sensitive, but further more detailed studies are needed to evaluate it.

Corticomotor threshold

This parameter has been less systematically studied, but abnormalities of the corticomotor threshold have led to a pathophysiological hypothesis. Eisen and colleagues[14] found that cortical threshold in ALS varied considerably and that there was a linear correlation between threshold and disease duration, so that early in the disease the corticomotor threshold was normal and later in the disease the motor cortex could not be stimulated. Early normal corticomotor threshold could be related to corticomotoneuron hyperexcitability induced by glutamate.

Mills and Nithi[6] confirmed that the corticomotor threshold is reduced early in ALS, favoring early abnormal cortical hyperexcitability. They found that in the muscles of patients who present no upper or lower motor neuron involvement, the threshold is elevated. In studies of patients with ALS as a group, corticomotor threshold is usually found to be higher in ALS than in controls.[15,16]

Cortical silent period

In patients with ALS, Triggs and colleagues[17] observed a silent period without a preceding MEP. This could indicate that:

(a) this inhibition is not dependent on inhibition of Renshaw cells or by muscle twitch reafferences; or

(b) in ALS, the excitatory effects of TMS are involved without abnormalities of the inhibition effects.

The duration of the silent period has been shown to be significantly shorter in ALS than in normal subjects.[11,16] Prout and Eisen[18] noted that the silent period was highly dependent on the intensity of the stimulus and that in 19 patients with ALS it was not significantly different from the normal group, even if the maximum silent period was shorter early in the disease. This shortening could be attributed to glutamate-induced corticomotoneuronal excitotoxicity. Desiato and Caramia[15] found a shortening of the silent period in a group of 47 patients with ALS; furthermore, the duration did not increase proportionally to stimulation intensity, as it did in normals. They considered this abnormal silent period as a potential neurophysiological marker of ALS because it is not observed in central motor involvement by other diseases, such as multiple sclerosis. These inconsistent results about the duration of the silent period in ALS need further studies to clarify this abnormality in different groups of ALS patients and during follow-up.

Paired TMS

The technique of paired TMS has been used to study ipsilateral corticocortical inhibition of the motor cortex in ALS. Yokota and colleagues[19] observed an attenuation of the normal early inhibition. Because there was a normal effect of the conditioning TMS on the H reflex, they assumed an impairment of the intracortical inhibitory mechanism in ALS. The same effects were observed by Ziemann and colleagues[20] in 14 ALS patients in whom the control responses were generate by I waves. Hanajima and colleagues[21] noted a normal inhibition at short intervals but no facilitation at long intervals in patients with motor neuron disease. Using paired TMS to study the motor interhemispheric influences, Salerno and Georgesco[22] observed a reduction of inhibitory effects in patients with ALS for short and long delays, implying probable distinct cortical circuitries.

Corticobulbar tract study by TMS

Recordings from the tongue and orofacial muscles in 30 patients with ALS, Urban and colleagues[23] demonstrated corticobulbar tract dysfunction in the orofacial muscles in 57% of the patients, in the tongue in 50% (70% following recording at both sites) but clinical evidence of upper motor neuron involvement in the cranial nerves in only 7%. Recording from the masseter muscles of the same number of patients, Trompetto and colleagues[24] observed abnormal MEPs in 63%, both in patients with clinical bulbar signs (78%) and those without (42%). Thus, TMS seems to be a sensitive technique for investigating the corticobulbar tract, which is usually difficult to study.

Influence of TMS on individual motor units

The influence of TMS on motor unit firing using a peristimulus time histogram (PSTH) can be utilized to study corticomotoneuronal function (see Chapter 8). Briefly, the excitatory peak is abnormally increased early in the disease and may reflect glutamate-induced excitotoxicity.[25–28] These abnormalities indicate primary dysfunction of the corticomotoneuronal projection system and are independent of functional changes in spinal motor neurons.[29–31] Loss of inhibition can also be demonstrated in ALS.[32]

Conclusion

Use of TMS in patients with ALS has made a great contribution to the assessment of central motor system dysfunction in this disease. Decreased cortical threshold and increased excitatory peak, as revealed by PSTH, during the early phase of the disease can be interpreted as the manifestation of glutamate-induced cortical hyperexcitability. Later in the disease, an increased cortical threshold and a decreased central MEP amplitude are markers of the loss of corticomotoneurons. Decreased cortical silent period and attenuation of inhibition when using paired TMS indicate an impairment of cortical inhibitory mechanisms that is probably different from the excitatory ones. When combining TMS parameters (i.e. relative MEP amplitude cortical threshold, and cortical silent period duration) a grading of MEP abnormalities can be defined and a strong correlation is observed between clinical evaluation of pyramidal involvement and MEP grading.[33] Moreover, TMS can contribute to the differentiation of the pyramidal syndrome of ALS from multiple sclerosis or cervical myelopathy, in which central motor conduction time is much more impaired.[34]

Most of the studies implicating TMS in ALS have demonstrated these significant abnormalities in groups of ALS patients in comparison with control groups or other pathological groups. Future series have to be studied in order to demonstrate that TMS can be considered as a sensitive test for subclinical upper motor neuron involvement in individual patients.

References

1. Merton PA, Morton HB. Stimulation of the cerebral cortex in intact human subject. *Nature* 1980; **285**: 227.
2. Barker AT, Jalinous R, Freeston IL. Noninvasive magnetic stimulation of the human motor cortex. *Lancet* 1985; **10**: 1106–1107.
3. Patton HD, Amassian VE. Single and multiple unit analysis of cortical stage of pyramidal tract activation. *J Neurophysiol* 1954; **17**: 345–363.
4. Claus D. Central motor conduction: method and normal results. *Muscle Nerve* 1990; **13**: 1125–1132.
5. Eisen A, Shtybel W. AAEM minimonograph 35: clinical experience with transcranial magnetic stimulation. *Muscle Nerve* 1990; **13**: 995–1011.
6. Mills KR, Nithi KA. Corticomotor threshold is reduced in early sporadic amyotrophic lateral sclerosis. *Muscle Nerve* 1997; **20**: 1137–1141.
7. Berardelli A, Inghilleri M, Formisano R et al. Stimulation of motor tracts in motor neuron disease. *J Neurol Neurosurg Psychiatry* 1987; **50**: 732–737.
8. Hugon J, Labeau M, Tabaraud F et al. Central motor conduction in motor neuron disease. *Ann Neurol* 1987; **22**: 544–546.
9. Shriefer TN, Hess CW, Mills KR, Murray NM. Central motor conduction studies using magnetic brain stimulation. *Electroencephalogr Clin Neurophysiol* 1989; **74**: 431–437.
10. Eisen A, Shytbel W, Murphy K, Hoirch M. Cortical magnetic stimulation in amyotrophic lateral sclerosis. *Muscle Nerve* 1990; **13**: 146–151.
11. Uozumi T, Tsuji S, Murai Y. Motor potentials evoked by magnetic stimulation of the motor cortex in normal subjects and patients with motor disorders. *Electroencephalogr Clin Neurophysiol* 1991; **81**: 251–256.

12. Claus D, Brunholzl C, Kerling FP, Henschel S. Transcranial magnetic stimulation as a diagnostic and prognostic test in amyotrophic lateral sclerosis. *J Neurol Sci* 1995; **129** (**suppl**): 30–34.

13. Mills KR, Nithi KA. Peripheral and central motor conduction in amyotrophic lateral sclerosis. *J Neurol Sci* 1998; **159**: 82–87.

14. Eisen A, Pant B, Stewart H. Cortical excitability in amyotrophic lateral sclerosis: a clue to pathogenesis. *Can J Neurol Sci* 1993; **20**: 11–16.

15. Desiato MT, Caramia MD. Towards a neurophysiological marker of amyotrophic lateral sclerosis as revealed by changes in cortical excitability. *Electroencephalogr Clin Neurophysiol* 1997; **105**: 1–7.

16. Salerno A, Carlander B, Camu W, Georgesco M. Motor evoked potentials (MEPs): evaluation of the different types of responses in amyotrophic lateral sclerosis and primary lateral sclerosis. *Electromyogr Clin Neurophysiol* 1996; **36**: 361–368.

17. Triggs WJ, Macdonell RA, Cros D, Chiappa KH, Shahani BT, Day BJ. Motor inhibition and excitation are independent of magnetic cortical stimulation. *Ann Neurol* 1992; **32**: 345–351.

18. Prout AJ, Eisen A. The cortical silent period and amyotrophic lateral sclerosis. *Muscle Nerve* 1994; **17**: 217–223.

19. Yokota T, Yoshino A, Inaba A, Saito Y. Double cortical stimulation in amyotrophic lateral sclerosis. *J Neurol Neurosurg Psychiatry* 1996; **61**: 596–600.

20. Ziemann U, Winter M, Reimers CD, Reimers K, Tergau F, Paulus W. Impaired cortex inhibitionin patients with amyotrophic lateral sclerosis. Evidence from paired transcranial magnetic stimulation. *Neurology* 1997; **49**: 1262–1268.

21. Hanajima R, Ugawa T, Terao Y, Ogata K, Kanazawa I. Ipsilateral cortico-cortical inhibition of the motor cortex in various neurological disorders. *J Neurol Sci* 1996; **140**: 109–116.

22. Salerno A, Georgesco M. Double magnetic stimulation of the motor cortex in amyotrophic lateral sclerosis. *Electroencephalogr Clin Neurophysiol* 1988; **107**: 133–139.

23. Urban PP, Vogt T, Hopf HC. Corticobulbar tract involvement in amyotrophic lateral sclerosis. A transcranial magnetic stimulation study. *Brain* 1998; **121**: 1099–1108.

24. Trompetto C, Caponenetto C, Buccolieri A, Marchese R, Abbruzzese G. Responses of masseter muscles to transcranial magnetic stimulation in patients with amyotrophic lateral sclerosis. *Electroencephalogr Clin Neurophysiol* 1998; **109**: 309–314.

25. Awiszus F, Feistner H. Abnormal EPSPs evoked by magnetic brain stimulation in hand muscle motoneurons of patients with amyotrophic lateral sclerosis. *Electroencephalogr Clin Neurophysiol* 1993; **89**: 408–414.

26. Eisen A, Entezari-Taher M, Stewart H. Cortical projections to spinal motoneurons: changes with aging and amyotrophic lateral sclerosis. *Neurology* 1996; **46**: 1396–1404.

27. Kohara N, Kaji R, Kojima Y et al. Abnormal excitability of the corticospinal pathway in patients with amyotrophic lateral sclerosis: a single motor unit study using transcranial magnetic stimulation. *Electroencephalogr Clin Neurophysiol* 1996; **101**: 32–41.

28. Nakajima M, Eisen A, Stewart H. Diverse abnormalities of corticomotoneuronal projections in individual patients with amyotrophic lateral sclerosis. *Electroencephalogr Clin Neurophysiol* 1997; **105**: 451–457.

29. Awiszus F, Feistner H. Comparison of single motor unit responses to transcranial magnetic and peroneal nerve stimulation in the tibialis anterior muscle of patients with amyotrophic lateral sclerosis. *Electroencephalogr Clin Neurophysiol* 1995; **97**: 90–95.

30. Nakajima M, Eisen A, McCarthy R et al. reduced corticomotoneuronal excitatory postsynaptic potentials (EPSPs) with normal Ia afferent EPSPs in amyotrophic lateral sclerosis. *Neurology* 1996; **47**: 1555–1561.

31. Nakajima M, Eisen A, Stewart H. Comparison of corticomotoneuronal EPSPs and macro-MUPs in amyotrophic lateral sclerosis. *Muscle Nerve* 1998; **21**: 18–24.

32. Enterzari-Taher M, Eisen A, Stewart H, Nakajima M. Abnormalities of cortical inhibitory neurons in amyotrophic lateral sclerosis. *Muscle Nerve* 1997; **20**: 65–71.

33. Trefouret S, Azulay JP, Peretti P, Pouget J.

Comparative evaluation of pyramidal tract by MRI and magnetic stimulation in amyotrophic lateral sclerosis and primary lateral sclerosis. *Neurology* 1997; **48**(**Suppl 2**): A129.

34. Trefouret S, Azulay JP, Bouillot P, Grisoli F, Peragut JC, Pouget J. Motor evoked potentials by magnetic stimulation in amyotrophic lateral sclerosis and cervical myelopathy. *Neurology* 1998; **50**(**Suppl 4**): A165.

10

Imaging in amyotrophic lateral sclerosis
Erik P Pioro

Introduction

Neuroimaging plays an essential role in evaluating the patient with suspected amytrophic lateral sclerosis (ALS) for two main reasons:

(a) first, and most importantly, is the identification of treatable conditions that mimic ALS by producing combined upper motor neuron (UMN) and lower motor neuron (LMN) dysfunction;

(b) secondly, and of increasing clinical importance, is the observation of parenchymal changes in the central nervous system (CNS) that are relatively specific for ALS and assist in making this diagnosis.

Additionally, imaging modalities that are now used for research purposes in ALS may become clinically relevant, depending on the results of ongoing studies.

The imaging modalities that are most useful in the investigation of patients with suspected ALS are magnetic resonance imaging (MRI) and computed tomography (CT), including post-myelography CT. These are now the first line of neuroimaging techniques, having supplanted the older techniques of plain film X-ray, spinal myelography, and angiography, although the last-named two are still used in certain circumstances. Their utility in studying patients suspected of having combined UMN and LMN dysfunction are included in a policy statement by the World Federation of Neurology in their El Escorial criteria for the diagnosis of ALS.[1] The statement outlines specific findings required for the diagnosis of ALS and those that are inconsistent with it (*Tables 10.1 and 10.2*). Anatomic changes in the brains and spinal cords of patients with ALS that probably represent neurodegeneration can be identified by MRI because of its ability to reveal parenchymal detail. Some of these neuroimaging changes, such as increased signal along the corticospinal tract on T2-weighted and proton density MRI (see below), are relatively specific for ALS.

Nuclear medicine imaging techniques that provide metabolic information on brain activity include positron emission tomography (PET) and single photon emission computed tomography (SPECT); they have revealed neural hypometabolism in ALS, especially in the setting of dementia. Another research technique used to study ALS brain is proton magnetic resonance spectroscopy (^{1}H-MRS), which allows in vivo measurement of certain neurochemicals, including markers of neuronal health.

Other specialized MRI techniques, such as diffusion-weighted MRI (DWI), functional MRI (fMRI), and magnetization transfer MRI (MTI), have recently been applied to patients with ALS to explore any diagnostic advantage over routine MRI. Although still limited in

Minimal or no bony abnormalities of the skull or spinal canal evident on plain X-rays

Minimal or no abnormalities on head or spinal cord MRI without compression of spinal cord or nerve roots

Minimal or no abnormalities on spinal cord myelography with post-myelography CT showing no spinal cord or root compression

Table 10.1
Neuroimaging features that support the diagnosis of ALS. (From World Federation of Neurology,[1] with permission.)

Significant bony abnormalities visible on plain X-rays of the skull or spinal canal that might explain the clinical findings

Significant abnormalities of head or spinal cord MRI suggesting intraparenchymal processes or arteriovenous malformations; compression of the brainstem, cranial nerves, spinal cord or spinal nerve roots by bony abnormalities, tumors, etc.

Significant abnormalities of spinal cord myelography with or without CT or on CT alone suggesting the lesions noted above.

Significant abnormalities on spinal cord angiography suggesting arteriovenous malformations

Table 10.2
Neuroimaging features that are inconsistent with the diagnosis of ALS. (From World Federation of Neurology,[1] with permission.)

number, studies with these modalities in ALS have provided novel information and may become useful in the clinical work-up of such patients. In the future, there may need to be revision of the statement by the World Federation of Neurology in their El Escorial criteria for the diagnosis of ALS that 'there are no neuroimaging tests which confirm the diagnosis of ALS'.[1]

This chapter presents the ways in which neuroimaging can identify pathologies that produce ALS-like clinical features, reveal lesions of the motor pathway that support the diagnosis of ALS, and provide novel informa-tion about ALS through research techniques including nuclear medicine and MRI-based applications.

Identifying conditions that resemble ALS

The primary role of neuroimaging in evaluating patients with symptoms and signs of ALS is to identify treatable or curable conditions. *Table 10.3* lists some of the more common structurally based pathologies that can produce UMN- or LMN-predominant deficits with a focal or more generalized distribution.

Type of ALS	Non-ALS lesion
Generalized (LMN-predominant) ALS	Multiple-level radiculopathies (cervical, lumbosacral or both) (e.g. spondylosis, carcinomatous meningitis) Radiculomyelopathy (e.g. intradural and extradural spinal cord tumors) Syringomyelia
Generalized (UMN-predominant) ALS	Cervical myelopathy Ischemia (e.g. strokes)
Generalized (UMN-predominant) ALS ± bulbar involvement	Multiple sclerosis
Bulbar-onset ALS	Craniocervical junction (e.g. foramen magnum lesions, syringobulbia, syringomyelia, Chiari I malformation)
Lower extremity onset ALS	Parasagittal intracranial lesions (e.g. meningioma, vascular malformation)
LMN, lower motor neuron; UMN, upper motor neuron.	

Table 10.3
Radiologically identifiable lesions producing ALS-like conditions.

Whether the patient has symptoms that are typical for ALS (*Table 10.4*) or atypical (*Table 10.5*) will help the physician to select the anatomic site to be imaged and to determine which conditions should be included in the differential diagnosis. In general, patients suspected of having ALS should undergo well-performed neuroimaging studies (preferably MRI), at least of the brain and cervical spinal cord, unless the diagnosis is certain.

The spinal cord is frequently the site of such lesions, which can be compressive, demyelinating, inflammatory, or ischemic. Spondylitic stenosis of the cervical spinal cord frequently causes deficits resembling UMN-predominant ALS by producing myelopathy alone (*Fig. 10.1*) or myelopathy in combination with radiculopathy (*Fig. 10.2*). The patient shown in *Fig. 10.1* with severe cervical myelopathy had been thought to have primary lateral sclerosis, a pure UMN disorder, until MRI of the cervical spine was performed. Extradural tumors (*Fig. 10.3*) or ligamentous hypertrophy (*Fig. 10.4*) causing spinal cord compression can result in similar clinical presentations. In the absence of neck or limb pain, these lesions may elude diagnosis until neuroimaging is performed. Lesions within the spinal cord (e.g. intradural tumors, syringomyelia) can result in muscle weakness and atrophy at the level of the lesion and spasticity below it (*Fig. 10.5*). Other regions of the CNS where lesions can produce ALS-like clinical findings include the junction of the brainstem and spinal cord (the

Clinical feature	Regions of CNS to image	Non-ALS pathology
UMN-predominant or pure UMN	Brain; spinal cord (cervical, thoracic)	Demyelinating disease (e.g. multiple sclerosis) Ischemia (e.g. strokes) Parasagittal mass (e.g. meningioma, vascular malformation) Retroviral myelopathy Spondylitic myelopathy Subacute combined degeneration of the spinal cord
Bulbar-onset	Brainstem; base of skull	Chiari I malformation Demyelinating disease (e.g. multiple sclerosis in brainstem) Mass (e.g. tumor, vascular malformation) in brainstem or at foramen magnum Syringobulbia Ischemia (e.g. of brainstem)
Unilateral	Brain; spinal cord (cervical or thoracic)	Inflammation (e.g. multiple sclerosis, transverse myelitis) Ischemia (e.g. stroke) Mass (e.g. tumor, vascular malformation) Radiculopathies (cervical, limbosacral)

LMN, lower motor neuron; UMN, upper motor neuron.

Table 10.4
Typical clinical features for ALS resulting from look-alike conditions.

Clinical feature	Regions of CNS to image	Non-ALS pathology
Recovering ± relapsing	Brain	Multiple sclerosis (relapsing–remitting form)
Bladder involvement	Spinal cord (e.g. thoracolumbar)	Demyelination (e.g. multiple sclerosis) Inflammation (e.g. transverse myelitis) Mass (e.g. tumor, vascular malformation)
Sensory loss and/or pain	Spinal cord (e.g. cervical)	Radiculopathy, radiculomyelopathy Syringomyelia

Table 10.5
Atypical clinical features of ALS resulting from look-alike conditions.

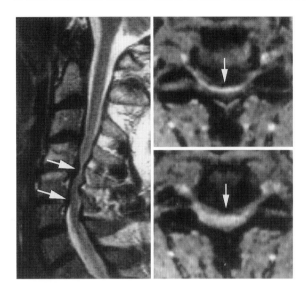

Figure 10.1
Severe canal stenosis produced ribbon-thin compression of the cervical spinal cord primarily at the C4–C5 intervertebral space (upper right; arrow) but also at the C5–C6 intervertebral levels (lower right; arrow) in a 47-year-old man who presented with a 7-year history of progressive gait difficulty. The patient's handwriting began deteriorating 6 months before evaluation and the jaw jerk was found to be very brisk. A diagnosis of primary lateral sclerosis, a pure UMN disease, was suspected until cervical spondylosis was found by MRI.

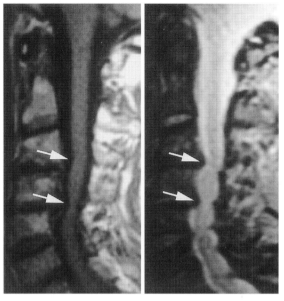

Figure 10.2
Compression of the cervical spinal cord is noted at the C3–C4 and C4–C5 intervertebral levels (arrows) on T1-weighted MRI (left) and T2-weighted MRI (right) in a 55-year-old man who presented with upper extremity weakness and muscle atrophy as well as leg spasticity. He was thought to have classic ALS until MRI revealed spondylomyeloradiculopathy.

cervicomedullary or craniocervical junction) (*Fig. 10.6*), the lower brainstem (pons and medulla) (*Fig. 10.7*), and the cerebral hemispheres (the parasagittal cortex or multifocally in the subcortical white matter) (*Fig. 10.8*).

It is essential to identify treatable causes promptly, not only to maximize the chances of successful therapy but also to minimize the emotional toll of diagnostic uncertainty. However, the existence of a condition causing ALS-like symptoms does not exclude the co-occurrence of true ALS. This is particularly true for cervical

spondylitic radiculomyelopathy, which, like ALS, tends to occur more frequently with increasing age. Not uncommonly, one is faced with an elderly patient who has cervical stenosis on MRI and clinical findings that could be attributable to either radiculomyelopathy or early ALS; progressive deterioration after decompressive laminectomies reveals the true nature of the underlying pathology. A discussion of potentially treatable conditions that should be included in the differential diagnosis of ALS can also be found in Chapter 1.

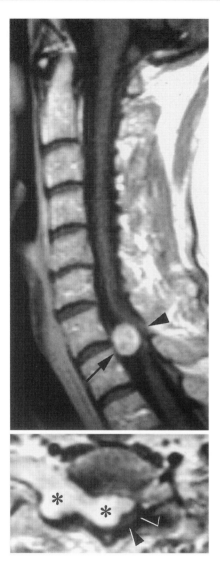

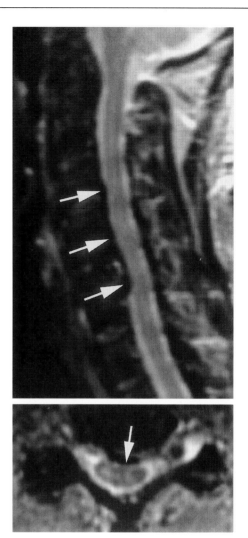

Figure 10.3

A 65-year-old man who had unilateral atrophy and weakness of intrinsic hand muscles and progressive leg spasticity was found to have a gadolinium-enhancing tumor on T1-weighted MRI at the C7–C8 intervertebral level (top; arrow) compressing the spinal cord (arrowhead). A transverse view at this level (bottom) reveals a 'dumb-bell-shaped' intradural neurinoma of the nerve root (asterisks) invading the spinal canal and severely compressing the spinal cord (arrowheads).

Figure 10.4

Multilevel compression of the anterior spinal cord (arrows) at C3–C6 vertebral levels is due to ossification of the posterior longitudinal ligament in a 75-year-old man who developed progressive gait difficulty, limb spasticity, and weakness. Associated lumbar canal stenosis (not shown) produced superimposed LMN signs, further suggesting ALS.

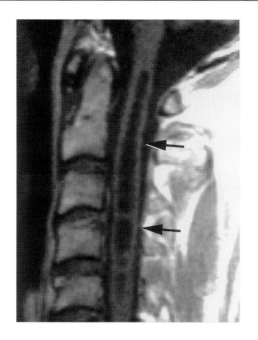

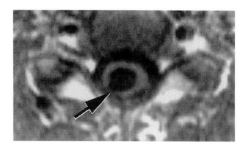

Figure 10.5
Syringomyelia of the cervical spinal cord (arrows) in a 49-year-old woman is evident by T1-weighted MRI in the sagittal plane (top) and the coronal plane (bottom). The patient had weakness and atrophy of the intrinsic hand muscles, which was initially thought to represent LMN-predominant ALS.

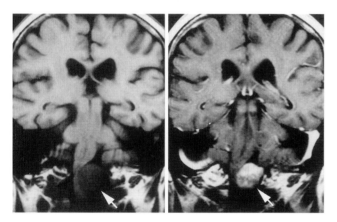

Figure 10.6
A 63-year-old woman with unilateral tongue atrophy, as well as arm and leg spasticity and weakness, was discovered to have a meningioma of the foramen magnum. This was noted (arrows) to cause severe lateral displacement and compression of the cervicomedullary junction on coronal MRI before (left) and after (right) gadolinium enhancement.

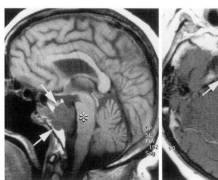

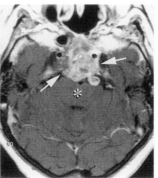

Figure 10.7
Compression of the basis pontis (asterisks) in a 74-year-old woman resulted from a clival chordoma (arrows) as seen in pre- (left) and post- (right) gadolinium T1-weighted images. The tumor caused lower extremity spasticity, facial weakness, and a subsequent abducens nerve palsy (which prompted the MRI).

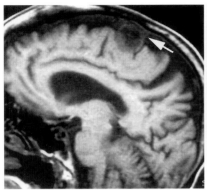
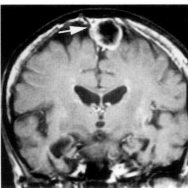

Figure 10.8
A 60-year-old woman with progressive leg weakness, initially thought to be due to UMN-predominant ALS, presented with a focal motor seizure. MRI in the sagittal (left) and coronal (right) planes reveals a meningioma arising from the falx cerebri (arrows), which enhanced after gadolinium administration (right; arrow).

Specific MRI abnormalities in ALS

Atrophy of brain and spinal cord

Brain and spinal cord atrophy have been reported anecdotally in ALS but few studies have carefully compared its frequency in patients and age-matched controls. Most studies, but not all, report some degree of atrophy in patients with motor neuron disease.[2–8] This is consistent with post mortem analyses, which have revealed varying degrees of atrophy.[9]

Brain atrophy

In one early CT study,[7] up to 64% of patients with all types of ALS (n = 50) were found to have cortical atrophy compared to 12% of controls (n = 50). It was bilateral and mild to moderate in degree, and it did not correlate with duration of disease. Interestingly, cortical atrophy was noted in 75% of patients with classic or bulbar ALS (n = 35) but only in 44% of patients with UMN-predominant ALS (n = 9). Even 16% of patients with no evidence of UMN pathology (n = 6) showed some degree of atrophy. The frontal cortex was only the

third most severely atrophied region (32%), after the parietal (50%) and insular (38%) cortices. These regions contribute in varying degrees to the corticospinal tract.

The corpus callosum has also been found to be atrophic anteriorly in 25 consecutive right-handed patients with ALS compared to 25 age- and sex-matched right-handed control subjects.[5] Five of the patients had cognitive decline and psychiatric symptoms. T1-weighted MRI revealed severe atrophy of the anterior fourth of the corpus callosum in the patients with higher cortical dysfunction.

A prospective CT and MRI study[6] of patients with ALS documented that cerebral atrophy first appeared in the frontal and anterior temporal lobes, next in the pre-central gyrus (primary motor cortex), and finally in the post-central gyrus (primary sensory cortex), cingular gyrus, and corpus callosum. Frontotemporal atrophy occurred most rapidly in patients with early respiratory failure and severe ophthalmoplegia but was absent in the three patients who survived 10–20 years without ventilatory support. This is in contrast to a case report of four patients with juvenile familial ALS and mean disease duration of 27 years.[3] All four patients had moderate or severe dementia and the patient undergoing MRI (who had been symptomatic for 21 years) had moderately severe atrophy of the cerebrum and brainstem.

This discrepancy between the two studies may be attributable to the presence of dementia. In an MRI planimetric study of 74 consecutive patients with sporadic ALS,[2] the subgroup with significant neuropsychologic impairment (n = 45) had significant atrophy compared to the subgroup with intact short-term memory and normal frontal lobe function. Another study of 26 patients with ALS documented frontal atrophy only in the subgroup (n = 14) with cognitive impairment.[4] Therefore, pooling ALS patients with and without neuropsychologic impairment may account for conflicting results in other earlier studies of cerebral atrophy.

Spinal cord atrophy

Visualization of spinal cord anatomy is much better with MRI than CT but is still limited on 1.5 T imaging systems. Several studies have reported the MRI appearance of the spinal cord in ALS but atrophy has been rarely documented.[8] Mild atrophy of the cervical spinal cord was reported in a 51-year-old woman with bulbar-onset ALS and prominent UMN signs.[10] However, the atrophy was minor compared to hyperintensity of the lateral and ventral corticospinal tracts seen on T2-weighted sequences. Corticospinal tract hyperintensity in ALS has been described primarily intracranially and is discussed below. The most convincing changes in spinal cord atrophy have been demonstrated in patients with benign focal amyotrophy (monomelic amyotrophy or juvenile amyotrophy of the distal arms).[11] This is a slowly progressive focal motor neuron disease in which there is degeneration of anterior horn cells, usually in the lower cervical cord,

with resulting spinal cord atrophy. Demonstrating spinal cord atrophy in such patients may help differentiate this relatively benign condition from the early stages of juvenile-onset ALS.

Corticospinal tract hyperintensity

The increasing use of MRI to evaluate the CNS of patients with suspected ALS is revealing parenchymal pathology not previously detected by CT. Bilateral, usually symmetrical, hyperintensity (increased signal) of the corticospinal (or pyramidal) tract on T2- and proton density-weighted MRI is the most characteristic neuroimaging finding in ALS.[8,12–18] It probably represents wallerian degeneration of the corticospinal tract[19] and is visualized more frequently in the cerebrum than the spinal cord. Although it is not pathognomonic of ALS, its occurrence in the appropriate clinical setting and without structural abnormalities makes the diagnosis very likely.

Intracranial hyperintensity

Since the first MRI report in 1988 of subcortical white matter hyperintensity in two patients with ALS,[20] this observation has been confirmed by many groups.[8,12,14–18,21] Hyperintensity of the corticospinal tract has been documented primarily by T2-weighted MRI at 1.5 T at almost every level along its intracranial trajectory from beneath the primary motor cortex, through the centrum semiovale, the posterior limb of the internal capsule, and the cerebral peduncles, into the pons (*Figs 10.9* and *10.10*). This abnormality is most easily identified in the internal capsules and cerebral peduncles but it is almost never seen in the medulla, possibly because of technical limitations. A combined neuroimaging and pathologic study showed that the hyperintensity corresponded to the demyelination and degen-

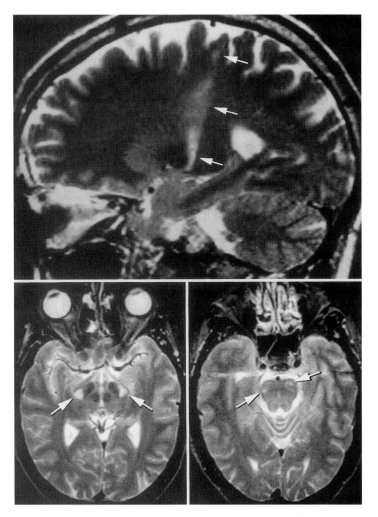

Figure 10.9
Corticospinal tract hyperintensity in a 35-year-old man with ALS is noted on T2-weighted MR brain images to extend from the subcortical white matter and internal capsule (top; arrows) to the cerebral peduncles (bottom left; arrows) and basis pontis (bottom right; arrows).

eration of the large-caliber corticospinal tract fibers.[19] Hyperintense signal has also been observed in the middle third of the corpus callosum in ALS,[14,16] where post mortem study has revealed a discrete bundle of degenerated fibers,[9] which probably represents homotopic fiber connections between the precentral gyri.

The reported frequency of such corticospinal tract hyperintensity in patients with ALS ranges from 17% to 100% (median 40%), depending on the study.[8] Similar findings have been reported in other forms of motor neuron degeneration, including primary lateral sclerosis, familial ALS, and juvenile-onset ALS.[22] Its relatively frequent occurrence may represent the better detection of these changes by modern-day MRI or it may reflect a referral bias in the patient population studied. However, it is possible that corticospinal tract hyperintensity occurs in a specific subset

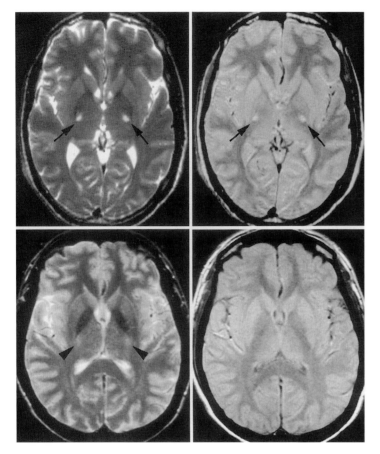

Figure 10.10
Prominent hyperintensities can be seen (arrows) in the posterior third of the posterior limb of the internal capsule on T2-weighted MRI (top left) and proton density-weighted MRI (top right) in patients with ALS. Healthy subjects occasionally have faint hyperintensities here on T2-weighted MRI (bottom left) but not on proton density-weighted MRI (bottom right).

of patients with motor neuron disease. Based on published descriptions and in comparison to those with no MRI abnormality, these patients tend to be female and younger and to have prominent UMN features (e.g. spasticity, hyper-reflexia, and a Babinski reflex) and a shorter duration of disease, which may be more rapidly progressive. Analysis of pooled data from such studies (*t* test assuming unequal variances) revealed no statistically significant differences between the two groups for most of these features.[8] However, ALS patients with corticospinal tract hyperintensities were significantly ($p < 0.001$) younger

(50.7 ± 11.0 years, mean $\pm$ standard deviation; n = 42) than those without such MRI abnormalities (59.0 ± 10.7 years, n = 74). Although the likelihood of detecting corticospinal tract hyperintensities in younger patients with ALS may be greater simply because they will undergo MRI more readily, they may represent a subgroup with earlier disease onset.

Not infrequently, healthy subjects also have a region of hyperintensity in the posterior limb of the internal capsule detected by T2-weighted MRI (see *Fig. 10.10*).[8,12,17,23] Depending on the report, between 53% and 76%

(median 57%) of normal subjects have a relatively faint, circumscribed hyperintensity that is not visualized beyond the internal capsule and upper cerebral peduncle levels. It probably arises from the aggregated, myelinated, large-diameter axons of the normal corticospinal tract in this location.[19] Most importantly, this hyperintensity in normal subjects is visible only on T2-weighted and FLAIR (fluid attenuated inversion recovery)[14] sequences and not on proton-density MRI (see *Fig. 10.10*).[8,17,23] Therefore, proton density-weighted sequences should be included in the imaging protocol because they are more specific than T2-weighted sequences in revealing the abnormal hyperintensities in the corticospinal tracts of ALS patients.

In addition to T2-related corticospinal tract hyperintensity, one group has reported its visualization on T1-weighted sequences.[21] This was speculated to arise from cellular pathological changes occurring in ALS, including accumulation of lipid-laden macrophages, neurofilaments, and toxic metals. These T1-weighted hyperintensities were more common in the anterolateral columns of the spinal cord (67%) than intracranially (24%) (see below).

Spinal cord hyperintensity

The demonstration of hyperintense signal in the corticospinal tract of the spinal cord on T2-weighted MRI scans is relatively rare. This may be due either to technical limitations of detection by MRI or a real difference in corticospinal tract pathology at the spinal cord level. It has been reported in only 16 patients with ALS, most of whom also had intracranial hyperintensities.[8,14,21] As with intracranial corticospinal tract hyperintensities, those in the spinal cord probably result from axonal degeneration and demyelination.

As mentioned above, T1-weighted hyperintensities have been described in the anterolat-eral columns of the spinal cord in some ALS patients. Of 21 patients studied, 14 (67%) had this change while only seven showed T2-related hyperintensities.[21] No definite relationship was observed between the T1-related spinal cord hyperintensities and clinical features such as symptom duration or severity of UMN signs. It will be notable if other groups report similar T1-weighted hyperintensities in brain or spinal cord of patients with ALS.

Neocortical hypointensity

Another T2-weighted MRI abnormality reported in the brains of 35–93% (median = 52%) of patients with ALS is a hypointensity (diminished signal) of the neocortical gray matter.[8,13–15,18] This has been observed bilaterally, primarily in the pre-central gyrus but also in the post-central gyrus. Some patients with ALS show both cortical hypointensity and corticospinal tract hyperintensity. The ribbon-like hypointensity is rather obvious because of the hyperintense signal of cerebrospinal fluid in adjacent sulci (*Fig. 10.11*). It probably arises from neuronal degeneration and accumulation of a paramagnetic substance based on finding iron-laden astrocytes and macrophages in the pre-central cortex of such brains post mortem.[24]

Although this MRI abnormality occurs in a proportion of patients with typical ALS, its observation in some patients with Alzheimer's disease[8] and even in healthy subjects[14,18,25] limits its usefulness as a neuroimaging sign in isolation. Nevertheless, a diminished signal in the primary motor cortex on T2-weighted MRI scans of patients presenting with features of ALS supports the diagnosis of ALS.

Brain hypometabolism in ALS

PET and SPECT are nuclear medicine techniques that have been used to assess cerebral

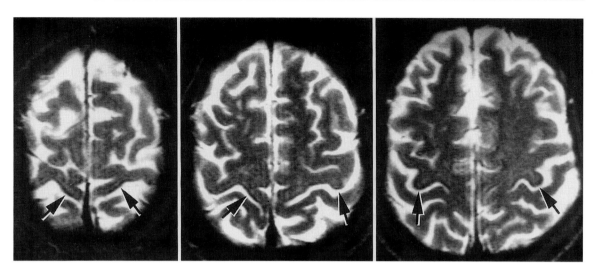

Figure 10.11
A 54-year-old man with ALS is found on T2-weighted MRI to have a thin ribbon-like band of hypointensity along the posterior margin of the pre-central gyrus (the primary motor cortex) shown here at three transverse levels (arrows).

blood flow and neuronal metabolism in various disease states, including ALS.[8,26–28] Patients with motor neuron disease, particularly ALS, have decreased cerebral blood flow and, therefore, diminished neuronal metabolism, primarily in sensorimotor regions. There are usually no changes on routine neuroimaging although some of these patients have hyperintensity of the corticospinal tract revealed by T2- and proton density-weighted MRI (*Fig. 10.12*). Cerebral blood flow abnormalities in extra-motor regions have also been detected by PET and SPECT in some ALS patients with clinical or subclinical dementia. Although these nuclear medicine techniques have been used primarily for research purposes, they may assist in the clinical diagnosis of motor neuron disease, particularly in cases associated with dementia.

PET

Results from PET studies in ALS patients have been somewhat inconsistent, at least in part because of differences in technique and analysis of statistical data.[8,26–32] Various radiolabeled isotopes have been utilized: [^{18}F]2-fluoro-2-deoxy-D-glucose (FDG) for measurements while the subject is at rest, and oxygen-15 gas (^{15}O) or oxygen-15-labeled carbon dioxide (C^{15}O$_2$) primarily for studies while the subject performs certain motor tasks. The latter studies have provided information on the dynamic state of brain activation in ALS and revealed abnormalities when measurements at rest were normal.

PET studies at rest
In general, non-demented patients with ALS at rest appear to have at least a trend towards

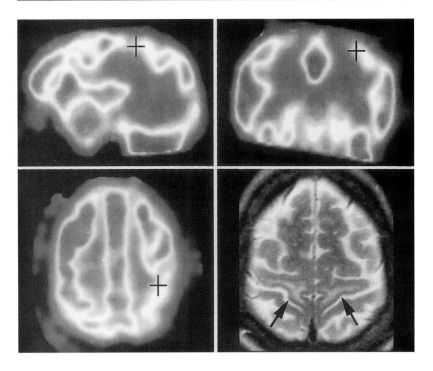

Figure 10.12
PET reveals diminished metabolism of [^{18}F]2-fluoro-2-deoxy-D-glucose in subcortical frontoparietal regions (next to cross) in the sagittal plane (upper left), the coronal plane (upper right), and the transverse plane (lower left) from a 55-year-old woman with ALS. T2-weighted MRI of the equivalent brain level (bottom right) reveals diffuse hyperintensity at the origin of the corticospinal tract (arrows) in the subcortical white matter of the pre-central gyrus (the primary motor cortex).

diminished brain glucose metabolism in the sensorimotor cortex and basal ganglia.[26] Patients who are demented or have neuro-psychological dysfunction of the frontal lobes have more significant FDG hypometabolism in frontal (superior and inferior) and temporal (superior and mesial) cortical regions.[27] The regional distribution of hypometabolism in ALS patients with dementia is the opposite to that of patients with Alzheimer's dementia, the latter having metabolism that is low in the parietal cortex and normal in the frontal lobes. The association of ALS with parkinsonism (e.g. Guamanian ALS) prompted 6-fluorodopa PET studies in patients with sporadic ALS.[31] Compared to age-matched controls, striatal 6-fluorodopa uptake progressively decreased as the ALS progressed.

PET studies with activation

Results of PET studies using ^{15}O and C^{15}O$_2$ to measure regional cerebral blood flow and oxygen metabolic rate in patients with ALS making freely selected joystick movements suggested cortical reorganization and abnormal recruitment of non-primary motor areas as a result of motor neuron loss.[29] Stereotyped movements in ALS patients revealed impaired activation in frontal lobe regions, suggesting underlying frontal lobe cognitive deficits even though none of the patients was clinically demented. Similar activation PET studies of five patients with LMN-predominant ALS have uncovered cortical dysfunction (anterior insular cortex) even when no abnormalities were detectable at rest.[30] Abnormal activation of this perisylvian area was thought to reflect recruitment of an accessory sensorimotor area in response to limb weakness. Testing of verbal fluency and executive frontal lobe function have identified other extramotor neuronal deficits, especially along a thalamofrontal association pathway in some patients with ALS.[32]

SPECT

Unlike PET studies, SPECT studies do not measure cerebral blood flow, although values in ALS are usually expressed relative to blood flow in regions not affected (e.g. cerebellum).[4,8] The potential clinical usefulness of SPECT over PET arises from several differences:

(a) more widely available machines and familiarity of technique;
(b) less complex technical support; and
(c) less expensive and more stable radiochemicals (e.g. ^{123}I-iodoamphetamine, [^{99m}Tc]-D, L-hexamethyl-propylene-amineoxime

The majority of studies have revealed regional cerebral hypoperfusion in motor and pre-motor areas of many patients with ALS. Those with superimposed dementia have more widespread hypoperfusion, including hypoperfusion of regions anterior and often inferior to the primary motor cortex. As with PET studies at rest, SPECT abnormalities were not found in patients with LMN-predominant ALS.

New imaging modalities in ALS

Several relatively novel neuroimaging modalities are being employed to study the brains of patients with ALS. These modalities are all based on magnetic resonance technology and include:

(a) ^{1}H-MRS;
(b) fMRI;

(c) DWI; and
(d) MTI.

All techniques are possible on clinically available 1.5 T strength magnets, although higher field strength magnets (e.g. 3 T) may be advantageous for most of these modalities. Experience with these techniques is limited in ALS except for ^{1}H-MRS,[33] which was the first of these magnetic resonance technologies to be explored in studying this disease. Much remains to be learned about how useful each of these modalities will be in furthering our understanding of ALS. Only an abbreviated introduction is given for each of these methodologies; the interested reader is referred to articles dealing with the specific techniques for details.

^{1}H-MRS

^{1}H-MRS non-invasively measures certain proton-containing, non-water compounds that may be altered in various diseases.[34] The most easily detected are the *N*-acetyl (NA) groups (e.g. *N*-acetyl aspartate (NAA) and *N*-acetyl aspartyl glutamate (NAAG)), which, in the mature brain, are found only in neurons. In the cerebrum, most of the NA groups are composed of NAA, whereas in the brainstem, the contribution from NAAG is significant. Therefore, the NAA resonance can be used as a surrogate marker of neuronal integrity (including axonal and dendritic integrity), at least in the cerebrum. Other prominent metabolites include choline (Cho), a component of lipid in cell membranes that does not appear to be significantly altered in ALS[33,35,36] and creatine phosphocreatine (Cr), compounds involved in energy metabolism that are distributed relatively evenly in all brain cells and are used to normalize the signal from the other metabolites. A decrease in the resonance intensity of NAA relative to Cr can therefore be an in vivo

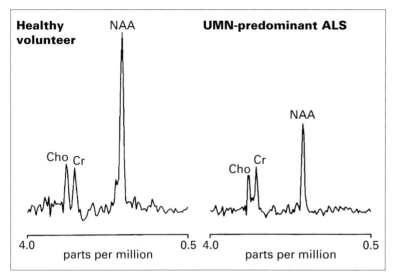

Figure 10.13

Compared to proton magnetic resonance spectra from the primary motor cortex of a healthy volunteer (left), a patient with UMN-predominant ALS (right) has a lower N-acetylaspartate (NAA) signal relative to creatine (Cr). There is no significant change in the choline (Cho) signal intensity. (Adapted from Pioro et al.[35])

index of neuronal loss or dysfunction, as shown in a patient with UMN-predominant ALS (*Fig. 10.13*). Therefore, ^{1}H-MRS could potentially assess the existence and degree of UMN pathology in ALS, which is difficult to do objectively.

The first ^{1}H-MRS study of patients with motor neuron disease revealed evidence of neuronal loss or damage in the neocortex and subjacent white matter of patients with ALS but not of patients with progressive muscular atrophy.[35] Because the spectra in this study were simultaneously acquired from multiple volume elements (voxels), data from multiple cortical gyri could be analysed. Compared with healthy controls, patients with ALS had the lowest NAA-to-Cr ratios in the primary sensorimotor cortex; lesser but still significant decreases were found in the posterior pre-motor and superior parietal gyrus–precuneate regions. No abnormalities were detected in the most anterior portion of the superior frontal gyrus. Patients with definite UMN signs ('classic' ALS; n = 12) had lower NAA-to-Cr ratios than those with promi-

nent LMN signs who had probably upper motor neuron signs (ALS-PUMNS; n = 12) (*Fig. 10.14*) Evidence that a decreased NAA-to-Cr ratio represents pathology of the corticomotoneuron (at least) includes the presence of normal ratios in patients with progressive muscular atrophy who had no UMN signs and of lower ratios in patients with more prominent UMN signs (classic ALS) compared to those with ALS-PUMNS. Furthermore, continued decline of the NAA-to-Cr ratio in the sensorimotor cortex of a patient who underwent repeat ^{1}H-MRS after 8 months of clinical deterioration was consistent with progressive neuronal dysfunction or loss. This and most of the subsequent ^{1}H-MRS studies, which have confirmed and expanded upon the aforementioned findings, utilized a long echo-time (TE), which reveals the three major metabolites studied in ALS (i.e. NAA, Cho, and Cr).[33] Short TE ^{1}H-MRS, on the other hand, allows visualization of additional metabolites, including myo-inositol, glutamate (Glu) and glutamine (Gln) which are of potential interest in ALS.

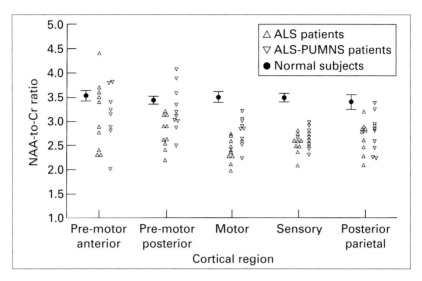

Figure 10.14

Scatterplot of individual ratios of N-acetylaspartate (NAA) to creatine (Cr) in five cortical regions of patients with classic ALS (n = 12) and with ALS-PUMNS (n = 12). Compared to the means (± SEM) from healthy age-matched controls (n = 10), statistically significant decreases occur in both patient groups in the primary motor and primary sensory cortices (p < 0.05). NAA-to-Cr ratios are significantly lower in the posterior portion of the pre-motor cortex and posterior parietal cortex only in ALS patients and are not different from normal subjects in more anterior regions. Statistical analysis was by Wilcoxon rank sum test. (Data from Pioro et al.[35])

A preliminary short TE ¹H-MRS study of the medulla oblongata revealed a diminished NA-to-Cr ratio ($p < 0.05$) in patients with definite or probable ALS (n = 6), as defined by the El Escorial criteria,[1] compared to healthy individuals (n = 6).[33] This is consistent with the pathology, which occurs in lower cranial nerve nuclei and corticospinal (pyramidal) tracts in ALS, sometimes before more rostral regions are affected.[9] Of particular interest, these patients had an abnormally increased Glu + Gln signal ($p < 0.05$) providing the first in vivo evidence of disturbed Glu metabolism in ALS. Whether this is primary or secondary to the neuronal (and axonal) degeneration, however, requires further study.

More recently, a long TE ¹H-MRS study at 3 T in the brainstem (upper medulla and pontine tegmentum) in patients with probable or definite ALS (n = 12) revealed significantly decreased NA-to-Cr ratios compared to healthy controls (n = 17).[36] An inverse relationship was observed between the NA-to-Cr ratio in the brainstem and the severity of spasticity or bulbar weakness.

A multislice multinoxel ¹H-MRS analysis of frontoparietal cortex and subcortical corticospinal tract pathways revealed regional reductions in the NAA-to-Cho + Cr ratio in 10 patients with definite or probable ALS compared to nine normal subjects.[37] Reductions in this ratio ranged between 16% and

19% and were significant ($p = 0.02$) only in the motor cortex and related subcortical corticospinal tract regions. Significant positive correlation was noted between the cortical NAA-to-Cho + Cr ratios and maximum finger-tap rate ($r = 0.80$; $p = 0.01$), suggesting that the reduction in cortical signal was a surrogate marker of corticomotoneuron loss in ALS.

Both long and short TE were used in a single-voxel ^{1}H-MRS study of the pre-central gyrus in 33 patients with motor neuron disease and 24 healthy controls.[38] NAA-to-Cr ratios and NAA-to-Cho ratios were both significantly lower in the ALS patient, especially in the subgroup with definite UMN signs; the Cho-to-Cr ratio was increased, but only in the latter subgroup. Follow-up scans, which were obtained in nine patients up to 2 years later, revealed progressive reduction primarily in NAA-to-Cho ratios. This decrease was most dramatic in patients with the most normal ratios on initial investigation, such as one patient initially thought to have a pure LMN syndrome but who subsequently developed UMN signs.

^{1}H-MRS at 4.7 T has also been used to examine an animal model of motor neuron disease, the wobbler mouse, for evidence of cerebral neuronal pathology.[39] Compared to healthy littermates ($n = 5$), 8–12-week-old mutant animals ($n = 5$) were found to have significantly decreased ($p < 0.006$) NAA-to-Cr ratios, but not Cho-to-Cr ratios, in the cortex and subcortex. Included in the 63 μl voxel analysed were neocortex, caudate–putamen, thalamus, and hippocampus (*Fig. 10.15*), any of which could have contributed to the reduced NAA-to-Cr ratio. Immunocytochemical markers of neuronal pathology, as present in ALS (e.g. phosphorylated heavy neurofilament, ubiquitin), were found only in neocortical regions of the wobbler mice.

Other magnetic resonance modalities

Relatively little has been done to date in ALS using other magnetic resonance-related techniques, such as DWI, fMRI, and MTI. Except for a few published reports, other studies have been presented either in abstract form or as discussions at a workshop sponsored by the ALS Association ('New NMR Science and ALS') on 21–22 May 1998 in Warrenton, Virginia, USA.

DWI

DWI is based on visualizing the random movement of water molecules in and among various tissue components and how this movement is influenced in health and in disease states.[40] The extent of such movement, or 'diffusion', is restricted by normal structures (e.g. neurons, neuroglia, and axons in the CNS); this produces the apparent diffusion coefficient (ADC). There is normal variability in the ADC because of structural heterogeneity, especially in white matter tracts such as the corticospinal tract. The ADC is higher along their length and less across it revealing an asymmetry which is termed 'anistrophy'. In circumstances in which the ADC is not asymmetric (e.g. in the cortex), there is isotropy. Various pathologies (e.g. edema, demyelination, wallerian degeneration) can alter the ADC and anisotropy, resulting in regional changes in image appearance. Because diffusion in three dimensions cannot be adequately expressed as a single ADC, the motion is characterized in mathematical terms by the 'diffusion tensor'. The 'trace' of the diffusion tensor is also useful because it is independent of diffusion gradient orientation and provides an image related to mean diffusivity.[41]

In a study of 18 patients with ALS, 20 healthy controls, and 25 neurologic controls (stroke patients), no differences were noted in

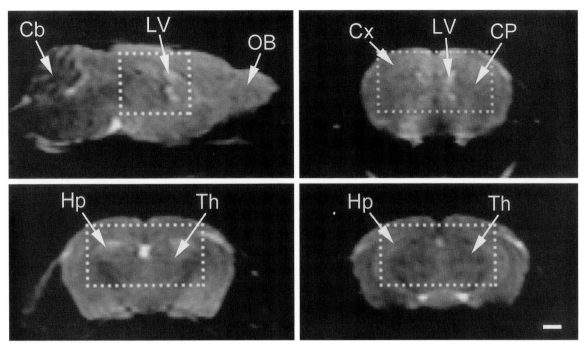

Figure 10.15
One sagittal T2-weighted brain image (upper left) and three coronal T2-weighted brain images from a wobbler mouse (1.0 mm thick and 0.5 mm interslice gap) demonstrate structures within the volume of interest undergoing ^{1}H-MRS: parasagittal cortex (Cx), caudate–putamen (CP), hippocampus (Hp), and thalamus (Th). The dimensions of the volume of interest are 3.0 mm craniocaudal, 6.0 mm left to right, and 3.5 mm anteroposterior. Cb, cerebellum; LV, lateral ventricle; OB, olfactory bulb. Scale bar = 1 mm.

the diffusion coefficients perpendicular to the corticospinal tract in the posterior limb of the internal capsule. However, in five patients who had discrete paraventricular lesions, diffusion coefficients of this region were increased in all directions and anisotropy was therefore lost. This suggested that the pathology in the paraventricular region was different from that in the internal capsule.[42]

Of relevance to examining corticospinal tract degeneration in ALS, a preliminary DWI study using diffusion tensor (and trace) and diffusion anisotropy identified wallerian degeneration in the brainstem of patients with

chronic unilateral stroke (n = 10) compared to healthy subjects (n = 8).[43] The midbrain and medulla clearly showed wallerian degeneration (increased signal on trace, decreased anisotropy). Paradoxical findings in the pons of an apparent change in the orientation of the descending corticospinal tract fibers were probably related to the remaining pontine fibers, which are transversely oriented.

fMRI

Activation of the cerebral cortex results in increased regional blood flow, which in turn results in a relative local decrease in blood deoxyhemoglobin. Differences in the magnetic field characteristics of deoxyhemoglobin and oxyhemoglobin in activated areas result in increased signal intensity on fMRI.[44]

Only a limited number of fMRI studies have been reported on patients with ALS. Based on a preliminary report[45] and the author's own observations, performance of a simple motor paradigm (e.g. finger tapping) results in activation of regions outside the normal sensorimotor cortex area. This expanded somatopic representation is similar to what has been reported in earlier PET studies of patients with ALS (see above). However, an unexpected observation was the alteration of cortical activation following sensory stimulation of the hand and foot of patients with ALS compared to controls. In the patients with ALS, mechanical stimulation of the palm resulted in diminished activation of sensorimotor cortex. Plantar stimulation (to elicit a Babinski response), in contrast, resulted in increased ipsilateral and extrasensorimotor cortex activation in the patients with ALS.

MTI

Cross-relaxation between free ('mobile') water protons and restricted protons in macromolecules is the basis of MTI. This technique serves to enhance contrast or itself provide a novel contrast mechanism, which allows quantification of structural or biochemical changes in certain pathologic states.[46] MTI shows significant promise in the study of CNS lesions in multiple sclerosis, but its use in ALS has been very limited.

Magnetization transfer measurements were performed in the brains of patients with ALS (n = 9) and control subjects (n = 9).[47] Magnetization transfer ratios (MTRs) of a 3 mm diameter circular region were obtained from the posterior third of the posterior limb of the internal capsule (the location of the corti-

cospinal tract) as well as from widespread gray and white matter areas. Only the region of the corticospinal tract in the posterior limb of the internal capsule revealed a significantly lower mean MTR in patients compared to controls ($p < 0.0007$). This decrease was proposed to represent degeneration of the corticospinal tract. It is of note that all patients had MTRs below the normal mean, although only three (33%) had T2-weighted corticospinal tract hyperintensity in this location. This suggests that MTI may be able to detect earlier stages of corticospinal tract degeneration. However, no relationships were observed between MTR and ALS scores, duration of illness, or signal intensity on T2-weighted images.

References

1. Brooks, BR. El Escorial World Federation of Neurology. Criteria for the diagnosis of amytrophic lateral sclerosis. *J Neurol Sci* 1994; **124 (suppl)**: 96–107.
2. Frank B, Haas J, Heinze HK et al. Relation of neuropsychological and magnetic resonance findings in amyotrophic lateral sclerosis: evidence for subgroups. *Clin Neurol Neurosurg* 1997; **99**: 79–86.
3. Otero Siliceo E, Arriada-Mendicoa N, Balderrama J. Juvenile familial amyotrophic lateral sclerosis: four cases with long survival. *Dev Med Child Neurol* 1998; **40**: 425–428.
4. Abe K, Fujimura H, Toyooka K et al. Cognitive function in amyotrophic lateral sclerosis. *J Neurol Sci* 1997; **148**: 95–100.
5. Yamauchi H, Fukuyama H, Ouchi Y et al. Corpus callosum atrophy in amyotrophic lateral sclerosis. *J Neurol Sci* 1995; **134**: 189–196.
6. Kato S, Hayashi H, Yagishita A. Involvement of the frontotemporal lobe and limbic system in amyotrophic lateral sclerosis: as assessed by serial computed tomography and magnetic resonance imaging. *J Neurol Sci* 1993; **116**: 52–58.
7. Poloni M, Mascherpa C, Faggi L et al. Cere-

bral atrophy in motor neuron disease evaluated by computed tomography. *J Neurol Neurosurg Psychiatry* 1982; **45**: 1102–1105.

8. Mitsumoto H, Chad DC, Pioro EP. *Amyotrophic Lateral Sclerosis*. Philadelphia: FA Davis, 1997, 134–150.

9. Brownell B, Oppenheimer DR, Hughes JT. The central nervous system in motor neurone disease. *J Neurol Neurosurg Psychiatry* 1970; **33**: 338–357.

10. Friedman DP, Tartaglino LM. Amyotrophic lateral sclerosis: hyperintensity of the corticospinal tracts on MR images of the spinal cord. *Am J Radiol* 1993; **160**: 604–606.

11. Biondi A, Dormont D, Weitzner IJ et al. MR imaging of the cervical cord in juvenile amyotrophy of distal upper extremity. *AJNR* 1989; **10**: 263–268.

12. Abe K, Fujimura H, Kobayashi Y et al. Degeneration of the pyramidal tracts in patients with amyotrophic lateral sclerosis. A premortem and postmortem magnetic resonance imaging study. *J Neuroimaging* 1997; **7**: 208–212.

13. Waragai M, Shinotoh H, Hayashi M, Hattori T. High signal intensity on T1 weighted MRI of anterolateral column of the spinal cord in amyotrophic lateral sclerosis. *J Neurol Neurosurg Psychiatry* 1997; **62**: 88–91.

14. Thorpe JW, Moseley IF, Hawkes CH et al. Brain and spinal cord MRI in motor neuron disease. *J Neurol Neurosurg Psychiatry* 1996; **61**: 314–317.

15. Waragai M, Takaya Y, Hayashi M. Serial MRI and SPECT in amyotrophic lateral sclerosis: a case report. *J Neurol Sci* 1997; **148**: 117–120.

16. Van Zandijcke M, Casselman J. Involvement of corpus callosum in amyotrophic lateral sclerosis shown by MRI. *Neuroradiology* 1995; **37**: 287–288.

17. Hofmann E, Ochs G, Pelzl A, Warmuth-Metz M. The corticospinal tract in amyotrophic lateral sclerosis: an MRI study. *Neuroradiology* 1998; **40**: 71–75.

18. Fazekas G, Kleinert G, Schmidt R et al. Magnetic resonance tomography of the brain in amyotrophic lateral sclerosis. *Wien Med Wochensch* 1996; **146**: 204–206.

19. Yagishita A, Nakano I, Oda M, Hirano A. Location of the corticospinal tract in the internal capsule at MR imaging. *Radiology* 1994; **191**: 455–460.

20. Goodin DS, Rowley HA, Olney RK. Magnetic resonance imaging in amyotrophic lateral sclerosis. *Ann Neurol* 1988; **23**: 418–420.

21. Waragai M. MRI and clinical features in amyotrophic lateral sclerosis. *Neuroradiology* 1997; **39**: 847–851.

22. Midani H, Truwit CL, Parry GJ. MRI in juvenile ALS: a patient report. *Neurology* 1998; **50**: 1879–1881.

23. Guermazi A. Is high signal intensity in the corticospinal tract a sign of degeneration (letter)? *AJNR* 1996; **17**: 801–802.

24. Oba H, Araki T, Ohtomo K et al. Amyotrophic lateral sclerosis: T2 shortening in motor cortex at MR imaging. *Radiology* 1993; **189**: 843–846.

25. Iwasaki Y, Ikeda K, Shiojima T et al. Clinical significance of hypointensity in the motor cortex on T2-weighted images. *Neurology* 1994; **44**: 1181.

26. Hoffman JM, Mazziotta JC, Hawk TC, Sumida R. Cerebral glucose utilization in motor neuron disease. *Arch Neuro* 1992; **49**: 849–854.

27. Levine RL, Brooks BR, Matthews CG et al. Frontotemporal hypometabolism in amyotrophic lateral sclerosis–dementia complex. *J Neuroimaging* 1993; **3**: 234–241.

28. Tanaka M, Kondo S, Hirai S et al. Cerebral blood flow and oxygen metabolism in progressive dementia associated with amyotrophic lateral sclerosis. *J Neurol Sci* 1993; **120**: 22–28.

29. Kew JJ, Leigh PN, Playford ED et al. Cortical function in amyotrophic lateral sclerosis. A positron emission tomography study. *Brain* 1993; **116**: 655–680.

30. Kew JJ, Brooks DJ, Passingham RE et al. Cortical function in progressive lower motor neuron disorders and amyotrophic lateral sclerosis: a comparative PET study. *Neurology* 1994; **44**: 1101–1110.

31. Takahashi H, Snow BJ, Bhatt MH et al. Evidence for a dopaminergic deficit in sporadic amyotrophic lateral sclerosis on positron emission scanning. *Lancet* 1993; **342**: 1016–1018.

32. Abrahams S, Goldstein LH, Kew JJ et al. Frontal lobe dysfunction in amyotrophic lateral sclerosis. A PET study. *Brain* 1996; **119**: 2105–2120.

33. Pioro EP. MR spectroscopy in amyotrophic lateral sclerosis/motor neuron disease. *J Neurol Sci* 1997; **152 (suppl 1)**: S49–S53.

34. Castillo M, Kwock L, Mukherji SK. Clinical applications of proton MR spectroscopy. *AJNR* 1996; **17**: 1–15.

35. Pioro EP, Antel JP, Cashman NR, Arnold DL. Detection of cortical neuron loss in motor neuron disease by proton magnetic resonance spectroscopic imaging in vivo. *Neurology* 1994; **44**: 1933–1938.

36. Cwik VA, Hanstock C, Allen PS. Martin MRW. Estimation of brainstem neuronal loss in ALS with in vivo proton MR spectroscopy. *Neurology* 1998; **50**: 72–77.

37. Rooney WD, Miller RG, Gelinas D et al. Decreased N-acetylaspartate in motor cortex and corticospinal tract in ALS. *Neurology* 1998; **50**: 1800–1805.

38. Block W. Karitzky J, Traber F et al. Proton magnetic resonance spectroscopy of the primary motor cortex in patients with motor neuron disease: subgroup analysis and follow-up measurements. *Arch Neurol* 1998; **55**: 931–936.

39. Pioro EP, Wang Y, Moore JK et al. Neuronal pathology in the wobbler mouse brain revealed by in vivo proton magnetic resonance spectroscopy and immunocytochemistry. *NeuroReport* 1998; **9**: 3041–3046.

40. Le Bihan D, Breton E, Aubin ML. MR imaging of intravoxel incoherent motions: application to diffusion and perfusion in neurologic disorders. *Radiology* 1986; **161**: 401–407.

41. Basser PJ, Mattiello J, Le Bihan D. MR diffusion tensor spectroscopy and imaging. *Biophys J* 1994; **66**: 259–267.

42. Segawa F, Kishibayashi J, Kamada K et al. MRI of paraventricular white matter lesions in amyotrophic lateral sclerosis — analysis by diffusion-weighted images. *Brain Nerve* 1994; **46**: 835–840.

43. Pierpaoli C, Barnett A, Virta A et al. Diffusion MRI of wallerian degeneration. A new tool to investigate neuronal connectivity in vivo (abstract)? *Prac Intl Soc Magn Res Med* 1998: 1247.

44. Ogawa S, Menon RS, Kim SG, Ugurbil K. On the characteristics of functional magnetic resonance imaging of the brain. *Annu Rev Biophys Biomol Struct* 1998; **27**: 447–474.

45. Khan A, Fernandez-Schmidt D, Bushara K et al. Differential sensorimotor cortex (SMC) activation following cutaneous stimulation of the hand and foot in amyotrophic lateral sclerosis (ALS) — the effect of the Babinski response: a functional magnetic resonance imaging (fMRI) study (abstract). *Neurology* 1998; **50 (suppl 4)**: A316–A317.

46. Finelli DA. Magnetization transfer in neuroimaging *MRI Clinics of North America*, 1998; **6**: 31–52.

47. Kato Y, Matsumura K, Kinosada Y et al. Detection of pyramidal tract lesions in amyotrophic lateral sclerosis with magnetization-transfer measurements. *AJNR* 1997; **18**: 1541–1547.

SECTION IV

PATHOGENESIS

11

Oxidative stress in amyotrophic lateral sclerosis: pathogenic mechanism or epiphenomenon?

Wim L Robberecht and JMB Vianney de Jong

Reactive oxygen species (ROS) are generated in many biological oxidation reactions. ROS can induce lethal cellular damage through oxidation and peroxidation of proteins, lipids, and nucleic acids. Therefore, cells and tissues are provided with antioxidant defence systems. Various enzyme systems (e.g. superoxide dismutase, catalase, and glutathion peroxidase) convert ROS into (more) innocent molecules, and compounds such as vitamin E and vitamin C are ROS scavengers.

If the generation of ROS outweighs the scavenging capacity of the cell, because of increased ROS production or loss of cellular antioxidant defence systems, oxidative stress emerges. This process is thought to contribute to a variety of processes such as aging, ischemic cell death, and neurodegenerative disease. Oxidation-induced damage has been demonstrated in human sporadic and familial amyotrophic lateral sclerosis (ALS) and in transgenic mice overexpressing a mutant *SOD1* gene (mt*SOD1*). The mechanism of this damage and its pathogenic significance remain unclear.

Evidence for increased generation of ROS in ALS

Mutations in the *SOD1* gene on chromosome 21 are present in about 15–20% of families with familial ALS.[1] This gene encodes the cytosolic copper- and zinc-dependent superoxide dismutase (SOD1), an enzyme that acts as a homodimer and converts superoxide anions into hydrogen peroxide, which is then further metabolized by glutathion peroxidase and catalase.[2]

The available evidence suggests that the mutant SOD1 (mtSOD1) gains a novel cytotoxic activity. This 'gain of function' may involve oxidative stress as a crucial pathophysiological process (*Fig. 11.1*).

One possible explanation is that the mutations affect the protein's conformation so that the copper in the active center of the mutant molecule becomes accessible to substrates other than superoxide. Two possible substrates have been suggested: hydrogen peroxide and peroxynitrate ($ONOO^-$).

In several[3,4] but not all[5] biochemical studies, mtSOD1 was found to have enhanced peroxidase activity, through which the enzyme converts hydrogen peroxide into toxic hydroxyl radicals. The mutated enzyme would thus be a source of toxic ROS rather than a scavenger. It has proven to be difficult to demonstrate such ROS-generating activity in intact cells. PC12 cells transduced with mtSOD1 with the A4V and V148G mutation (mtSOD1^{A4V} and mtSOD1^{V148G}) showed enhanced superoxide production when stressed with hydrogen per-

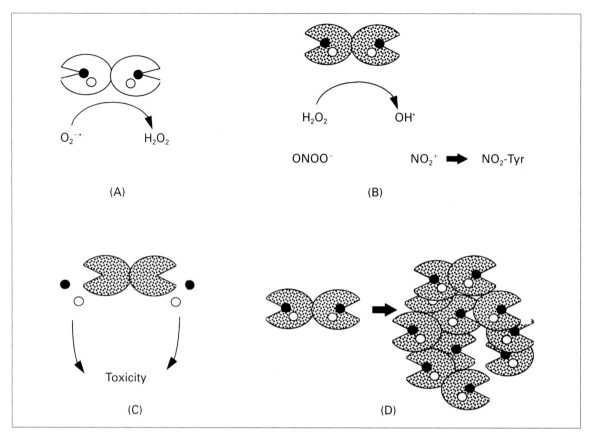

Figure 11.1
Possible mechanisms through which mtSOD1 gains a neurotoxic function. (A) Normal SOD1 function. (B) Aberrant biochemical activity of the mt SOD1. (C) Copper – or Zinc – induced toxicity. (D) Abnormal tendency of mt SOD1 to aggregate.

oxide.[6] In vivo, Bogdanov and colleagues[7] and Liu and colleagues[8] were able to demonstrate enhanced free-radical production in the brain or spinal cord of mtSOD1[G93A] mice. This abnormality was present before the onset of motor neuron loss, making it likely that oxidative radicals at least contribute to the degeneration of motor neurons. Bruijn and colleagues[9] did not find similar abnormalities in mtSOD1[G37R] mice.

On the other hand, Beckman and colleagues[10] have suggested that mtSOD1 becomes more accessible for ONOO⁻, from which it generates nitronium ions. This ONOO⁻ is formed from the reaction of nitric oxide with superoxide. Nitronium ions may nitrosylate tyrosine residues and thus oxidatively damage proteins. Loss of zinc from the mutated protein, owing to a decreased affinity for this metal, has been reported to enhance the nitronium-generating activity.[11] Support for this hypothesis comes from studies demonstrating the presence of nitrotyrosines in spinal cord from mtSOD1^{G93A} and mtSOD1^{G37R} mice and in post mortem tissue from mtSOD1-related familial ALS patients, using analytical and immunocytochemical methods.[9,12,13] Interestingly, similar increased staining for nitrotyrosines has also been observed in sporadic ALS spinal cord.[12,14]

Biochemical studies have suggested that neurofilaments, and especially neurofilament-L, are targets for nitrosylation,[15] but no evidence for the presence of nitrosylated neurofilament protein has so far been found in mice or humans.[9,16]

It should be mentioned that the nitrotyrosines that have been observed appear not to be protein-bound. The significance of free nitrotyrosines is uncertain. It is of course possible that nitrosylated proteins in the cell are quickly degraded, so that they escape detection.

If mtSOD1-catalysed conversion of ONOO$^-$ into nitronium ions plays a role in ALS, the formation of nitric oxide synthase (NOS) becomes of pathogenic importance. A role for this enzyme in motor neuron degeneration has been suggested because of the co-localization of inducible nitric oxide synthase (iNOS) with SOD1 in inclusions in motor neurons.[17,18] Almer and colleagues[19] reported up-regulation of iNOS in the spinal cord of mtSOD1^{G93A} mice, which also showed marked glial and microglial proliferation. Since these changes only became apparent after onset of clinical signs, the authors suggested a secondary pathogenic role for NOS.

Eliminating neuronal nitric oxide synthase (nNOS) expression in mtSOD1^{G93A} mice, through crossbreeding with nNOS knock out mice (nNOS$^{-/-}$), did not affect disease course in a study by Facchinetti and colleagues.[20] Some residual nNOS activity appears to remain present in nNOS$^{-/-}$ mice because of expression of alternative nNOS splice products. Since these nNOS$^{-/-}$ mice were resistant to other nitric oxide-dependent brain insults, the authors thought that this remaining nNOS activity was unlikely to explain the negative findings.

In several pharmacological studies, the possible role of nitric oxide has been investigated. Treatment of mtSOD1^{G93A} mice with non-specific NOS inhibitors nitro-L-arginine methyl ester (L-NAME), relatively nNOS-selective NOS inhibitors (7-nitroindazole), and highly nNOS-selective NOS inhibitors (AR-R17338 and AR-R18512) did not affect disease onset or duration.[20,21] Surprisingly, the selective nNOS inhibitor AR-R17477 did modestly prolong survival in mtSOD1^{G93A} mice;[20] the inconsistency of this finding remains to be explained.

A key study testing the possible involvement of peroxidase or ONOO$^-$-converting activity of mtSOD1 was performed by Bruijn and colleagues.[22] These authors manipulated the cellular wild type SOD1 (wtSOD1) content by eliminating or increasing expression of the wtSOD1 in mtSOD1^{G85R} mice. This did not affect the onset or course of the motor neuron disease of these mice. The authors concluded that it is unlikely that superoxide or ONOO$^-$ are pathogenic factors. However, as pointed out by Brown,[23] it should be noted that, even when wtSOD1 is eliminated, hydrogen peroxide that is generated through other processes in the cell could be sufficient to induce oxidative stress.

Bruijn and colleagues[22] also reported the consistent presence of mtSOD1-containing aggregates in motor neurons from mtSOD1^{G37R}, mtSOD1^{G85R}, and mtSOD1^{G93A} mice. Inclusions had already been observed in neurons and astrocytes of mtSOD1^{G37R} mice,[24] and neuronal inclusions can be abundant in human mtSOD1-associated familial ALS.[25,26]

Therefore, an abnormal tendency to aggregate may explain the cytotoxic activity of the mtSOD1. Support for this comes from the finding that mtSOD1 overexpressed in cultured motor neurons after intranuclear injection of the mtSOD1[G41R], mtSOD1[G93A], and mtSOD1[N139K] genes, forms aggregates in a glutamate-receptor-dependent and calcium-dependent fashion.[27,28]

The formation of aggregates in mtSOD1 neurons does not exclude a key role for oxidative stress in motor neuron degeneration induced by the mutant protein. Oxidative stress could initiate or enhance aggregation of mtSOD1,[29-31] and the aggregates themselves may induce neurotoxicity through the generation of ROS.

If the affinity of mtSOD1 for zinc and copper is decreased, a relative excess of these metals may emerge and result in toxicity that involves the formation of free radicals. Reduced zinc affinity of purified mtSOD1 has been reported,[11] but most mtSOD1 molecules appear to bind copper normally.[32] Furthermore, no evidence for increased copper or zinc levels were found in fibroblasts of patients with mtSOD1-associated familial ALS.[33]

Indirect evidence for the involvement of copper comes from the observation that treatment of PC12 cells with D-penicillamine, a copper chelator, attentuates cell death induced by the mtSOD1[V148G] introduced into these cells using a viral vector.[6] Furthermore, treatment of mtSOD1[G93A] mice with D-penicillamine delayed disease onset and extended survival.[34] The idea that these beneficial effects in vitro and in vivo may well be exerted through the copper-chelating properties of this compound is suggested by the finding that it reversed the pro-apoptotic effect of mtSOD1[A4V] and mtSOD1[G93A] in a neural cell line, and inhibited the enhanced peroxidase activity of the mutant enzyme.[3]

Evidence for oxidatively-induced damage in familial ALS and sporadic ALS

In several studies, oxidation-induced damage to DNA, lipids, and proteins or sensitivity of mtSOD1-containing cells to oxidative damage has been reported. However, no specific indication as to the origin or mechanism of such damage was provided by these studies. Staining for 8-hydroxy-2'-deoxyguanosine, an index of oxidation-induced modification of nucleic acids, has been found to be increased in spinal motor neurons of patients with mtSOD1-associated and non-mtSOD1-associated familial and sporadic ALS.[13] Activation of DNA repair systems has been studied as well. Treatment of NSC34, a motor neuron cell line, with hydrogen peroxide or ONOO$^-$ results in cell death associated with the activation of poly(ADP-ribose)polymerase,[35] which results in the depletion of nicotinamide adenine dinucleotide and ATP.[36] Inhibitors of PARP resulted in an attenuation of NSC34 cell death.[35] Point mutations[37] and an allelic frequency that is different from controls[38] in the APEX nuclease gene have been reported in patients with sporadic ALS. This gene encodes APE1, an endonuclease that removes apurinergic and apyrimidinergic sites. The activity and the level of this enzyme have been reported to be decreased in sporadic ALS brain tissue.[39]

Increased levels of carbonyl protein, a measure of oxidative damage to proteins, have been found in the spinal cord of SOD1[G93A] trangenic mice, but only clearly so in the later stages of the disease.[40] A similar increase has been reported in the motor cortex or spinal cord of sporadic ALS patients.[13,41,42]

Increased immunocytochemical staining of malondialdehyde-modified proteins, a marker for oxidative damage to lipids, has been found in motor neurons in familial ALS and sporadic ALS patients[13] and of $SOD1^{G93A}$ transgenic mice.[43] Levels of malondialdehyde were increased in the spinal cord of $SOD1^{G93A}$ transgenic mice,[43] but not in $SOD1^{G37R}$ transgenic mice[9] or in the motor cortex of familial ALS patients.[13] 4-hydroxynonenal, a lipid peroxidation product of fatty acids, was found to be increased in the cerebrospinal fluid of sporadic ALS patients.[44] Furthermore, the content of protein modified by 4-hydroxynonenal in the spinal cord of sporadic ALS patients was reported to be increased.[45]

Cell lines overexpressing a mutant $SOD1$ gene are known to show enhanced sensitivity to oxidative stress induced by serum withdrawal or growth factor deprivation.[46] In primary cultures of nigral neurons from $SOD1^{G93A}$ transgenic mice, increased sensitivity to exogenously-induced oxidative stress has been demonstrated.[47] To avoid the possibly confounding effect of the overexpression of the mutant gene in these models, we studied primary fibroblast cultures from patients with $SOD1$-associated familial ALS (mt$SOD1^{L38V}$, mt$SOD1^{D90A}$ and mt$SOD1^{G93C}$) and found these cells to be more sensitive to hydrogen peroxide and 3-morpholinosydnonimine hydrochloride, but not to serum withdrawal or treatment with nitroprussate.[48] Fibroblasts from sporadic ALS patients were even more sensitive to this exogenously-induced oxidative stress. In a study on fibroblasts of patients with familial ALS not associated with SOD1, no biochemical evidence for oxidative stress was found.[49]

In conclusion, many studies have demonstrated evidence for oxidative damage in both mt$SOD1$-associated familial ALS and sporadic ALS. None of these studies, however, has provided compelling evidence for the primary role of ROS in motor neuron death.

Some authors have argued that the similar presence of oxidative damage in both mt$SOD1$-familial ALS and sporadic ALS suggests that sporadic ALS is caused by a nonhereditary abnormality of SOD1.[50] No exonic mutations in the $SOD1$ gene in sporadic ALS have been found (apart from the few so-called 'apparently sporadic ALS patients'), and the activity of SOD1 in the red blood cells and motor cortex of sporadic ALS patients is normal.[41,51] Somatic mutations of the $SOD1$ gene appear to be absent in sporadic ALS motor cortex.[52] However, the SOD1 activity in (aged) motor neurons has not been measured, and pathogenic post-translational modifications of the SOD1[50] await further attention.

Evidence that neurons in ALS up-regulate their antioxidant defence systems

Indirect evidence for oxidative stress in ALS comes from the observation that cellular free radical scavenging enzyme systems are up-regulated in this disease. In glial cells, an up-regulation of SOD1, manganese superoxide dismutase, and catalase has been observed immunocyochemically[53] but not biochemically.[41,54,55] For glutathione peroxidase, both an increase[54] and a decrease[55] in activity has been found. Staining for heme oxygenase-1 has been reported to be increased in motor neurons of human familial and sporadic ALS[13] but not in $SOD1^{G93A}$ transgenic mice.[56] Similarly, increased metallothionine immunoreactivity has been found in ALS spinal cord.[57] Finally, the normal age-related increase in vitamin E levels in the brain is absent in mt$SOD1^{G93A}$ transgenic mice, suggesting that $SOD1^{G93A}$ transgenic mice exhaust their antioxidant vitamin E capacity.[58]

Antioxidants protect against ALS-associated cell death

Evidence that oxidative stress plays a pathogenic role in motor neuron death in mtSOD1-associated ALS also comes from studies demonstrating an effect of antioxidants on the course of the disease. PC12 cells transduced with mtSOD1[V148G] and mtSOD1[A4V] were at least partially protected by antioxidants from cell death induced by the mtSOD1 gene.[6] No such effect was found in motor neuron cultures in which mtSOD1 was overexpressed after intranuclear injection.[28]

Treatment with vitamin E and selenium delays the onset of clinical disease in SOD1[G93A] transgenic mice without modifying disease progression.[58] Furthermore, treatment with carboxyfullerenes delays disease onset.[59] Circumstantial support also comes from the finding that disease onset in SOD1[G93A] transgenic mice is delayed by the overexpression of Bcl-2, which is thought to exert its anti-apoptotic effects through an antioxidant mechanism.[60]

Few studies investigating the effect of antioxidants have been performed in humans. N-acetylcysteine is a strong antioxidant, which has been evaluated in a prospective double-blind, placebo-controlled study in 111 patients who were treated for 12 months with daily subcutaneous injections (50 mg/kg). Although the drug had no beneficial effect overall, a trend towards a positive effect on survival was apparent in a subgroup of 81 patients with limb-onset ALS.[61]

Link of oxidative stress to excitotoxicity

Evidence is growing that glutamate-induced excitotoxicity plays a primary or secondary role in the pathogenesis of ALS (see Chapter 14). Several lines of evidence suggest a link between oxidative stress induced by mtSOD1 and glutamate-induced cell death (Fig. 11.2).

First, mtSOD1-containing motor neurons may be more vulnerable to excitotoxicity. In pathological studies,[62–65] mitochondria are the first, or at least among the first, targets for the deleterious effects of mtSOD1. Mitochondrial damage results in a decreased production of ATP and an increased production of free radicals. The activation of poly (ADP ribose) polymerase (PARP) induced by DNA damage (see above) enhances this ATP deficit. The resulting energy failure jeopardizes the function of ATP-requiring ionic pumps that maintain the electrochemical gradients across neuronal plasmamembranes. Insufficient clearance of calcium ions that entered the cell through stimulation of glutamate receptors induces a rise in cytosolic calcium levels, which initiates a variety of enzymatic processes that lead to cell death.

Increased cytosolic calcium concentrations have been observed in SH-SY5Y cells transfected with mtSOD1[G93A] and in peripheral blood lymphocytes from patients with sporadic ALS.[66,67] Furthermore, small vacuoles filled with calcium have been observed in spinal motor neurons of mtSOD1[G93A] mice[68] and increased intracellular calcium has been observed in the motor terminals of patients with sporadic ALS.[69]

Secondly, mtSOD1-induced damage may induce excessive glutamergic stimulation, owing to insufficient clearance of glutamate from the extracellular space by the glial glutamaat transporter, excitatory amino acid transporter (EAAT)2. A loss of EAAT2 has been observed in ALS post mortem tissue and in the spinal cord of mtSOD1[G85R] mice. Evidence suggests that the loss of EAAT2 is due to oxidative damage induced by the mtSOD1. This protein is known to be particularly

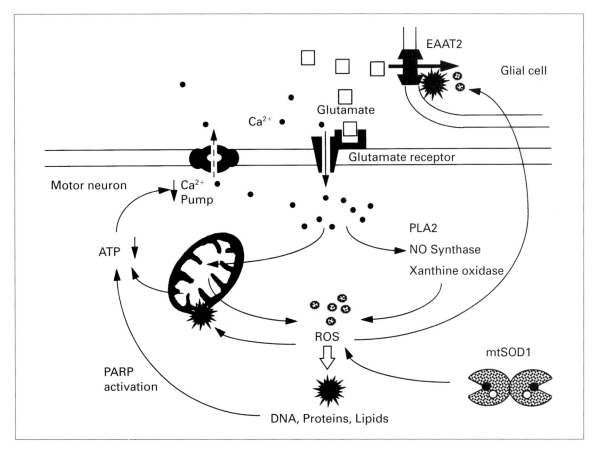

Figure 11.2
Possible link between oxidative stress induced by mtSOD1 and glutamate-induced excitotoxicity.

vulnerable to oxidative stress, and immuno-precipitations studies have revealed that EAAT2 is one of the proteins oxidatively damaged by 4-hydroxynonenal.[45] More direct evidence comes from a recent study by Trotti and colleagues,[70] who found that mtSOD1 directly impairs glutamate transport by EAAT2 through an effect on the C-terminal part of this protein. This suggests that oxidative stress leads to the formation of toxic intermediates

(such as 4-hydroxynonenal), which impairs glutamate transport and thus induces (secondary) excitotoxic motor neuron degeneration.

Finally the formation of aggregates of mtSOD1 observed in cultured motor neurons injected with mt*SOD1*, seems to be dependent upon calcium entry induced by glutamate stimulation,[28] providing a further link between these two mechanisms.

Selectivity of motor neuron death

If oxidative stress induced by the mtSOD1 plays a pathogenic role in ALS, it remains to be explained why only motor neurons die in a disease caused by a mutation in an ubiquitously expressed gene. The susceptibility of motor neurons to glutamate-induced cell death and their limited calcium-buffering capacity are thought to contribute (see Chapter 14). It has not definitely been settled whether the abundance of SOD1 expression predicts vulnerability.[71-73] Although SOD1 mRNA content seems to be higher in the susceptible neurons,[71] the protein levels of SOD1, although high, seem not to be significantly different from other, non-vulnerable neurons.[71-73] However, the half-life of SOD1 in motor neurons may be higher than has been estimated on the basis of the findings in cell lines, in which the stability of the mutant enzyme is clearly decreased.[74,75] Factors such as the antioxidant capacity of motor neurons as compared with other neurons or of the astrocytes that surround motor neurons have not so far been assessed.

Significance of oxidative stress as a disease mechanism in ALS

The significance of the presence of oxidative damage in ALS motor neurons is unclear. The presence of very similar oxidative damage in familial ALS and sporadic ALS suggests two possibilities:

(a) the mechanism of motor neuron degeneration may involve oxidative stress, independent of the primary etiology; or
(b) the signs of oxidative damage are epiphenomena of motor neuron death without pathogenic significance.

It should be noted that the finding of oxidative stress in ALS is by no means specific for this disease. In Alzheimer's disease, the findings are similar to those in ALS. Up-regulation of heme oxygenase-1, an increased content of nitrotyrosins, and oxidative damage to nucleic acids, protein, and lipids have all been found in Alzheimer's disease brain, and β-amyloid itself is thought to represent a source of ROS.[76] Nigral cell death, characteristic of Parkinson's disease, may at least in part be mediated by oxidative stress.[77] This hypothesis is especially tempting as monoamine metabolism is generally accepted to be a source of ROS. Similar findings are emerging in dementia with Lewy bodies, inclusion body myopathy, and other diseases. This does not necessarily mean that oxidative stress is pathogenically irrelevant. It may be part of a final, albeit secondary, common pathway through which degenerative diseases evolve. Such a scenario could explain the age-dependency of clinical presentation of most of these diseases and their progressive nature.

Acknowledgments

Wim Robberecht is a Clinical Investigator of the Fund for Scientific Research (FWO) Flanders.

References

1. Rosen DR, Siddique T, Patterson D et al. Mutations in Cu/Zn superoxide dismutase gene are associated with familial amyotrophic lateral sclerosis. *Nature* 1993; **362**: 59–62.
2. Fridovich I. Superoxide dismutases. *Adv Enzymol* 1986; **58**: 61–97.
3. Wiedau-Pazos MW, Goto JJ, Rabizadeh S et al. Altered reactivity of superoxide dismutase in familial amyotrophic lateral sclerosis. *Science* 1996; **271**: 515–518.
4. Yim MB, Kang JH, Yim HS et al. A gain-of-

function of an amyotrophic lateral sclerosis-associated Cu,Zn-superoxide dismutase mutant: an enhancement of free radical formation due to a decrease in k_m for hydrogen peroxide. *Proc Natl Acad Sci USA* 1996; **93**: 5709–5714.

5. Singh RJ, Karoui H, Gunther MR et al. Reexamination of the mechanism of hydroxyl radical adducts formed from the reaction between familial amyotrophic lateral sclerosis-associated Cu,Zn superoxide dismutase mutants and H_2O_2. *Proc Natl Acad Sci USA* 1998; **95**: 6675–6680.

6. Ghadge GD, Lee JP, Bindokas VP et al. Mutant superoxide dismutase 1-linked familial amyotrofic lateral sclerosis: molecular mechanisms of neuronal death and protection. *J Neurosci* 1997; **17**: 8756–8766.

7. Bogdanov MB, Ramos LE, Xu Z, Beal MF. Elevated 'hydroxyl radical' generation in vivo in an animal model of amyotrofic lateral sclerosis. *J Neurochem* 1998; **71**: 1321–1324.

8. Liu R, Althaus JS, Ellerbrock BR et al. Enhanced oxygen radical production in a transgenic mouse model of familial amyotrofic lateral sclerosis. *Ann Neurol* 1998; **44**: 763–770.

9. Bruijn LI, Beal MF, Becher MW et al. Elevated free nitrotyrosine levels, but not protein-bound nitrotyrosine or hydroxyl radicals, throughout amyotrophic lateral sclerosis (ALS)-like disease implicate tyrosine nitration as an aberrant in vivo property of one familial ALS-linked superoxide dismutase 1 mutant. *Proc Natl Acad Sci USA* 1997; **94**: 7606–7611.

10. Beckman JS, Carson M, Smith CD, Koppenol WH. ALS, SOD and peroxynitrite. *Nature* 1993; **364**: 584.

11. Crow JP, Sampson JB, Zhuang Y et al. Decreased zinc affinity of amyotrophic lateral sclerosis-associated superoxide dismutase mutants leads to enhanced catalysis of tyrosine nitration by peroxynitrite. *J Neurochem* 1997; **69**: 1936–1944.

12. Beal MF, Ferrante RJ, Browne SE et al. Increased 3-nitrotyrosine in both sporadic and familial amyotrophic lateral sclerosis. *Ann Neurol* 1997; **42**: 644–654.

13. Ferrante RJ, Browne SE, Shinobu LA et al. Evidence of increased oxidative damage in both sporadic and familial amyotrophic lateral sclerosis. *J Neurochem* 1997; **69**: 2064–2074

14. Abe K, Pan LH, Wantanabe M et al. Induction of nitrotyrosine-like immunoreactivity in the lower motor neuron of amyotrophic lateral sclerosis. *Neurosci Lett* 1995; **199**: 152–154.

15. Crow JP, Ye YZ, Strong M et al, Superoxide dismutase catalyzes nitration of tyrosines by peroxynitrite in the rod and head domains of neurofilament-L. *J Neurochem* 1997; **69**: 1945–1953.

16. Strong MJ, Stopper NM, Crow JP et al. Nitration of the low molecular weight neurofilament is equivalent in sporadic amyotrophic lateral sclerosis and control cervical spinal cord. *Biochem Biophys Res Comm* 1998; **248**: 157–164.

17. Chou SM, Wang HS, Komai K. Colocalization of NOS and SOD1 in neurofilament accumulation within motorneuronen of ALS: an immunohistochemical study. *J Chem Neuroanat* 1996; **10**: 249–258.

18. Chou SM, Wang HS, Taniguchi. A role of SOD-1 and nitric oxide-cyclic GMP cascade on neurofilament aggregation in ALS/MND. *J Neurol Sci* 1996; **139** (suppl): 16–26.

19. Almer G, Slobodanka V, Romero N, Przedborski S. Inducible nitric oxide synthase upregulation in a transgenic mouse model of familial amyotrophic lateral sclerosis. *J Neurochem* 1999; **72**: 2415–2425.

20. Facchinetti F, Sasaki M, Cutting FB et al. Lack of involvement of neuronal nitric oxide synthase in the pathogenesis of a transgenic mouse model of familial amyotrophic lateral sclerosis. *Neuroscience* 1999; **90**: 1483–1492.

21. Upton-Rice MN, Cudkowicz ME, Mathew RK et al. Administration of nitric oxide synthase inhibitors does not alter disease course of amyotrophic lateral sclerosis SOD1 mutant transgenic mice. *Ann Neurol* 1999; **45**: 413–414.

22. Bruijn LI, Houseweart MK, Kato S et al. Aggregation and motor neuron toxicity of an ALS-linked SOD1 mutant independent from wild-type SOD1. *Science* 1998; **281**: 1851–1854.

23. Brown RH. SOD1 aggregates in ALS: cause, correlate or consequence? *Nature Med* 1998; **4**: 1362–1364.

24. Bruijn LI, Becher MW, Lee MK et al. ALS-

linked SOD1 mutant G85R mediates damage to astrocytes and promotes rapidly progressive disease with SOD1-containing inclusions. *Neuron* 1997; **18**: 327–338.

25. Shibata N, Hirano A, Kobayashi M et al. Intense superoxide dismutase-1 immunoreactivity in intracytoplasmic hyaline inclusions of familial amyotropic lateral sclerosis with posterior column involvement. *J Neuropath Exp Neurol* 1996; **55**: 481–490.

26. Ince PG, Tomkins J, Slade JY et al. Amyotrophic lateral sclerosis associated with genetic abnormalities in the gene encoding Cu/Zn superoxide dismutase: molecular pathology of five new cases, and comparison with previous reports and 73 sporadic cases of ALS. *J Neuropath Exp Neurol* 1998; **57**: 895–904.

27. Durham HD, Roy J, Dong L, Figlewicz DA. Aggregation of mutant Cu/Zn superoxide dismutase proteins in a culture model of ALS. *J Neuropath Exp Neurol* 1997; **56**: 523–530.

28. Roy J, Minotti S, Dong L, Figlewicz DA, Durham HD. Glutamate potentiates the toxicity of mutant Cu/Zn-superoxide dismutase in motor neurons by postsynaptic calcium-dependent mechanisms. *J Neurosci* 1998; **18**: 9673–9684.

29. Berlett B, Stadtman E. Protein oxidation in aging, disease and oxidative stress. *J Biol Chem* 1997; **272**: 20313–20316.

30. Kwon OJ, Lee SM, Floyd RA, Park JW. Thiol-dependent meta-catalyzed oxidation of copper, zinc superoxide dismutase. *Biochim Biophys Acta* 1998; **1387**: 249–256.

31. Friguet B, Szweda LI. Inhibition of the multicatalytic proteinase (proteasome) by 4-hydroxy-2-nonenal cross-linked protein. *FEBS Lett* 1997; **405**: 21–25.

32. Corson LB, Strain JJ, Culotta VC, Cleveland DW, Chaperone-facilitated copper binding is a property common to several classes of familial amyotrophic lateral sclerosis-linked superoxide dismutase mutants. *Proc Natl Acad Sci USA* 1996; **95**: 6361–6366.

33. Radunovic A, Delves HT, Robberecht W et al. Copper and zinc levels in familial amyotrophic lateral sclerosis patients with CuZnSOD gene mutations. *Ann Neurol* 1997; **42**: 130–131.

34. Hottinger AF, Fine EG, Gurnery ME et al. The copper chelator D-penicillamine delays onset of disease and extends survival in a transgenic mouse model of familial amyotrophic lateral sclerosis. *Eur J Neurosci* 1997; **9**: 1548–1551.

35. Cookson MR, Ince PG, Shaw PJ. Peroxynitrite and hydrogen peroxide-induced cell death in the NSC34 neuroblastoma × spinal cord cell line. *J Neurochem* 1998; **72**: 501–508.

36. Szabo C, Dawson VL. Role of poly (ADP-ribose) synthetase in inflammation and ischemia–reperfusion. *Trends Pharmacol Sci* 1998; **19**: 287–297.

37. Olkowski ZL. Mutant AP endonuclease in patients with amyotrophic lateral sclerosis. *NeuroReport* 1998; **9**: 239–242.

38. Hayward C, Colville S, Swingler RJ, Brock DJ. Molecular genetic analysis of the APEX nuclease gene in amyotrophic lateral sclerosis. *Neurology* 1999; **52**: 1899–1901.

39. Kisby GE, Milne J, Sweatt C. Evidence of reduced DNA repair in amyotrophic lateral sclerosis brain tissue. *NeuroReport* 1997; **8**: 1337–1340.

40. Andrus PK, Fleck TJ, Gurney ME, Hall ED. protein oxidative damage in a transgenic mouse model of familial amyotrofic lateral sclerosis. *J Neurochem* 1998; **71**: 2041–2048.

41. Bowling AC, Schulz JB, Brown RH Jr, Beal MF. Superoxide dismutase activity, oxidative damage and mitochondrial energy metabolism in familial and sporadic amyotrophic lateral sclerosis. *J Neurochem* 1993; **64**: 2366–2369.

42. Shaw PJ, Ince PG, Falkous G, Mantle D. Oxidative damage to protein in sporadic motor neuron disease spinal cord. *Ann Neurol* 1995; **38**: 691–695.

43. Hall ED, Andrus PK, Oostveen JA et al. Relationship of oxygen radical-induced lipid peroxidative damage to disease onset and progression in a transgenic model of familial ALS. *J Neurosci Res* 1998; **53**: 66–77.

44. Smith RG, Henry YK, Mattson MP, Appel SH. Presence of 4-hydroxynonenal in cerebrospinal fluid of patients with sporadic amyotrophic lateral sclerosis. *Ann Neurol* 1998; **44**: 696–699.

45. Pedersen WA, Fu W, Keller JN et al. Protein modification by the lipid peroxidation product 4-hydoxynonenal in the spinal cords of amyotrofic lateral sclerosis patients. *Ann Neurol*

1998; **44**: 819–824.

46. Rabizadeh S, Gralla EB, Borchelt DR et al. Mutations associated with amyotrophic lateral sclerosis convert superoxide dismutase from an antiapoptotic gene to a proapoptotic gene: studies in yeast and neural cells. *Proc Natl Acad Sci USA* 1995; **92**: 3024–3028.

47. Mena MA, Khan U, Togasaki DM et al. Effects of wild-type and mutated copper/zinc superoxide dismutase on neuronal survival in postnatal midbrain culture. *J Neurochem* 1997; **69**: 21–33.

48. Aguirre T, Van Den Bosch L, Goetschalckx K et al. Increased sensitivity of fibroblasts from ALS patients to oxidative stress. *Ann Neurol* 1998; **43**: 452–457.

49. Jansen GA, Wanders RJA, Jöbsis GJ et al. Evidence against increased oxidative stress in fibroblasts from patients with non-superoxide-dismutase-1 mutant familial amyotrophic lateral sclerosis. *J Neurol Sci* 1996; **139** (suppl): 91–94.

50. Bredesen DE, Ellerby LM, Hart PJ et al. Do posttranslational modificaitons of CuZnSOD lead to sporadic amyotrophic lateral sclerosis? *Ann Neurol* 1997; **42**: 135–138.

51. Robberecht W, Sapp P, Viaene MK et al. Cu/Zn superoxide dismutase activity in familial and sporadic amyotrophic lateral sclerosis. *J Neurochem* 1994; **62**: 384–387.

52. Shaw PJ, Tomkins J, Salde JY et al. CNS tissue Cu/Zn superoxide dismutase (SOD1) mutations in motor neurone disease (MND). *NeuroReport* 1997; **8**: 3923–3927.

53. Shaw PJ, Chinnery RM, Thagesen H et al. Immunocytochemical study of the distribution of free radical scavenging enzymes Cu/Zn superoxide dismutase (SOD1), Mn superoxide dismutase (Mn SOD) and catalase in normal human spinal cord and in motor neuron disease. *J Neurol Sci* 1997; **147**: 115–125.

54. Ince PG, Shax PJ, Candy JM et al. Iron, selenium and glutathion peroxidase activity are elevated in sporadic motor neuron disease. *Neurosci Lett* 1994; **182**: 87–90.

55. Przedborski S, Donaldson D, Jakowec M et al. Brain superoxide dismutase, catalase and glutathione peroxidase activities in amyotrophic lateral sclerosis. *Ann Neurol* 1996; **39**: 158–165.

56. Dwyer BEZ, Lu SY, Nishimura RN. Heme oxygenase in the experimental ALS mouse. *Exp Neurol* 1998; **150**: 206–212.

57. Sillevis Smitt PAE, Blaauwgeers HGT, Troost D, de Jong JMBV. Metallothionine immunoreactivity is increased in the the spinal cord of patients with ALS. *Neurosci Lett* 1992; **144**: 107–110.

58. Gurney ME, Cutting FB, Zhai P et al. Benefit of vitamin E, riluzole, and gabapentin in a transgenic model of familial amyotrophic lateral sclerosis. *Ann Neurol* 1996; **39**: 147–157.

59. Dugan LL, Turetsky DM, Du C et al. Carboxyfullerenes as neuroprotective agents. *Proc Natl Acad Sci U S A* 1997; **94**: 9434–9439.

60. Kostic V, Jackson-Lewis V, de Bilbao F et al. Bcl-2: prolonging life in a transgenic model of familial amyotrofic lateral sclerosis. *Science* 1997; **277**: 559–562.

61. Louwerse ES, Weverling GJ, Bossuyt PMM et al. Randomized, double-blind controlled trial of acetylcysteine in amyotrophic lateral sclerosis. *Arch Neurol* 1995; **52**: 559–564.

62. Kong J, Xu Z. Massive mitochondrial degeneration in motor neurons triggers the onset of amyotrophic lateral sclerosis in mice expressing a mutant SOD1. *J Neurosci* 1998; **18**: 3241–3250.

63. Dal Canto MC, Gurney ME. Development of central nervous system pathology in a murine transgenic model of human amyotrophic lateral sclerosis. *Am J Pathol* 1994; **145**: 1271–1279.

64. Gurney ME, Pu H, Chiu AY et al. Motor neuron degeneration in mice that express a human Cu, Zn Superoxide Dismutase Mutation. *Science* 1994; **64**: 1772–1775.

65. Wong PC, Pardo CA, Borchelt DR et al. An adverse property of a familial ALS-linked SOD1 mutation causes motor neuron disease characterized by vacuolar degeneration of mitochondria. *Neuron* 1995; **14**: 1105–1116.

66. Carri MT, Ferri A, Battistoni A et al. Expression of a Cu, Zn superoxide dismutase typical of familial amyotrophic lateral sclerosis induces mitochondrial alteration and increase of cytosolic Ca^{2+} concentration in transfected neuroblastoma SH-SY5Y cells. *FEBS Lett* 1997; **414**: 365–368.

67. Curti D, Malaspina A, Facchetti G et al. Amy-

otrophic lateral sclerosis: oxidative energy metabolism and calcium homeostasis in peripheral blood lymphocytes. *Neurology* 1996; **47**: 1061–1064.

68. Siklos L, Engelhardt J, Harati Y et al. Ultrastructural evidence for altered calcium in the motor nerve terminals in amyotrophic lateral sclerosis. *Ann Neurol* 1996; **39**: 203–219.

69. Siklos L, Engelhardt JL, Alexiany ME et al. Intracellular calcium parallels motorneuron degeneration in SOD-1 mutant mice. *J Neuropath Exp Neurol* 1998; **57**: 571–587.

70. Trotti D, Rolfs A, Danbolt NC et al. SOD1 mutants linked to amyotrophic lateral sclerosis selectively inactivate a glial glutamate transporter. *Nature Neurosci* 1999; **2**: 427–433.

71. Tsuda T, Munthasser S, Fraser PE et al. Analysis of the functional effects of a mutation in SOD1 associated with familial amyotrophic lateral sclerosis. *Neuron* 1994; **13**: 727–736.

72. Pardo CA, Xu ZS, Borchelt DR et al. Superoxide dismutase is an abundant component in cell bodies, dendrites and axons of motor neurons and in a subset of other neurons. *Proc Natl Acad Sci USA* 1995; **92**: 954–958.

73. Bergeron C, Petrunka C, Weyer L. Copper/zinc superoxide dismutase expression in the human central nervous system: correlation with selective neuronal vulnerability. *Am J Pathol* 1996; **148**: 273–279.

74. Borchelt DR, Lee MK, Slunt HS et al. Superoxide dismutase 1 with mutations linked to familial amyotrophic lateral sclerosis possesses significant activity. *Proc Natl Acad Sci USA* 1994; **91**: 8292–8296.

75. Borchelt DR, Wong PC, Becher MW et al. Axonal transport of mutant superoxide dismutase 1 and focal axonal abnormalities in the proximal axons of transgenic mice. *Neurobiol Dis* 1998; **5**: 27–35.

76. Markesberry WR, Carney JM. Oxidative alterations in Alzheimer's disease. *Brain Pathol* 1999; **9**: 133–146.

77. Dunnett SB, Björklund A. Prospects for new restorative and neuroprotective treatments in Parkinson's disease. *Nature* 1999; **399 (suppl)**: A32–A39.

12

Genetics of amyotrophic lateral sclerosis: an overview

Peter M Andersen, Mitsuya Morita and Robert H Brown, Jr

Introduction

Amyotrophic lateral sclerosis (ALS) remains one of the most devastating of human disorders. The cause of the progressive degeneration of motor neurons in this disease remains unknown. In a subset of cases, it is apparent that the disease is inherited, often as a dominant trait. It should therefore be possible to use the power of modern genetic analysis to define the cause of the motor neuron cell death in such cases. Moreover, because the clinical and pathological characteristics of familial ALS (FALS) and sporadic ALS (SALS) are almost identical, it is reasonable to hypothesize that an understanding of the molecular defects that trigger FALS will provide insights into the pathogenesis of both FALS and SALS. Furthermore, because some rare forms of FALS are complex, with involvement of non-motor systems in the nervous system, genetic analyses of such FALS families may also illuminate the pathogenesis of neurodegenerative conditions such as dementia. With this perspective, this chapter provides an overview of the spectrum of inherited motor neuron diseases and summarizes important lessons learned from studies of the molecular pathogenesis of some of these diseases.

The epidemiology of FALS

The concept that ALS can be inherited dates to the earliest descriptions of the disease. Of the 11 patients reported by Aran in 1850,[1] one (number seven) was a 43-year-old sea captain who presented with cramps followed by the development of wasting and paresis in the upper extremities and then the lower extremities. He died 2 years after onset. Aran commented that one of the patient's three sisters and two maternal uncles had died from a similar disease. Although Aran described this as a case of progressive muscular atrophy (PMA) later evaluations[2,3] have considered this to be a case of ALS. None of the 20 patients reported by Charcot[4] in the 1860s were recognized as familial cases, and for a long time Charcot denied that ALS could be a hereditary disease. In 1880, William Osler[5] described progressive muscular atrophy in 13 adults in two generations of the Farr family of Vermont; additional cases from this family were later added by Brown in 1951[6] and then by Cudkowicz and colleagues in 1997.[7] Cudkowicz also reported that the disease in this Farr family is caused by the A4V mutation in the gene encoding the protein cytosolic copper–zinc superoxide dismutase (CuZn–SOD).

Charcot's view that ALS is not hereditary was generally accepted until Kurland and Mulder reported six new FALS pedigrees in 1955.[8] On the basis of this experience, they proposed that ALS could be inherited as a Mendelian dominant trait and that a dominant inheritance pattern might account for a significant proportion of all cases. Subsequent studies[9,10] confirmed that FALS can be inherited as an autosomal trait with high penetrance. These studies noted that an earlier age of onset distinguishes FALS from SALS, but that such cases are otherwise clinically indistinguishable. Williams and colleagues[11] studied nine Australian families with an autosomal-dominant mode of inheritance. Only one of these families showed high disease penetrance. This family had a significantly lower mean age of onset (47.8 years) than the eight families with diminished penetrance (60.8 years). Williams and colleagues argued that the incidence of FALS is likely to be underestimated by the exclusion of apparently sporadic cases in which the familial disease has low penetrance. Other rare reports have also described pedigrees with autosomal-dominant inheritance and diminished penetrance.[8,12–15]

However, FALS pedigree with high penetrance predominate in the literature, probably because they are easily recognized and recorded. Perhaps because most ALS epidemiological studies have been retrospective, FALS cases with low penetrance are rarely described. Other factors may lead to under-representation of FALS cases, including:

(a) inadequate recording of family history in the patient's records;
(b) loss of contact between different branches of a family;
(c) reluctance of a family to acknowledge an inherited disorder such as ALS;
(d) early death from usual causes of individuals in the family, who transmit the gene defect but do not develop the disease;
(e) misdiagnosis of ALS; or
(f) illegitimacy.

A number of pedigrees have been described in which the children developed ALS before their parents.[10,11,13,16] The author has encountered FALS pedigrees in which sons develop the disease while their mothers, who are obligatory carriers, remain disease-free.

Epidemiological studies in different populations usually report a FALS frequency of 5–10% (*Table 12.1*). These percentages should be judged with the aforementioned limitations in mind. It must also be recalled that the diagnostic criteria used and the methods of collecting data varied widely among the listed studies. It is our experience that FALS is often underdiagnosed, most frequently because of diminished disease penetrance and the doctor's inattention to family history. In a study of the prevalence of CuZn–SOD mutations among Scandinavian ALS patients, blood samples were randomly collected from neurological departments and the refering neurologist was specifically asked if the patient had a family history of ALS. Seventy-two (16.9%) of the 427 ALS patients from whom blood samples were collected reportedly had a family history of ALS.[17]

There is general agreement[7–10,18–20] that FALS is clinically and neuropathologically indistinguishable from SALS, suggesting that FALS and SALS share common final pathways for motoneuron degeneration.

Intrafamilial variation in site of onset is common in FALS pedigrees.[8,21–23] Within the same family, cases of PMA, classical ALS progressive bulbar palsy, and even primary lateral sclerosis may be found,[8,21,24–31] The intrafamilial variation of phenotype suggests that different types of FALS may share a common, hereditary pathogenetic mechanism.[29] Some studies find the intrafamilial differences to be less than the interfamilial differences.[15] Only rarely is the same site of onset found consistently in all members of a FALS family.[17,30,32–36] Some studies find more frequent onset in the lower extremities in FALS than in SALS,[9,10]

Study	Year	n	% FALS	Area studied
Haberlandt[167]	1959	251	13.5	Germany
Murray et al.[168]	1974	52	5.8	Nova Scotia, Canada
Jokelainen[72]	1977	255	0.8	Finland
Rosen[118]	1978	668	4.9	U.S.A
Gunnarsson and Palm[169]	1984	89	5.6	Wärmland, Sweden
Forsgren et al.[117]	1983	128	4.7	Northern Sweden
Giagheddu et al.[170]	1983	182	4.4	Sardinia
Li et al.[19]	1988	580	5	England
Højer-Petersen et al.[126]	1989	186	2.7	Jutland, Denmark
Murros and Fogelholm[123]	1983	36	11.6	Finland
Haverkamp et al.[119]	1995	1200	9.5	U.S.A.
Fong et al.[122]	1996	84	1.2	Hong Kong

n = total number of cases

Table 12.1
Selected epidemiological studies of FALS.

but Li and colleagues[19] reported lower extremity onset in 37% of both SALS and FALS patients. In this study, bulbar onset was present in 19% of SALS and 15% of FALS cases.

The mean age of onset in FALS pedigrees with high penetrance is usually about 10–14 years earlier than in SALS.[19,28] Intrafamilial variation in age at onset of ALS of the order of 15–25 years is a common finding in many families,[8,23,28] but a few families with small variation have been reported.[1,15,35,37,38] Only one family has shown evidence suggestive of anticipation.[19]

It has been reported that there is considerable variation in the rate of disease progression within FALS families,[39,41] although some FALS pedigrees consistently appear to show either rapid or slow progression.[8,15,23,37] Espinoa and colleagues[42] detailed a family in which several female patients survived for more than 10 years (one for more than 30 years), whereas the two male siblings had more rapid progression of the illness.

Strong and colleagues[28] reviewed the world literature on FALS (84 families with 249 cases in 1989) and found that in contrast to the age-dependent incidence of SALS, the age of onset of FALS was normally distributed about a mean of 45.7 years (standard deviation ± 11.3 years). Survival curves for FALS are markedly skewed, with 74% surviving at 1 year, 48% at 2 years and 23% at 5 years. In that review, only the age of onset was found to predict survival: as the age at onset increased, survival decreased. No relationship was detected between variables such as age of onset, sex and site of disease onset.

Mulder and colleagues[10] studied 103 patients from 72 families and found a mean age of onset of 48.3 years and a median survival time of 2.4 years (range 4 months to 36 years). This study concluded that survival time did not correlate with age at onset or sex, but that it did differ with site of onset. Moreover, patients with onset in upper extremities survived longer than patients with onset in the oropharynx or legs.

Genes known to cause ALS

In 1991 a collaborative group reported that some FALS families are genetically linked to chromosome 21q22.1–22.2. This investigation clearly established that there is genetic heterogeneity in FALS, since only about 50% of the families showed linkage to this locus (*Table 12.2*).[43] In 1993, Rosen and colleagues[44] reported that this linkage arises because of mutations in the CuZn–SOD (SOD1; EC 1.15.1.1, superoxide:superoxide oxidoreductase) gene at this locus. The initial report described 11 missense mutations in the CuZn–SOD gene in 13 of 18 investigated North American FALS pedigrees.

CuZn–SOD is a cytoplasmic homodimeric enzyme. Each subunit consists of 153 amino acids coded by five small exons. Because the two subunits are tightly packed and held together by strong hydrophobic interactions, the enzyme is extremely stable.[45] CuZn–SOD is ubiquitously expressed in eukaryotic cells. It is abundant, making up about 0.5–2% of the soluble proteins in the human brain.[46,47] The enzyme catalyses the conversion of the superoxide free radical anions $O_2 \cdot^-$ to hydrogen peroxide and dioxygen:

$$O_2 \cdot^- + O_2 \cdot^- + 2H^+ \xrightarrow{\text{SOD}} H_2O_2 + O_2$$

Despite numerous investigations over the past 6 years, the molecular mechanism for the neurotoxicity of mutant CuZn–SOD protein is

Mendelian inheritance			Non-mendelian inheritance (possible risk factor, modifying genes or loci)	
Locus	Inheritance	Gene	Locus	Gene
Adult onset			2	Neuron-specific kinesin heavy chain
21q22	AD, AR	CuZn–SOD	5q13	SMN and/or NAIP
X$_{centromere}$	XD	u	6q25	Mn SOD
			9p13	CNTF receptor
			11p13	EAAT2
Juvenile onset			11q12	CNTF
2q33	AR	u	14q11	APEX nuclease
9q34	AD	u	17q21	Tau
15q15	AR	u	19q13	ApoE
			22q12	NF-H
			Mitochondrial	Cytochrome *c* Oxidase

Abbreviations: AD, autosomal dominant; APEX nuclease, apurinic–apyrimidinic endonuclease; Apo E, apolipoprotein E; AR, autosomal recessive; CNTF, ciliary neutrotrophic factor; EAAT, excitory amino acid transporter-2; NAIP, neuronal apoptosis inhibitory protein; NF-H, neurofilament heavy chain; SMN, survival motor neuron; SOD, superoxide dismutase; u, unknown gene; XD, X-linked dominant.

Table 12.2
Genes and loci in ALS.

not well understood, nor has the basis for the delayed onset and the motor neuron selectivity of cell death in CuZn–SOD FALS been clearly defined. The collective evidence suggests that a loss of dismutation activity is not the cause of neurodegeneration in ALS. Rather, the mutated CuZn–SOD molecule has acquired one or more cytotoxic functions.

At present, 67 mutations have been reported world-wide in patients with CuZn–SOD ALS (*Table 12.3*). These are widely scattered over the gene[41] with a preponderance of mutations in exons 4 and 5. A highly conserved glycine at codon 93 is mutated to all six possible alternative amino acid residues. This residue is probably critical for the conformational stability of the CuZn–SOD backbone. The paucity of mutations in exon 3 (codons 56 to 79) is unexplained.

Fifty-nine of the 67 mutations in the CuZn–SOD gene are missense changes. The remaining eight are nonsense, deletions or insertions. No true null mutation has been found. Eight mutations are predicted to decrease the length of the resulting polypeptide. These lie between codons 118 and 133 and include two splice mutations in the 3'-terminal end of intron 4. No truncation mutations have been found in the final 20 codons of CuZn–SOD.

Perhaps surprisingly, there are no obvious clinical differences between contrasting classes of mutations. Moreover, FALS patients with CuZn–SOD mutations are clinically indistinguishable from FALS or SALS patients without a known CuZn–SOD mutation.[7,20] In the aggregate, patients with CuZn–SOD mutations show the same phenotypic variability in the site of onset (limb, truncal or bulbar), disease progression rate, and survival time as patients without a CuZn–SOD mutation, although it has been suggested that bulbar onset is rare among patients with a CuZn–SOD mutation.[41] Clinical details associated with most mutations are relatively sparse,[41] but cases with bulbar onset have been reported for six mutations (see *Table 12.3*). Large intra- and interfamilial phenotypic differences have been reported as well as pedigrees with diminished disease penetrance.[41] For some mutations, the phenotype is less variable. Thus, the A4V mutation, found in about half of all North American families with a CuZn–SOD mutation,[7,48] reproducibly causes an aggressive course with a survival time of rarely more than 2 years (mean duration ± standard deviation: 1.4 ± 0.9 years, n = 84).[7] Furthermore, A4V patients have almost exclusively lower motor neuron involvement, both clinically and at autopsy.[49] A4V autopsies also reveal more non-motor pathology than in SALS.[49,50] Formally, most A4V cases might therefore be most accurately described as progressive muscular atrophy. A4V is associated with almost complete penetrance[7,49] although a few elderly unaffected obligate gene carriers are known. All of these carriers are women.

Contrasting the rapid course in A4V ALS, the disease is far slower in patients with some other CuZn–SOD mutations, including E21G,[51] G37R,[7,48] G41D,[7] H46R,[30,48] D90A,[17] G93C,[7] G93V,[7] I104F,[52] L144S,[48,53] and I151T.[54] Patients with these mutations may survive for more than 10–15 years.

Of the 67 CuZn–SOD mutations, only the D90A is inherited as a recessive trait. In northern Sweden and Finland, the D90A CuZn–SOD mutation exists as a polymorphism; 1–5% of the population are heterozygous for the D90A allele. It is estimated that there are 99,000 D90A heterozygous carriers in Finland alone.[16,17,36] Presently, some 70 FALS and SALS patients who are homozygous for the D90A CuZn–SOD mutation have been found in Scandinavia. All these patients show a characteristic, diphasic phenotype. In the early,

Nr	Codon	Amino acid change	Genotype	Sequence change	Country found	Comments	Principal references
Missense and nonsense mutations:							
1	4	Ala–Val	A4V	GCC to GTC	Italy, Sweden, USA	Most common mutation in USA. Very aggressive phenotype. PBP	Deng et al., 1993[171]
2	4	Ala–Thr	A4T	GCC to ACC	Cyprus, Japan, USA, Cyprus		Nakano et al., 1994[172]
3	6	Cys–Phe	C6F	TGC to TTT	Japan		Morita et al., 1998[173]
4	7	Val–Glu	V7E	GTG to GAG	Japan		Hirano et al., 1994[174]
5	8	Leu–Gln	L8Q	CTG to CAG	Austria	PBP	Bereznai et al., 1997[175]
6	12	Gly–Arg	G12R	GGC to CGC	Italy		Riggio et al., 1999[176]
7	12	Gly–Ala	G12A	GGC to CGC	Italy		Peuco et al., 1999[66]
8	14	Val–Met	V14M	GTG to ATG	USA		Deng et al., 1995[177]
9	14	Val–Gly	V14G	GTG to GGG	Sweden	Single SALS case	Andersen et al., 1997[55]
10	16	Gly–Ser	G16S	GGC to AGC	Japan	SALS	Kawamata et al., 1997[178]
11	21	Glu–Lys	E21K	GAG to AAG	Scotland	SALS	Jones et al., 1994[162]
12	21	Glu–Gly	E21G	GAG to GGG	France		Boukaftane et al., 1998[51]
13	37	Gly–Arg	G37R	GGA to AGA	Spain, Turkey, USA	Transgenic mouse model	Rosen et al., 1993[44]
14	38	Leu–Val	L38V	CTG to GTG	Australia, Belgium, USA		Rosen et al., 1993[44]
15	38	Leu–Arg	L38R	CTG to CGG	France		Boukaftane et al., 1998[51]
16	41	Gly–Ser	G41S	GGC to AGC	Italy, USA		Rosen et al., 1993[44]
17	41	Gly–Asp	G41D	GGC to GAC	USA		Rosen et al., 1993[44]
18	43	His–Arg	H43R	CAT to CGT	Australia	Very large pedigree	Rosen et al., 1993[44]
19	45	Phe–Cys	F45C	TTC to TGC	Italy		Riggio et al., 1997[176]
20	46	His–Arg	H46R	CAT to CGT	Japan, USA	Uniform, mild phenotype	Aoki et al., 1993[179]
21	48	His–Glu	H48Q	CAT to CAG	United Kingdom		Enayat et al., 1995[180]
22	49	Glu–Lys	E49K	GAG to AAG	France		Boukaftane et al., 1998[51]
23	67	Leu–Arg	L67R	CTA to CGA	France		Boukaftane et al., 1998[51]
24	72	Gly–Ser	G72S	GGT to AGT	England	SALS	Shaw et al., 1998[60]
25	76	Asp–Tyr	D76Y	GAT to TAT	Denmark	SALS, PBP	Andersen et al., 1997[55]
26	84	Leu–Phe	L84F	TTG to TTC	France, United Kingdom	Single homozygous ALS in France	Shaw et al., 1998[60]
27	84	Leu–Val	L84V	TTG to GTG	Japan, USA		Deng et al., 1995[177]
28	85	Gly–Arg	G85R	GGC to CGC	USA	Transgenic mouse model	Rosen et al., 1993[44]
29	86	Asn–Ser	N86S	AAT to AGT	Japan, Scotland (Pakistan), Norway	Pakistani family living in Scotland	Maeda et al., 1997[181]
30	90	Asp–Ala	D90A	GAC to GCC	Australia, Belgium, Canada, Estonia, Finland, France, Germany, Italy, Norway, Sweden, UK, USA	Recessive or dominant inheritance in different populations. Several SALS cases. PBP.	Andersen et al., 1995[16]
31	90	Asp–Val	D90V	GAC to GTC	Japan	Transgenic mice model	Morita et al., 1998[182]

Table 12.3
Copper–zinc superoxide dismutase mutations associated with ALS

Nr	Codon	Amino acid change	Genotype	Sequence change	Country found	Comments	Principal references
32	93	Gly–Ala	G93A	GGT to GCT	USA	Transgenic mouse model	Rosen et al., 1993[44]
33	93	Gly–Cys	G93C	GGT to TGT	USA		Rosen et al., 1993[44]
34	93	Gly–Arg	G93R	GGT to CGT	United Kingdom		Orrell et al., 1995[183]
35	93	Gly–Asp	G93D	GGT to GAT	USA		Esteban et al., 1994[184]
36	93	Gly–Ser	G93S	GGT to AGT	Iceland, Japan, USA		Kawata et al., 1997[185]
37	93	Gly–Val	G93V	GGT to GTT	USA, UK		Hosler et al., 1996[186]
38	100	Glu–Gly	E100G	GAA to GGA	New Zealand, UK, USA		Rosen et al., 1993[44]
39	100	Glu–Lys	E100K	GAA to AAA	Afro-American	SALS	Siddique et al., 1996[187]
40	101	Asp–Asn	D101N	GAT to AAT	Asia, UK		Jones et al., 1994[164]
41	101	Asp–Gly	D101G	GAT to GGT	United Kingdom		Yulug et al., 1995[188]
42	104	Iso–Phe	I104F	ATC to TTC	Japan	Very variable phenotype	Abe et al., 1996[30]
43	106	Leu–Val	L106V	CTC to GTC	Japan, USA		Rosen et al., 1993[44]
44	108	Gly–Val	G108V	GGA to GTA	United Kingdom		Orrell et al., 1997[189]
45	112	Ile–Thr	I112T	ATC to ACC	USA		Esteban et al., 1994[184]
46	113	Ile–Thr	I113T	ATT to ACT	Australia, Canada, France, UK, USA	Incomplete penetrance in several populations. Many SALS cases	Rosen et al., 1993[44]
47	115	Arg–Gly	R115G	CGC to GGC	Germany		Kostrzewa et al., 1994[190]
48	118	Val–Lys . . . stop	V118 KTGPX	delGInsAAAAC	United Kingdom	Frameshift mutation, 121 amino acids long. Single SALS case	Jackson et al., 1997[58]
49	124	Asp–Val	D124V	GAT to GTT	Australia, USA		Hosler et al., 1998[186]
50	125	Asp–His	D125H	GAC to CAC	United Kingdom		Enayat et al., 1995[180]
51	126	Leu–. . .	L126 GQRWKX	TTG to **G	Japan	2 bp deletion causing frameshift. 130 amino acids long	Pramatarova et al., 1994[191]
52	126	Leu–stop	L126X	TTG to TAG	USA	125 amino acids long	Siddique et al., 1996[187]
53	127	Gly–. . .stop	G127GG QRWKX	ins TGGG after bp 1450	Denmark	4 bp addition with frameshift. 132 amino acids long. Transgenic mouse model	Hansel et al., 1998[192]
54	132	Gly–Aspstop	E132DX	insTT	United Kingdom	2 bp addition causing frameshift, 132 amino acids long	Orrell et al., 1997[20]
55	133	Glu–	E133 deltaE	delGAA	USA	3 bp deletion, 152 amino acids long. Single SALS	Hosler et al., 1996[186]
56	134	Ser–Asn	S134N	AGT to AAT	Japan		Watanabe et al., 1997[193]
57	139	Asn–Lys	N139K	AAC to AAA	USA		Pramatarova et al., 1995[194]
58	144	Leu–Phe	L144F	TTG to TTC	USA, Yugoslavia		Deng et al., 1993[171]
59	144	Leu–Ser	L144S	TTG to TCG	USA		Sapp et al., 1995[53]

Table 12.3 (cont.)
Copper–zinc superoxide dismutase mutations associated with ALS.

Nr	Codon	Amino acid change	Genotype	Sequence change	Country found	Comments	Principal references
60	145	Ala–Thr	A145T	GCT to ACT	USA		Sapp et al., 1995[53]
61	146	Cys–Arg	C146R	TGT to CGT	Japan		Siddique et al, 1996[187]
62	148	Val–Gly	V148G	GTA to GGA	USA		Deng et al, 1993[71]
63	148	Val–Ile	V148I	GTA to ATA	Japan	PBP	Ikeda et al., 1995[195]
64	149	Ile–Thr	I149T	ATT to ACT	UK, USA		Pramatarova et al., 1995[194]
65	151	Ile–Thr	I151T	ATC to ACC	Germany	PBP	Kostrzewa et al., 1996[54]
66	intron 4			T to G 10 bp before exon 5	USA	Add Phe–Leu–Gin to 5′ end of exon 5. 156 amino acids long	Sapp et al., 1995[53]
67	intron 4			A to G 11 bp before exon 5	USA	Frameshift and add Phe–Phe–Thr–Gly–Pro–stop. 123 amino acids long	Siddique et al., 1996[187]
Silent Mutations:							
1	10	Gly	G10G	GGC to GGT	United Kingdom	SALS	Jackson et al., 1997[58]
2	59	Ser	S59S	AGT to AGC	USA	SALS	Hosler et al., 1996[186]
3	116	Thr	T116T	ACA to ACG	New Zealand	Healthy relative	Calder et al., 1995[196]
4	139	Asn	D139D	AAC to AAT	Sweden	SALS	Andersen et al. 1997[55]
5	140	Ala	A140A	GCT to GCA	Sweden, USA	FALS, SALS	Hosler et al., 1996[186]
6	153	Gln	Q153Q	CAA to CAG	Norway	SALS	Andersen et al., 1997[55]

Abbreviations: PBP, bulbar onset; bp, base pair; aa, amino acids.

Table 12.3 (cont.)
Copper–zinc superoxide dismutase mutations associated with ALS.

preparetic phase, patients complain of a burning or aching pain in the lower back, hips, or knees, a sensation of unsteadiness and clumsiness, stiffness, and occasionally cramps in the muscles in the lower limbs. Non-opiate analgesics have little effect on the pain but vitamin E has a surprisingly good effect at high doses.

Neurological examination and EMG in this preparetic phase reveals few abnormalities, though the Achilles reflexes may be affected. The preparetic phase is seen in at least two-thirds of affected D90A cases and lasts from months to a few years. It is followed by a paretic phase with slowly ascending weakness that always begins in the lower limbs (usually in the leg that was most symptomatic in the preparetic phase). At the onset of the paretic phase, a few patients have demonstrated slight ataxia of a spinocerebellar type. The sequential development of abnormal reflexes is characteristic. Initially, when leg weakness is slight, the Achilles reflexes are very weak or absent whereas the patellar reflexes are brisk. A pattern of initially brisk deep tendon reflexes followed by hypoactive to absent deep tendon reflexes is seen as the disease slowly spreads to the upper extremities and after a mean of 5.4 years, to the bulbar muscles.[17,55] Extensor plantar response have been noted in most patients, but this may disappear with disease progression even before muscular wasting is pronounced. Urgency of micturition or difficulty initiating urination has been found in more than two-thirds of patients.

Neurophysiologically, the disease is characterized by moderate to marked prolongation of central motor conduction times with normal amplitudes following transcranial magnetic stimulation. These features have been found in all examined patients and in different stages of the disease.[17,31] It remains to be seen whether the unusually prolonged central motor conduction time is unique to patients who are homozygous for D90A; analogous findings have been seen in patients with the D76Y[31] and K12A mutation.[56]

The median survival time for D90A homozygous cases from onset of the paretic phase is 11.7 years. Surprisingly, the mean age at onset does not differ from cases with the aggressive A4V mutation (44 years versus 46 years), which suggests that factors that determine the age at onset act independently of those that determine survival time (a two-hit model).[31,55]

Recently, rare cases of homozygous D90A patients with a clinical picture typical of D90A patients in northern Scandinavia have been identified in isolated populations in southern France, southern Italy, Germany, and North America. A few SALS and FALS patients who are heterozygous for D90A have also been found in central France, Belgium, and Great Britain; these patients are not of Scandinavian origin. These patients show a more variable phenotype and usually a faster disease progression than the D90A homozygous patients (Camu W, personal communication, 1997).[57,58]

It has been hypothesized that homozygosity for the D90A mutation is associated with a tightly linked genetic factor that ameliorates the effect of the D90A mutant CuZn–SOD protein. This modifying effect is absent in non-Scandinavian D90A heterozygous cases.[17] Consistent with this is the observation that all studied D90A homozygous patients from different countries share the same founder haplotype, which apparently arose some 43 generations ago.[59] The D90A heterozygotes with more typical ALS do not share this founder haplotype. This has been interpreted as indicating that the D90A heterozygote ALS patients have not inherited the modifying gene and thus are more vulnerable to the cytotoxic effects of the D90A-mutated protein.[60] The

D90A polymorphism is the only known CuZn–SOD polymorphism. Studies in different countries have found CuZn–SOD mutations to be very rare in the general population. Only a few silent mutations and intronic variants have been found.[41]

In a screening study of CuZn–SOD mutations among Scandinavian ALS patients, 41 (9.6%) of 427 patients carried CuZn–SOD mutations.[55] This is the highest prevalence of ALS with CuZn–SOD mutations reported anywhere in the world and can be attributed to the D90A polymorphism; 34 of the 41 patients were homozygous for D90A. In the same study, 23.5% of patients with recognized FALS had a CuZn–SOD mutation. This is comparable to studies on FALS populations in the USA, UK, and France, which have revealed that 23.4%,[7] 20–21%,[20,60] and 14.3%,[51] respectively, carry mutations in the CuZn–SOD gene.

Other genes and loci with possible primary involvement in ALS

To date, the only well-established ALS gene is CuZn–SOD. However, mutational analyses suggest the existence of at least five additional genes whose defects can give rise to ALS or an ALS-like phenotype with Mendelian inheritance (see *Table 12.2*). Moreover, other ALS loci have been defined by linkage analysis.

In 1990, Hamida and colleagues[61] described a juvenile-onset form of ALS in 17 Tunisian families. This was characterized by the early onset (mean 12 years), recessive inheritance, and very slowly disease progression. Thus far, the neuropathological features of these cases have not been described. Hamida delineated three clinical subtypes. Type 1 is the most prevalent form and is clinically characterized by distal weakness and wasting associated with a mild spasticity of all limbs and very long survival. Type 1 was recently mapped to 15q15.1–q21.1.[62] Type 2 is an intermediate type between ALS and spastic paraplegia. Type 3 is distinguished by the predominance of spasticity of facial and limb muscles, whereas the amyotrophy of hands and peroneal muscles is mild or absent. Type 3 has been mapped to 2q33–q35.[63] Hosler and colleagues[64] narrowed this region to approximately 1.7 cM between D2S116 and D2S2237. The locus on 2q33 has not been linked to any pedigree with adult-onset FALS.[7]

A phenotypically different ALS-like disorder with juvenile onset (mean age 17 years) and normal lifespan has been described in a large Anglo-American pedigree. The phenotype is characterized by very slow progression with distal limb amyotrophy and pyramidal tract signs. The disease is inherited as an autosomal dominant trait with complete penetrance and has been linked to 9q34, between D9S1831 and D9S164.[65,66]

X-linked dominant ALS have been found in a single large American pedigree with typical clinical and neuropathological ALS features. The causative gene has yet to be found.[67]

In general, FALS (like SALS) is clinically distinct from other neurodegenerative disorders. Nonetheless, numerous case reports indicate that FALS may sometimes arise concurrently with parkinsonism or dementia, usually of frontotemporal distribution without typical features of Alzheimer's disease.[3,38,68–78] Dementia has not been reported in any ALS case with a CuZn–SOD mutation, and no association between dementia and ALS has been found in pedigrees with the D90A CuZn–SOD mutation.[17] However, in a FALS family with D76Y, Alzheimer-type dementia was diagnosed in an obligate gene carrier and her two siblings.[55] Neuropathology studies on cases with different CuZn–SOD mutations have showed multisystem pathology, with a predilection for the motor system.[49,79]

Other genes that are rarely causative in ALS

Autopsy studies have revealed aggregation and abnormal assembly of neurofilaments in the perikarya and axons of motor neurons in both SALS[80–82] and FALS with posterior column and spinocerebellar tract involvement.[83] Similar findings have been reproduced in transgenic mice with different neurofilament mutations (see Chapters 5 and 18). These findings raise the hypothesis that primary mutations in the neurofilament (NF) genes might occur in FALS. Investigations of this possibility by Figlewicz and colleagues[84] revealed deletions in the NF heavy subunit genes. The tail of the neurofilament heavy chain (NF-H) consists of repetitive lysine–serine–proline (KSP) motifs; there are two known polymorphisms with either 43 or 44 KSP-repeat motifs. Figlewicz and colleagues[84] discovered deletion mutations in this KSP-repeat domain in NF-H in five unrelated SALS patients. Four of these patients had the same 3 bp deletion, and the fifth had a 102 bp deletion. No KSP-changes were found in another 351 SALS cases or in 306 controls.

Al-Chalabi and colleagues[85] searched for mutations in the NF-H gene in 207 ALS cases from the UK and 323 Scandinavian ALS cases and found three different novel deletions in the KSP-repeat motif in two UK SALS patients and one Scandinavian SALS patient, as well as a novel KSP-deletion in a single Swedish FALS patient and the patient's brother, who has developed a non-progressive lower motor neuron syndrome with paraparesis. Twenty-two of the ALS cases included in this study had a

CuZn–SOD mutation, including three heterozygotes and nine homozygotes for the D90A mutation. There was no association between CuZn–SOD genotype, NF-H genotype, and phenotype. In this study, two young unaffected controls were found to have a KSP mutation and 444 other controls were without mutations.

In a study of 164 UK ALS cases, Tomkins and colleagues[86] found a 84 bp insertion containing four KSP repeat motifs in a single SALS case with classical ALS features. None of the remaining 163 patients or 209 controls carried a NF-H mutation.

Vechio and colleagues,[87] using single-strand conformational polymorphism (SSCP), coupled with DNA sequencing, found no mutations in the entirety of NF-L, NF-M, and NF-H genes in 100 FALS cases (without CuZn–SOD mutations) and 75 SALS cases. Rooke and colleagues[88] failed to find any KSP mutations in the NF-H gene in 75 FALS cases.

These findings support the argument that NF-H tail deletions may be the primary defects in rare cases of typical ALS. The potential importance of neurofilaments and the cytoskeleton in ALS is underscored by the observation that marked neurofilamentous pathology is evident in FALS patients with A4V,[83] I113T,[89] and D48Q mutations[90] in CuZn–SOD as well as in transgenic mice with the human G85R[91] and G93A mutations.[92]

Glutamate excitotoxity has been implicated as a major pathophysiological mechanism in ALS (see Chapter 14). In one study, variant mRNA transcripts for the astroglial glutamate transporter excitatory amino acid transporter-2 (EAAT2) (glutamate transporter-1 (GLT-1)) were detected in affected central nervous system tissue of 60% of autopsied SALS patients.[93] In vitro analyses indicate that the variant transcripts reduce expression of the EAAT2 protein and thereby augment glutamate activity at synapses. As yet, these findings have not been duplicated in other studies.[94,95] To examine the possibility that primary mutations in the EAAT2 gene might cause some cases of FALS, genetic linkage analysis and mutational screening was undertaken in a large series of FALS and SALS cases. With one exception, no germline mutations were detected in the EAAT2 gene. The single exception was in a patient with a mis-sense mutation that alters a glycosylation site. The functional significance of this mutation remains unclear.[96] In another study, Meyer and colleagues[95] failed to find any EAAT2 sequence variants in 55 ALS patients. These data argue convincingly that genomic mutations in EAAT2 are rare in ALS.

Spinal muscular atrophy (SMA) is a recessively inherited motor neuron syndrome that is customarily divided into four subtypes on clinical grounds: type 1 is a severe infantile form (Werdnig–Hoffman disease), whereas types 2, 3, and 4 are less severe types of infantile, juvenile and adolescent onset. All three types map to chromosome 5q13 and are associated with defects in a gene that encodes a protein described as 'survival motor neuron' (SMN).[97] The SMN gene is present in at least two copies, one telomeric (SMNt) and one centromeric (SMNc). The SMNt gene is homozygously deleted in more than 90% of patients with type 1 SMA. In adult-onset SMA (type 4), SMNt deletions are less frequent.[98,99] In the same locus as SMN is a gene for the neuronal apoptosis inhibitory protein (NAIP). NAIP is commonly deleted in SMA cases (67% of type 1 SMA patients, 42% in other types).[100] However, in contrast to SMN mutations, NAIP mutations are not uniformly detected in SMA. In SMA, the NAIP deletion usually coexists with the SMNt deletion.[101] The functions and interactions of SMN and NAIP and mutations in these genes are incompletely understood. Orrell and colleagues[102] found no

mutations of the SMN or NAIP genes in 54 SALS and 10 FALS cases. Moulard and colleagues[99] studied the SMNt and SMNc genes in 66 FALS patients, 177 SALS patients, and 14 patients with sporadic pure lower motor neuron features. Only in the last group were mutations found: two patients had homozygous SMNt deletions and five patients had homozygous SMNc deletions. Jackson and colleagues[103] searched for SMN and NAIP mutations in 130 SALS patients, five patients with Kennedy's disease, and 17 FALS cases; the only pathological finding was a homozygous deletion of NAIP exon 5 in an SALS patient with typical ALS features. Parboosingh and colleagues[104] failed to find any mutations in the NAIP and SMN genes in 69 FALS patients (without CuZn–SOD mutations) and 194 SALS patients.

Gangliosidmyelin (GM2) gangliosidosis is caused by hexosaminidase A and B deficiency and is inherited as an autosomal recessive trait. The classical phenotype is an infantile encephalopathy with dementia and visual loss, but several cases have been reported with variable phenotypes, including juvenile and adult encephalopathies, cerebellar ataxia, dystonia, Charcot–Marie–Tooth-like disorder, or with mental illness. Rare cases have resembled SMA types 3 and 4 or ALS (both juvenile and adult-onset cases have been described); individual cases often combine motor weakness with extra motor features such as tremor and psychosis.[105–111] The author is unaware of any epidemiological study of the frequency of motor neuron disease features in patients with GM2 gangliosidosis. However, GM2 gangliosidosis has been screened for in more than 100 patients with combined upper and lower motor neuron findings. No defects in hexosaminidase A or B activity have been identified.

High incidence foci of motor neuron disease

have been reported among the Chamorros of the Mariana Island, the Japanese of the Kii Peninsula, and the Auyu and Jakai of southern West New Guinea. In the 1960s, the prevalence rate of motor neuron disease in these areas was estimated at about 100 per 100,000 of the population, between 50 and 100 times in excess of the prevalence elsewhere in the world.[112] In the Mariana Islands and the Kii Peninsula the patients with motor neuron disease are clinically indistinguishable from patients with SALS. However, at autopsy these cases show widespread neurofibrillary degeneration with prominent involvement of subcortical areas, a pattern that is distinctly unlike conventional ALS. Parkinsonism–dementia complex also occurs with a high incidence in the Mariana Islands, and ALS and parkinsonism–dementia complex are suggested to have the same etiology because they share some pathological and epidemiological features.[113] In New Guinea, the phenotype of motor neuron disease is clinically akin to ALS, but the progression of the disease is very slow.[114] Although ALS in the Mariana Islands and West New Guinea is often familial, the inheritance pattern does not appear to be Mendelian. Attempts to identify genetic markers, including mutations in the CuZn–SOD gene, have been negative. Since 1970, a dramatic fall in the incidence of motor neuron disease has been observed in all three areas,[115,116] which is consistent with the possibility that environmental factors contribute more to the disease than a pure genetic defect.

Modifying or predisposing genes

In any given ALS case, the clinical phenotype may be a consequence of several, combined predisposing environmental and genetic factors. The genetic factors are predicted to be either allelic variants of known ALS genes or novel modifying genes. Two epidemiological observations argue for the existence of one or more sex-linked modifying or predisposing genes in ALS. First, there is a marked male preponderance among the younger patients, contrasting with a relative female preponderance in patients above 60 years of age. Before the age of 60–65 years, the male-to-female ratio has been reported as 1.1:1,[117] 1.2:1,[72] 1.4:1,[118] 1.7:1,[119] 1.9:1,[120] and 2.5:1[121] in different population studies. The sex ratio decreases, until after age 65–70 years the male-to-female ratio approaches unity.[72,118,119,122] Familial ALS with high penetrance has a male-to-female ratio of 1:1.[9,11,19] The author is unaware of any study of sex differences in age or site of onset in high penetrance FALS pedigrees or of sex differences in FALS pedigrees with low disease penetrance.

A second observation argues that there are predisposing genes in ALS. In SALS, the frequency of sites of onset differs between male and female patients. Moreover, patients with bulbar onset tend to be a few years older than patients with limb onset[7,118,120,123,124] and to have a relative female preponderance compared to patients with truncal or limb onset.[125,126] In two studies from Denmark, nearly half the female patients had bulbar onset.[120,126] As yet, there is no biological explanation for these epidemiological findings.

One potential risk factor for the development of ALS is the status of apolipoprotein E (ApoE). ApoE is the major serum protein involved with cholesterol storage, transport, and metabolism and exists in three major forms, $\epsilon2$, $\epsilon3$, and $\epsilon4$. This protein has a crucial role in the facilitation of growth and maintenance of myelin and axonal membranes,[127] making it plausible that ApoE may be involved in other neurodegenerative diseases. Indeed, it is well established that the presence of the ApoE ε4 allele is a risk factor for sporadic and familial late-onset Alzheimer's disease.[128] It is also associated with earlier onset of Alzheimer's disease.[129]

Four studies have evaluated the hypothesis that ApoE ε4 alleles might modify the phenotype in ALS.[130–133] Al-Chabali and colleagues[130] found an association between the ApoE ε4 allele with bulbar-onset among 124 UK ALS cases. Moulard and colleagues[131] found among 130 French SALS cases an association both with bulbar onset and earlier onset for patients carrying the ApoE ε4 allele. Possession of the ApoE ε2 allele was associated with both longer survival and limb onset. In contrast, Mui and colleagues[132] found no differences in ApoE allele frequencies between a North American ALS population and the general population, nor were there any differences between age at onset or the duration of FALS and the inheritance of ApoE ε4. Similarly, Smith and colleagues[133] found no significant differences in distribution of ApoE alleles for patients with bulbar-onset ALS among 155 North American SALS patients.

Allelic variants of genes involved in other neurodegenerative diseases could potentially also be involved in ALS or ALS-plus syndromes (e.g. ALS–dementia, ALS–parkinsonism). One gene of particularly interest in this regard is the *tau* gene, as *tau* mutations can produce autosomal-dominantly inherited degenerative syndromes with frontotemporal dementia, features of amyotrophy, and parkinsonism (FTDP-17). *tau* mutations have also been implicated (but not documented) in progressive supranuclear paresis and corticobasal degeneration.[134] To date, no cases of pure ALS have been associated with primary *tau* gene mutations. Other candidate risk genes might include presenilin genes 1 and 2 (with mutations linked to early-onset Alzheimer's disease)

and alpha-synuclein[135] and parkin[136] (both linked to Parkinson's disease). Interestingly, the amino terminus of parkin matches many different ubiquitin proteins. However, to date no studies have implicated these proteins in the ALS syndrome.

Expansion of a cytosin, adenin and guanin (CAG)-trinucleotide repeat in the androgen receptor gene causes X-linked spinobulbar muscular atrophy (Kennedy's syndrome).[137] Patients with Kennedy's disease occasionally present with symptoms reminiscent of ALS.[138,139] However, no CAG-expansion in the androgen receptor gene have been found in ALS (author's unpublished results).[138]

Kinesins are microtubule-anchored motor proteins involved in the intracellular transport of organelles and chromosomes during cell division. Mutations of the gene that encode the microtubule motor subunit kinesin heavy chain in *Drosophilia melanogaster* disrupt fast axonal transport and cause progressive distal paralysis in larvae.[140] Toyoshima and colleagues[141] found massive accumulation of kinesin in spheroids in the spinal cord of five patients with motor neuron disease, which co-localized with highly phosphorylated neurofilaments. The gene for the neuron-specific kinesin heavy chain have been mapped to chromosome 2 and the genes for neuron-specific kinesin light chain to 19q13.2–q13.3. These loci do not correspond to any known ALS loci. At this time, there have been no investigations of mutations in these genes in ALS.

Hereditary spastic paraplegia is a degenerative disorder that is characterized clinically by progressive lower extremity weakness and spasticity. There are at least seven loci for hereditary spastic paraplegia mapped to chromosomes 8q and 16q (both with autosomal-recessive inheritance); chromosomes 2p, 8q, 10q, 12q, 14q, and 15q (all autosomal dominant inheritance), and the X chromosome

Disease		Gene	Locus	Mode of inheritance
Hereditary spastic paresis	SPG1	L1CAM	Xq28	XR
	SPG2	Proteolipid protein	Xq22	XR
	SPG3	u	14q	AD
	SPG4	u	2p	AD
	SPG5A	u	8q12	AR
	SPG5B	Paraplegin	16q24	AR
	SPG6	u	15q	AD
	SPG8	u	8q	AD
	SPG9	u	10q	AD
	SPG10	u	12q	AD
Spinobulbar muscular atrophy (Kennedy's syndrome)	SMBA	Androgen receptor	Xq11	XR
Spinal muscular atrophy (SMA)	SMA1-3(4)	SMN, NAIP	5q13	AR
GM2 gangliosidosis		Hexosaminidase A	15q23	AR
		Hexosaminidase B	5q13	AR

Abbreviations: AD, autosomal dominant; AR, autosomal recessive, NAIP, neuronal apoptosis inhibitory protein; SMN, survival motor neuron; u, unknown gene; XR, x-linked recessive; SPG, spastic paraplegia.

Table 12.4
Genes and loci in motor neuron diseases other than ALS.

(*Table 12.4*). Specific mutations that cause hereditary spastic paraplegia have been defined in the genes that encode paraplegin (16q), L1CAM (Xq28), and proteolipid (PLP) (Xq22).[142] The gene defects at the other loci are still not determined.[143] The authors have also encountered rare instances of adrenoleukodystrophy presenting as adult-onset hereditary spastic paraplegia with distal sensory loss. Thus, there are several candidate genes to screen in cases of motor neuron disease presenting primarily with spasticity. However, no studies to date indicate that these genes are implicated in ALS with both lower and upper motor neuron features.

Ciliary neurotrophic factor (CNTF) has a powerful survival-promoting effect on motor neurons. Inactivation of the CNTF gene causes progressive loss of motor neurons in adult mice with a mild phenotype.[144] Two studies have failed to find a causal relation between a null mutation (resulting in a truncated protein lacking biological activity) in the CNTF gene and ALS even in patients who are homozygous for the mutation.[145,146] Similarly, screening for causal mutations in the CNTF receptor α gene has proved negative.[147]

Numerous studies[148,149] suggest there is subtle mitochondrial dysfunction in ALS pathogenesis. A single case of motor neuron disease has been reported with a heteroplasmic 5 bp deletion in the mitochondrial DNA-encoded subunit I of cytochrome *c* oxidase.[150] The mutation was associated with a predominantly upper motor neuron phenotype, although some signs of spinal involvement were detected. Two muscle biopsies revealed ragged red fibers with 47% and 68.7% mutant mitochondrial DNA, respectively. The patient died 5 years after onset, at the age of 34 years. DNA and muscle biopsy analysis of the healthy mother and three sisters were normal. Recently, a male patient with typical ALS features was found to have the MELAS syndrome with the A3243G point mutation of the mitochondrial tRNA(Leu) gene and ragged red fibers on muscle biopsy (Somer H, personal communication).

Using single-strand conformational polymorphism (SSCP), Parboosingh and colleagues[151] screened 66% (exons 3-5) of the gene that encodes the mitochondrial manganese-containing superoxide dismutase (Mn–SOD) in 73 FALS cases and found no mutations. Tomblyn and colleagues[152] sequenced the entire coding region of Mn–SOD in 20 SALS patients and 10 controls in the USA and found only a structural dimorphism A9V in the mitochondrial targeting sequence in the Mn SOD gene. Replacing Ala with Val has been predicted to cause a complete loss of the α-helical segment, thereby impairing the regulation of mitochondrial transport of Mn–SOD. Homozygosity for the V9 allele was over-represented among the SALS patients in Tomblyn's study.[152] By contrast, homozygosity for the A9 allele was a significant risk factor for ALS (especially in females) in a study that compared 72 Swedish SALS patients with 136 controls.[153] A caveat of the study by Tomblyn and colleagues[152] is the very small groups and the absence of Hardy–Weinberg equilibrium in the study group.

The apurinic–apyrimidinic endonuclease (APEX nuclease) is a DNA repair enzyme, and the gene is mapped to 14q11.2–q12. Recently, it was reported that APEX nuclease levels and activity in the frontal cortex was significantly lower in 11 SALS patients than in six controls.[154] Olkowski[155] identified mis-sense mutations in the APEX nuclease gene in eight of 11 ALS patients, but not in five controls. In contrast, Hayward and colleagues[156] examined 117 SALS patients and 36 FALS patients and only identified a four-base deletion in a single SALS patient and silent mutation in three SALS patients. They also found the frequency of the D148E polymorphism in this gene to be significantly different in sporadic ALS patients compared with controls. These results suggest that mutations in the APEX gene might contribute to the etiology of ALS. Further studies are needed to clarify the role of mutations in the Mn–SOD and APEX nuclease genes in ALS.

Does genetics contribute to sporadic ALS?

Beyond the above studies, additional findings support the hypothesis that genetic factors are important in the genesis of SALS. Three epidemiological studies found that ALS affects genetically predisposed individuals. Longitudinal analysis of ALS mortality in the USA,[157] Norway,[158] and Sweden[159] concluded that the mortality curves for ALS are consistent with deaths being confined to an inherently susceptible population subset.

Few twin studies have been done on ALS populations, but Hawkes and Graham[160] found evidence of a genetic component in SALS based on twin analysis.

Williams and colleagues[11] studied the disease penetrance in nine FALS pedigrees and found that in eight pedigrees with diminished penetrance the age at onset was significantly higher than in the single pedigree with complete penetrance. This makes it more likely that gene carriers in those families will die from other causes before developing ALS, thereby masking the familial disposition for ALS. In the eight pedigrees with dominant inheritance but reduced penetrance, the mean age of onset was comparable to that reported in most epidemiological studies for SALS.

Presently, 10 mutations in the CuZn–SOD gene have been found in apparent SALS cases (see *Table 12.3*). In two reports, only extensive genealogical research revealed distant relatives with ALS.[55,161] The three apparent SALS cases with the I113T found in Scotland have been linked in a haplotype study to three known I113T Scottish FALS pedigrees,[41,162] suggesting that not all carriers of CuZn–SOD mutations develop disease. Cudkowicz and colleagues[7] estimated the disease penetrance by age 70 years in the USA for I113T to be 100% (four pedigrees), as was also estimated for pedigrees with E100G (two families with 26 patients) and L38V (two families with 14 patients), and 91% for A4V (27 families with 87 patients). Other reported figures for penetrance in FALS are 50% by the age of 47 years (in the ALS CuZn–SOD population),[48] 82% by the age of 55 years (in the general FALS population),[9] and 80% at age 85 years (in the general FALS population.[163] Penetrance for D90A homozygous ALS patients is estimated to be 94% at the age of 70 years.[17] However, it should be noted that most of the pedigree used in these estimations are those with high penetrance collected for genetic linkage analysis (i.e. families with symptomatic disease in multiple generations). It is the author's experience from investigating FALS families in Scandinavia that there may be a significant group of FALS pedigrees with very low penetrance, such that patients in these families are usually diagnosed as SALS cases.

Three groups have studied the frequency of

CuZn–SOD mutations in SALS populations and found that 4% (14 patients out of 335),[55] 3% (five patients out of 175),[58] and 7% (four patients out of 56)[164] of SALS cases are carriers. Although the number of apparent SALS cases with a CuZn–SOD mutation is small, analysis of these cases may give clues to causes of incomplete penetrance and the disease mechanism.

In northern Scandinavia, the widespread occurrence of the D90A CuZn–SOD polymorphism as the genetic background for recessive ALS, and thereby some cases of SALS, is an excellent precedent for allelic variants in other genes that cause low penetrance, recessively inherited FALS. This invites the speculation that some cases of SALS may be caused by two independently segregating autosomal loci. If homozygosity is required at both loci for developing SALS (a 'double recessive' model), only one of 16 siblings would be homozygous for both disease alleles. Such an individual would most likely show up as an SALS patient. To elaborate further, if the two disease alleles exist as polymorphisms with allele frequencies of $p1 = 0.55$ and $p2 = 0.06$, this simple mathematical model can explain all SALS cases (assuming complete penetrance, random mating, and no new mutations or migration).

Should new, suspected ALS cases undergo genetic testing?

At present there is essentially no effective therapy for ALS (whether SALS or FALS). Accordingly, it is difficult to justify extensive (and expensive) DNA testing in ALS patients. However, in practice the authors often obtain DNA studies simply because the patients request that all reasonable tests be completed to define the cause of the problem. If the patient belongs to an ALS family with a known

CuZn–SOD DNA mutation, detection of that specific mutation in a new patient can hasten the diagnosis and, depending on the mutation, allow some prognostic projections (see *Table 12.3*).

If the patient's phenotype corresponds to that predicted for homozygous D90A ALS cases, confirmation of the D90A homozygous genotype has diagnostic, prognostic, and counseling value.

Genetic counseling in ALS

Although most FALS pedigrees in the literature show high if not complete penetrance for ALS by the age of 70–80 years, a number of pedigrees with or without mutations in the CuZn–SOD gene have been reported to have diminished penetrance. The diminished penetrance can make it difficult if not impossible to give adequate genetic counseling to the question often asked by patients: are my children also going to become affected?

Before any counseling, a pedigree containing at least four generations (to great grandparents) should be constructed and information about number of siblings, age, and cause of death should be obtained for all members in the previous generations. Also, the utmost should be done to verify the diagnosis of ALS. The author encountered a pedigree of seemingly FALS with atypical features and reduced penetrance in both the maternal and paternal lines. Analysis showed the index patient to be the carrier of a paternally inherited CuZn–SOD mutation *and* a maternally inherited CAG-expansion in the androgen receptor gene. The reported maternal relatives with ALS in fact had Kennedy's disease.

In FALS pedigrees with well documented high or complete penetrance and autosomal-dominant inheritance, the probability of the children having inherited the gene and becom-

ing affected will be close to 50%. The risk for unaffected siblings will depend on their age and the age-dependent penetrance in that particular family.

In FALS pedigrees with diminished penetrance, it is difficult to provide genetic counseling. Only if it is possible to construct a pedigree of at least four or five generations and to document critical clinical details on the age and cause of death of all individuals in previous generations is it possible to estimate the risk in a FALS pedigree with reduced penetrance. In the authors' experience, this information is rarely available. The clinician is therefore often left to tell the patient and the anxious spouse that the probability of ALS is less than 50% but more than that of the background population (1:1000),[112] reminding the family that most relatives have died of other causes at an advanced age.

In mono-generation FALS pedigrees in which genealogy has failed to find any cases of ALS in the previous three generations and in which a recessive trait can therefore be suspected (excluding non-genetic causes), the risk for the siblings of being homozygous is 25% and their actual disease risk depends on the disease penetrance and the age of the individual. The only known mutation that causes adult-onset, recessive ALS is the D90A CuZn–SOD mutation, which has an estimated penetrance of 94% at the age of 70 years,[17] but studies of other mono-generational FALS pedigrees without a CuZn–SOD mutation make it possible and perhaps likely that as yet unknown FALS genes can show recessive inheritance.[31]

In SALS patients for whom reliable information is available about the previous three generations, the risk for the children is most likely to be the same as that of the background population. In the rare SALS patients who are homozygous for D90A CuZn–SOD, the children are obligate mutation carriers and their risk of being homozygous for D90A will depend on the genotype of the spouse. In an anonymous study of spouses of D90A homozygous ALS cases in Finland and Sweden, two of eighteen spouses were heterozygous for the D90A mutation.[31]

The discovery of mutations in the CuZn–SOD gene in some cases of ALS opens up the potential for performing pre-natal and pre-symptomatic diagnostic testing of at-risk individuals (siblings and children of patients). Presently, pre-symptomatic testing have been performed in pedigrees with the A4V CuZn–SOD mutation (in the USA), The H43R CuZn–SOD mutation (in Australia), and the D90A CuZn–SOD mutation (in Sweden). It is probably advisable that blood samples from relatives that have been collected for ALS research purposes should not be used for pre-symptomatic testing. Rather, the generally accepted guidelines established for pre-symptomatic testing in familial cancer diseases and for Huntington's disease should be followed.[165,166] Only at-risk individuals from families with well established, high-penetrance FALS should be tested. Presymptomatic testing of first- or even second-degree relatives from FALS pedigrees with low or uncertain disease penetrance or of SALS patients should be avoided. The main exception to this guideline is relatives of SALS patients who are homozygous for D90A CuZn–SOD. In these rare cases, establishing the genotype of the spouse is often less psychologically demanding and easier than actually testing the children. Also, siblings of D90A-homozygous SALS cases can undergo pre-symptomatic testing following the Huntington's disease guidelines. In all cases, adequate professional and community resources should be available to deal with the impact of test results in subjects and their relatives.

References

1. Aran FA. Recherches sur une maladie non encore décrite du système musculaire atrophie musculaire progressive. *Arch Gén Méd* 1850; **24**: 5–35; 172–214.

2. Norris FH. Adult spinal motor neurone disease. In: Vinken PJ, Brujn GW, eds. *Handbook of Clinical Neurology, System Disorders and Atrophies* vol 22. New York: John Wiley, 1975.

3. Mulder DW. Clinical limits of amyotrophic lateral sclerosis. In: Rowland, LP, ed. *Human Motor Neuron Diseases*. New York: Raven Press, 1982.

4. Charcot J-M. Leçons sur les maladies du système nerveux. IInd series, collected by Bourneville 1873. In: Charcot J-M. *Lectures on the Diseases of the Nervous System* vol 2, series 2. London: New Sydenham Society, 1881, 163–204.

5. Osler W. On heredity in progressive muscular atrophy as illustrated in the Farr family of Vermont. *Arch Med* 1880; **4**: 316–320.

6. Brown MR. 'Wetherbee Ail': The inheritance of progressive muscular atrophy as a dominant trait in two New England families. *N Engl J Med* 1951; **245**: 645.

7. Cudkowicz ME, McKenna-Yasek D, Sapp PE et al. Epidemiology of mutations in superoxide dismutase in amyotrophic lateral sclerosis. *Ann Neurol* 1997; **41**: 210–221.

8. Kurland KT, Mulder DW. Epidemiological investigations of amyotrophic lateral sclerosis. Familial aggregations indicative of dominant inheritance. Part I & II. *Neurology* 1955; **5**: 182–267.

9. Emery AEH, Holloway S. Familial motor neuron diseases. In: Rowland LP, ed. *Human Motor Neuron Diseases*. New York: Raven Press, 1982, 139–145.

10. Mulder DW, Kurland LT, Offord KP, Beard CM. Familial adult motor neuron disease: amyotrophic lateral sclerosis. *Neurology* 1986; **36**: 511–517.

11. Williams DB, Floate DA, Leicester J. Familial motor neuron disease: differing penetrance in large pedigrees. *J Neurol Sci* 1988; **86**: 215–230.

12. Bernhardt M. Ueber eine heriditäre form der

progressiven spinalen mit bulbärparalyse complicirten muskelatrophie. *Virchows Arch A Pathol Anat Physiol* 1889; **115**: 197–216.

13. Gardner JH, Feldmahn A. Heriditary adult motor neuron disease. *Trans Am Neurol Assoc* 1966; **91**: 239–241.

14. Husquinet H, Franck G. Hereditary amyotrophic lateral sclerosis transmitted for five generations. *Clin Genet* 1980; **18**: 109–115.

15. Chio A, Brignolio F, Meineri P, Schiffer D. Phenotypic and genotypic heterogeneity of dominantly inherited amyotrophic lateral sclerosis. *Acta Neurol Scand* 1987; **75**: 277–282.

16. Andersen PM, Nilsson P, Ala HV et al. Amyotrophic lateral sclerosis associated with homozygosity for an Asp90Ala mutation in CuZn-superoxide dismutase. *Nat Genet* 1995; **10**: 61–66.

17. Andersen PM, Forsgren L, Binzer M et al. Autosomal recessive adult-onset ALS associated with homozygosity for Asp90Ala CuZn-superoxide dismutase mutation. A clinical and genealogical study of 36 patients. *Brain* 1996; **119**: 1153–1172.

18. Tandan R, Bradley WG. Amyotrophic lateral sclerosis: Part 2. Etiopathogenesis. *Ann Neurol* 1985; **18**: 419–431.

19. Li TM, Alberman E, Swash M. Comparison of sporadic and familial disease amongst 580 cases of motor neuron disease. *J Neurol Neurosurg Psychiatry* 1988; **51**: 778–784.

20. Orrell RW, Habgood JJ, Gardiner I et al. Clinical and functional investigation of 10 missense mutations and a novel frameshift insertion mutation of the gene for copper-zinc superoxide dismutase in UK families with amyotrophic lateral sclerosis. *Neurology* 1997; **48**: 746–751.

21. Engel WK, Kurland LT, Klatzo I. An inherited disease similar to amyotrophic lateral sclerosis with a pattern of posterior column involvement. An intermediate form? *Brain* 1959; **82**: 203–220.

22. Takahashi K, Nakamura H, Okada E. Hereditary amyotrophic lateral sclerosis. Histochemical and electron microscopic study of hyaline inclusions in motor neurons. *Arch Neurol* 1972; **27**: 292–299.

23. Veltema AN, Roos RA, Bruyn GW. Autosomal dominant adult amyotrophic lateral sclerosis. A six generation Dutch family. *J Neurol Sci* 1990; **97**: 93–115.

24. Hamilton AS. Familial progressive muscular atrophy in adults. *J Nerv Ment Dis* 1918; **48**: 127–150.

25. Myrianthopoulos NC, Brown IA. A genetic study of progressive spinal muscular atrophy. *Am J Hum Genet* 1954; **6**: 387–411.

26. Thomson AF, Alvarez FA. Hereditary amyotrophic lateral sclerosis. *J Neurol Sci* 1968; **8**: 101–110.

27. Nakano T, Tsukada N, Yanagisawa N et al. Familial motor neuron disease with cases of amyotrophic lateral sclerosis and spinal muscular atrophy. *Rinsho Shinkeigaku* 1985; **25**: 1119–1125.

28. Strong MJ, Hudson AJ, Alvord WG. Familial amyotrophic lateral sclerosis, 1850–1989: a statistical analysis of the world literature. *Can J Neurol Sci* 1991; **18**: 45–58.

29. Appelbaum JS, Roos RP, Salazar-Grueso EF et al. Intrafamilial heterogeneity in hereditary motor neuron disease. *Neurology* 1992; **42**: 1488–1492.

30. Abe K, Aoki M, Ikeda M et al. Clinical characteristics of familial amyotrophic lateral sclerosis with Cu/Zn superoxide dismutase gene mutations. *J Neurol Sci* 1996; **136**: 108–116.

31. Andersen PM. Amyotrophic Lateral Sclerosis and CuZn-Superoxide Dismutase. A clinical, genetic and enzymatic study. Doctoral thesis Umeå University: Umeå, Sweden 1997.

32. Robinson GW. The spinal type and family form of progressive muscular atrophy as appearing in adults. *J Nerv Ment Dis* 1917; **45**: 401.

33. Hirano A, Kurland LT, Sayre GP. Familial amyotrophic lateral sclerosis. A subgroup characterized by posterior and spinocerebellar tract involvement and hyaline inclusions in the anterior horn cells. *Arch Neurol* 1967; **16**: 232–243.

34. Amick LD, Nelson JW, Zellweger H. Familial motor neuron disease, non-Chamorro type: report of kinship. *Acta Neurol Scand* 1971; **47**: 341–349.

35. Hestnes A, Mellgren SI. Familial amyotrophic

lateral sclerosis. Report of a family with predominant upper limb pareses and late onset. *Acta Neurol Scand* 1980; **61**: 192–199.

36. Keränen M-L, Ala-Hurula V-M, Saarinen A, Andersen PM, Marklund SL. Familiaalinen amyotrofinen lateraaliskleroosi Pohjois-Suomessa. *Duodecim* 1996; **112**: 2026–2030.

37. Roe PF. Familial motor neurone disease. *J Neurol Neurosurg Psychiatry* 1964; **27**: 140–143.

38. Alter M, Schaumann B. A family with amyotrophic lateral sclerosis and Parkinsonism. *J Neurol* 1976; **212**: 281–284.

39. Alajouanine MM, Nick J. Sur trois cas familiaux de sclérose latérale amyotrophique survenue dans la même fratrie. *Rev Neurol* 1959; **100**: 490–492.

40. Giménez-Roldán S, Esteban A. Prognosis in hereditary amyotrophic lateral sclerosis. *Arch Neurol* 1977; **34**: 706–708.

41. Radunovic A, Leigh PN. Cu/Zn superoxide dismutase gene mutations in amyotrophic lateral sclerosis: Correlation between genotype and clinical features. *J Neurol Neurosurg Psychiatry* 1996; **61**: 565–572.

42. Espinosa RE, Okihiro MM, Mulder DW, Sayre GP. Hereditary amyotrophic lateral sclerosis. A clinical and pathologic report with comments on classification. *Neurology* 1962; **12**: 1–7.

43. Siddique T, Figlewicz DA, Pericak-Vance MA et al. Linkage of a gene causing familial amyotrophic lateral sclerosis to chromosome 21 and evidence of genetic-locus heterogeneity. *N Engl J Med* 1991; **324**: 1381–1384.

44. Rosen DR, Siddique T, Patterson D et al. Mutations in CuZn superoxide dismutase gene are associated with familial amyotrophic lateral sclerosis. *Nature* 1993; **362**: 59–62.

45. Forman HJ, Fridovich I. On the stability of bovine superoxide dismutase. The effects of metals. *J Biol Chem* 1973; **248**: 2645–2649.

46 Pardo CA, Xu Z, Borchelt DR et al. Superoxide dismutase is an abundant component in cell bodies, dendrites, and axons of motor neurons and in a subset of other neurons. *Proc Natl Acad Sci USA 1995;* **92**: 954–958.

47. Bowling AC, Barkowski EE, McKenna-Yasek D et al. Superoxide dismutase concentration and activity in familial amyotrophic lateral sclerosis. *J Neurochem* 1995; **64**: 2366–2369.

48. Juneja T, Pericak VM, Laing NG et al. Prognosis in familial amyotrophic lateral sclerosis: Progression and survival in patients with glu100gly and ala4val mutations in Cu,Zn superoxide dismutase. *Neurology* 1997; **48**: 55–57.

49. Cudkowicz ME, McKenna-Yasek D, Chen C et al. Limited corticospinal tract involvement in amyotrophic lateral sclerosis subjects with the A4V mutation in the copper/zinc superoxide dismutase gene. *Ann Neurol* 1998; **43**: 703–710.

50. Shibata N, Hirano A, Kobayashi M et al. Intense superoxide dismutase-1 immunoreactivity in intracytoplasmic hyaline inclusions of familial amyotrophic lateral sclerosis with posterior column involvement. *J Neuropathol Exp Neurol* 1996; **55**: 481–490.

51. Boukaftane Y, Khoris J, Moulard B et al. Identification of six novel SOD1 gene mutations in familial amyotrophic lateral sclerosis. *Can J Neurol Sci* 1998; **25**: 192–196.

52. Ikeda M, Abe K, Aoki M et al. Variable clinical symptoms in familial amyotrophic lateral sclerosis with a novel point mutation in the Cu/Zn superoxide dismutase gene. *Neurology* 1995; **45**: 2038–2042.

53. Sapp PC, Rosen DR, Hosler BA et al. Identification of three novel mutations in the gene for Cu/Zn superoxide dismutase in patients with familial amyotrophic lateral sclerosis. *Neuromuscul Disord* 1995; **5**: 353–357.

54. Kostrzewa M, Damian MS, Muller U. Superoxide dismutase 1: identification of a novel mutation in a case of familial amyotrophic lateral sclerosis. *Human Genetics* 1996; **98**: 48–50.

55. Andersen PM, Nilsson P, Keränen M-L et al. Phenotypic heterogeneity in MND-patients with CuZn-superoxide dismutase mutations in Scandinavia. *Brain* 1997; **10**: 1723–1737.

56. Penco S, Schenone A, Bordo D et al. A SOD1 gene mutation in a patient with slowly progressing familial ALS. *Neurology* 1999; **53**: 404–406.

57. Robberecht W, Aguirre T, Van et al. D90A heterozygosity in the SOD1 gene is associated with familial and apparently sporadic amyotrophic lateral sclerosis. *Neurology* 1996; **47**: 1336–1339.

58. Jackson M, Al CA, Enayat ZE et al. Copper/zinc superoxide dismutase 1 and sporadic amyotrophic lateral sclerosis: analysis of 155 cases and identification of a novel insertion mutation. *Ann Neurol* 1997; **42**: 803–807.

59. Al-Chalabi A, Andersen PM, Chioza B et al. Recessive amyotrophic lateral sclerosis families with the D90A SOD1 mutation share a common founder: evidence for a linked protective factor. *Hum Mol Genet* 1998; **7**: 2045–2050.

60. Shaw CE, Enayat ZE, Chioza BA et al. Mutations in all five exons of SOD-1 may cause ALS. *Ann Neurol* 1998; **43**: 390–394.

61. Ben Hamida M, Hentati F, Ben Hamida C. Hereditary motor system diseases (chronic juvenile amyotrophic lateral sclerosis). Conditions combining a bilateral pyramidal syndrome with limb and bulbar amyotrophy. *Brain* 1990; **113**: 347–363.

62. Hentati A, Ouahchi K, Pericak-Vance MA et al. Linkage of a common locus for recessive amyotrophic lateral sclerosis (abst) *Am J Hum Genet* 1997; **61** (**suppl**): A279.

63. Hentati A, Bejaoui K, Pericak VM et al. Linkage of recessive familial amyotrophic lateral sclerosis to chromosome 2q33-q35. *Nat Genet* 1994; **7**: 425–428.

64. Hosler BA, Sapp PC, Berger R et al. Refined mapping and characterization of the recessive familial amyotrophic lateral sclerosis locus (ALS2) on chromosome 2q33. *Neurogenetics* 1998; **2**: 34–42.

65. Chance PF, Rabin BA, Ryan SG et al. Linkage of the gene for an auotosomal dominant form of juvenile amyotrophic lateral sclerosis to chromosome 9q34. *Am J Hum Genet* 1998; **62**: 633–640.

66. Rabin BA, Griffin JW, Crain BJ et al. Autosomal dominant juvenile amyotrophic lateral sclerosis. *Brain* 1999; **122**: 1539–1550.

67. Siddique T, Hong ST, Brooks BR et al. X-linked dominant locus for late-onset familial amyotrophic lateral sclerosis. Abstract 1785 *Am Soc Hum Genet Meeting*, 48th Annual meeting, October 27–31, 1998, Denver, Colorado.

68. Robertson EE. Progressive bulbar paralysis showing heredofamilial incidence and intellectual impairment. *Arch Neurol Psychiatry* 1953; **69**: 197–207.

69. Brait K, Fahn S, Schwarz GA. Sporadic and familial parkinsonism and motor neuron disease. *Neurology* 1973; **23**: 990–1002.

70. Finlayson MH, Martin JB. Cerebral lesions in familial amyotrophic lateral sclerosis and dementia. *Acta Neuropathol (Berl)* 1973; **26**: 237–246.

71. Pinsky L, Finlayson MH, Libman I, Scott BH. Familial amyotrophic lateral sclerosis with dementia – a second Canadian family. *Clin Genet* 1975; **7**: 187.

72. Jokelainen M. Amyotrophic lateral sclerosis in Finland. II: Clinical characteristics. *Acta Neurol Scand* 1977; **56**: 194–204.

73. Burnstein MH, Ananth J. Amyotrophic lateral sclerosis, dementia and psychosis: report of a family and discussion. *Psychiatric J of the University of Ottawa* 1980; **3**: 166–167.

74. Appel SH. A unifying hypothesis for the cause of amyotrophic lateral sclerosis, parkinsonism, and Alzheimer's disease. *Ann Neurol* 1981; **10**: 499–505.

75. Hudson AJ. Amyotrophic lateral sclerosis and its association with dementia, parkinsonism and other neurological disorders: a review. *Brain* 1981; **104**: 217–247.

76. Schmitt HP, Emser W, Heimes C. Familial occurrence of amyotrophic lateral sclerosis, parkinsonism, and dementia. *Ann Neurol* 1984; **16**: 642–648.

77. Neary D, Snowden JS, Mann DM et al. Frontal lobe dementia and motor neuron disease. *J Neurol Neurosurg Psychiatry* 1990; **53**: 23–32.

78. Gunnarsson LG, Dahlbom K, Strandman E. Motor neuron disease and dementia reported among 13 members of a single family. *Acta Neurol Scand* 1991; **84**: 429–433.

79. Ince PG, Tomkins J, Slade JY et al. Amyotrophic lateral sclerosis associated with genetic abnormalities in the gene encoding Cu/Zn superoxide dismutase: molecular pathology of five new cases, and comparison with previous reports and 73 sporadic cases of ALS. *J Neuropathol Exp Neurol* 1998; **57**: 895–904.

80. Carpenter S. Proximal axonal enlargement in motor neuron disease. *Neurology* 1968; **18**: 841–851.

81. Munoz DG, Greene C, Perl DP, Selkoe DJ. Accumulation of phosphorylated neurofilaments in anterior horn motoneurons of amyotrophic lateral sclerosis patients. *J Neuropathol Exp Neurol* 1988; **47**: 9–18.

82. Manetto V, Sternberger NH, Perry G et al. Phosphorylation of neurofilaments is altered in amyotrophic lateral sclerosis. *J Neuropathol Exp Neurol* 1988; **47**: 642–653.

83. Hirano A, Nakano I, Kurland LT et al. Fine structural study of neurofibrillary changes in a family with amyotrophic lateral sclerosis. *J Neuropathol Exp Neurol* 1984; **43**: 471–480.

84. Figlewicz DA, Krizus A, Martinoli MG et al. Variants of the heavy neurofilament subunit are associated with the development of amyotrophic lateral sclerosis. *Hum Mol Genet* 1994; **3**: 1757–1761.

85. Al-Chalabi A, Andersen PM, Nilsson P et al. Deletions of the heavy neurofilament subunit tail in amyotrophic lateral sclerosis. *Hum Mol Genet* 1999; **8**: 157–164.

86 Tomkins J, Usher P, Slade JY et al. Novel insertion in the KSP region of the neurofilament heavy gene in amyotrophic lateral sclerosis (ALS). *Neuroreport* 1998; **9**: 3967–3970.

87. Vechio JD, Bruijn LI, Xu Z et al. Sequence variants in human neurofilament proteins: Absence of linkage to familial amyotrophic lateral sclerosis. *Ann Neurol* 1996; **40**: 603–610.

88. Rooke K, Figlewicz DA, Han FY, Rouleau GA. Analysis of the KSP repeat of the neurofilament heavy subunit in familiar amyotrophic lateral sclerosis. *Neurology* 1996; **46**: 789–790.

89. Rouleau GA, Clark AW, Rooke K et al. SOD1 mutation is associated with accumulation of neurofilaments in amyotrophic lateral sclerosis. *Ann Neurol* 1996; **39**: 128–131.

90. Shaw CE, Enayat ZE, Powell JF et al. Familial amyotrophic lateral sclerosis. Molecular pathology of a patient with a SOD1 mutation. *Neurology* 1997; **49**: 1612–1616.

91. Bruijn LI, Becher MW, Lee MK et al. ALS-linked SOD1 mutant G85R mediates damage to astrocytes and promotes rapidly progressive disease with SOD1-containing inclusions. *Neuron* 1997; **18**: 327–338.

92. Tu PH, Raju P, Robinson KA et al. Transgenic mice carrying a human mutant superoxide dismutase transgene develop neuronal cytoskeletal pathology resembling human amyotrophic lateral sclerosis lesions. *Proc Natl Acad Sci USA* 1996; **93**: 3155–3160.

93. Lin CL, Bristol LA, Jin L et al. Aberrant RNA processing in a neurodegenerative disease: the cause for absent EAAT2, a glutamate transporter, in amyotrophic lateral sclerosis. *Neuron* 1998; **20**: 589–602.

94. Nagai M, Abe K, Okamoto K, Itoyama Y. Identification of alternative splicing forms of GLT-1 mRNA in the spinal cord of amyotrophic lateral sclerosis patients. *Neurosci Lett* 1998; **244**: 165–168.

95. Meyer T, Munch C, Volkel H et al. The EAAT2 (GLT-1) gene in motor neuron disease: absence of mutations in amyotrophic lateral sclerosis and a point mutation in patients with hereditary spastic paraplegia. *J Neurol Neurosurg Psychiatry* 1998; **65**: 594–596.

96. Aoki M, Lin CL, Rothstein JD et al. Mutations in the glutamate transporter EAAT2 gene do not cause abnormal EAAT2 transcripts in amyotrophic lateral sclerosis. *Ann Neurol* 1998; **43**: 645–653.

97. Lefebvre S, Burglen L, Reboullet S et al. Identification and characterization of a spinal muscular atrophy-determining gene. *Cell* 1995; **80**: 155–165.

98. Brahe C, Servidei S, Zappata S et al. Genetic homogeneity between childhood-onset and adult-onset autosomal recessive spinal muscular atrophy. *Lancet* 1995; **346**: 741–742.

99. Moulard B, Salachas F, Chassande B et al. Association between centromeric deletions of the SMN gene and sporadic adult-onset lower motor neuron disease. *Ann Neurol* 1998; **43**: 640–644.

100. Roy N, Mahadevan MS, McLean M et al. The gene for neuronal apoptosis inhibitory protein is partially deleted in individuals with spinal muscular atrophy. *Cell* 1995; **80**: 167–178.

101. Rodrigues NR, Owen N, Talbot K et al. Gene deletions in spinal muscular atrophy. *J Med Genet* 1996; **33**: 93–96.

102. Orrell RW, Habgood JJ, de Belleroche JS,

Lane RJ. The relationship of spinal muscular atrophy top motor neuron disease: investigation of SMN and NAIP gene deletions in sporadic and familial ALS. *J Neurol Sci* 1997; **145**: 55–61.

103. Jackson M, Morrison KE, Al CA et al. Analysis of chromosome 5q13 genes in amyotrophic lateral sclerosis: homozygous NAIP deletion in a sporadic case. *Ann Neurol* 1996; **39**: 796–800.

104. Parboosingh JS, Meininger V, McKenna-Yasek D et al. Deletions causing spinal muscular atrophy do not predispose to amyotrophic lateral sclerosis. *Arch Neurol* 1999; **56**: 710–712.

105. Le Coz P, Assouline E, Vanier MT et al. GM2-Gangliosidosis variant B1 disclosed during adolescence by an isolated multisystemic involvement of the central and peripheral nervous systems. *Rev Neurol (Paris)* 1994; **1**: 61–66.

106. Banerjee P, Siciliano L, Oliveri D et al. Molecular basis of an adult form of beta-hexosaminidase B deficiency with motor neuron disease. *Biochem Biophys Res Commun* 1991; **181**: 108–115.

107. Mondelli M, Rossi A, Palmeri S et al. Neurophysiological study in chronic GM2 gangliosidosis (hexosaminidase A and B deficiency), with motor neuron disease phenotype. *Ital J Neurol Sci* 1989; **10**: 433–439.

108. Rubin M, Karpati G, Wolfe LS et al. Adult onset motor neuronopathy in the juvenile type of hexosaminidase A and B deficiency. *J Neurol Sci* 1988; **87**: 103–119.

109. Cashman NR, Antel JP, Hancock LW et al. N-acetyl-beta-hexosaminidase beta locus defect and juvenile motor neuron disease: a case study. *Ann Neurol* 1986; **19**: 568–572.

110. Hancock LW, Horwitz AL, Cashman NR et al. N-acetyl-beta-hexosaminidase B deficiency in cultured fibroblasts from a patient with progressive motor neuron disease. *Biochem Biophys Res Commun* 1985; **130**: 1185–1192.

111. Mitsumoto H, Sliman RJ, Schafer IA et al. Motor neuron disease and adult hexosaminidase A deficiency in two families: evidence for multisystem degeneration. *Ann Neurol* 1985; **17**: 378–385.

112. Bobowick AR, Brody JA. Epidemiology of motor-neuron diseases. *N Engl J Med* 1973; **288**: 1047–1055.

113. Ahlskog JE, Waring SC, Petersen RC et al. Olfactory dysfunction in Guamanian ALS, parkinsonism, and dementia. *Neurology* 1998; **51**: 1672–1677.

114. Gajdusek DC. Motor-neuron disease in natives of New Guinea. *N Engl J Med* 1963; **268**: 474–476.

115. Yoshida S, Uebayashi Y, Kihira T et al. Epidemiology of motor neuron disease in the Kii Peninsula of Japan, 1989–1993: active or disappearing focus? *J Neurol Sci* 1998; **155**: 146–155.

116. Garruto RM, Yanagihara R, Gajdusek DC. Disappearance of high-incidence amyotrophic lateral sclerosis and parkinsonism-dementia on Guam. *Neurology* 1985; **35**: 193–198.

117. Forsgren L, Almay BG, Holmgren G, Wall S. Epidemiology of motor neuron disease in northern Sweden. *Acta Neurol Scand* 1983; **68**: 20–29.

118. Rosen AD. Amyotrophic lateral sclerosis. Clinical features and prognosis. *Arch Neurol* 1978; **35**: 638–642.

119. Haverkamp LJ, Appel V, Appel SH. Natural history of amyotrophic lateral sclerosis in a database population. Validation of a scoring system and a model for survival prediction. *Brain* 1995; **118**: 707–719.

120. Kristensen O, Melgaard B. Motor neuron disease. Prognosis and epidemiology. *Acta Neurol Scand* 1977; **56**: 299–308.

121. Mackay RP. Course and prognosis in amyotrophic lateral sclerosis. *Arch Neurol* 1963; **8**: 117–127.

122. Fong KY, Yu YL, Chan YW et al. Motor neuron disease in Hong Kong Chinese: epidemiology and clinical picture. *Neuroepidemiology* 1996; **15**: 239–245.

123. Murros K, Fogelholm R. Amyotrophic lateral sclerosis in Middle-Finland: an epidemiological study. *Acta Neurol Scand* 1983; **67**: 41–47.

124. Jablecki CK, Berry C, Leach J. Survival prediction in amyotrophic lateral sclerosis. *Muscle Nerve* 1989; **12**: 833–841.

125. Rosati G, Pinna L, Granieri E et al. Studies

on epidemiological, clinical, and etiological aspects of ALS disease in Sardinia, Southern Italy. *Acta Neurol Scand* 1977; **55**: 231–244.

126. Højer-Pedersen E, Christensen PB, Jensen NB. Incidence and prevalence of motor neuron disease in two Danish counties. *Neuro-epidemiology* 1989; **8**: 151–159.

127. Mahley RW. Apolipoprotein E: cholesterol transport protein with expanding role in cell biology. *Science* 1988; **240**: 622–630.

128. Corder EH, Saunders AM, Strittmatter WJ et al. Gene dose of apolipoprotein E type 4 allele and the risk of Alzheimer's disease in late onset families. *Science* 1993; **261**: 921–923.

129. Borgaonkar DS, Schmidt LC, Martin SE et al. Linkage of late-onset Alzheimer's disease with apolipoprotein E type 4 on chromosome 19. *Lancet* 1993; **342**: 625.

130. Al-Chalabi A, Enayat ZE, Bakker MC et al. Association of apolipoprotein E epsilon 4 allele with bulbar-onset motor neuron disease. *Lancet* 1996; **347**: 159–160.

131. Moulard B, Sefiani A, Laamri A et al. Apolipoprotein E genotyping in sporadic amyotrophic latreal sclerosis: evidence for a major influence on the clinical presentation and prognosis. *J Neurol Sci* 1996; **139**: 34–37.

132. Mui S, Rebeck GW, McKenna-Yasek D et al. Apolipoprotein E epsilon 4 allele is not associated with earlier age at onset in amyotrophic lateral sclerosis. *Ann Neurol* 1995; **38**: 460–463.

133. Smith RG, Haverkamp LJ, Case S et al. Apolipoprotein E epsilon 4 in bulbar-onset motor neuron disease. *Lancet* 1996; **348**: 334–335.

134. Hutton M, Lendon CL, Rizzu P et al. Association of missense and 5'-splice-site mutations in tau with the inherited dementia FTDP-17. *Nature* 1998; **393**: 702–705.

135. Polymeropoulos MH, Lavedan C, Leroy E et al. Mutation in the alpha-synuclein gene identified in families with Parkinson's disease. *Science* 1997; **276**: 2045–2047.

136. Kitada T, Asakawa S, Hattori N et al. Mutations in the parkin gene cause autosomal recessive juvenile parkinsonism. *Nature* 1998; **392**: 605–608.

137. Andrew SE, Goldberg YP, Hayden MR. Rethinking genotype and phenotype correlations in polyglutamine expansion disorders. *Hum Mol Genet* 1997; **6**: 2005–2010.

138. Parboosingh JS, Figlewicz DA, Krizus A et al. Spinobulbar muscular atrophy can mimic ALS: The importance of genetic testing in male patients with atypical ALS. *Neurology* 1997; **49**: 568–572.

139. Shaw PJ, Thagesen H, Tomkins J et al. Kennedy's disease: unusual molecular pathologic and clinical features. *Neurology* 1998; **51**: 252–255.

140. Hurd DD, Saxton WM. Kinesin mutations cause motor neuron disease phenotypes by disrupting fast axonal transport in Drosophila. *Genetics* 1996; **144**: 1075–1085.

141. Toyoshima I, Sugawara M, Kato K et al. Kinesin and cytoplasmic dynein in spinal spheroids with motor neuron disease. *J Neurol Sci* 1998; **159**: 38–44.

142. Fink JK, Heiman-Patterson T, Bird T et al. Hereditary spastic paraplegia: advances in genetic research. Hereditary Spastic Paraplegia Working group. *Neurology* 1996; **46**: 1507–1514.

143. Hedera P, Rainier S, Alvarado D et al. Novel Locus for Autosomal Dominant Hereditary Spastic Paraplegia, on Chromosome 8q. *Am J Hum Genet* 1999; **64**: 563–569.

144. Masu Y, Wolf E, Holtmann B et al. Disruption of the CNTF gene results in motor neuron degeneration. *Nature* 1993; **365**: 27–32.

145. Takahashi R, Yokoji H, Misawa H et al. A null mutation in the human CNTF gene is not causally related to neurological diseases. *Nat Genet* 1994; **7**: 79–84.

146. Giess R, Goetz R, Schrank B et al. Potential implications of a ciliary neurotrophic factor gene mutation in a German population of patients with motor neuron disease. *Muscle Nerve* 1998; **21**: 236–238.

147. Imura T, Shimohama S, Kawamata J, Kimura J. Genetic variation in the ciliary neurotrophic factor receptor alpha gene and familial amyotrophic lateral sclerosis. *Ann Neurol* 1998; **43**: 275.

148. Bowling AC, Schulz JB, Brown RJ, Beal MF. Superoxide dismutase activity, oxidative damage, and mitochondrial energy metabo-

lism in familial and sporadic amyotrophic lateral sclerosis. *J Neurochem* 1993; **61**: 2322–2325.

149. Browne SE, Bowling AC, Baik MJ et al. Metabolic dysfunction in familial, but not sporadic, amyotrophic lateral sclerosis. *J Neurochem* 1998; **71**: 281–287.

150. Comi GP, Bordoni A, Salani S et al. Cytochrome c oxidase subunit I microdeletion in a patient with motor neuron disease. *Ann Neurol* 1998; **43**: 110–116.

151. Parboosingh JS, Rouleau GA, Meninger V et al. Absence of mutations in the Mn superoxide dismutase or catalase genes in familial amyotrophic lateral sclerosis. *Neuromuscul Disord* 1995; **5**: 7–10.

152. Tomblyn M, Kasarskis EJ, Xu Y, St Clair DK. Distribution of MnSOD polymorphisms in sporadic ALS patients. *J Mol Neurosci* 1998; **10**: 65–66.

153. Van Landeghem GF, Tabatabaie, Beckman L, Beckman G, Andersen PM. Mn-SOD Signal Sequence Polymorphism Associated with Sporadic Motor Neuron Disease. *Eur J Neurol* 1999 (in press).

154. Kisby GE, Milne J, Sweatt C. Evidence of reduced DNA repair in amyotrophic lateral sclerosis brain tissue. *Neuroreport* 1997; **8**: 1337–1340.

155. Olkowski ZL. Mutant AP endonuclease in patients with amyotrophic lateral sclerosis. *Neuroreport* 1998; **9**: 239–242.

156. Hayward C, Colville S, Swingler RJ, Brock DJ. Molecular genetic analysis of the APEX nuclease gene in amyotrophic lateral sclerosis. *Neurology* 1999; **52**: 1899–1901.

157. Riggs JE. Longitudinal Gompertzian analysis of amyotrophic lateral sclerosis mortality in the U.S., 1977–1986: evidence for an inherently susceptible population subset. *Mech Ageing Dev* 1990; **55**: 207–220.

158. Neilson S, Robinson I, Nymoen EH. Longitudinal analysis of amyotrophic lateral sclerosis mortality in Norway, 1966–1989: evidence for a susceptible subpopulation. *J Neurol Sci* 1994; **122**: 148–154.

159. Neilson S, Gunnarsson LG, Robinson I. Rising mortality from motor neurone disease in Sweden 1961–1990: the relative role of increased population life expectancy and environmental factors. *Acta Neurol Scand* 1994; **90**: 150–159.

160. Graham AJ, Hawkes CH. Twin study using mortality data: a new sampling method. *Int J Epidemiol* 1995; **24**: 758–762.

161. Suthers G, Laing N, Wilton S, Dorosz S, Waddy H. 'Sporadic' motoneuron disease due to familial SOD1 mutation with low penetrance. *Lancet* 1994; **344**: 1773.

162. Jones CT, Swingler RJ, Brock DJ. Identification of a novel SOD1 mutation in an apparently sporadic amyotrophic lateral sclerosis patient and the detection of Ile113Thr in three others. *Hum Mol Genet* 1994; **3**: 649–650.

163. de Belleroche J, Orrell R, King A. Familial amyotrophic lateral sclerosis/motor neurone disease (FALS): a review of current developments. *J Med Genet* 1995; **32**: 841–847.

164. Jones CT, Shaw PJ, Chari G, Brock DJ. Identification of a novel exon 4 SOD1 mutation in a sporadic amyotrophic lateral sclerosis patient. *Molecular & Cellular Probes* 1994; **8**: 329–330.

165. Scourfield J, Soldan J, Gray J et al. Huntington's disease: psychiatric practice in molecular genetic prediction and diagnosis. *Br J Psychiatry* 1997 Feb; **170**: 146–149.

166. de Wert G. Ethics of predictive DNA-testing for hereditary breast and ovarian cancer. *Patient Educ Couns* 1998; **1**: 43–52.

167. Haberlandt WF. Genetic aspects of amyotrophic lateral sclerosis and progressive bulbar paralysis. *Acta Genet Med Gemell* 1959; **8**: 369–373.

168. Murray TJ, Pride S, Haley G. Motor neuron disease in Nova Scotia. *Can Med Assoc J* 1974; **110**: 814–817.

169. Gunnarsson L-G, Palm R. Motor neuron disease and heavy manual labor: an epidemiologic survey of Värmland County, Sweden. *Neuroepidemiology* 1984; **3**: 195–206.

170. Giagheddu M, Puggioni G, Masala C et al. Epidemiologic study of amyotrophic lateral sclerosis in Sardinia, Italy. *Acta Neurol Scand* 1983; **68**: 394–404.

171. Deng HX, Hentati A, Tainer JA et al. Amyotrophic lateral sclerosis and structural defects in Cu, Zn superoxide dismutase. *Science* 1993; **261**: 1047–1051.

172. Nakano R, Sato S, Inuzuka T et al. A novel mutation in Cu/Zn superoxide dismutase gene in Japanese familial amyotrophic lateral sclerosis. *Biochem Biosphys Res Commun* 1994; **200**: 695–703.

173. Morita M, Aoki M, Abe K et al. A novel two-base mutation in the Cu/Zn superoxide dismutase gene associated with familial amyotrophic lateral sclerosis in Japan. *Neurosci Lett* 1996; **205**: 79–82.

174. Hirono M, Fujii J, Nagai Y et al. A new variant Cu/Zn superoxide dismutase (Val17→Glu) deduced from lymphocyte mRNA sequences from Japanese patients with familial amyotrophic lateral sclerosis. *Biochem Biophys Res Commun* 1994; **204**: 572–577.

175. Bereznai B, Winkler A, Borasio GD, Gasser T. A novel SOD1 mutation in an Austrian family with amyotrophic lateral sclerosis. *Neuromuscul Disord* 1997; **7**: 113–116.

176. Riggio MC, Botti S, Gellera C et al. SOD1 Gene: Molecular Screening in Amyotrophic Lateral Sclerosis in Italian families. Abstract European Neurological Society Conference, Milan, Italy, June 1999.

177. Deng HX, Tainer JA, Mitsumoto H et al. Two novel SOD1 mutations in patients with familial amyotrophic lateral sclerosis. *Hum Mol Genet* 1995; **4**: 1113–1116.

178. Kawamata J, Shimohama S, Takano S et al. Novel G16S (GGC-AGC) mutation in the SOD-1 gene in a patient with apparently sporadic young-onset amyotrophic lateral sclerosis. *Hum Mutat* 1997; **9**: 356–358.

179. Aoki M, Ogasawara M, Matsubara Y et al. Mild ALS in Japan associated with novel SOD mutation. *Nat Genet* 1993; **5**: 323–324.

180. Enayat ZE, Orrell RW, Claus A et al. Two novel mutations in the gene for copper zinc superoxide dismutase in UK families with amyotrophic lateral sclerosis. *Hum Mol Genet* 1995; **4**: 1239–1240.

181. Maeda T, Kurahashi K, Matsunaga M et al. [On intra-familial clinical diversities of a familial amyotrophic lateral sclerosis with a point mutation of Cu/Zn superoxide dismutase (Asn 86-Ser)]. *No Shinkei Geka* 1997; **49**: 847–851.

182. Morita M, Abe K, Takahashi M et al. A novel mutation Asp90Val in the SOD1 gene associated with Japanese familial ALS. *Eur J Neurol* 1998; **5**: 389–392.

183. Orrell R, Debelleroche J, Marklund S et al. A novel SOD mutant and ALS. *Nature* 1995; **374**: 504–505.

184. Esteban J, Rosen DR, Bowling AC et al. Identification of two novel mutations and a new polymorphism in the gene for Cu/Zn superoxide dismutase in patients with amyotrophic lateral sclerosis. *Hum Mol Genet* 1994; **3**: 997–998.

185. Kawata A, Kato S, Hayashi H, Hirai S. Prominent sensory and autonomic disturbances in familial amyotrophic lateral sclerosis with a Gly93Ser mutation in the SOD1 gene. *J Neurol Sci* 1997; **153**: 82–85.

186. Hosler BA, Nicholson GA, Sapp PC et al. Three novel mutations and two variants in the gene for Cu/Zn superoxide dismutase in familial amyotrophic lateral sclerosis. *Neuromuscul Disord* 1996; **6**: 361–366.

187. Siddique T, Deng H-X. Genetics of amyotrophic lateral sclerosis. *Hum Mol Genet* 1996; **5**: 1465–1470.

188. Yulug IG, Katsanis N, Debelleroche J et al. An improved protocol for the analysis of SOD1 gene mutations, and a new mutation in exon 4. *Hum Mol Genet* 1995; **4**: 1101–1104.

189. Orrell RW, Habgood JJ, Shepherd DI et al. A novel mutation of SOD-1 (Gly 108 Val) in familial amyotrophic lateral sclerosis. *Eur Neurol* 1997; **4**: 48–51.

190. Kostrzewa M, Burck-Lehmann U, Muller U. Autosomal dominant amyotrophic lateral sclerosis: A novel mutation in the Cu/Zn superoxide dismutase-1 gene. *Hum Mol Genet* 1994; **3(12)**: 2261–2262.

191. Pramatarova A, Goto J, Nanba E et al. A two basepair deletion in the SOD 1 gene causes familial amyotrophic lateral sclerosis. *Hum Mol Genet* 1994; **3(11)**: 2061–2062.

192. Hansen C, Gredal O, Werdelin L et al. Novel 4-bp Insertion in the CuZn-Superoxide Dismutase (SOD1) gene Associated With Familial Amyotrophic Lateral Sclerosis. *Hum Mutat* 1998; Suppl 1: S327–S328.

193. Watanabe M, Aoki M, Abe K et al. A novel missense point mutation (S134N) of the

Cu/Zn superoxide dismutase gene in a patient with familial motor neuron disease. *Hum Mutat* 1997; **9**: 69–71.

194. Pramatarova A, Figlewicz DA, Krizus A et al. Identification of new mutations in the Cu/Zn superoxide dismutase gene of patients with familial amyotrophic lateral sclerosis. *Am J Hum Genet* 1995; **56**: 592–596.

195. Ikeda M, Abe K, Aoki M et al. A novel point mutation in the Cu/Zn superoxide dismutase gene in a patient with familial amyotrophic lateral sclerosis. *Hum Mol Genet* 1995; **4**: 491–492.

196. Calder VL, Domigan NM, George PM et al. Superoxide dismutase (glu100→gly) in a family with inherited motor neuron disease: detection of mutant superoxide dismutase activity and the presence of heterodimers. *Neurosci Lett* 1995; **189**: 143–146.

13

Transgenic animal models of amyotrophic lateral sclerosis

Mark E Gurney

Introduction

Recent successes in using transgenic mouse technology to produce animal models of neurodegenerative diseases is rapidly advancing our understanding of pathogenic mechanisms and facilitating the search for effective therapeutics. These models are based on the expression in mice of mutant human genes that cause familial amyotrophic lateral sclerosis (FALS),[1-3] Alzheimer's disease,[4,5] Huntington's disease,[6] and other neurodegenerative diseases.[7-9] The use of transgenic technology has allowed the creation of genetically exact models of the human disease. Since disease is initiated by a mutant human protein, such models open a window to the exploration and ultimately to the understanding of complex disease processes that in patients would otherwise remain closed.

With respect to FALS, the generation of a transgenic model was based on the finding of autosomal-dominant mutations of the SOD1 gene that encodes the enzyme copper–zinc superoxide dismutase (SOD) in patients with FALS.[10] Over 60 different point mutations have been documented in the SOD1 gene. For the most part, these are missense mutations that substitute one amino acid for another in the polypeptide backbone of copper–zinc SOD.[11]

Only a single copy of a mutant human SOD1 gene is sufficient to cause disease in patients. Thus, disease could be due to hap-loinsufficiency, to negative dominant mutations, which would decrease SOD activity levels in tissues still further, or to gain-of-function mutations, which cause the protein to become toxic (*Table 13.1*). Initial studies in patient material indicated that copper–zinc SOD activity was decreased in red blood cells and in brain tissue at autopsy.[11,12] This decrease could be due to lower intrinsic enzymatic activity in the mutant protein, to a decrease in protein stability, or to a combination of the two effects.[13] The absence of deletions in the SOD1 gene in FALS patients argued against haploinsufficiency as a genetic mechanism in the disease. Instead, the discovery of so many missense mutations argues that the presence of the mutant protein is required for pathogenesis. This suggests that the SOD1 mutations may cause a gain-of-function in copper–zinc SOD, which is toxic to upper and lower motor neurons.

The gain-of-function hypothesis received support from experiments in transgenic mice. Transgenic technology allows the genome of an organism to be manipulated in specific ways. An exogenous disease gene can be introduced and expressed in a tissue-specific manner, or alternatively, an endogenous gene can be mutated or deleted. The mouse has been the organism that is most tractable to transgenic manipulation. Exogenous genes are introduced by microinjection of purified DNA

Loss-of-function
Nominally ruled out in FALS patients with SOD1 mutations owing to autosomal-dominant pattern of inheritance.

In addition, SOD1 mutations linked to FALS are primarily point mutations that substitute one amino acid for another.[11]

If disease was due to a loss-of-function with haploinsufficiency, one would expect to find deletions of the SOD1 gene in FALS. Such mutations have not been reported in patients.

Haploinsufficiency
Implies that a 50% reduction in tissue copper–zinc SOD activity causes disease. This theory received initial support from the finding that many FALS patients had decreased copper–zinc SOD activity in red blood cells[11] and in brain tissue at autopsy.[12]

Negative dominant
Implies that heterodimers formed from mutant and wild-type copper–zinc SOD subunits have decreased stability or decreased superoxide dismutase activity in comparison to wild-type homodimers.

Gain-of-function
Implies that the mutant protein had acquired a novel, toxic activity.

Table 13.1
Genetic mechanisms in neurodegenerative disease.

into the male pronucleus of the fertilized mouse egg *(Fig. 13.1)*. Integration of the foreign DNA is random, with multiple copies of the DNA usually integrating at a single site. Pronuclear microinjection is especially useful to study dominant traits or to characterize the in vivo activity of gene promoters. Endogenous genes are manipulated in embryonic stem cells, which are pluripotent cells that will contribute to the formation of the embryo when reintroduced into a mouse blastula. Manipulation of embryonic stem cells makes it possible to target DNA to specific chromosomal sites by homologous recombination. This makes it possible to inactivate an endogenous gene or to introduce specific mutational modifications. The pronuclear microinjection technique was used to create transgenic mice carrying human SOD1 genes incorporating FALS-linked mutations.[1–3,14] The normal function of the SOD1 gene was investigated by using the embryonic stem cell technique to inactivate copper–zinc SOD expression by deleting a portion of the endogenous gene.[15]

Expression of the human copper–zinc SOD containing the mutations G93A, G37R, or G85R at sufficient levels in transgenic mice causes a progressive paralytic disease, which in its essential features resembles human amyotrophic lateral sclerosis *(Fig. 13.2)*.[1–3] Since control mice expressing wild-type human copper–zinc SOD remain clinically normal,[1] this implies that the mutations cause the protein to be pathogenic in mice and presumably in humans as well. The comparison of mice that express mutant forms of human copper-zinc

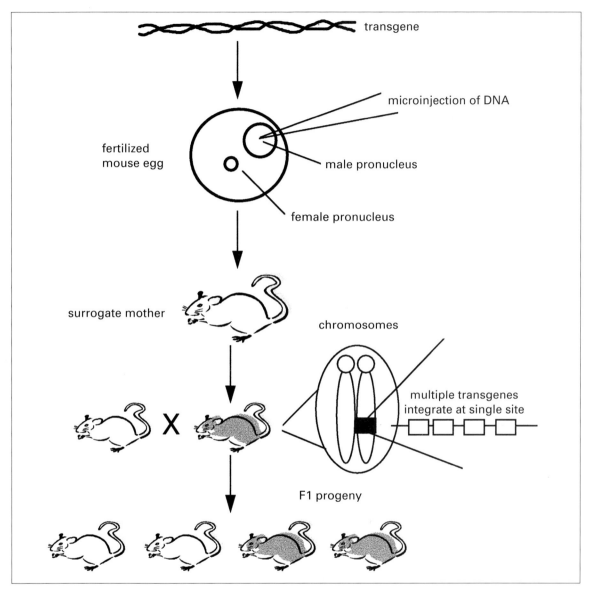

Figure 13.1
Transgenic mice are produced by microinjection of cloned DNA comprising a synthetic or natural gene into the male pronucleus of a fertilized mouse egg. The injected eggs are implanted into a surrogate mother to allow development to term. Generally, multiple copies of the synthetic gene integrate into the host chromosome at a single location or locus. The transgene locus is inherited in a Mendelian fashion on breeding of the founder transgenic mouse to a nontransgenic mouse.

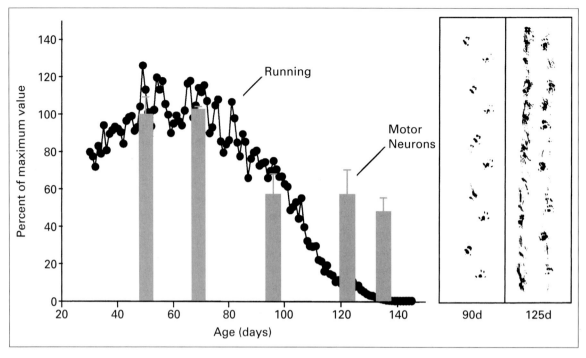

Figure 13.2

Clinical and pathological features of motor neuron disease in SOD1–G93A mice. SOD1–G93A mice are outwardly normal until about 3 months of age.[16] At that time they develop a subtle shaking in their limbs, which is most evident when the animal is lifted into the air by the base of its tail, as well as other more subtle motor abnormalities.[1,16,42] In addition to the shaking or trembling, the animals are hyper-reflexive and display crossed spread of spinal reflexes, suggesting a loss of descending inhibitory inputs within the spinal cord ventral horn. Nightly running in a wheel averages 7–11 km per night until about 3 months of age.[19,41] Thereafter, there is a slow decline in running, owing to increasing paralysis. By about 4 months of age, progressive paralysis mainly affecting the rear legs becomes evident on clinical examination. This results in a shortening of stride measured on an inclined plane.[1,16].

SOD1–G93A mice survive until about 5 months of age, at which time complete paralysis with inability to forage for food and water necessitates that they be killed.[16,17,39] The earliest sign of pathology within the spinal cord ventral horn occurs in some mice by 1 month of age, well in advance of clinical signs.[43] This pathology consists of vacuolar changes within the proximal axons of spinal motor neurons where they enter the ventral roots. By 2 months of age, pathology has spread to the motor neuron cell body and includes fragmentation of the golgi apparatus,[44] vacuolar changes involving the smooth endoplasmic reticulum,[45] and an unusual swelling of the mitochondrial intermembrane space.[3,45] Denervation of muscle is also apparent before evidence of clinical disease,[16] as are functional changes in the motor unit.[46] Motor neuron loss is not evident until 3 months of age, when clinical signs of disease become apparent.[16] In late-stage disease, neurofilaments accumulate in the motor neuron cell body[43,44,47] cytoplasmic staining for ubiquinated material increases,[47] and axonal spheroids are seen in the ventral horn.[46] Slow axonal transport is also impaired.[48] Data on motor neuron loss are from Chiu et al[16] and average counts in the cervical and lumbar segments. Both nightly running and motor neuron counts have been normalized to 100%.

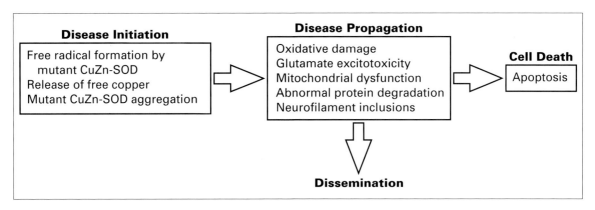

Figure 13.3
Initiators and propagators of disease in FALS.

SOD with those that express wild-type human copper–zinc SOD is an important control since the G93A and G37R mutant forms of SOD enzyme have essentially wild-type dismutase activity towards superoxide.[1,13] Thus, merely elevating superoxide dismutase activity in the spinal cord does not cause disease. Pathogenicity is an intrinsic property of the mutant enzyme.

Neuroprotection studies in FALS transgenic mice

The molecular events whereby mutations in copper–zinc SOD cause motor neuron disease are just beginning to be unraveled. Possible pathophysiological mechanisms in FALS are outlined in *Fig. 13.3*. Studies of potential therapeutics, principally in the SOD1–G93A transgenic model, lend support to the hypothesis that distinct pathological mechanisms underlie disease initiation and propagation. Symptomatic disease in this model coincides with the period of motor neuron loss (see *Fig. 13.2*).[16] This assumes that the timing to onset of clinical disease is a measure of the process con-

tributing to disease initiation, whereas the duration of symptomatic disease reflects the rate of disease propagation. Contributing to this concept was the observation in multiple lines of SOD1–G93A mice that the timing of disease onset varied with transgene dosage from 3 months of age to as late as 8 months of age, whereas the duration of symptomatic disease was roughly similar in all lines and lasted about 1.5 months.[17]

Neuroprotective strategies that should ameliorate oxidative damage, at least in theory (copper chelation therapy,[16] dietary antioxidants,[19,20] and co-expression of bcl-2[21]), all delay disease onset yet do not affect the duration of symptomatic disease. In contrast, drugs that are proposed to inhibit glutamate excitotoxicity[19] and genetic manipulations that interfere with apoptosis[22] have no effect on disease onset, but they do extend survival by extending the duration of symptomatic disease. Thus, oxidative mechanisms appear to be associated with disease initiation, while glutamate-mediated excitotoxicity and apoptotic mechanisms are associated with disease propagation and motor neuron death (*Table 13.2*). Which of

Treatment	Transgenic line	Onset	Survival	Duration	Reference
D-penicillamine (100 mg/kg by gavage)	TgN(SOD1–G93A)1Gur	Delayed	Increased	No change	18
Vitamin E plus selenium (vitamin E 50 IU/kg, selenium 2 μg/kg in diet)	TgN(SOD1–G93A)1Gur	Delayed (by 15%)	No change	Decreased	19
Carboxyfullerene (15 mg/kg by osmotic minipump)	TgN(SOD1–G93A)1Gur	Delayed (by 10%)	Increased (7%)	No change	20
Co-expression of bcl-2	TgN(SOD1–G93A)1Gur^dl	Delayed (by 19%)	Increased (15%)	No change	20
Riluzole (24 mg/kg in diet or 50 mg/kg through the drinking water)	TgN(SOD1–G93A)1Gur	No change	Increased (10%)	Increased (28%)	19, 41
Gabapentin (7.5 g/kg in the diet)	TgN(SOD1–G93A)G1L	No change	Increased (5%)	Increased (20%)	19
Co-expression of ICE-C285G	TgN(SOD1–G93A)1Gur^dl	No change	Increased (8%)	Increased (45%)	22

The two lines of SOD1–G93A transgenic mice are available through the Induced Mutant Resource of the Jackson Laboratory. They differ in transgene copy number and consequently in the timing of disease onset and survival. TgN(SOD1–G93A)1Gur mice have a lifespan of 132 ± 12 days compared to a lifespan of 251 ± 28 days for TgN(SOD1–G93A)1Gur^dl mice.[39] Drug dosages tabulated are the estimated dose of drug delivered per kg mouse body weight per day.

Table 13.2
Neuroprotective strategies in mutant SOD1 transgenic mice. Treatments that potentially inhibit oxidative mechanisms (copper chelation, dietary antioxidants, and co-expression of bcl-2) delay disease onset but do not affect disease duration. Conversely treatments that inhibit glutamate-mediated excitotoxicity or apoptotic mechanisms (drugs that decrease glutamate release, co-expression of a negative-dominant inhibitor of caspase-1, ICE-C285G) do not affect disease onset, but they do extend disease duration. Thus, the two types of therapies appear to target distinct pathogenic mechanisms that underlie disease initiation and disease propagation in the transgenic model.

these mechanisms also contribute to the dissemination of disease along the length of the spinal cord is unclear. In patients, disease appears to disseminate across spinal segments more rapidly than along the length of the cord, such that clinical involvement of the arms or legs is frequently symmetric.

What is the pathogenic gain-of-function in mutant copper–zinc SOD?

The discovery of SOD1 mutations in FALS[10] led to the initial hypothesis that such mutations decreased copper–zinc SOD enzymatic activity, thereby leading to the accumulation of O_2^{0} and other reactive oxygen species, with consequent induction of motor neuron death.[11] Induction of neuronal death in cell culture by targeting copper–zinc SOD expression with antisense oligonucleotides lend credence to this hypothesis,[23,24] but knock-out of the SOD1 gene in mice by homologous recombination in embryonic stem cells failed to induce motor neuron degeneration.[15]

Instead, induction of motor neuron disease in mice by transgenic expression of mutant, but not wild-type, human copper–zinc SOD has argued persuasively that disease is due to gain-of-function mutations in the enzyme. This has been borne out by subsequent cell culture experiments that have compared the effects of expressing mutant or wild-type human copper–zinc SOD in primary neurons or neural cell lines.[25-27] Expression of mutant human copper–zinc SOD provides a pro-apoptotic signal while expression of the wild-type enzyme generally is antiapoptotic. Since a variety of cultured cells are vulnerable to the toxic effects of mutant copper–zinc SOD, such experiments do not address the issue of selective motor neuron vulnerability; nor do they provide compelling evidence that vulnerable neurons die in vivo through an apoptotic mechanism, since in culture virtually any cell can be induced to undergo apoptosis by selecting an appropriate noxious stimulus. Nonetheless, adenoviral expression of SOD1–A4V or SOD1–V148G in differentiated pheochromocytoma (PC12) cells with consequent induction of apoptotic death shows close parallels with the pathophysiology of motor neuron death in the transgenic FALS model.[27]

Acute expression of mutant human copper–zinc SOD in differentiated PC12 cells induces apoptotic cell death.[27] This can be attenuated by manipulations that blunt the deleterious effects of oxygen free radicals such as antioxidants (e.g. vitamin E, glutathione, and the SOD mimetics, EUK-8 and EUK-134) and bcl-2, a negative regulator of an oxygen

radical-mediated pathway of apoptotic cell death.[28,29] Consistent with these findings, basal rates of oxygen radical production are increased in cells expressing mutant, but not wild-type, copper–zinc SOD.[27] A copper chelator, tetraethylenepentamine, also attenuates cell death in the culture model, presumably by reducing the copper loading of the mutant enzyme.

These results parallel data collected in the FALS transgenic model. D-penicillamine, a copper chelator used clinically for the management of Wilson's disease, a copper storage disease, delays the onset of clinical symptoms in SOD1–G93A mice and proportionately extends survival.[18] The same effect has been obtained with at least two antioxidants and with bcl-2 overexpression. The combination of vitamin E and selenium,[19] and carboxyfullerenes ((Carbon 60) C60) 'Buckyballs' modified with malonic acid substituents[20]) also delay the onset of clinical symptoms in SOD1–G93A mice. Vitamin E and selenium were also shown to maintain wheel running performance but had negligible effect on survival, while the carboxyfullerenes extended survival in proportion to the delay in disease onset.

What is the gain-of-function in copper–zinc SOD that initiates motor neuron disease? The experiments discussed above suggest that disease is initiated by free radical-mediated attack on vulnerable neurons. Copper–zinc SOD possesses a narrow, positively charged, active-site channel, which normally limits the access of reactants to the copper redox center, and thus locks away much of the natural chemistry of copper.[30] Copper(II) and copper(I) ions are relatively toxic to the cell because they catalyse the oxidation of lipids, proteins, and nucleic acids. The copper in copper–zinc SOD normally exists as copper(II) ions, yet its reduction to copper(I) ions allows the enzyme to react with hydrogen peroxide via the Fenton reaction to generate hydroxyl radical.[31] This normally leads to inactivation of the enzyme owing to oxidation of one or more of the histidine residues that co-ordinate copper in the active site.[32,33] It can also lead to a generation of secondary free radicals by reaction of the hydroxyl radical with other oxidizable substrates within the active site. In vitro biochemical studies of the G93A and other copper–zinc SOD mutations linked to FALS indicate that the mutations enhance catalysis of a Fenton-like reaction, with consequent production of damaging free radicals.[34,35] Since more than 50 missense mutations of copper–zinc SOD linked to FALS alter residues that are located primarily in the polypeptide backbone of the enzyme,[11] they probably relax the conformation of the protein and allow the copper catalytic center greater access to solvent. In support of this hypothesis, FALS-linked mutations alter the zinc site and the redox behavior of copper–zinc SOD.[36]

A pathological feature that FALS shares with Alzheimer's disease, Huntington's disease, and Parkinson's disease is the formation of protein aggregates within the cell body of vulnerable neurons. Aggregates of mutant copper–zinc SOD have been described in patients,[37] in cultured neurons expressing mutant copper–zinc SOD,[26] and also in the SOD1–G85R mice.[14] This has led to the hypothesis that aggregation of mutant copper–zinc SOD also plays a role in disease causation. If copper is retained within such aggregates, then disease may still involve the free radical mechanisms discussed above. On the other hand, formation of cytosolic protein aggregates may cause disease through effects on intracellular protein trafficking, integrity of intracellular organelles, or by interfering with axon transport. It may be possible to use transgenic technology to distinguish between these two alternatives. Within the cell, a specific copper chaperone protein is necessary for the delivery of copper to the SOD apoenzyme, even though the apoenzyme can be metallated quite readily in vitro.[38]

Cellular copper chaperone systems

Copper(I) and copper(II) ions can be toxic at low concentrations by catalysing the auto-oxidation of lipids, proteins, and nucleic acids. Yet copper is an essential co-factor for metalloenzymes such as copper–zinc SOD, dopamine β-hydroxylase, monoamine oxidase, cytochrome C oxidase, ceruloplasmin, and extracellular SOD. Specialized copper transporters exist within the cell that transfer copper into copper-containing enzymes (*Fig. 13.4*). A single copper uptake protein in the plasma membrane (CTR1) passes copper to one of the three copper chaperones, the copper chaperone for SOD (CCS), COX17, and ATX1, which target copper to cytosolic, mitochondrial, or vesicular pathways.[38,39] CCS is required in yeast for the delivery of copper to copper–zinc SOD.[38] The amino terminus of CCS contains the consensus copper binding motif MHCXXC, which also is present in the copper transporting ATPases. Remarkably, CCS is a copper–zinc SOD paralog. A carboxyl terminal domain of 141 amino acids has 50% identity to copper–zinc SOD, with conservation of three of the four histidine residues that, in copper–zinc SOD, co-ordinate copper(II) in the active site. CCS does not rescue the phenotype of SOD1 null yeast, so it lacks intrinsic superoxide dismutase activity.[38] If the sole function of CCS is to load copper into cytosolic copper–zinc SOD, the targeted deletion of the CCS gene should have the same minimal phenotype as deletions of the SOD1 gene. By crossing one of the mutant SOD1 transgenes into a CCS null mouse, the hypoth-

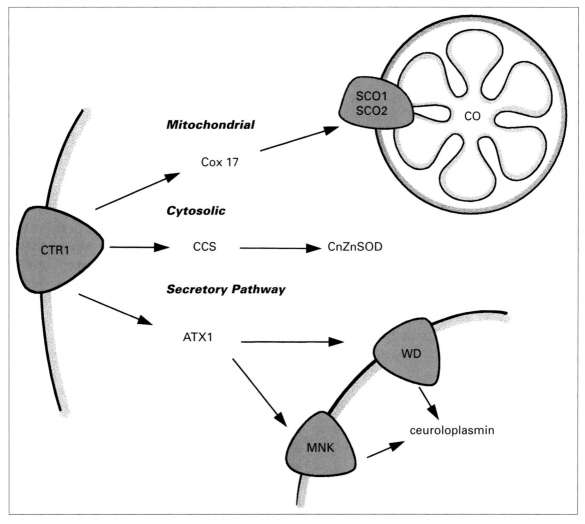

Figure 13.4
The intracellular transport pathways for copper to the mitochondria, cytosolic enzymes, and secretory pathways, utilizes specialized protein carriers. CCS, the copper chaperone for SOD, is needed for the loading of copper into the copper site of copper-zinc SOD.[38]

esis that copper loading of mutant copper–zinc SOD is necessary for induction of motor neuron disease can be put to a critical test.

If CCS null mice are viable, it will be of considerable interest to assess the pathogenicity of a mutant SOD1 transgene on the CCS null background. Since this should prevent the delivery of copper to the SOD apoenzyme, it should delay or prevent disease if disease indeed is due to generation of toxic free radicals by the mutant enzyme.

References

1. Gurney ME, Pu H, Chiu AY et al. Motor neuron degeneration in mice that express a human CuZn superoxide dismutase mutation. *Science* 1994; **264**: 1772–1775.

2. Ripps ME, Huntley GW, Hof PR et al. Transgenic mice expressing an altered murine superoxide dismutase gene provide an animal model of amyotrophic lateral sclerosis. *Proc Natl Acad Sci U S A* 1995; **92**: 689–693.

3. Wong PC, Pardo CA, Borchelt DR et al. An adverse property of familial ALS-linked SOD1 mutation causes motor neuron disease characterized by vacuolar degeneration of mitochondria. *Neuron* 1995; **14**: 1105–1116.

4. Games D, Adams D, Alessandrini R et al. Alzheimer-type neuropathology in transgenic mice overexpressing V717F beta-amyloid precursor protein. *Nature* 1995; **373**: 523–527.

5. Hsiao K, Chapman P, Nilsen S et al. Correlative memory deficits, A-β elevation, and amyloid plaques in transgenic mice. *Science* 1996; **274**: 99–102.

6. Mangiarini L, Sathasivam K, Seller M et al. Exon 1 of the HD gene with an expanded CAG repeat is sufficient to cause a progressive neurological phenotype in transgenic mice. *Cell* 1996; **87**: 493–506.

7. Hsiao KK, Scott M, Foster D et al. Spontaneous neurodegeneration in transgenic mice with mutant prion protein. *Science* 1990; **250**: 1587–1590.

8. Burright EN, Clark HB, Servadio A et al. SCA1 transgenic mice: a model for neurodegeneration caused by an expanded CAG trinucleotide repeat. *Cell* 1995; **82**: 937–948.

9. Ikeda H, Yamaguchi M, Sugai S et al. Expanded polyglutamine in the Machado–Joseph disease protein induces cell death in vitro and in vivo. *Nat Genet* 1996; **13**: 196–202.

10. Rosen DR, Siddique T, Patterson D et al. Mutations in CuZn superoxide dismutase gene are associated with familial amyotrophic lateral sclerosis. *Nature* 1993; **362**: 59–62.

11. Deng HX, Hentati A, Tainer JA et al. Amyotrophic lateral sclerosis and structural defects in CuZn superoxide dismutase. *Science* 1993; **261**: 1047–1051.

12. Bowling AC, Schultz JB, Brown RH Jr, Beal MF. Superoxide dismutase activity, oxidative damage and mitochondrial energy metabolism in familial and sporadic amyotrophic lateral sclerosis. *J Neurochem* 1993; **61**: 2322–2325.

13. Borchelt DR, Lee MK, Slunt HS et al. Superoxide dismutase 1 with mutations linked to familial amyotrophic lateral sclerosis possesses significant activity. *Proc Natl Acad Sci U S A* 1994; **91**: 8292–8296.

14. Brujin LI, Becher MW, Lee MK et al. ALS-linked SOD1 mutant G85R mediates damage to astrocytes and promotes rapidly progressive disease with SOD1-containing inclusions. *Neuron* 1997; **18**: 327–338.

15. Reaume AG, Elliott JL, Hoffman EK et al. Motor neurons in Cu/Zn superoxide dismutase-deficient mice develop normally but exhibit enhanced cell death after axonal injury. *Nat Genet* 1996; **13**: 43–47.

16. Chiu AY, Zhai P, Dal Canto MC et al. Age dependent penetrance of disease in a transgenic mouse model of familial amyotrophic lateral sclerosis. *Mol Cell Neurosci* 1995; **6**: 349–362.

17. Gurney ME. Transgenic animal models of familial amyotrophic lateral sclerosis. *J Neurol* 1997; **244 (suppl 2)**: S15–S20.

18. Hottinger AF, Fine EG, Gurney ME et al. The copper chelator D-penicillamine delays onset of disease and extends survival in a transgenic mouse model of familial amyotrophic lateral sclerosis. *Eur J Neurosci* 1997; **9**: 1548–1551.

19. Gurney ME, Cutting FB, Zhai P et al. Benefit of vitamin E, riluzole and gabapentin in a transgenic model of familial amyotrophic lateral sclerosis. *Ann Neurol* 1996; **39**: 147–157.

20. Dugan LL, Turetsky DM, Du C et al. Carboxyfullerenes as neuroprotective reagents. *Proc Natl Acad Sci U S A* 1997; **94**: 9434–9439.

21. Kostic V, Jackson-Lewis V, de Bilbao F et al. Bcl-2: prolonging life in a transgenic model of familial amyotrophic lateral sclerosis. *Science* 1997; **277**: 559–562.

22. Friedlander RM, Brown RH Jr, Gagliardini V et al. Inhibition of ICE slows ALS in mice. *Nature* 1997; **388**: 31.

23. Troy CM, Shelanski ML. Down-regulation of copper/zinc superoxide dismutase causes apoptotic death in PC12 neuronal cells. *Proc Natl Acad Sci U S A* 1994; **91**: 6384–6387.

24. Rothstein JD, Bristol LA, Hosler B et al. Chronic inhibition of superoxide dismutase produces apoptotic death of spinal neurons. *Proc Natl Acad Sci U S A* 1994; **91**: 4155–4159.

25. Rabizadeh S, Gralla EB, Borchelt DR et al. Mutations associated with amyotrophic lateral sclerosis convert superoxide dismutase from an antiapoptotic gene to a proapoptotic gene: studies in yeast and neural cells. *Proc Natl Acad Sci U S A* 1995; **92**: 3024–3028.

26. Durham HD, Roy J, Dong L, Figlewicz DA. Aggregation of mutant Cu/Zn superoxide dismutase proteins in a culture model of ALS. *J Neuropathol Exp Neurol* 1997; **56**: 523–530.

27. Ghadge GF, Lee JP, Bindokas VP et al. Mutant superoxide dismutase-1-linked familial amyotrophic lateral sclerosis: molecular mechanisms of neuronal death and protection. *J Neurosci* 1997; **17**: 8756–8766.

28. Hockenbery DM, Oltvai ZN, Yin XM et al. Bcl-2 functions in an antioxidant pathway to prevent apoptosis. *Cell* 1993; **75**: 241–251.

29. Kane DJ, Sarafian TA, Anton R et al. Bcl-2 inhibition of neural death: decreased generation of reactive oxygen species. *Science* 1993; **262**: 1274–1277.

30. Getzoff ED, Cabelli DE, Fisher CL et al. Faster superoxide dismutase mutants designed by enhancing electrostatic guidance. *Nature* 1992; **358**: 347–351.

31. Hodgson EK, Fridovich I. The interaction of bovine erythrocyte superoxide dismutase with hydrogen peroxide: inactivation of the enzyme. *Biochemistry* 1975; **14**: 5294–5299.

32. Yim MB, Chock PB, Stadtman ER. Copper zinc superoxide dismutase catalyzes hydroxyl radical production from hydrogen peroxide. *Proc Natl Acad Sci U S A* 1990; **87**: 5006–5010.

33. Yim MB, Chock PB, Stadtman ER. Enzyme function of copper zinc superoxide dismutase as a free radical generator. *J Biol Chem* 1993; **268**: 4099–4105.

34. Wiedau-Pazos M, Goto JJ, Rabizadeh S et al. Altered reactivity of superoxide dismutase in familial amyotrophic lateral sclerosis. *Science* 1996; **271**: 515–518.

35. Yim MB, Kang JH, Yim HS et al. A gain-of-function of an amyotrophic lateral sclerosis-associated CuZn-superoxide dismutase mutant: an enhancement of free radical formation due to a decrease in K_m for hydrogen peroxide. *Proc Natl Acad Sci U S A* 1996; **93**: 5709–5714.

36. Lyons TJ, Liu H, Goto JJ et al. Mutations in copper-zinc superoxide dismutase that cause amyotrophic lateral sclerosis alter the zinc binding site and redox behavior of the protein. *Proc Natl Acad Sci U S A* 1996; **93**: 12240–12244.

37. Shibata N, Asayama K, Hirano A, Kobayashi M. Immunohistochemical study on superoxide dismutase in spinal cords from autopsied patients with amyotrophic lateral sclerosis. *Dev Neurosci* 1996; **18**: 492–498.

38. Culotta VC, Klomp LWJ, Strain J et al. The copper chaperone for superoxide dismutase. *J Biol Chem* 1997; **272**: 23469–23472.

39. Gurney ME. The use of transgenic models of amyotrophic lateral sclerosis in preclinical drug studies. *J Neurol Sci* 1997; **152** (**suppl 1**): S67–S73.

40. Pufahl RA, Singer CP, Peariso KL et al. Metal ion chaperone function of soluble Cu(I) receptor Atx1. *Science* 1997; **278**: 853–856.

41. Gurney ME, Fleck TJ, Himes CS, Hall ED. Riluzole preserves motor function in a transgenic model of familial amyotrophic lateral sclerosis. *Neurology* 1998; **50**: 62–66.

42. Barneoud P, Lolivier J, Sanger DJ et al. Quantitative assessment in FALS mice: a longitudinal study. *NeuroReport* 1997; **8**: 2861–2865.

43. Dal Canto MC, Gurney ME. Neuropathological changes in two lines of mice carrying a transgene for mutant human CuZn SOD and in mice overexpressing wild type human SOD: a model of familial amyotrophic lateral sclerosis FALS. *Brain Res* 1995; **676**: 25–40.

44. Mourelatos Z, Gonatas NK, Stieber A et al. The Golgi apparatus of spinal cord motor neuron in transgenic mice expressing mutant CuZn superoxide dismutase becomes fragmented in early preclinical stages of the disease. *Proc Natl Acad Sci U S A* 1996; **93**: 5472–5477.

45. Dal Canto MC, Gurney ME. The development of CNS pathology in a murine transgenic model of human ALS. *Am J Path* 1994; **145**: 1271–1279.

46. Azzouz M, Le Clerc N, Gurney M et al. Progressive motor neuron impairment in an animal model of familial amyotrophic lateral sclerosis. *Muscle Nerve* 1997; **20**: 45–51.

47. Tu PH, Raju P, Robinson KA et al. Transgenic mice carrying a human mutant superoxide dismutase transgene develop neuronal cytoskeletal pathology resembling human amyotrophic lateral sclerosis. *Proc Natl Acad Sci U S A* 1996; **93**: 3155–3160.

48. Zhang B, Tu PH, Abtahian F et al. Neurofilaments and orthograde transport are reduced in ventral root axons of transgenic mice that express human SOD1 with a G93A mutation. *J Cell Biol* 1997; **139**: 1–9.

14

Excitotoxicity in amyotrophic lateral sclerosis

Mandy Jackson and Jeffrey D Rothstein

Introduction

Many hypotheses have been put forward to account for the selective neurodegeneration of motor neurons in amyotrophic lateral sclerosis (ALS).[1] These hypotheses include the involvement of environmental factors, autoimmune phenomena, oxidative stress, excitotoxicity, cytoskeletal abnormalities, and loss of trophic factor support, all of which are discussed in other chapters. Any theory, however, must explain the mechanism and processes that lead to neuronal cell death, the selectivity for motor neurons, and the late onset of disease. In fact, it is very likely that ALS may be caused by a variety of different primary insults, all of which culminate in the final phenotype of upper and lower motor neuron degeneration that is characteristic of ALS. At least two different pathways already exist, as to date copper-zinc superoxide (SOD1) gene mutations have only been found in 15–20% of all familial ALS patients[2,3] and have only been detected in a small proportion of apparently 'sporadic' cases.[4–6] Thus, other mutations or risk factors must exist to account for the remaining familial and sporadic patient population.

Over the past few years, evidence has accumulated that supports the hypothesis that exitotoxic damage contributes to selective motor neuronal death. This chapter outlines the molecular mechanisms of excitotoxicity and sum-marizes the experimental evidence that supports the involvement of exitotoxic mechanisms in the pathogenesis of ALS.

Glutamate

Glutamate is the major excitatory neurotransmitter in the mammalian central nervous system (CNS). When the pre-synaptic terminal is depolarized, glutamate is released in a calcium-dependent process.[7] It then diffuses across the synaptic cleft, where it can activate two main categories of receptor: the ionotropic receptors and the metabotropic receptors. The ionotropic receptors are ligand-gated cation channels and the metabotropic receptors are coupled through G-proteins to second messenger systems. Within each family, numerous receptor subtypes have been identified (*Fig. 14.1*).[8]

Glutamate receptors

The ionotropic receptors are divided into three classes according to the pharmacological specificity of their preferred agonist:

(a) *N*-methyl-D-aspartate (NMDA) receptors;
(b) α-amino-3-hydroxy-5-methyl-4-isoxazole propionic acid (AMPA) receptors; and
(c) kainate receptors.

The AMPA and kainate receptors are thought to be the primary mediators of fast,

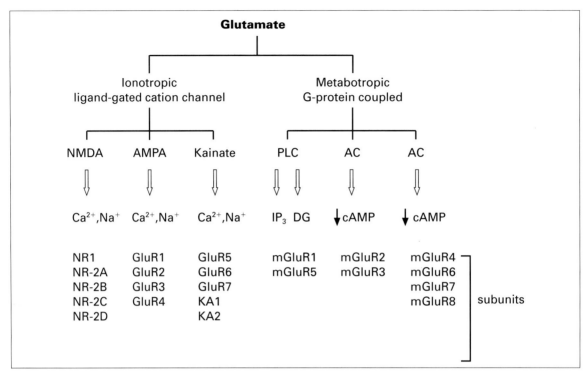

Figure 14.1
Two main categories of mammalian glutamate receptors have been identified — ionotropic and metabotropic. Within each family there are several subtypes. The ionotropic subunits combine to form heteromeric assemblies. Each metabotropic subunit can form a functional receptor by itself. PLC, phospholipase C; AC, adenylate cyclase; IP$_3$, inositol-1,4,5-triphosphate; DG, diacylglycerol; NMDA, N-methyl-$_D$-asparate; AMPA, α-amino–3–hydroxy-5-methyl-4-isoxazole proprionic acid.

excitatory neurotransmission. To date, no antagonist has been developed that blocks only AMPA or only kainate receptors, and so kainate and AMPA receptors are usually referred to as non-NMDA receptors. The AMPA receptors are heteromeric complexes formed from four different subunits (GluR1–GluR4) that can assemble in various combinations to form functional receptors.[9,10] The majority of these receptors are permeable only to the monovalent cations sodium and potassium; however, channel assemblies lack-

ing GluR2 subunits are also permeable to calcium ions.[11] The kainate receptor subunits are termed GluR5–GluR7, KA1 and KA2.[12,13] The latter two subunits form high-affinity binding sites for kainate when expressed with members of the GluR5–7 family.

Endogenous NMDA receptors are thought to be formed as a pentameric subunit assembly consisting of subunits of two genes, NR1 (eight isoforms) and NR2 (four isoforms).[14] NR1 subunits can self-assemble to form functional receptors, but the four types of NR2 subunit are not active when expressed without NR1.[12] All NMDA receptors have a very high calcium conductance[15] and many agents alter the activity of the NMDA receptor.[16–18] These agents include:

(a) glycine, which is required for receptor activation;
(b) polyamines such as spermine and spermidine, which can enhance NMDA receptor responses;
(c) zinc, which can potentiate or inhibit receptor activation; and
(d) protons, which are a potent inhibitor of the NMDA receptor.

In addition, the NMDA receptor is not only ligand-gated, but also voltage-gated. At resting membrane potential, the ion channel is blocked by extracellular magnesium ions, which prevents ion transduction even if glutamate and glycine are bound to the receptor. Since this blockade is voltage-dependent, post-synaptic depolarization facilitates NMDA receptor activation. As a result, the NMDA receptor is activated only under conditions of coincident agonist binding and post-synaptic depolarization.

The metabotropic receptors have been subdivided into three classes depending on the second messenger system that is activated.[19] Class I activates phospholipase C, increases the production of inositol 1, 4, 5-triphosphate and the release of calcium from internal stores,[20] and leads to the formation of diacylglycerol, which then might activate protein kinase C. Class II and III receptors are negatively coupled to adenylate cyclase and reduce the intracellular amount of cAMP.[21] Class II and III receptors differ in their pharmacological profile against specific agonists. The role of metabotropic receptors in normal physiological conditions remains somewhat of a mystery owing to the lack of potent and specific metabotropic receptor agonists.

Glutamate transporters

The normal function of glutamate in excitatory synaptic transmission is rapidly terminated by the efficient removal of glutamate from the synapse. This is achieved by high-affinity, sodium-dependent glutamate transporters, which are capable of concentrating intracellular glutamate up to 10,000-fold compared with the extracellular environment.[22] The transport of each glutamate anion is accompanied by two sodium ions, with potassium and hydroxyl ions being countertransported.[23] In addition, certain transporters have a high conductance for chloride anions. Within the glial cells, glutamate is either transaminated by glutamine synthetase to form glutamine or metabolized to α-ketoglutarate by glutamate dehydrogenase. The astrocyte then supplies the nerve terminal with glutamine, α-ketoglutarate, or both; these serve as precursors of the neurotransmitter glutamate. In this way, glutamate is recycled from nerve terminal to glial cells and back to nerve terminal.

To date, five human glutamate transporters have been cloned, based on the original cloning of the analogous proteins in animals (*Table 14.1*), and these have been termed excitatory amino acid transporter (EAAT)1, glutamate/asparate transporter (GLAST), EAAT2 (GLT-1), EAAT3((excitatory amino acid carrier) (EAAC1),[24] EAAT4,[25] and EAAT5.[26] The last-named two function both as transporters and as glutamate-gated chloride channels. The localization of these proteins was subsequently determined using highly specific antibodies. Both GLAST(EAAT1) and GLT-2(EAAT2) are astroglial-specific, while EAAC1(EAAT3) is specific for neurons, including cortical motor neurons.[27] EAAT4 is also neuron-specific but is expressed predominantly in the cerebellum, almost exclusively in Purkinje cells.[28]

Name	Location	Number of amino acids	Transmembrane domains	Glycosylation sites	Phosphorylation sites	EC_{50} (μM)
EAAT1 (GLAST)	Astrocytes	543	>6	2	2 PKC	77
EAAT2 (GLT-1)	Astrocytes	573	8–9	2	2 cAMP 2 PKC	1
EAAT3 (EAAC1)	Neurons	524	10	4	9 PKC	12
EAAT4	Neuronal (Purkinje cells)	548		3		2.5
EAAT5	Neuronal (retinal cells)	560		1		64

EAAT, excitatory amino acid transporter; PKC, protein kinase; EC_{50}, effective concentration that gives 50% maximal velocity.

Table 14.1
Characteristics of cloned human and animal high-affinity glutamate transporters.

Excitotoxicity

The neurotoxic properties of glutamate were first shown 30 years ago by Lucas and Newhouse.[29] While screening compounds that might ameliorate retinal dystrophy, they discovered that systemic injection of glutamate destroys the inner neural layers of the immature mouse retina. Subsequently Olney and Ho[30] showed that systemic injection of certain excitatory amino acids into immature animals caused neuronal degeneration in areas of the CNS that are not protected by the blood–brain barrier. Further work demonstrated a direct correlation between glutamate-induced neurotoxicity and activation of excitatory amino acid receptors,[31] and the term 'excitotoxicity' was coined to describe the neurodegeneration resulting from exposure to excitatory amino acids.

In the subsequent 20 years, progress has been made in understanding the mechanisms that mediate excitotoxicity. The post-receptor mechanisms of excitotoxicity have not yet been fully elucidated, but it is thought that two distinct phases may be involved (*Fig. 14.2*). First, there is neuronal swelling caused by depolarization-mediated influx of sodium and chloride ions and water,[32] and secondly, owing to the overstimulation of the excitatory amino acid receptors, there is an excessive influx of calcium ions.[33] This in turn leads to depolarization of the cell, which triggers the activation of voltage-dependent sodium and calcium channels, thus amplifying and spreading the depolarization and calcium influx. The subsequent loss of calcium homeostasis results in the initiation of a complex cascade of events, including the activation of calcium-dependent enzymes such as nitric oxide synthase, xanthine oxidase, and phospholipases, thus enhancing the formation of nitric oxide, peroxynitrite, hydroxyl radicals, and superoxide anions. These products can damage the neuron by causing lipid peroxidation, mitochondrial dysfunction, and decreased energy production.[34] Eventually, cell

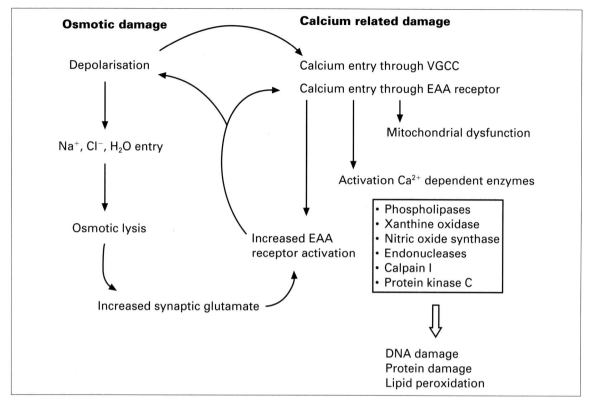

Figure 14.2
Proposed mechanism of excitatory amino acid neurotoxicity. EAA, excitatory amino acid; VGCC, voltage-dependent calcium channels.

lysis occurs, releasing the contents of the cell, including glutamate, which can then act on neighboring neurons and set in motion further neuronal damage.

Numerous studies, however, have documented the ability of normal concentrations of glutamate to be neurotoxic when a neuron is metabolically compromised.[35,36] Therefore, excitotoxicity can also be a secondary disease mechanism, termed 'slow' or 'weak' excitotoxicity. This may occur as a consequence of a defect in energy metabolism, resulting in reduced ATP production. Maintenance of the membrane potential and ion gradients under resting conditions is achieved by the enzyme sodium–potassium ATPase, which requires ATP. Thus the activity of this enzyme is greatly impaired under conditions of reduced ATP, leading to membrane depolarization and ionic disturbances. This could lead to the elimination of the normal voltage-dependent magnesium block of the NMDA receptor channel, with resulting overactivation of NMDA receptors by normal endogenous glutamate levels.[37,38]

It is evident, therefore, that there are several initial triggers that could lead to excito-

Event	Initial result	Secondary result
Excess glutamate ↑ release abnormal production impaired uptake	↑ Excitatory amino acid receptor activation	↑ Intracellular calcium and sodium
Altered EAA receptor number or density distribution affinity	↑ Excitatory amino acid receptor activation	↑ Intracellular calcium and sodium
Inability to buffer calcium	↑ Intracellular calcium	
ATP depletion	↓ Sodium–potassium ATPase activity Membrane depolarization	Relief of magnesium blockade ↑ NMDA receptor activation Activation of voltage-gated calcium channel ↑ Intracellular calcium
	↓ Sodium extrusion from cytosol	↓ Sodium dependent glutamate uptake and calcium extrusion ↑ Synaptic glutamate and intracellular calcium
	↓ Calcium sequestration in endoplasmic reticulum	↑ Cytosolic calcium
Mitochondrial dysfunction	↑ Free radicals	Protein damage Membrane depolarization
	Mitochondrial depolarization	↓ Calcium uptake by mitochondria ↑ Cytosolic calcium

Table 14.2
Possible mechanisms of excitotoxicity.

toxicity (*Table 14.2*). To date there is no direct evidence to support the concept that the loss of glutamate transport or even excess extracellular glutamate are the primary defects in ALS that lead to excitotoxicity. Nonetheless, there are a series of studies, which are discussed below, that do suggest that glutamate could contribute to, and propagate, the process of selective motor neuron degeneration in ALS.

Defects in glutamate metabolism in ALS

The first evidence that glutamate could participate in the pathogenesis of ALS came from the discovery that there was an increase in gluta-mate levels in plasma and cerebrospinal fluid (CSF) from ALS patients.[39,40] These investigations documented a three-fold increase in mean CSF glutamate and aspartate levels in CSF from ALS patients compared with age-matched controls and disease control patients. Results from different laboratories have not consistently reproduced these findings, perhaps because of technical factors.[41] However, a recent study confirmed the observed increase in CSF glutamate levels in ALS patients, but it was only detected in a subset (49%) of ALS patients, indicating the heterogeneity of the ALS population.[42]

The elevation of these two excitatory amino acids could reflect the degeneration of motor neurons, but if this was the case then one would also expect other amino acids with high intracellular concentrations to be elevated. Instead, there is selective elevation of these two excitatory amino acids. Interestingly, both glutamate and aspartate are cleared from the extracellular space by the same transporter protein, the glutamate transport carrier. This led to the hypothesis that there may be a defect in glutamate transport.

Abnormalities of glutamate transport

Glutamate transport function is typically evaluated by measuring the accumulation of radio-labeled glutamate into brain membrane preparations. Glutamate transport was measured in ALS post mortem tissue from a variety of brain and spinal cord regions.[43] It was found that the maximal velocity was reduced by 59% in the motor cortex and spinal cord in ALS cases compared to controls. Since these regions are the most neuropathologically affected brain regions, these changes may be a result of cellular degeneration; however, no changes were observed in the same regions from Huntington's chorea and Alzheimer's disease brains. Furthermore, the loss of transport was specific for the sodium-dependent glutamate carrier, since the transport of both phenylalanine and γ-aminobutyric acid were normal in ALS motor cortex. A subsequent study, which determined the distribution and destiny of glutamate transport sites in the spinal cord, supports the finding that there is a loss of glutamate transport.[44] In ALS patients, a reduction in the density of [^{3}H]D-aspartate binding was observed compared both to normal controls and a neurological disease control group.

In order to test the hypothesis that chronic loss of glutamate transport could lead to a slow loss of motor neurons, organotypic spinal cord cultures were used as a model system.[45] These are cultures prepared from 8-day-old rats in which thin slices of lumbar spinal cord can be maintained morphologically intact. To mimic the loss of glutamate transport in ALS, drugs that non-selectively block all glutamate transport subtypes were added. Chronic blockade of glutamate transport in vitro led to increased extracellular glutamate and a slow selective loss of motor neurons, which could be prevented by co-administration of specific glutamate receptor antagonists.[45] From these results it appears that a defect in glutamate transport can produce selective motor neuron degeneration.

Further evidence for an abnormality of glutamate transport has come from immunoblot and immunohistochemical analysis of multiple brain regions and spinal cord tissue from ALS patients using the specific glutamate transporter protein antibodies.[46] There were no statistical changes in either the neuronal subtype EAAC1 (EAAT3) or the glial subtype GLAST (EAAT1), but there was a large decrease in immunoreactive protein for GLT-1 (EAAT2) in ALS motor cortex and spinal cord but not in other brain regions. This loss was not merely due to a loss of astroglia, since the glial marker, glial fibrillary acidic protein (GFAP), and the other astroglial glutamate transporter, GLAST, were not decreased in ALS motor cortex.

To address the question of whether the loss of GLT-1 (EAAT2) alone can produce motor neuron degeneration or lead to increased extracellular glutamate, molecular knock-out studies were used. When antisense oligonucleotides to individual glutamate transporters were administered intraventricularly to rats, it was found that the loss of glial transporter subtypes GLAST (EAAT1) and GLT-1 (EAAT2) had much greater neurotoxic consequences than the loss of the neuronal transporter.[47] The loss of either of these astroglial glutamate transporters produced elevated extracellular glutamate levels, neurodegeneration that is characteristic of excitotoxicity, and a progressive paralysis beginning in the hind limbs. The loss of the neuronal glutamate transporter EAAC1 (EAAT3) did not elevate extracellular glutamate in the striatum but did produce mild neurotoxicity and resulted in epilepsy.

These results indicate that the bulk of glutamate clearance occurs through the astroglial transporters. Additional evidence to support this conclusion is provided by immunoprecipitation experiments.[48] It was shown that anti-GLT antibodies removed more than 90% of the glutamate transport activity, demonstrating that GLT-1 (EAAT2) is the dominant glutamate transporter in the brain. Finally, homozygous mice deficient in EAAT2 show elevated levels of residual glutamate in the synaptic cleft and selective neuronal degeneration,[49] providing a further link between transporter dysfunction, excitotoxicity, and motor neuron degeneration. Taken together, these results indicate that the increase in CSF glutamate levels and the loss of tissue glutamate transport in ALS patients are due to the selective loss of the EAAT2 protein.

Selective loss of EAAT2

There are several possible mechanisms that could lead to the selective loss of one glutamate transporter subtype. For example, as motor neurons degenerate, alterations in glutamatergic neurotransmission could lead to a down-regulation of the glutamate transporters. This has been tested in a rat model in which, following cortical ablation, glutamate transport does decrease, but the decrease is only transient — by 1 month after the lesion, functional transport returns to normal.[50] Thus, glial transporters demonstrate interesting injury responses, but these changes do not

explain the persistent loss of EAAT2 in ALS. It is unlikely that a loss of mRNA in ALS motor cortex is responsible for the selective loss of EAAT2 since there was no significant change in the mRNA levels of EAAT1, EAAT2, and EAAT3 from ALS patients.[51] This does not rule out the possibility of point mutations, which could lead to reduced protein stability and subsequent protein loss. However, mutational analysis provided no evidence for genomic mutations of EAAT2 in familial ALS or sporadic ALS.[52] An independent study also revealed no mutations within the genomic sequence of EAAT2 in 151 ALS patients, of which 128 were sporadic cases and 23 familial cases.[53] Interestingly, a mutation of a putative glycosylation site on EAAT2 has been found in one case of sporadic ALS, but the functional significance of this abnormality is not yet known.[52]

Other explanations for a loss of EAAT2 could involve defects in translation or post-translational mechanisms, such as oxidative damage from peroxynitrite, superoxide anions, and hydroxyl radicals. In fact, it has already been demonstrated that glutamate transporters can be irreversibly damaged by peroxynitrite and hydrogen peroxide.[54] Furthermore, several groups have documented evidence for oxidative damage in sporadic ALS by detecting increased protein carbonyls in the motor cortex and the spinal cord.[55,56] It has been shown that oxidation of EAAT2 leads to irreversible cross-linking of oligomer complexes,[48] and so the selective reduction in EAAT2 in ALS patients may be due to the internalization of these damaged proteins.

Recently, abnormal EAAT2 mRNA species have been identified in 65% of patients with sporadic ALS using accurate quantitative methods.[57] They were detected in the neuropathologically affected areas of the brain but not in other brain regions, and they have not been observed in other neurodegenerative disorders such as Huntington's disease, Alzheimer's disease, and spinal muscular atrophy. In vitro expression studies indicate that the proteins translated from these aberrant mRNA species may undergo rapid degradation and exert a dominant negative effect on the wild-type protein, resulting in loss of protein activity. The loss of EAAT2 protein in ALS is therefore likely to be due to the presence of these aberrant mRNA species. However, the origin of these species is unclear. The presence of multiple mRNA species most likely indicates that aberrant RNA processing or degradation may be occurring in ALS. Interestingly, the gene responsible for spinal muscular atrophy, *SMN*, was recently found to code for an essential protein in RNA metabolism.

In summary, the experimental studies demonstrate that the chronic loss of glutamate transport in organotypic spinal cord cultures can be selectively toxic to motor neurons. Since there is a selective loss of the glutamate transporter EAAT2 in ALS patients, it has been hypothesized that a loss of tissue glutamate transport is responsible for motor neuron degeneration in ALS. The selective loss of EAAT2 may be due to the presence of aberrant RNA species or to oxidative damage. It would be very simplistic, however, to believe that glutamate toxicity is the sole cause of ALS. As discussed above, it is very likely that multiple different insults that result in increased intracellular calcium ions (*Fig. 14.3*; see *Table 14.2*) may intersect leading to the common phenotype of motor neuron death. For example, both glutamate excess and anticalcium antibodies could lead to increased intracellular calcium.

Once an initial factor generates a rise in intracellular calcium ions, calcium-dependent enzymes are activated and electron leakage from the respiratory chain is stimulated. Both events lead to enhanced production of reactive oxygen species. The free radicals thus generated may further damage the mitochondria, leading to membrane depolarization and increased influx of calcium ions through voltage-gated calcium channels and NMDA receptors. In addition, the free radicals may damage cellular proteins such as neurofilaments, resulting in blockage of axonal transport and glutamate transporters, which would further augment the excitotoxic process. The relative importance of the different routes in increasing calcium in disease pathogenesis is however, likely to vary from individual to individual. For example, in cases of familial ALS, which possess a SOD1 mutation, free radical damage may be the predominant factor, though the different routes are not likely to be independent but mutually propagating.

Therefore, the slowly developing and spreading pattern of motor neuron degeneration in ALS may reflect a multistep process of an initiating event and a propagating series of cyclic cascades. If the hypothesis of initiator and propagators is correct, then drugs may be designed against ALS that interfere with either step. As diagnosis of ALS is often made well into the disease process, drugs that block the initiating steps may not be as effective at halting the disease propagation as those directed toward altering the cyclical, propagating steps. Recent experiments with familial ALS transgenic mice suggest this hypothesis may have merit.[58] The mice were treated with the antioxidant, vitamin E, or with the antiglutamate agents, riluzole and gabapentin. Interestingly, vitamin E was able to delay disease onset but not overall survival, whereas both antiglutamate agents were ineffective at altering disease onset but were able to prolong survival. Thus, these mice may provide evidence for a multistep process in motor neuron degeneration.

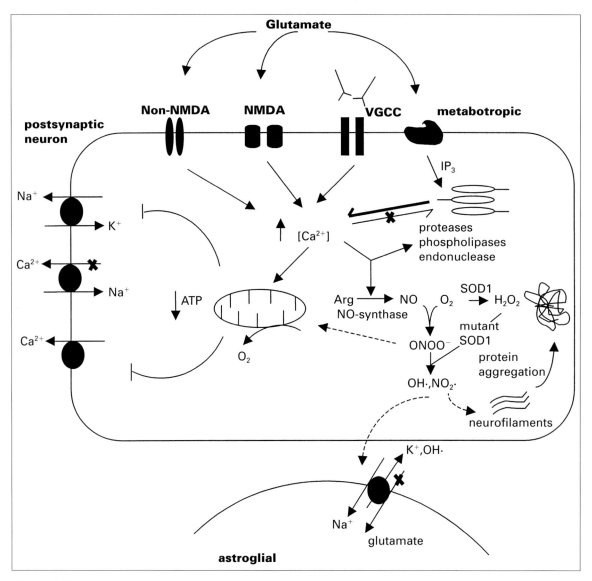

Figure 14.3

Mechanisms of motor neuron degeneration. Both glutamate excess, by the activation of glutamate receptors, and anti-calcium channel antibodies could lead to increase in intracellular calcium. This in turn would lead to activation of calcium dependent enzymes and electron leakage from the respiratory chain, resulting in the generation of free radicals and a decreased production of ATP. Increased production of free radical species may damage neurofilaments, leading to their accumulation, or may damage glutamate transporters, leading to excess glutamate and excitotoxicity and additional oxidative stress. The decreased neuronal ATP results in impaired sodium–potassium ATPase activity and neuronal depolarization, leading to enhanced NMDA receptor activation and increased activation of voltage-dependent calcium channels (VGCC). Decreased sodium–potassium ATPase activity also dissipates the sodium gradient and impairs sodium-dependent glutamate uptake and calcium extrusion. Decreased ATP levels also impairs the ATP-dependent sequestration of calcium in the endoplasmic reticulum. NMDA, N-methyl-ᴅ-asparate; VGCC, voltage-dependent calcium channels.

Selective motor neuron degeneration

Whatever the underlying genetic or environmental factor or factors in the pathogenesis of ALS may turn out to be, any theory must ultimately explain the selectivity of the disease process to motor neurons and why certain motor neuron populations (oculomotor neurons[59] and Onuf's nuclei[60]) are spared. It is possible that motor neurons are more susceptible to glutamate toxicity than other spinal neurons. One contributing factor may be differences in the ability to buffer calcium, since motor neurons are unusual in that they do not contain the calcium-buffering proteins, parvalbumin and calbindin D-28K.[61] Interestingly, the exceptions are those in the oculomotor tract and Onuf's nucleus, which are the motor neurons spared in ALS. Additional evidence to provide a role for calcium-binding proteins in motor neuron vulnerability comes from a study in which calbindin D-28K was expressed in motor neuron hybrid cells and shown to prevent ALS IgG-induced toxicity.[62] Treatment of these differentiated infected cells with calbindin D-28K antisense oligodeoxynucleotides significantly decreased the expression of calbindin D-28K and enhanced the sensitivity to ALS IgG-mediated toxicity.

Motor neurons may also contain an unusual complement of glutamate receptors. In most neuronal types, toxicity to glutamate is mediated principally by the NMDA receptor subtype, whereas in motor neurons, the AMPA–kainate receptor subtype appears to be more important.[43] This was shown by the fact that non-NMDA antagonists could effectively prevent neuronal degeneration induced by the inhibition of glutamate transport, whereas NMDA antagonists were not neuroprotective. Recently it was shown by in situ hybridization that the GluR2 AMPA–kainate receptor subunit is absent from human spinal motor neurons.[63] In AMPA receptors the GluR2 subunit is important in regulating the permeability of calcium ions. The result is that the absence of this subunit renders the non-NMDA receptors on motor neurons permeable to calcium ions. This is corroborated by earlier work using a cobalt-based stain on spinal cord organotypic cultures.[64] Using this histochemical method, it was shown that the most sensitive population of neurons that are permeable to calcium via non-NMDA glutamate receptors were the ventral motor neurons, those affected in ALS. Thus, the localization of calcium-permeable non-NMDA glutamate receptors on motor neurons may make them selectively vulnerable to excitotoxicity.

Alternatively, because motor neurons possess very high levels of SOD1 mRNA,[65] they may become susceptible targets for adverse effects if free radical scavenging mechanisms are defective. These neurons are very large and have long axons; they are therefore dependent on axonal transport mechanisms for maintaining their integrity. It is these energy-requiring transport mechanisms that may be critically sensitive to oxidative damage, since it is likely to lead to aberrant accumulation of neurofilaments and subsequent blockage of axonal transport. This may explain why, in the human disease, it is the largest-caliber, neurofilament-rich motor axons that are lost and the smallest axons with lower neurofilament content that are spared.

In short, the challenge of elucidating the mechanism of neurodegeneration in ALS still remains. Progress is being made and, as reviewed above, substantial evidence suggests that an interplay between elevated extracellular glutamate levels and intracellular calcium ion concentration play a pivotal role in the pathogenesis of ALS. This has led to the implementation of a variety of therapeutic approaches, namely those that inhibit the release of glutamate and excitatory amino acid antagonists, but in the future the ability to increase calcium-binding proteins may provide therapeutic benefits in ALS. So far, promising results have been obtained only with riluzole, which blocks glutamatergic neurotransmissions in the CNS.[66]

The mechanism of action of riluzole seems to differ from that of a pure excitatory amino acid antagonist. It appears to activate a G-protein-dependent process that leads to the inhibition of glutamate acid release and the blockade of some of the post-synaptic events mediated by the activation of NMDA receptors, including mobilization of calcium.[67] The neuroprotective activity of riluzole may be due to these various mechanisms acting in synergy to block excitotoxicity.

In two placebo-controlled studies[68,69] there was a beneficial impact upon the progress of ALS in over 1,100 patients. Both studies demonstrated a 35% decrease in risk of death or tracheostomy over an 18-month period for patients given riluzole 100 mg/day compared with placebo, but there was no effect on muscle strength. As a result of these studies, riluzole has been approved and marketed for the treatment of ALS in many countries, lending support to the hypothesis that glutamate excitotoxicity is an important mechanism in the pathogenesis of ALS.

References

1. Rowland LP. Ten central themes in a decade of ALS research. In: Rowland LP, ed. *Advances in Neurology* vol 56. New York: Raven Press, 1991, 3–23.

2. Rosen DR, Siddique T, Patterson D et al. Mutations in Cu/Zn superoxide dismutase are associated with familial amyotrophic lateral sclerosis. *Nature* 1993; **362**: 59–62.

3. Siddique T, Nijhawan D, Hentati A. Molecular genetic basis of familial ALS. *Neurology* 1996; **47 (suppl 2)**: S27–S35.

4. Jones CT, Shaw PJ, Chari G, Brock DJ. Identification of a novel exon 4 SOD-1 mutation in a sporadic amyotrophic lateral sclerosis patient. *Mol Cell Probes* 1994; **8**: 329–330.

5. Jackson M, Al-Chalabi A, Enayat ZE et al. Copper/zinc superoxide dismutase 1 and sporadic amyotrophic lateral sclerosis: analysis of 155 cases and identification of a novel insertion mutation. *Ann Neurol* 1997; **42**: 803–807.

6. Robberecht W, Aguirre T, Van Den Bosch L et al. D90A heterozygosity in the SOD1 gene is associated with familial and apparently sporadic amyotrophic lateral sclerosis. *Neurology* 1996; **47**: 1336–1339.

7. McMahon HT, Nicholls DG. Transmitter glutamate release from isolated nerve terminals: evidence for biphasic release and triggering by localised Ca^{2+}. *J Neurochem* 1991; **56**: 86–94.

8. Monaghan DT, Bridges RJ, Cotman CW. The excitatory amino acid receptors: their classes, pharmacology and distinct properties in the function of the central nervous system. *Annu Rev Pharmacol Toxicol* 1989; **29**: 365–402.

9. Hollman M, O'Shea-Greenfield A, Rogers SW, Heinemann S. Cloning by functional expression of a member of the glutamate receptor family. *Nature* 1989; **342**: 643–648.

10. Keinanen K, Wisden W, Sommer B et al. A family of AMPA-selective glutamate receptors. *Science* 1990; **249**: 556–560.

11. Hollmann M, Hartley M, Heinemann S. Ca^{2+} permeability of KA-AMPA gated glutamate receptor channels depends on subunit composition. *Science* 1991; **252**: 851–853.

12. Hollman M, Heinemann S. Cloned glutamate receptors. *Annu Rev Neurosci* 1994; **17**: 31–108.

13. Seeburg PH. The molecular biology of mammalian glutamate receptor channels. *Trends Neurosci* 1993; **16**: 359–365.

14. Nakanishi N, Axel R, Shneider NA. Alternative splicing generates functionally distinct N-methyl-D-aspartate receptors. *Proc Natl Acad Sci U S A* 1992; **89**: 8552–8556.

15. McBain CJ, Mayer ML. N-methyl-D-aspartic acid receptor structure and function. *Physiol Rev* 1994; **74**: 723–760.

16. Ascher P, Johnson JW. The NMDA receptor, its channel and its modulation by gycine. In: Watkins JC, Collingridge GL, eds. *The NMDA Receptor*. Oxford: Oxford University Press, 1989, 109–121.

17. Burnasheve N, Schoepfer R, Monyer H et al. Control by asparagine residues of calcium permeability and magnesium blockade of the NMDA receptor. *Science* 1992; **257**: 1415–1419.

18. Williams K, Zappia AM, Pritchett DB et al. Sensitivity of the N-methyl-D-aspartate receptor to polyamines is controlled by NR2 subunits. *Mol Pharmacol* 1994; **45**: 803–809.

19. Pin JP, Duvoisin R. The metabotropic glutamate receptors: structure and functions. *Neuropharmacology* 1995; **34**: 1–26.

20. Miller RJ. Metabotropic excitatory amino acid receptors reveal their true colours. *Trends Pharmacol Sci* 1991; **12**: 365–367.

21. Tanabe S, Nomura A, Masu M et al. Signal transduction, pharmacological properties, and expression patterns of two rat metabotropic glutamate receptors, mGluR3 and mGluR4. *J Neurosci* 1993; **13**: 1372–1378.

22. Nicholls DG, Attwell D. The release and uptake of excitatory amino acids. *Trends Pharmacol Sci* 1990; **11**: 462–468.

23. Bouvier M. Szatkowski M, Amato A, Attwell D. The glial cell glutamate uptake carrier countertransports pH-changing anions. *Nature* 1992; **306**: 471–474.

24. Arriza JL, Fairman WA, Wadiche JI et al. Functional comparisons of three glutamate transporter subtypes cloned from human motor cortex. *J Neurosci* 1994; **14**: 5559–5569.

25. Fairman WA, Vandenberg RJ, Arriza JL et al. An excitatory amino acid transporter with properties of a ligand-gated chloride channel. *Nature* 1995; **375**: 599–603.

26. Arriza JL, Eliasof S, Kavanaugh MP, Amara SG. Excitatory amino acid transporter 5, a retinal glutamate transporter coupled to a chloride conductance. *Proc Natl Acad Sci U S A* 1997; **94**: 4155–4160.

27. Rothstein JD, Martin L, Levey AI et al. Localization of neuronal and glial glutamate transporters. *Neuron* 1994; **13**: 713–725.

28. Furuta A, Martin LJ, Lin C-LG et al. Cellular and synaptic localization of the neuronal glutamate transporters excitatory amino acid transporter 3 and 4. *Neuroscience* 1997; **81**: 1031–1042.

29. Lucas DR, Newhouse JP. The toxic effect of sodium L-glutamate on the inner layers of the retina. *Arch Ophthalmol* 1957; **58**: 193–204.

30. Olney JW, Ho OL. Brain damage in infant mice following oral intake of glutamate, aspartate or cysteine. *Nature* 1970; **227**: 609–610.

31. Olney JW, Sharpe LG, Feigin RD. Glutamate-induced brain damage in infant primates. *J Neuropathol Exp Neurol* 1972; **31**: 464–488.

32. Choi DW. Ionic dependence of glutamate neurotoxicity in cortical cell culture. *J Neurosci* 1987; **7**: 369–379.

33. Miller RJ, Murphy SN, Glaum SR. Neuronal Ca^{2+} channels and their regulation by excitatory amino acids. *Ann N Y Acad Sci* 1989; **568**: 149–158.

34. Meldrun B, Garthwaite J. Excitatory amino acid neurotoxicity and neurodegenerative disease. *Trends Pharmacol Sci* 1990; **11**: 379–387.

35. Novelli A, Reilly JA, Lysko PG, Henneberry RC. Glutamate becomes neurotoxic via the N-methyl-D-aspartate receptor when intracellular energy levels are reduced. *Brain Res* 1988; **451**: 205–212.

36. Zeevalk GD, Nicklas WJ. Mechanisms underlying initiation of excitotoxicity associated with metabolic inhibition. *J Pharmacol Exp Ther* 1991; **257**: 870–878.

37. Beal MF. Does impairment of energy metabolism result in excitotoxic neuronal death in neurodegenerative illness? *Ann Neurol* 1992; **31**: 119–130.

38. Beal MF. Role of excitotoxicity in human neurological disease. *Curr Opin Neurol* 1992; **2**: 657–662.

39. Plaitakis A, Caroscio JT. Abnormal glutamate metabolism in amyotrophic lateral sclerosis. *Ann Neurol* 1987; **22**: 575–579.

40. Rothstein JD, Tsai G, Kuncl RW et al. Abnormal excitatory amino acid metabolism in amyotrophic lateral sclerosis. *Ann Neurol* 1990; **28**: 18–25.

41. Spink C, Martin DL. Excitatory amino acids in amyotrophic lateral sclerosis (letter). *Ann Neurol* 1991; **29**: 110.

42. Shaw PJ, Forrest V, Ince PG et al. CSF and plasma amino acid levels in motor neuron disease: elevation of CSF glutamate in a subset of patients. *Neurodegeneration* 1995; **4**: 209–216.

43. Rothstein JD, Martin LJ, Kuncl RW. Decreased glutamate transport by the brain and spinal cord in amyotrophic lateral sclerosis. *N Engl J Med* 1992; **22**: 1464–1468.

44. Shaw PJ, Chinnery RM, Ince PG. [³H]D-Aspartate binding sites in the normal human spinal cord and changes in motor neuron disease, a quantitative autoradiographic study. *Brain Res* 1994; **655**: 195–201.

45. Rothstein JD, Jin L, Dykes-Hoberg M, Kuncl RW. Chronic glutamate uptake inhibition produces a model of slow neurotoxicity. *Proc Natl Acad Sci U S A* 1993; **90**: 6591–6595.

46. Rothstein JD, Van Kammen M, Levey AI et al. Selective loss of glial glutamate transporter GLT-1 in amyotrophic lateral sclerosis. *Ann Neurol* 1995; **38**: 73–84.

47. Rothstein JD, Dykes-Hoberg M, Pardo CA et al. Knockout of glutamate transporters reveals a major role for astroglial transport in excitotoxicity and clearance of glutamate. *Neuron* 1996; **16**: 675–686.

48. Haugeto O, Ullensvang K, Levy LM et al. Brain glutamate transporter proteins form homomultimers. *J Biol Chem* 1996; **271**: 27715–27722.

49. Tanaka K, Watase K, Manabe T et al. Epilepsy and exacerbation of brain injury in mice lacking the glutamate transporter GLT-1. *Science* 1997; **276**: 1699–1702.

50. Ginsburg S, Martin L, Rothstein JD. Regional deafferentation down regulates subtypes of glutamate transporters. *J Neurochem* 1995; **65**: 2800–2803.

51. Bristol LA, Rothstein JD. Glutamate transporter gene expression in amyotrophic lateral sclerosis motor cortex. *Ann Neurol* 2996; **39**: 676–679.

52. Aoki M, Lin CLG, Rothstein JD et al. Mutations in the glutamate transporter EAAT2 gene do not cause abnormal transcripts in ALS. *Ann Neurol* 1998; **43**: 645–653.

53. Jackson M, Steers G, Leigh N, Morrison KE. Polymorphisms in the glutamate transporter gene EAAT2 in European ALS patients. *J Neurol* 1999; in press.

54. Trotti D, Rossi D, Gjesdal O et al. Peroxynitrite inhibits glutamate transporter subtypes. *J Biol Chem* 1996; **271**: 5976.

55. Bowling AC, Schultz JB, Brown RH, Beal MF. Superoxide dismutase activity, oxidative damage, and mitochondrial energy metabolism in familial and sporadic amyotrophic lateral sclerosis. *J Neurochem* 1993; **61**: 2322–2325.

56. Shaw PJ, Ince PG, Falkous G, Mantle D. Oxidative damage to protein in sporadic motor neuron disease spinal cord. *Ann Neurol* 1995; **38**: 691–695.

57. Lin CLG, Bristol LA. Jin L et al. Aberrant RNA processing in a neurodegenerative disease: a common cause for loss of glutamate transport EAAT2 protein in sporadic amyotrophic lateral sclerosis. *Neuron* 1998; **20**: 589–602.

58. Gurney ME, Cutting FB, Zhai P et al. Benefit of vitamin E, riluzole and gabapentin in a transgenic model of familial amyotrophic lateral sclerosis. *Ann Neurol* 1996; **39**: 147–157.

59. Hughes JT. Pathology of amyotrophic lateral sclerosis. *Adv Neurol* 1982; **36**: 61–73.

60. Mannen T, Iwata M, Toyokura Y, Nagashima K. Preservation of a certain motoneurone group of the sacral cord in amyotrophic lateral sclerosis: its clinical significance. *J Neurol Neurosurg Psychiatry* 1977; **40**: 464–469.

61. Alexianu ME, Ho BK, Mohamed H et al. The role of calcium-binding proteins in selective motoneuron vulnerability in amyotrophic lateral sclerosis. *Ann Neurol* 1994; **36**: 846–858.

62. Ho BK, Alexianu ME, Colom LV et al. Expression of calbindin D-28K in motoneuron hybrid cells after retroviral infection with calbindin D-28K cDNA prevents amyotrophic lateral sclerosis IgG-mediated cytotoxicity. *Proc Natl Acad Sci U S A* 1996; **93**: 6796–6801.

63. Williams TL, Day NC, Ince PG et al. Calcium permeable α-amino-3-hydroxy-5-methyl-4-isoxazole propionic acid receptors: a molecular determinant of selective vulnerability in amyotrophic lateral sclerosis. *Ann Neurol* 1997; **42**: 200–207.

64. Pruss RM, Akeson RL, Racke MM, Wilburn JL. Agonist activated cobalt uptake identifies divalent cation-permeable kainate receptors on neurons and glial cells. *Neuron* 1991; **7**: 509–518.

65. Tsuda T, Munthasser S, Fraser PE et al. Analysis of the functional effects of a mutation in SOD-1 associated with familial amyotrophic lateral sclerosis. *Neuron* 1994; **13**: 727–736.

66. Martin D, Thompson MA, Nadler JV. The neuroprotective agent riluzole inhibits release of glutamate and aspartate from slices of hippocampal area CA1. *Eur J Pharmacol* 1993; **250**: 473–476.

67. Hubert JP, Delumeau JC, Glowinski J et al. Antagonism by riluzole of entry of calcium evoked by NMDA and veratridine in rat cultured granule cells: evidence for a dual mechanism of action. *Br J Pharmacol* 1994; **113**: 261–267.

68. Miller RG, Bouchard JP, Duquette P et al. Clinical trials of riluzole in patients with ALS. *Neurology* 1996; **47** (**suppl 2**): S86–S92.

69. Lacomblez L, Bensimon G, Leigh PN et al. A confirmatory dose ranging study of riluzole in ALS. ALS/Riluzole Study Group II. *Neurology* 1996; **47** (**suppl 4**): S242–S250.

15

Exogenous neurotoxins
Michael J Strong

Introduction

In the century following the classical descriptions of amyotrophic lateral sclerosis (ALS) by Aran[1,2] and Charcot,[3] little knowledge was gained regarding the pathogenesis of this devastating disorder. In contrast, significant advances have been made in our understanding of the biology of ALS in the most recent decades. Concomitant with this rapid acquisition of knowledge has been the recognition that classical sporadic ALS is not a discrete disease entity, but rather a clinical phenotype of motor neuron degeneration marked by progressive muscle loss and upper motor neuron dysfunction. This multiplicity of etiologies for the disease process is most convincingly illustrated by the familial variants of ALS (FALS), in which some pedigrees possess linkage to mutations in the copper–zinc superoxide dismutase gene (SOD1), while others do not.[4,5] Even amongst FALS pedigree expressing a mutant SOD1, considerable heterogeneity exists in both clinical manifestations (e.g. disease duration) and in the neuropathological features of non-motor system involvement.[6–9] Similarly, otherwise classical forms of sporadic ALS are now recognized to be associated with frontotemporal dementia — a process previously held to be uncommon in ALS.[10,11] The hyperendemic focus of ALS in the western Pacific, now resolving through dietary inter-vention, yielded yet another variant of ALS that, for the most part, was largely indistinguishable clinically from the more common sporadic ALS.[12,13]

Hence, a discussion of exogenous neurotoxins in the etiology of sporadic ALS is colored by the recognition that ALS cannot be a single disease entity, but rather must be a collection of clinical, electrophysiological, and neuropathological characteristics to which we apply the descriptive term of ALS. Viewed in this light, there should be little surprise that ALS might be considered as a disorder of multiple etiologies in which the final common pathway is the progressive degeneration of motor neurons. This chapter reviews the potential role of exogenous neurotoxins in either inducing or modifying this process.

Sporadic ALS

A common theme in the epidemiology of ALS is the observation of increasing incidence and prevalence rates attributed to the occurrence of an, as yet, unidentified exogenous toxin or process. There are, however, several factors that need to be considered in this analysis. The most consistent observation is that ALS is an age-dependent disease in which increased incidence rates are observed amongst the elderly. Whether these increases in the incidence rates of ALS exceed those that would be predicted solely on the basis of aging of the population is the critical question. In an analysis of over 9,000 deaths from ALS from 1968 to 1982, Durrleman and Alperovitch[14] observed increasing ALS mortality rates in the years 1968–1971 and 1979–1982. The authors postulated that an increase in the disease frequency, particularly in the elderly, could be attributed to an exogenous factor through either a more prolonged exposure to such an agent, or a greater susceptibility to it. Similarly, Lilienfeld and colleagues[15] found an increase in age-specific mortality rates, particularly in the elderly, and postulated an exogenous factor as the basis for this. Increases in the annual mortality rates from ALS in Sweden have also been observed, leading to the postulate of either an increase in the number of individuals living to higher ages, or, given that all ages classes demonstrated an increased rate, an influence of an environmental factor that was most prominently expressed in the elderly.[16,17] Buckley and colleagues[18] similarly found increases in the age- and sex-adjusted incidence rates of motor neuron disease in the years from 1959–1979, with the increase most apparent in women over the age of 45 years and men over the age of 60 years. The theme of increasing age-specific incidence rates has also been observed amongst the elderly population in Israel,[19] the UK,[20] and south-western Ontario, Canada.[21]

However, the observation of a global increase in ALS incidence over time irrespective of age is not replicated in all studies — thus leading to an inherent difficulty in attempting to conclude that an environmental agent is responsible, in some way, for the disease process. For instance, Kristensen and Melgaard[22] concluded that there had been no significant change in the incidence rates in Funen County, Denmark, for the years 1948–72. This conclusion was echoed in an

analysis of the Mayo Clinic patient registry for the years 1925–1984, although the age-dependency of incidence rates was confirmed.[23] Kondo and Minowa[24] proposed that ALS mortality rates were actually declining in Japan. However, the authors postulated that this was related to the elimination of the traditional rural life in Japan that had contained 'risk factors' for the development of motor neuron disease. While Chiò and colleagues[25] also found an increase in the mortality rates for ALS in the Italian population for the interval from 1958 to 1987, these authors attributed this observation to changes in methodological and demographic variables rather than a true increase in the incidence rates.

Not withstanding the previous discussion, the epidemiological studies support, on balance, the conclusion that ALS is an age-dependent neurodegenerative process with a disproportionate increase in incidence rates amongst the elderly. If this is really true, then determining if environmental risk factors exist to which the aging population have been exposed, and which directly or indirectly increase the lifetime of developing ALS, is not a trivial task. Granieri and colleagues,[26] in an incidence, prevalence, and mortality survey of the Italian population from 1964 to 1982, observed ALS to be more common in males, in people aged 50–70 years, and in agricultural workers. More patients were observed in suburban areas, in rural farming communities, and in communities with fewer than 5,000 people. Prevalence rates were also shown to be higher among agricultural workers both in southern Italy[27] and in Sweden,[28] and among farmers and shepherds in Sardinia.[28] Bracco and colleagues[29] found no evidence for a specific increase in the prevalence of ALS among agricultural workers in Florence, Italy, but they did note a significant increase in incidence amongst farmers, non-specialized factory workers, maids, and athletes as a group. Heavy manual laborers were also over-represented in the study of Gunnarsson and Palm.[30] Hudson and colleagues[21] linked the observation of an increased incidence rate amongst industrial regions in south-western Ontario to the derivation of the water supply from regions with major chemical industry. Breland and Currier[31] observed a greater representation of heavy physical labor in ALS patients in contrast to a greater representation of professional labor in multiple sclerosis patients. In one of the few dissenting papers, Edgar and colleagues[32] observed no correlation between death rates and area of birth, although such an association existed in an analysis of multiple sclerosis. This latter observation suggested a lack of evidence for an exogenous factor in ALS.

Many studies have suffered from the lack of sufficient patient numbers to derive a statistically valid conclusion with regard to single toxicological events in the history of ALS patients. The reports, at various times, of the association of ALS with lead and mercury exposure,[33] solvent exposure,[34] athletic activity,[33] milk ingestion,[33] and employment in the textile industry[35] fall subject to such difficulties. Recently, a statistically significant increased risk in those exposed to welding or soldering has been reported.[36] Similarly, an increased occurrence of mechanical trauma in ALS compared to controls has been observed by a number of authors.[29,37,38] Of interest, the observation of an increased occurrence of ALS amongst those with an occupational exposure in the manufacture of plastics many find pathogenic support through the experimental modeling of ALS.[39,40]

The role of electrical injury in the etiology of ALS remains controversial, particularly with regard to the latency interval between the occurrence of the electrical insult and the onset of the disease process. Gawel and colleagues[41] in a case control study of 63 ALS patients and 61 control subjects referred to a neurology clinic, found an increased incidence of antecedent electric shock, although the latency between the occurrence of the shock and the development of ALS was not discussed. Although an increased risk of the development of ALS in people in occupations at risk of electrical exposure has been described by Deapen and Henderson[39] and Schulte and colleagues,[42] Kondo and Tsubaki[37] failed to find such an association.

Hence, although limitations exist with regard to the interpretation of the epidemiological studies, the overall analysis suggests that sALS is increasing in incidence, with the most significant increases occurring amongst the elderly, and that geographic risk factors such as rural or farming exposure may contribute to this process. Antecedent electrical injury and an exposure to plastics industry may contribute to this.

Western Pacific variant of ALS

The prototypic example of an environmental agent playing a causative role in the occurrence of ALS is the hyperendemic foci of ALS of the western Pacific, including the Kii peninsula, Guam, and Papua New Guinea.[43] Although the exact environmental agent and the extent of its role in the induction of the disease remains uncertain, it seems relatively clear that the occurrence of ALS in this population is directly related to an exogenous neurotoxin.

Epidemiology

The epidemiological data in support of such a conclusion is relatively strong. With the westernization of the region, rendering the population less dependent on traditional native foodstuffs, the incidence rates declined dramatically to values approximating those of the North American population.[44] Although population studies initially suggested a prominent genetic component to these incidence rates,[45,46] to date, linkage to the mutant SOD1 enzyme observed in FALS has not been observed.[47] A recent segregation analysis, incorporating all patients suffering from either ALS or parkinsonism–dementia or both, excluded a two-allele additive major locus hypothesis as accounting for the disorder.[48]

These findings are, however, not inconsistent with an underlying genetic susceptibility that is endemic to the population, with a superimposed exogenous factor functioning as an unique trigger for the disease process. Two major environmental hypotheses have arisen with regard to the nature of this exogenous factor — either the chronic aluminium intoxication invoked by dietary calcium deficiency, or the exposure to a neurotoxic metabolite of the false sago palm (*Cycas circinalis*).

Aluminium hypothesis

One unifying geographic feature amongst all three hyperendemic foci of ALS in the western Pacific is the unique composition of the soil and its effect upon the water supply and crops in yielding a diet deficient in calcium and magnesium and rich in bioavailable aluminium compounds.[49,50] Studies undertaken while the area was still a hyperendemic focus of ALS demonstrated the induction of a secondary hyperparathyroid state based on chronic calcium deficiency.[51–53] The small nuclear radius of aluminium, although a trivalent cation, leads to its enhanced absorption in lieu of calcium. A number of varying techniques have demonstrated either elevated tissue levels of aluminium or the co-localization of aluminium

silicates with intraneuronal aggregates within degenerating neurons.[54–61] Although a recent analysis of contemporary cases of western Pacific ALS failed to replicate the elevated tissue levels of aluminium discussion,[62] this is not unexpected given the reduction in the incidence rates within this population concomitant with the alteration in the dietary habits. Presumably, ALS that continues to occur is more akin to that of the Western cultures, and is no longer a reflection of heightened aluminium exposure. Indeed, the failure to find such evidence in current Guamanian ALS cases fully supports the concept that the hyperendemic focus of ALS in Guam reflected an additive, two-insult process.

For there to be a potential etiological relationship between an environmental neurotoxin and the ultimate development of a motor neuron disorder, there needs to be some evidence that the neurotoxin can experimentally produce some semblance of the disease process.[63] Clearly, aluminium is a potent neurotoxin. When administered to susceptible species, in either organic or inorganic forms and by a variety of routes, aluminium induces a fulminant neurotoxicological process marked by widespread neurofilamentous aggregate formation or a process marked by physiological pathology in the absence of aggregate formation.[64] It is the induction of neurofilamentous pathology that is of direct relevance to understanding the role of aluminium as an exogenous agent in the induction of ALS.

Based on the western Pacific ALS findings, Garruto and colleagues[65] and Yase and colleagues[66] undertook studies of chronic calcium deficiency with or without magnesium deficiency, with dietary aluminium supplementation in non-human primates. Both groups observed widespread motor neuron degeneration marked by intraneuronal aggregates of neurofilament. Other groups subsequently observed that repeated monthly intracisternal sublethal inoculums of aluminium chloride to young adult New Zealand white rabbits would induce a progressive motor neuron disorder marked by intraneuronal neurofilamentous aggregates with neuropathological features similar to those observed in ALS.[67,68] In studies of acute aluminium chloride neurotoxicity, the author has demonstrated that aluminium chloride induces phosphatase-resistant high molecular weight neurofilament (NFH) and a modification in NFH–tubulin binding characteristics.[69,70] These studies suggested that the induction of neuropathological changes following aluminium exposure related to a post-translational modification in NFH.

Hence, although there is no evidence that chronic aluminium exposure is relevant to the occurrence of sporadic ALS, there is sufficient evidence that it is active as a neurotoxicant in the western Pacific focus of ALS and that it can experimentally induce a disease process identical to that of ALS. Moreover, the author's studies of the neurochemistry of aluminium neurotoxicity clearly demonstrate the potential for this agent to induce a post-translational modification in NFH sufficient to induce the disease process. Whether such a process is occurring in ALS remains to be determined.

Cycas circinalis *hypothesis*

The second exogenous toxin of potential relevance to the induction of the western Pacific variant of ALS involves the ingestion or use of the neurotoxic seed of *Cycas circinalis* (cycad).[71] First recognized by Margorie Whiting, the seed of *Cycas circinalis* (the false sago palm) was utilized as a dietary supplement (e.g. a source of flour) in the western Pacific during times of drought or as a medicinal poultice.[72,73] Although detoxified through repeated washings, trace levels of α-amino-β-

methylaminopropionic acid (L-BMAA) and of methyl-azomethanol β-D-glucoside (cycasin) were observed in the purified material.[74,75] Whether the levels of L-BMAA in the processed cycad are, however, sufficient to induce neuronal degeneration remains controversial.[76] However, as with the exogenous administration of aluminium to non-human primates, the administration of cycad to primates results in limb muscle atrophy, tremor, and a non-reactive degeneration of the anterior horns with a loss of pyramidal neurons in the motor cortex.[71] As discussed by Spencer and colleagues,[73] cycad, when improperly purified, contains the potent neurotoxin L-BMAA, which is converted to methyl-azoxymethanol, a potent DNA methylating compound.

Conclusions

The difficulty in determining whether an exogenous neurotoxin is responsible for inducing ALS is that the evidence available to reach such a conclusion is circumstantial at best. The intuitive feeling that ALS must be increasing, and thus must be related to an, as yet, ill-defined neurotoxin, simply defies proof. Nonetheless, the evidence — however circumstantial — is compelling. From the preceding review, it seems that the incidence of ALS is increasing and that this increase is most evident in the elderly. It can be argued that this population is at the greatest risk because of a cumulative exposure to an environmental agent. Most consistent amongst the epidemiological analysis are the over-representation of farmers, laborers, and those working with metals or plastics. The resolution of the traditional form of ALS amongst the inhabitants of the geographic foci in the western Pacific and the linkage to an environmental agent (regardless of its nature) is striking evidence that ALS can be associated with an environmental trigger. Causation has still, even in this focus, not been proven. Rather, a multi-insult process, in which an environmental agent plays a major role, is the most probable explanation. Finally, two examples (amongst many possible) were provided to demonstrate that exogenous neurotoxins, thought relevant to the induction of ALS, can induce motor system-selective degeneration in a variety of hosts.

On balance, it is not unreasonable to conclude that ALS can be associated with an environmental trigger. As alluded to at the introduction to this chapter, the challenge will remain to determine which of the phenotypically similar disease processes that we identify as ALS are in fact reflections of such a process.

Acknowledgements

The generous assistance of Dr Arthur Hudson in reviewing this manuscript is gratefully appreciated.

References

1. Aran FA. Recherches sur un maladie non encore décrite du systéme musculaire (atrophie musculaire progressive) (2e article – suite et fin). *Arch Gen Med* 1850; **24**: 172–214.
2. Aran FA. Recherches sur une maladie non encore décrite du systéme musculaire (atrophie musculaire progressive). *Arch Gen Med* 1850; **24**: 5–35.
3. Charcot JM, Joffroy A. Deux cas d'atrophie musculaire progressive avec lésions de la substance grise et des faisceaux antérolatéraux de la moelle épinière. *Arch Physiol Norm Pathol* 1869; **2**: 354–744.
4. Strong MJ, Hudson AJ, Alvord WG. Familial amyotrophic lateral sclerosis, 1850–1989: a statistical analysis of the world literature. *Can J Neurol Sci* 1991; **18**: 45–58.
5. Rosen DR, Siddique T, Patterson D et al. Mutations in Cu/Zn superoxide dismutase gene are associated with familial amyotrophic lateral sclerosis. *Nature* 1993; **362**: 59–62.
6. Ince PG, Shaw PJ, Slade JY et al. Familial amyotrophic lateral sclerosis with a mutation in exon 4 of the Cu/Zn superoxide dismutase gene: pathological and immunocytochemical changes. *Acta Neuropathol* 1996; **92**: 395–403.
7. Orrell RW, King AW, Hilton DA et al. Familial amyotrophic lateral sclerosis with a point mutation of SOD-1: intrafamilial heterogeneity of disease duration associated with neurofibrillary tangles. *J Neurol Neurosurg Psychiatry* 1995; **59**: 266–270.
8. Rouleau GA, Clark AW, Rooke K et al. SOD1 mutations associated with accumulation of neurofilaments in amyotrophic lateral sclerosis. *Ann Neurol* 1996; **39**: 128–131.
9. Takahashi H, Makifuchi T, Nakano R et al. Familial amyotrophic lateral sclerosis with a mutation in Cu/Zn superoxide dismutase gene. *Acta Neuropathol* 1994; **88**: 185–188.
10. Strong MR, Grace GM. Cognitive changes in amyotrophic lateral sclerosis. In: Kertesz A, Munoz DA, eds. *Pick's Disease and Pick Complex*. New York: John Wiley and Sons, 1998.
11. Strong MJ, Grace GM, Orange JB, Leeper HA. Cognition, language and speech in amyotrophic lateral sclerosis: a review. *J Clin Exp Neuropsychol* 1996; **18**: 291–303.
12. Rodgers-Johnson P, Garruto RM, Yanigahara R et al. Amyotrophic lateral sclerosis and parkinsonism–dementia on Guam: a 30-year evaluation of clinical and neuropathological trends. *Neurology* 1986; **36**: 7–13.
13. Garruto RM. Cellular and molecular mechanisms of neuronal degeneration: amyotrophic lateral sclerosis, parkinsonism–dementia, and Alzheimer disease. *Am J Human Biol* 1989; **1**: 529–543.
14. Durrleman S, Alperovitch A. Increasing trend of ALS in France and elsewhere: are the changes real? *Neurology* 1989; **39**: 768–773.
15. Lilienfeld DE, Ehland J, Landrigan PJ et al. Rising mortality from motoneuron disease in the USA, 1962–84. *Lancet* 1989; **i**: 710–713.
16. Neilson S, Gunnarsson LG, Robinson I. Rising mortality from motor neuron disease in Sweden 1961–1990: the relative role of increased population life expectancy and environmental factors. *Acta Neurol Scand* 1994; **902**:

150–159.

17. Gunnarsson LG, Lindberg G, Söderfelt B, Axelson O. The mortality of motor neuron disease in Sweden. *Arch Neurol* 1990; **47**: 42–46.

18. Buckley J, Warlow C, Smith P et al. Motor neuron disease in England and Wales, 1959–1979. *J Neurol Neurosurg Psychiatry* 1983; **46**: 197–205.

19. Kahana E, Zilber N. Changes in the incidence of amyotrophic lateral sclerosis in Israel. *Arch Neurol* 1984; **41**: 157–160.

20. Li TM, Swash M, Alberman E. Morbidity and mortality in motor neuron disease: comparison with multiple sclerosis and Parkinson's disease: age and sex specific rates and cohort analysis. *J Neurol Neurosurg Psychiatry* 1985; **48**: 320–327.

21. Hudson AJ, Davenport A, Hader WJ. The incidence of amyotrophic lateral sclerosis in southwestern Ontario, Canada. *Neurology* 1986; **36**: 1524–1528.

22. Kristensen O, Melgaard B. Motor neuron disease. Prognosis and epidemiology. *Acta Neurol Scand* 1977; **56**: 299–308.

23. Yoshida S, Mulder DW, Kurland LT et al. Follow-up study on amyotrophic lateral sclerosis in Rochester, Minn., 1925 through 1984. *Neuroepidemiology* 1986; **5**: 61–70.

24. Kondo K, Minowa M. Epidemiology of motor neuron disease in Japan: declining trends of the mortality rate. In: Tsubaki T, Yase Y, eds. *Amyotrophic Lateral Sclerosis.* Amsterdam: Elsevier, 1988, 11–16.

25. Chiò A, Magnani C, Schiffer D. Amyotrophic lateral sclerosis mortality in Italy, 1958 to 1987: a cross-sectional and cohort study. *Neurology* 1993; **43**: 927–930.

26. Granieri E, Carreras M, Tola R et al. Motor neuron disease in the province of Ferrara, Italy, in 1964–1982. *Neurology* 1988; **38**: 1604–1608.

27. Rosati G, Pinna L, Granieri E et al. Studies on epidemiological, clinical and etiological aspects of ALS disease in Sardinia, Southern Italy. *Acta Neurol Scand* 1977; **55**: 231–244.

28. Giagheddu M, Puggioni G, Biancu F et al. Epidemiological study of amyotrophic lateral sclerosis in Sardinia, Italy. *Acta Neurol Scand* 1983; **68**: 394–404.

29. Bracco L, Antuono P, Amaducci L. Study of epidemiological and etiological factors of amyotrophic lateral sclerosis in the province of Florence, Italy. *Acta Neurol Scand* 1979; **60**: 112–124.

30. Gunnarsson LG, Palm R. Motor neuron diseases and heavy manual labor: an epidemiological survey of Värmland County, Sweden. *Neuroepidemiology* 1984; **3**: 195–206.

31. Breland AE Jr, Currier RD. Multiple sclerosis and amyotrophic lateral sclerosis in Mississippi. *Neurology* 1967; **17**: 1011–1016.

32. Edgar AH, Brody JA, Detels R. Amyotrophic lateral sclerosis mortality among native-born and migrant residents of California and Washington. *Neurology* 1973; **23**: 48–51.

33. Felmus MT, Patten BM, Swanke L. Antecedent events in amyotrophic lateral sclerosis. *Neurology* 1976; **26**: 167–172.

34. Hawkes CH, Cavanagh JB, Fox AJ. Motoneuron disease: a disorder secondary to solvent exposure? *Lancet* 1989; **i**: 73–76.

35. Abarbanel JM, Herishanu YO, Osimani A, Frisher S. Motor neuron disease in textile factory workers. *Acta Neurol Scand* 1989; **79**: 347–349.

36. Strickland D, Smith SA, Dolliff G et al. Amyotrophic lateral sclerosis and occupational history. Arch Neurol 1996; **53**: 730–733.

37. Kondo K, Tsubaki T. Case-control studies of motor neuron disease. Association with mechanical injuries. *Arch Neurol* 1981; **38**: 220–226.

38. Sienko DG, Davis JP, Taylor JA, Brooks BR. Amyotrophic lateral sclerosis. A case-control study following detection of a cluster in a small Wisconsin community. *Arch Neurol* 1990; **47**: 38–41.

39. Deapen DM, Henderson BE. A case-control study of amyotrophic lateral sclerosis. *Am J Epidemiol* 1986; **123**: 709–799.

40. Strong MJ, Garruto RM, Wolff AV et al. N-Butyl benzenesulfonamide: a neurotoxic plasticizer inducing a spastic myelopathy in rabbits. *Acta Neuropathol* 1991; **81**: 235–241.

41. Gawel M, Zaiwalla Z, Clifford Rose F. Antecedent events in motor neuron disease. *J Neurol Neurosurg Psychiatry* 1983; **46**: 1041–1043.

42. Schulte PA, Burnett CA, Boeniger MF, Johnson J. Neurodegenerative diseases: occupational

occurrence and potential risk factors, 1982 through 1991. *Am J Public Health* 1996; **86:** 1281–1288.

43. Garruto RM. Pacific paradigms of environmentally-induced neurological disorders: clinical, epidemiological and molecular perspectives. *NeuroToxicology* 1991; **12:** 347–378.

44. Garrutto RM, Yanagihara R, Gajdusek DC. Disappearance of high-incidence amyotrophic lateral sclerosis and parkinsonism–dementia on Guam. *Neurology* 1985; **35:** 193–198.

45. Plato CC, Reed DM, Elizan TS, Kurland LT. Amyotrophic lateral sclerosis/Parkinsonism–dementia complex of Guam. IV. Familial and genetic studies. *Am J Hum Genet* 1967; **19:** 617–632.

46. Chen KM, Brody JA, Kurland LT. Patterns of neurological diseases on Guam. I. Epidemiological aspects. *Arch Neurol* 1968; **19:** 573–578.

47. Figlewicz DA, Garruto RM, Krizus A et al. The Cu/Zn superoxide dismutase gene in ALS and Parkinsonism–dementia of Guam. *NeuroReport* 1994; **5:** 557–560.

48. Bailey-Wilson JE, Plato CC, Elston RC, Garruto RM. Potential role of an additive genetic component in the cause of amyotrophic lateral sclerosis and Parkinsonism–dementia in the Western Pacific. *Am J Med Genet* 1993; **45:** 68–76.

49. Garruto RM, Yanagihara R, Gajdusek DC et al. Concentrations of heavy metals and essential minerals in garden soil and drinking water in the western Pacific. In: Chen KM, Yase Y, eds. *Amyotrophic Lateral Sclerosis in Asia and Oceania.* Taipei, Shyan-Fu Chou, National Taiwan University, 1983, 265–329.

50. Kimura K, Yase Y, Higashi Y et al. Epidemiological and geomedical studies on amyotrophic lateral sclerosis. *Dis Nerv Syst* 1963; **24:** 155–159.

51. Yanagihara R, Garruto RM, Gajdusek DC et al. Calcium and vitamin D metabolism in Guamanian Chamorros with amyotrophic lateral sclerosis and parkinsonism–dementia. *Ann Neurol* 1984; **15:** 42–48.

52. Plato CC, Garruto RM, Yanigahara R et al. Cortical bone loss and measurements of the second metacarpal bone. I. Comparisons between adult Guamanian Chamorros and American Caucasians. *Am J Phys Anthropol* 1982; **59:** 461–465.

53. Garruto RM, Plato CC, Yanagihara R et al. Bone mass in Guamanian patients with amyotrophic lateral sclerosis and parkinsonism–dementia. *Am J Phys Anthropol* 1989; **80:** 107–113.

54. Yoshimasu F, Yasui M, Yase Y et al. Studies on amyotrophic lateral sclerosis by neutron activation analysis: 3. Systematic analysis of metals on Guamanian ALS and PD cases. *Folia Psychiatry Neurol Jpn* 1982; **36:** 173–180.

55. Yasui M, Yase Y, Ota K, Garruto RM. Aluminium deposition in the central nervous system of patients with amyotrophic lateral sclerosis from the Kii Peninsula of Japan. *NeuroToxicology* 1991; **12:** 615–620.

56. Garruto RM, Swyt C, Yanagihara R et al. Intraneuronal co-localization of silicon with calcium and aluminium in amyotrophic lateral sclerosis and parkinsonism with dementia of Guam. *N Engl J Med* 1986; **315:** 711–712.

57. Garruto RM, Fukatsu R, Yanagihara R et al. Imaging of calcium and aluminium in neurofibrillary tangle-bearing neurons in parkinsonism–dementia of Guam. *Proc Natl Acad Sci U S A* 1984; **81:** 1875–1879.

58. Yoshida S, Yase Y, Iwata S et al. Comparative trace-elemental study on amyotrophic lateral sclerosis (ALS) and parkinsonism–dementia (PD) in the Kii Peninsula of Japan and Guam. *Wakayama Med Rep* 1988; **30:** 41–53.

59. Ikuta F, Makifuchi T. Distribution of aluminium in the spinal motor neurons of ALS, examined by wavelength-dispersive X-ray microanalysis. Annual Report of the Research Committee of Motor Neuron Disease. Tokyo: The Ministry of Health and Welfare of Japan, 1977, 66–69.

60. Yoshimasu F, Yasui M, Yase Y et al. Studies on amyotrophic lateral sclerosis by neutron activation analysis. 2. Comparative study of analytical results on Guam PD, Japanese ALS and Alzheimer disease cases. *Folia Psychiatr Neurol Jpn* 1980; **34:** 75–82.

61. Yase Y, Kumamotot T, Yoshimasu F, Shinjo Y. Amyotrophic lateral sclerosis studies using neutron activation analysis studies. *Neurology (India)* 1968; **16:** 46–59.

62. Ahlskog JE, Waring SC, Kurland LT et al. Guamanian neurodegenerative disease: investigation of the calcium metabolism/heavy metal hypothesis. *Neurology* 1995; **45**: 1340–1344.

63. Strong MJ, Garruto RM. Experimental paradigms of motor neuron degeneration. In: Woodruff ML, Nonneman A, eds. *Animal Models of Toxin-Induced Neurological Disorders*. New York: Plenum Press, 1994, 39–88.

64. Strong MJ. Aluminium-induced neurodegeneration with special reference to amyotrophic lateral sclerosis and dialysis encephalopathy. *Rev Biochem Toxicol* 1994; **11**: 75–115.

65. Garruto RM, Shankar SK, Yanagihara R et al. Low-calcium, high aluminium diet-induced motor neuron pathology in cynomolgus monkeys. *Acta Neuropathol* 1989; **78**: 210–219.

66. Yasui M, Yase Y, Ota K. Evaluation of magnesium, calcium, aluminium metabolism in rats and monkeys maintained on calcium-deficient diets (abstract). *NeuroToxicology* 1991; **12**: 139.

67. Strong MJ, Gaytan-Garcia S, Jakowec D. Reversibility of neurofilamentous inclusion formation following repeated sublethal intracisternal inoculums of AlCl₃ in New Zealand white rabbits. *Acta Neuropathol* 1995; **90**: 57–67.

68. Wakayama I, Nerurkar VR, Strong MJ, Garruto RM. Comparative study of chronic aluminium-induced neurofilamentous aggregates with intracytoplasmic inclusions of amyotrophic lateral sclerosis. *Acta Neuropathol* 1996; **92**: 545–554.

69. Strong MJ, Jakowec DM. 200 kDa and 160 kDa neurofilament protein phosphatase resistance following in vivo aluminium chloride exposure. *NeuroToxicology* 1994; **15**: 799–808.

70. Cunningham K, Sopper MM, Strong MJ. Enhanced ex vivo cosedimentation of high molecular weight neurofilament protein (NFH) with microtubules following in vivo aluminium chloride exposure. Inhibition of dephosphorylation-dependant dissociation. *NeuroToxicology* 1997; **18**: 355–362.

71. Spencer PS, Nunn PB, Hugon J et al. Guam amyotrophic lateral sclerosis–parkinsonism–dementia linked to a plant excitant neurotoxin. *Science* 1987; **237**: 517–522.

72. Whiting MG. Toxicity of cycads. *Econ Bot* 1963; **17**: 271–302.

73. Spencer PS, Ohta M, Palmer VS. Cycad use and motor neuron disease in Kii Peninsula of Japan. *Lancet* 1987; **ii**: 1462–1463.

74. Kisby GE, Ellison M, Spencer PS. Content of the neurotoxins cycasin (methylazoxymethanol-β-D-glucoside) and BMAA (b-N-methylamino-L-alanine) in cycad flour prepared by Guam Chamarros. *Neurology* 1992; **42**: 1336–1340.

75. Duncan MW, Kopin IJ, Crowley JS et al. Quantification of putative neurotoxin 2-amino-3-(methylamino)propanoic acid (BMAA) in cycadales: analysis of the seeds of some members of the family Cycadaceae. *J Anal Toxicol* 1989; **13**: 169–175.

76. Duncan MW, Kopin IJ, Garruto RM et al. 2-amino-3-(methylamino)-propionic acid in cycad-derived foods is an unlikely cause of amyotrophic lateral sclerosis/parkinsonism. *Lancet* 1988; **2**: 631–632.

16

Neurotrophic factors
Michael Sendtner

Developmental motor neuron cell death and neurotrophic factors

During development of higher vertebrates, motor neurons are generated in excess. After they have made functional contacts to skeletal muscle, a significant proportion of these cells degenerate. For example, from about 6,000 motor neurons in the lumbar spinal cord of rat embryos at embryonic day 15, about 50% are lost at post-natal day 3.[1,2] This process, which is called 'physiological motor neuron cell death', serves as a model for understanding the mechanisms underlying the degeneration of motor neurons in various forms of human motor neuron disease.

Experiments by Victor Hamburger[3,4] and others in the first half of the 20th century have shown that the developmental cell death of motor neurons is guided by influences from the target tissue. Removal of a limb bud in developing chick embryos massively enhances the extent of motor neuron cell death during development, and transplantation of an additional limb reduces the number of dying motor neurons. Thus, individual organisms have the capacity to react to deviations from genetically determined developmental programs, and this kind of plasticity might have contributed to the generation of a highly complex nervous system in higher vertebrates during evolution. On the other hand, the higher complexity offers many possibilities for disturbances, such as gene mutations and dysregulation of gene expression, which can be a cause of disease.

Since the discovery of nerve growth factor (NGF) as a prototypic target-derived neurotrophic molecule that regulates survival of paravertebral sympathetic neurons and subpopulations of sensory neurons, a variety of neurotrophic factors have been identified and characterized on a molecular level. In particular, the list of molecules that support motor neuron survival is still growing, and it is to be expected that this list will become even longer during the next few years. In the mean time, more than a dozen different neurotrophic factors with survival promoting activity for motor neurons have been identified (*Table 16.1*). This indicates that the regulation of motor neuron survival is a highly complex process that is influenced by more than one neurotrophic factor. Moreover, many of these molecules are only expressed postnatally, indicating that post-natal survival is also controlled by neurotrophic factors and that these factors serve additional functions for motor neurons (e.g. the regulation of functional properties such as transmitter synthesis, sprouting, synaptic stability, and activity).

Thus, it is not surprising that despite the variety of motor neuron survival factors that

	Receptor on motor neurons
Neurotrophins	
Brain-derived neurotrophic factor (BDNF)	p75^{NTR}, trk-B
Neurotrophin-3 (NT-3)	p75^{NTR}, trk-C
Neurotrophin-4/5 (NT-4/5)	p75^{NTR}, trk-B
Ciliary neurotrophic factor (CNTF) – leukemia inhibitory factor (LIF) family	
CNTF	CNTF receptor-α, LIF receptor-β, gp130
LIF	LIF receptor-β, gp130
Cardiotrophin-1 (CT-1)	LIF receptor-β, gp130 (and possibly another component)
Hepatocyte growth factor (HGF) (scatter factor)	c-met
Insulin-like growth factors (IGFs)	
IGF-I	IGF receptor-1
IGF-II	IGF receptor-1, mannose-6-phosphate receptor
Glial-derived neurotrophic factor (GDNF) and related factors	
GDNF	GDNF receptor-α, c-ret
Neurturin (NTR)	GDNF receptor-α-2, c-ret
Persephin	c-ret (and possibly another component)

Table 16.1
Neurotrophic factors for motor neurons and their receptors.

have been identified so far, those that serve the prototypic function (i.e. the control of survival during the period of physiological motor neuron cell death) have not yet been identified.

The assumption that the developing muscle plays a major role in regulating motor neuron survival during development has been recently challenged by the observation that mice deficient in erbB3, the receptor for glial growth factor (GGF), show a severe deficit of developing Schwann cells, and as a consequence, a significant reduction (79%) in motor neurons.[5] These data indicate that developing Schwann cells are at least as important for the develop-

ing motor neurons as skeletal muscle. However, the data do not rule out the possibility that the motor neurons first become dependent on muscle-derived neurotrophic support and then on Schwann cell-derived support. Moreover, neuregulin–glial growth factor, which is synthesized and secreted from developing motor neurons,[6,7] also regulates the expression of acetylcholine receptor subunits in developing muscle, and thus has received another name, acetylcholine receptor inducing agent (ARIA). The same receptor, erbB3, which mediates the effects of GGF–ARIA in Schwann cells, is also expressed in skeletal muscle[8–10] and could be responsible for proper development of neuromuscular synapses, which is possibly a prerequisite for the production and secretion of neurotrophic factors from muscle. Therefore, final conclusions on the relative importance of muscle-derived and Schwann cell-derived neurotrophic support for developing motor neurons cannot be drawn at the moment. Rather, we have to assume that neurotrophic support from various sources is necessary for proper function of motor neurons and that disturbances in such processes could represent pathomechanisms that underlie or propagate dysfunction and cell death in human motor neuron disease.

Pathomechanisms of human motor neuron disease and neurotrophic factors

A variety of gene defects, in particular the mutations in the superoxide dismutase (SOD1) gene, have been identified and characterized as underlying the inherited forms of amyotrophic lateral sclerosis (ALS) (see Chapter 12) and other forms of motor neuron disease in the adult. However, in contrast to spinal muscular atrophy in children and young adults, most forms of ALS are sporadic. This does not necessarily mean that they are not genetically determined. It is possible that at least a proportion of these disorders have a multigenetic origin, which means that the disease becomes apparent only when several gene defects come together. Such cases will not follow Mendelian rules of inheritance, and thus they could appear as sporadic cases. Moreover, such genetic predispositions together with epigenetic influences (e.g. toxins) could be responsible for ALS. Alterations in the genes for neurotrophic factors could be candidates for such genetic predispositions for the following reasons.

(a) Many neurotrophic factors share their receptors or receptor components with other members of the same gene families. Thus, in the case of genetic defects leading to reduced expression or lack of expression of one factor, other members of the same gene family could compensate for this deficiency, and significant functional deficits would occur only when more than one factor is lacking. Mice lacking both ciliary neurotrophic factor (CNTF) and leukemia inhibitory factor (LIF) (*Fig. 16.1*) provide an example of such conditions.[11]

(b) Most motor neurons express several receptors and are thus responsive to a variety of neurotrophic molecules. The signaling pathways downstream from these receptors show a high degree of overlap. Thus, motor neurons could receive support from other gene families of neurotrophic factors (e.g. glial-derived neurotrophic factor) if there is lack of signaling from other neurotrophic factors (e.g. neurotrophins).

(c) The antiapoptotic signaling by neurotrophic factors interferes with various pathomechanisms that could be responsible for motor neuron disease, in particular the induction of neuronal cell death through glutamate and free radicals.[12–14]

Thus, a lack of neurotrophic factors, even if it does not lead to motor neuron disease on its own, could be a component in its development if it coincides with other pathogenic processes.

A series of observations support this concept. Mutations in the genes for some neurotrophic factors are abundant. In 1995, a mutation close to the splice acceptor site of the second exon of the human *cntf* gene was identified; this mutation leads to a shift of the reading frame and thus to a truncated, biologically inactive CNTF protein.[15] This mutation is very abundant in the Asian and European

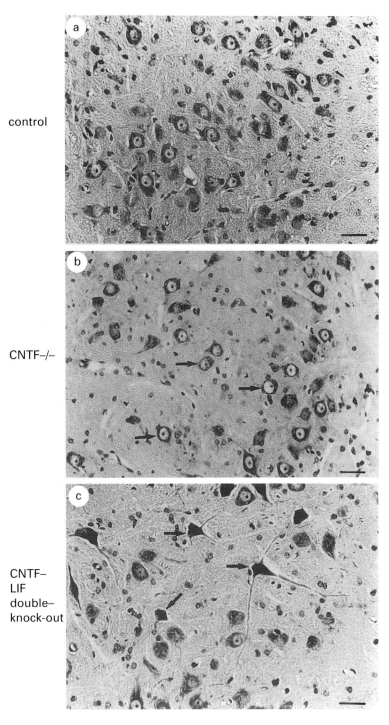

control

CNTF−/−

CNTF–
LIF
double–
knock-out

Figure 16.1
Morphology of facial motor neurons in mouse mutants that lack CNTF or LIF, or both. (a) Morphology of motor neurons in a 6-week-old control mouse. (b) Morphology of motor neurons in a 6-week-old CNTF −/− mouse. The arrows point to atrophic cells. The relative size of the cytoplasm in comparison to the nucleus has significantly decreased. (c) Morphology of motor neurons in a 6-week-old CNTF–LIF double knock-out mouse. A significant number of motor neurons is lost in these mice, and other motor neurons show morphological signs of atrophy and degeneration, in particular the loss of Nissl structure and decentralized nuclei. (Reproduced from Sendtner et al[11] with permission.)

	Healthy subjects (n = 151)	Patients with neurological disorders (n = 240)
Homozygous normal (N–N)	62.9%	—
Heterozygous mutant (N–M)	34.4%	—
Homozygous mutant (M–M)	2.6% (n = 4)	2.1% (n = 4)
Data from Takahashi et al.[15]		

Table 16.2
Ciliary neurotrophic factor genotypes in humans.

	Number of homozygous mutant subjects	Age
Healthy subjects	4/150	20, 30, 35, 50 years
Patients with neurological diseases	5/240	
ALS	2/47	Age of onset: 60, 71 years
Alzheimer's Disease	1/52	Age of onset: 63 years
Guillian Barre-Syndrome	1	Age of onset: 41 years
Peripheral neuropathy of unknown aetiology	1	Age of onset: 15 years
Data from Takahashi et al.[15]		

Table 16.3
Null mutation of the human ciliary neurotrophic factor gene.

population: about one-third of this population is heterozygous for this gene mutation (*Table 16.2*).

The number of CNTF-deficient people who could be identified in several studies is in the range of 1–3%.[15,16] The number of people with a CNTF −/− genotype appears to be similar in a group of healthy controls and in a group of patients with neurological disorders (see *Table 16.2*). Thus, it was concluded that deficiency of CNTF is not responsible for the development of neurological disorders. However, the average age of persons in the healthy control group (*Table 16.3*) was much lower than, for example, in the group of patients with motor neuron disorders. Therefore, large and optimally prospective studies are necessary to answer the question about a potential pathogenic role of this CNTF gene mutation.

Targeted mutation of the CNTF gene has been introduced in mice in order to determine the physiological role of this factor for motor neurons. Homozygous mutant mice show a loss of about 20% of their motor neurons during the first 6 post-natal months, corresponding to a small reduction (10%) in muscle strength at the same age.[17] Of course, the same scenario in humans would not be considered pathologic. It is believed that at least 50% of the motor neurons should be lost before motor neuron disease develops in humans.[18] Therefore, the findings in mice and in humans do not contradict each other.

Not very much is known about other gene defects in sporadic ALS. The author has found that polymorphisms in the gene for LIF exist and that these alterations could lead to loss of biological function of the LIF protein (Giess R and Sendtner M, unpublished observations). Nothing is known so far about mutations in the genes for cardiotrophin-1, glial-derived neurotrophic factor, neurturin, or persephin in ALS patients.

Such gene defects need not necessarily mimic the effects of homozygous gene knockout in mice. For most of these factors, transcription of the mRNA is driven from various promoters, or the primary transcripts are processed in a tissue-specific manner. Thus, there are many possibilities that could lead to dysregulation or lack of function of individual neurotrophic factors in ALS.

CNTF and related molecules

CNTF was originally identified and characterized as a component of chick eye extracts, and it was found to share many biological activities with a protein that was purified from rat sciatic nerves. After cloning and recombinant expression of rat CNTF,[19,20] it became apparent that this protein is a potent survival factor for developing motor neurons. Surprisingly, this factor is not expressed during embryonic development at a time when physiological cell

death of motor neurons occurs. CNTF acts through a tripartite receptor complex that is composed of a low-affinity binding subunit (CNTF receptor-α) and two transmembrane proteins (gp130 and LIF receptor-β).[21] The CNTF receptor-α exists both in a membrane-bound form, which is linked via a glycosylphosphatidylinositol (GPI) anchor to the cell membrane, and in a soluble form, which is apparently shed from synthesizing cells, most probably skeletal muscle. The two transmembrane components, gp130 and LIF receptor-β, show significant homologies, in particular in their intracellular domains.[22] Gp130 has originally been identified as a signal-transducing component of the interleukin (IL)-6 receptor, and LIF receptor-β as a low-affinity receptor component for LIF. Signaling of LIF requires both gp130 and LIF receptor-β, and thus CNTF and LIF share many cellular effects, particularly in motor neurons. These two transmembrane components of the CNTF receptor complex are also involved in receptors for oncostatin-M and cardiotrophin-1, thus allowing additional possibilities for receptor sharing between these different ligands.

CNTF is not expressed during embryonic development, but it is produced in very high quantities in differentiated myelinating Schwann cells. This protein, as well as cardiotrophin-1,[23] lacks a hydrophobic leader sequence and thus it is not released via the classical secretory pathway from producing cells. Very little CNTF is released from myelinating Schwann cells.[24] However, after nerve lesion or other conditions leading to leakage of the Schwann cell membrane, CNTF could be released and act on contacting neurons. In contrast to CNTF, which is constitutively expressed at high levels in myelinating Schwann cells, LIF mRNA levels are very low under physiological conditions, but they rapidly increase after peripheral nerve lesion,[25] so that significant quantities of this factor become available to lesioned motor neurons.

Mice with homozygous targeted disruption of the CNTF gene show a loss of about 20% of motor neurons. Mice lacking endogenous LIF do not exhibit any pathological signs in motor neurons.[11] However, mice that are double-deficient for CNTF and LIF show a more severe loss of motor neurons (more than 30%) (see *Fig. 16.1*), which corresponds to a significant reduction in muscle strength (about 30% in comparison to controls). After peripheral nerve lesion in the adult, lack of CNTF has only a very small effect on motor neuron survival, whereas lack of both CNTF and LIF leads to reduced survival of axotomized motor neurons (66% survival at 2 weeks after lesion).[11] These data indicate that both LIF and CNTF (and probably also other members of this ligand family for gp130 and LIFR-β) act together and at least partially compensate each other in case of deficiency due to gene mutations.

In contrast to mice that lack the individual ligands for this receptor complex, mice with targeted disruption of the genes for LIFR-β[26], receptor-α genes,[27] or gp130[28] show severe defects in the nervous system that are not compatible with life after birth. All these mouse mutants show enhanced cell death during the developmental period of physiological motor neuron cell death, indicating that at least one member of the CNFT–LIF gene family is involved in regulating cell survival during this period. A likely candidate is cardiotrophin-1, which is expressed in skeletal muscle, in contrast to CNTF and LIF, which are made available to motor neurons from Schwann cells.[23] However, cardtiotrophin-1 does not bind to CNTF receptor-α, and thus it cannot be responsible for the phenotype observed in CNTF receptor-α-deficient mice.[27] Therefore, it is assumed that there is an additional CNTF-like factor that is involved in the regulation and maintenance of motor neuron survival during embryonic development.

CNTF has been tested in a variety of mouse mutants for experimental treatment of motor neuron disease. Systemic administration of CNTF to progressive motor neuronopathy mice,[29,30] wobbler mice,[31,32] and motor neuron disease mice[33] shows significant effects on the course of the disease (see *Fig. 16.2*), although the mechanisms by which CNTF interferes with the pathogenic processes underlying these mouse mutants may be different. Chromosomal linkage data have shown that these mouse mutants are different from each other and are not related to mice with targeted disruption of the CNTF gene. Thus, one has to assume that endogenous expression of CNTF is normal in these mouse mutants. At least in the case of the progressive motor neuronopathy mouse, the levels of endogenous CNTF in peripheral nerves are much higher than the levels of CNTF that can be measured in the blood after pharmacological application.[24]

These data again suggest that very little CNTF becomes available under physiological conditions to motor neurons from myelinating Schwann cells. However, when a peripheral nerve is transected in progressive motor neuronopathy mice, significantly improved survival of the lesioned motor neurons can be observed. In contrast, progressive motor neuronopathy mice that lack endogenous CNTF do not show this significant improvement in motor neuron survival after nerve lesion, indicating that endogenous CNTF is indeed a lesion factor and can rescue motor neurons after release from lesioned Schwann cells.

Neurotrophins

The neurotrophins constitute a family of five proteins, which are related to nerve growth factor (NGF). At the moment, this family includes NGF, brain-derived neurotrophic factor (BDNF), neurotrophin (NT)-4/5, NT-3, and NT-6, which so far has been identified in lower vertebrates (fish) but not in mammals. Neurotrophins bind to a common low-affinity receptor (p75[NTR]) and specific high-affinity receptors: trk-A (specific for NGF), trk-B (specific for BDNF and NT-4/5) and trk-C (specific for NT-3).[34,35] The trk receptors are expressed in several splice variants.

Several lines of evidence indicate that the survival effects of neurotrophins are mediated through full-length variants of these receptors, including the cytoplasmic tyrosine kinase domains,[34,36–38] as well as other domains within the cytoplasmic part. The role of the p75 receptor is less clear. It is expressed at high levels during embryonic development, then down-regulated after birth,[39] but its expression can be reinduced after nerve lesion and in particular in ALS.[40,41] Developing motor neurons can bind and retrogradely transport NGF through this receptor but, again, this observation does not correlate with NGF having a function in survival of developing motor neurons. The p75[NTR] receptor is a member of the TNF/Fas receptor family, which can actively induce cell death in a variety of cell types. Indeed, death of developing retinal ganglion cells is actively induced through this receptor when NGF is present in high local quantities.[42,43] In newborn rats, the application of NGF increases the number of degenerating motor neurons after sciatic nerve lesion[44] and after facial nerve lesion.[45] It is very likely that these effects are mediated through the p75[NTR]. Current research focuses on the question of whether the p75[NTR] receptor expressed in motor neurons is a cell death receptor, or whether it is a component of high-affinity receptors for BDNF, NT-3, and NT-4/5. Such experiments will help to decide

whether p75[NTR] expressed at high levels in motor neurons of ALS patients is a cell death receptor that mediates proapoptotic effects of NGF, or whether it increases the sensitivity of these motor neurons to antiapoptotic effects of BDNF, NT-4/5, or NT-3.

Motor neurons express significant levels of full-length trk-B, and at least a subpopulation of motor neurons also expresses trk-C, which is a specific cellular receptor for NT-3.[46,47] The survival effects of BDNF and NT-3 were discovered when these proteins were applied to lesioned motor neurons[45,48] in newborn rats or to the allantoic membrane of developing chick embryos.[49] Although virtually all motor neurons express trk-B, only a subpopulation of about 50–60% of motor neurons can be maintained by BDNF in vivo or in vitro.[45,49] Therefore, additional cellular and extracellular signals might be involved in making the motor neurons responsive to BDNF or NT-3, or both.

NT-3 is the most abundantly expressed neurotrophin in skeletal muscle. Experiments with trk-C and NT-3 knock-out mice have shown that the γ-motor neurons innervating the muscle spindles are dependent on NT-3 for their development.[50,51] However, NT-3 also supports the survival of facial motor neurons,[45] a population that is lacking γ-motor neurons, indicating that subpopulations of α-motor neurons are also responsive to NT-3.

Moreover, NT-3 is expressed in significant quantities in developing motor neurons.[52] Autocrine functions of neurotrophins have been observed in other populations of neurons.[53] Thus, it is possible that NT-3 acts in an autocrine fashion in motor neurons. On the other hand, NT-3 from motor neurons could serve as a tropic molecule for proprioceptive neurons that invade the spinal cord through the dorsal horn and make contacts with the ventral motor neurons.[54] Moreover, NT-3 is a potent survival factor for upper motor neurons[55] and thus it could attract and guide their axons, at least in a subpopulation of corticospinal neurons that make direct contact with spinal motor neurons.

In contrast to NT-3, which is the most abundant neurotrophin in skeletal muscle, NT-4/5 expression in skeletal muscle is regulated by neuronal activity.[56] Denervation of muscle by nerve transection leads to a rapid decrease in NT-4/5 expression, and forced activity by electrical stimulation of motor nerves significantly up-regulates NT-4/5 expression.[47,56] Thus, neuronal activity at the neuromuscular end-plate has a significant influence on the expression of NT-4/5 and this neurotrophin could be involved in regulating efficacy at the neuromuscular synapse, as has been shown in co-cultures of Xenopus motor neurons and skeletal muscle after the addition of neurotrophins in vitro.[57]

Glial-derived neurotrophic factor and related molecules (neurturin and persephin)

The gene for glial-derived neurotrophic factor (GDNF) was cloned in 1993.[58] This molecule is a potent survival factor for midbrain dopaminergic neurons and rat motor neurons, both in cell culture and after peripheral nerve lesion in new-born rodents.[59] High levels of GDNF mRNA were found in skeletal muscle, E15 (embryonic day 15) hind limb, and Schwann cell cultures. Many populations of peripheral neurons, such as sympathetic or dorsal root sensory neurons, did not respond to GDNF. Therefore, this factor was considered an excellent candidate for specifically slowing down loss of function and degeneration of motor neurons in ALS.[59] Later work suggested that the specificity of GDNF for

motor neurons is only relative. Peripheral sympathetic neurons derived from new-born rat superior cervical ganglia also responded to GDNF when GDNF was added at higher concentrations.[60] This study also demonstrated that GDNF expression in Schwann cells is much higher than in skeletal muscle, and that GDNF mRNA expression is also increased after nerve lesion. Therefore, a function of GDNF as endogenous lesion factor for axotomized motor neurons was proposed, this function resembling very much the putative functions of endogenous LIF and CNTF.

GDNF acts through a receptor complex involving a low-affinity binding component (GDNF receptor-α),[61,62] which is bound to the membrane via a GPI anchor in a very similar manner to CNTF receptor-α. The cellular effects of GDNF and related molecules are mediated though the second receptor component, the transmembrane c-ret tyrosine kinase.[61–63]

Mice that lack endogenous GDNF show a small (20%) reduction in the number of spinal lumbar motor neurons.[64] The numbers of other populations of motor neurons, such as the facial motor neurons, are not reduced. Similar observations were made with mice that lack the c-ret tyrosine kinase receptor. This argues against a compensatory role of other members of the GDNF gene family, which so far includes two additional members: neurturin[65] and persephin.[66] Neurturin and persephin bind to low-affinity receptors that are related to GDNF receptor-α. Neurturin can also bind to GDNF receptor-α, although GDNF seems to be the preferred ligand for this receptor subunit. Three members of this receptor family are known so far (GFR-α-1, GFR-α-2, and GFR-α-3). GFR-α-1 and GFR-α-2 probably represent the specific binding subunits for GDNF and neurturin. Among these three ligands, persephin is the only one that is a specific survival factor for motor neurons and that does not support sensory or sympathetic neurons, even at very high concentrations. Thus, there may be a specific receptor subunit that is expressed only on lower motor neurons and not on dorsal root sensory neurons or paravertebral sympathetic neurons.[66] However, this specific binding component of the persephin receptor is not yet known. GFR-α-3 appears as an orphan receptor component in search of its ligand.[67]

These and other data indicate that there are probably more, as yet unidentified, ligands of the GDNF family, which could be of high importance for the physiological maintenance of motor neurons. Therefore, it is possible that the different members of the GDNF gene family compensate each other.

However, knock-out of the common transmembrane receptor component c-ret does not show enhanced motor neuron cell death in comparison to mice that lack GDNF. Recently, it was reported that the expression of the c-ret receptor is significantly decreased in motor neurons of post mortem spinal cord of ALS patients.[68] On the other hand, the number of motor neurons in which ret-immunoreactivity was detectable remained unchanged. Thus, pharmacological administration of GDNF or other members of this gene family of ligands has been suggested as a potential treatment for ALS.

Hepatocyte growth factor (scatter factor)

Hepatocyte growth factor (HGF) and its specific receptor, the c-met-receptor tyrosine kinase, together regulate the growth, motility, and morphogenesis of many cell types and organs. Originally, HGF was identified as a mitogen for developing hepatocytes. Its effect on the motility of cultured cells led to its independent discovery under the name 'scatter factor'. In addition, HGF was shown to promote survival of serum-deprived PC12 rat pheochromocytoma cells[69] and thus was brought into context with neuronal survival factors.

The effect of HGF on motor neurons first became apparent when researchers investigated its role in axon outgrowth.[70] It was found that HGF could attract motor axons and function as a chemoattractant from limb mesenchyme for the developing and growing motor axons. Mice in which the receptor for HGF was inactivated showed a severe defect in the migration of muscle precursor cells into the developing limb.[71] As a consequence, skeletal muscle did not form in the limb or the diaphragm. Thus, the HGF produced in limb mesenchyme could serve as a chemoattractant both for migrating muscle precursor cells and growing motor axons.

At later stages, when the myoblasts have migrated into the developing limbs and formed skeletal muscle, expression of HGF can be identified directly in skeletal muscle. Moreover, isolated motor neurons from 15-day-old rat embryos showed enhanced survival in the presence of HGF, which was in the same range as with other neurotrophic factors such as CNTF, BDNF, and GDNF.[71] These results were confirmed by other groups.[72,73]

Rat motor neurons express the c-met receptor at embryonic day 14, when the period of physiological motor neuron cell death begins.[72] The effect of HGF on motor neuron survival was shown to be synergistic with CNTF, and co-treatment with CNTF and HGF could protect cultured motor neurons from at least some of the toxic effects of vincristine. However, HGF acts only on a subpopulation (40%) of isolated motor neurons[73] that corresponds to a restricted expression of c-met in subgroups of motor neurons, in particular those motor neurons that innervate the upper and lower limbs. Around birth, c-met expression is markedly reduced in motor neurons, indicating that motor neurons respond to HGF only during this developmental period. Nevertheless, it would be interesting to know whether c-met expression and responsiveness to HGF can be reinduced in motor neurons under the pathophysiological conditions in ALS.

Insulin-like growth factors

Insulin-like growth factor (IGF)-I and IGF-II are members of a family that also includes insulin and relaxins.[74] In contrast to most other neurotrophic factors, IGFs are found in significant quantities in the circulation and have been shown to act as hormones. For example, IGF-I has been shown to be the effector of growth hormone actions in various tissues. Indeed, most cells express receptors for IGF-I and IGF-II, and the actions of these factors are not specific to motor neurons. The IGF-I receptor, which mediates the cellular effects of IGF-I and IGF-II, is highly expressed in developing brain but is down-regulated after birth. In contrast, most motor neurons maintain relatively high levels of IGF-I-receptor expression throughout life. The specific functions of IGF-I and IGF-II for motor neurons are not clear so far. The actions of IGFs are modulated by several binding proteins, and at least one of these binding proteins (IGF binding protein-5) is highly expressed in Schwann cells[75] and skeletal muscle. It is very likely that the actions of glial- and muscle-derived IGFs on motor neurons are modulated by such IGF-binding proteins. These findings have consequences for the potential therapeutic use of IGFs in patients with ALS, since such binding proteins influence the pharmacokinetics and availability of systematically injected IGFs.

Mice that lack IGF-I, IGF-II, or IGF receptor expression[76–78] have not been very helpful in defining the specific role of these molecules for developing motor neurons. These mice showed retarded growth and defects in many organs, so that a putative reduction in motor neuron survival could have many reasons, such as dysgenesis of Schwann cells and skeletal muscle. On the other hand, IGFs are potent survival factors for cultured motor neurons,[80] and injection of IGF into skeletal muscle or lesioned nerve stump shows distinct effects on motor neurons, in particular terminal sprouting at the motor end-plates and enhanced survival of motor neuron cell bodies.[79–82]

Therapeutic potential of neurotrophic factors for the treatment of ALS

A series of studies has been performed during recent years in order to assess the therapeutic potential of neurotrophic factors in ALS patients (see *Table 16.4*). In general, the results of these clinical trials have not been encouraging. The effects on disease progression were generally low or not significant, and side effects became apparent, particularly in the case of CNTF. These observations are not very surprising. Neurotrophic factors are normally produced in cells that are in direct contact with motor neurons and they reach the motor neurons within a microenvironment determined by the contact sites of the producing cell and the motor neuron. In this sense, the situation differs completely from that of other recombinant proteins that are successfully introduced as therapeutic agents, such as erythropoietin, a hormone that is secreted into the circulation and then enhances the generation of erythrocytes, or interferons, which are

Factor	Status	Number of patients	Dose	Duration	Application	Result	Reference
CNTF	Phase I	57	0.5–30 µg/kg every other day	2 weeks	Subcutaneous	Fever, weight loss	94
CNTF	Phase I	22	2–200 µg/kg daily	4 weeks	Subcutaneous	Herpes infection, stomatitis, skin reactions, fever, weight loss	95, 96
CNTF	Phase II/III	730	15, 30 µg/kg every other day	9 months	Subcutaneous	Side effects, no statistically significant effect	97
CNTF	Phase II	570	0, 5, 2, 5 µg/kg daily	6 months	Subcutaneously	Side effects, no effect on disease	98, 99
CNTF	Phase I	6	ca 0.5 µg/day	<3 months	Encapsulated cells, intrathecal	Well tolerated	90
CNTF	Phase I	4	8–192 µg/day	2 weeks	Intrathecal	Leg cramping, CSF pleocytosis, rise in CSF protein	100
BDNF	Phase I/II	283	10–300 µg/kg daily	6 months	Subcutaneous	Well tolerated	101
BDNF	Phase III	1150	25–100 µg daily	9 months	Subcutaneous	Well tolerated, no significant effect	
BDNF	Phase I	ca25	No data available		Intrathecal	No data available	
IGF-I	Phase III	266	50, 100 µg/kg daily	9 months	Subcutaneous	Well tolerated, ALS scores significantly different, no major effects	102
GDNF	Phase I	No data available			Intraventricular	No data available	

Table 16.4
Clinical trials with neurotrophic factors in patients with amyotrophic lateral sclerosis.

BDNF, brain-derived neurotrophic factor; CNTF, ciliary neurotrophic factor; GDNF, glial-derived neurotrophic factor; IGF, insulin-like growth factor.

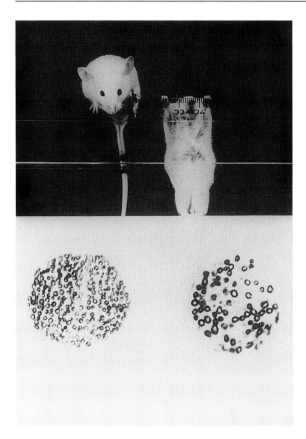

Figure 16.2
The effect of CNTF treatment in pmn mice. Two homozygous pmn mice were treated either with CNTF-secreting D3 cells (left) or untransfected control cells (right). The cells were injected intraperitoneally after the first symptoms could be detected in these mice at post-natal day 20. The mice shown are 36 days old. The CNTF-treated mice survived longer and showed improved motor performance.

Morphology of the phrenic nerve of a CNTF-treated pmn mouse and an untreated pmn mouse. In the CNTF-treated pmn mouse, more myelinated axons could be detected in the phrenic nerve, suggesting that the CNTF treatment not only maintained motor neuron cell bodies but also led to axonal preservation and regeneration. Reproduced with permission from Sendtner et al.[29]

produced in a variety of tissues, released into the blood and other body fluids, and thus influence cells of the immune system. Nevertheless, the positive effects of neurotrophic factors in mouse mutants serving as animal models for human motor neuron disease (*Fig. 16.2*) demonstrate that these molecules can interfere with apoptotic mechanisms that underlie the degeneration of motor neurons in human ALS.[83] Therefore, improved techniques for administration of these neurotrophic factors at sites where they can be taken up and retrogradely transported in motor neurons should be helpful in providing adequate conditions under which they could interfere with pathogenic processes in ALS.

At the moment, there are no clinically established means of administrating neuronotrophic factors in a way that resembles the physiological availability from Schwann cells or muscle cells. Viral gene transfer in Schwann cells and skeletal muscle[84,85] has shown promising results in progressive motor neuronopathy mice and in new-born rats after peripheral nerve lesion. In particular, survival in the presence of BDNF could be prolonged in comparison to experimental set-ups in which the factor is given systemically or repeatedly at high concentrations.[86–88]

Intrathecal administration, which is an established method of administering baclofen to spinal neurons, appears to be a promising technique to make these factors continuously available to ventral roots, where they can be taken up and retrogradely transported the short distance to the cell bodies of motor neurons[89] and produce cellular effects (*Fig. 16.3*). Alternatively, the implantation of encapsulated cells continuously releasing such neurotrophic factors in low, but physiologically relevant, concentrations[90] also appears straightforward for therapeutic administration of neurotrophic molecules.

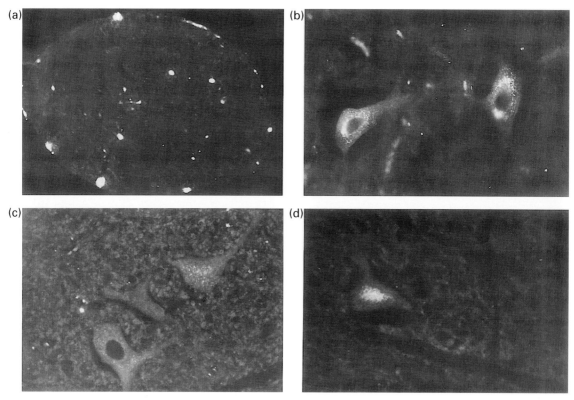

Figure 16.3

Distribution and effect of intrathecally administered BDNF in adult sheep. After chronic intrathecal infusion of BDNF, BDNF is (a) taken up in axons within the ventral root and (b) retrogradely transported to the motor neuron cell bodies, where it can be detected in vesicle-like structures around the nucleus. C-fos immunoreactivity in spinal motor neurons of (c) a control saline-treated sheep and (d) a sheep that was treated with BDNF for 7 weeks. Chronic infusion of BDNF led to an increase of c-fos immunoreactivity and a translocation to cellular compartments in or close to the nucleus. Reproduced with permission from Nature: Dittrich et al,[89] 358: 502–504 (1992) © 1992 Macmillan Magazines Ltd.

Not very much is known about how the availability and kinetics of pharmacologically administered neurotrophic factors is modified in vivo. In the case of IGF-I and IGF-II, there are several binding proteins that influence the biological functions of these molecules in vivo. Moreover, these factors differ from other neurotrophic factors by their capability to cross the blood–brain barrier.[91] Endogenous IGF-I is present in relatively high quantities in blood, but apparently this endogenous resource of IGF-I does not become available to the degenerating motor neurons in ALS patients. Similarly, BDNF is found at high concentrations in human platelets, and again, one has to assume that the degenerating motor neurons do not have access to BDNF from this circulating source. The physiological function of BDNF in platelets is not clear. Therefore, systemic BDNF administration could interfere with such unknown functions and cause side effects. Side effects are also expected when specific receptors for neurotrophic factors are expressed in many organs. For example, liver cells express the receptors for HGF and LIF, and therefore side effects are very likely if members of the CNTF family[92] or HGF are administered systemically. In addition, receptors for neurotrophins (p75^{NTR}, trk-C, and trk-B) are widely expressed in the peripheral nervous system, and specific side effects are to be expected even when these molecules are administered more locally, for example into the subarachnoidal space.

Experiments with isolated motor neurons in cell culture as well as data from in vivo experiments have shown that neurotrophic factors co-operate in supporting motor neuron survival. Some combinations even appear supraadditive. The combination of CNTF and IGF-I, for example, enhances survival of embryonic chick motor neurons in culture at a rate that is higher than the addition of the survival effects of each factor alone.[79,93] Such potentiating effects by combinations of neurotrophic molecules have been observed in many studies. It is to be expected that the technique of gene targeting in mice will lead to a better understanding of the individual function of each neurotrophic factor both on motor neuron survival and on distinct functional parameters, such as axon regeneration, dendrite growth, motor end-plate function, and synaptic activity. A better understanding of these functions together with a more detailed knowledge of the pathogenic processes underlying human ALS will help to redefine the therapeutic potential of these factors for treatment of this form of human motor neuron disease.

References

1. Oppenheim RW. The absence of significant postnatal motoneuron death in the brachial and lumbar spinal cord of the rat. *J Comp Neurol* 1986; **246**: 281–286.
2. Oppenheim RW. Naturally occurring cell death during neural development. *Trends Neurosci* 1985; **8**: 487–493.
3. Hamburger V. The effects of wing bud extirpation on the development of the central nervous system in chick embryos. *J Exp Zool* 1934; **68**: 449–494.
4. Hamburger V. Regression versus peripheral control of differentiation in motor hyperplasia. *Am J Anat* 1958; **102**: 365–410.
5. Rietmacher D, Sonnenberg-Rietmacher E, Brinkmann V et al. Severe neuropathies in mice with targeted mutations in the ErbB3 receptor. *Nature* 1997; **389**: 725–730.
6. Falls DL, Rosen KM, Corfas G et al. ARIA, a protein that stimulates acetylcholine receptor synthesis, is a member of the neu ligand family. *Cell* 1993; **72**: 801–815.
7. Marchionni MA, Goodearl ADJ, Chen MS et al. Glial growth factors are alternatively spliced erbB2 ligands expressed in the nervous system. *Nature* 1993; **263**: 312–318.
8. Altiok N, Bessereau JL, Changeux JP. ErbB3 and ErbB2/neu mediate the effect of heregulin on acetylcholine receptor gene expression in muscle: differential expression at the endplate. *EMBO J* 1995; **15**: 4258–4266.
9. Jo SA, Zhu X, Marchionni MA, Burden SJ. Neuregulins are concentrated at nerve–muscle synapses and activate ACh-receptor gene expression. *Nature* 1995; **373**: 158–161.
10. Tansey MG, Chu GC, Merlie JP. ARIA/HRG regulates AChR epsilon subunit gene expression at the neuromuscular synapse via activation of phosphatidylinositol 3-kinase and Ras/MAPK pathway. *J Cell Biol* 1996; **134**: 465–476.
11. Sendtner M, Götz R, Holtmann B et al. Cryptic physiological trophic support of motoneurons by LIF disclosed by double gene targeting of CNTF and LIF. *Curr Biol* 1996; **6**: 686–694.
12. Skaper SD, Negro A, Dal Toso R, Facci L. Recombinant human ciliary neurotrophic factor alters the threshold of hippocampal pyra-

midal neuron sensitivity to excitotoxin damage: synergistic effects of monosialogangliosides. *J Neurosci Res* 1992; **33**: 330–337.

13. Scala S. Wosikowski K, Giannakakou P et al. Brain-derived neurotrophic factor protects neuroblastoma cells from vinblastine toxicity. *Cancer Res* 1996; **56**: 3737–3742.

14. Benigni F, Villa P, Demitri MT et al. Ciliary neurotrophic factor inhibits brain and peripheral tumor necrosis factor production and, when coadministered with its soluble receptor, protects mice from lipopolysaccharide toxicity. *Mol Med* 1995; **1**: 568–575.

15. Takahashi R, Yokoji H, Misawa H et al. A null mutation in the human CNTF gene is not causally related to neurological diseases. *Nature Genet* 1994; **7**: 79–84

16. Giess R, Götz R, Schrank B et al. Potential implications of a ciliary neurotrophic factor gene mutation in a German population of patients with motor neuron disease. *Muscle Nerve* 1998; **21**: 236–238.

17. Masu Y, Wolf E, Holtmann B et al. Disruption of the CNTF gene results in motor neuron degeneration. *Nature* 1993; **365**: 27–32.

18. Munsat TL, Andres PL, Finison L et al. The natural-history of motoneuron loss in amyotrophic lateral sclerosis. *Neurology* 1988; **38**: 409–413.

19. Stöckli KA, Lottspeich F, Sendtner M et al. Molecular cloning, expression and regional distribution of rat ciliary neurotrophic factor. *Nature* 1989; **342**: 920–923.

20. Lin LFH, Mismer D, Lile JD et al. Purification, cloning, and expression of ciliary neurotrophic factor (CNTF). *Science* 1989; **246**: 1023–1025.

21. Stahl N, Yancopoulos GD. The tripartite CNTF receptor complex: activation and signalling involves components shared with other cytokines. *J Neurobiol* 1994; **25**: 1454–1466.

22. Gearing DP, Thut CJ, Vard de Bos T et al. Leukemia inhibitory factor receptor is structurally related to the IL-6 signal transducer, gp130. *EMBO J* 1991; **10**: 2839–2848.

23. Pennica D, Arce V, Swanson TA et al. Cardiotrophin-1, a cytokine present in embryonic muscle, supports long-term survival of spinal motoneurons. *Neuron* 1996; **17**: 63–74.

24. Sendtner M, Götz R, Holtmann B, Thoenen H. Endogenous ciliary neurotrophic factor is a lesion factor for axotomized motoneurons in adult mice. *J Neurosci* 1997; **17**: 6999–7006.

25. Banner LR, Patterson PH. Major changes in the expression of the mRNAs for cholinergic differentiation factor/leukemia inhibitory factor and its receptor after injury to adult peripheral nerves and ganglia. *Proc Natl Acad Sci USA* 1994; **91**: 7109–7113.

26. Li M, Sendtner M, Smith A. Essential function of LIF receptor in motor neurons. *Nature* 1995; **378**: 724–727.

27. De Chiara TM, Vejsada R, Poueymirou WT et al. Mice lacking the CNTF receptor, unlike mice lacking CNTF, exhibit profound motor neuron deficits at birth. *Cell* 1995; **83**: 313–322.

28. Yoshida K, Taga T, Saito M et al. Targeted disruption of gp130, a common signal transducer for the interleukin 6 family of cytokines, leads to myocardial and hematological disorders. *Proc Natl Acad Sci USA* 1996; **93**: 407–411.

29. Sendtner M, Schmalbruch H, Stöckli KA et al. Ciliary neurotrophic factor prevents degeneration of motor neurons in mouse mutant progression motor neuronopathy. *Nature* 1992; **358**: 502–504.

30. Sagot Y, Tan SA, Baetge E et al. Polymer encapsulated cell lines genetically engineered to release ciliary neurotrophic factor can slow down progressive motor neuronopathy in the mouse. *Eur J Neurosci* 1995; **7**: 1313–1322.

31. Mitsumoto H, Ikeda K, Holmlund T et al. The effects of ciliary neurotrophic factor on motor dysfunction in wobbler mouse motor neuron disease. *Ann Neurol* 1994; **36**: 142–148.

32. Mitsumoto H, Ikeda K, Klinkosz B et al. Arrest of motor neuron disease in wobbler mice cotreated with CNTF and BDNF. *Science* 1994; **265**: 1107–1110.

33. Helgren ME, Friedman B, Kennedy M et al. Ciliary neurotrophic factor (CNTF) delays motor impairments in the mnd mouse, a genetic model of motor neuron disease. *Neurosci Abstr* 1992; **267**: 618.

34. Bothwell M. Functional interactions of neurotrophins and neurotrophin receptors. *Annu*

Rev Neurosci 1995; **18**: 223–253.

35. Dechant G, Barde YA. Signalling through the neurotrophin receptor p75NTR. *Current Opin Neurobiol* 1997; **7**: 413–418.

36. Glass DJ, Yancopoulos GD. The neurotrophins and their receptors. *Trends Cell Biol* 1993; **3**: 262–268.

37. Kaplan DR, Stephens RM. Neurotrophin signal transduction by the Trk receptor. *J Neurobiol* 1994; **25**: 1404–1417.

38. Stephens RM, Loeb DM, Copeland TD et al. Trk receptors use redundant signal transduction pathways involving SHC and PLC-gamma 1 to mediate NGF responses. *Neuron* 1996; **3**: 691–705.

39. Ernfors P, Henschen A, Olson L, Persson H. Expression of nerve growth factor receptor mRNA is developmentally regulated and increased after axotomy in rat spinal cord motoneurons. *Neuron* 1989; **2**: 1605–1613.

40. Kerkhoff H, Jennekens FGI, Troost D, Veldman H. Nerve growth factor receptor immunostaining in the spinal cord and peripheral nerves in amyotrophic lateral sclerosis. *Acta Neuropathol (Berl)* 1991; **81**: 649—656.

41. Seeburger JL, Tarras S, Natter H, Springer JE. Spinal cord motoneurons express p75[NGFR] and p145[trkB] mRNA in amyotrophic lateral sclerosis. *Brain Res* 1993; **621**: 111–115.

42. Frade JM, Rodriguez Tebar A, Barde YA. Induction of cell death by endogenous nerve growth factor through its p75 receptor. *Nature* 1996; **383**: 166–168.

43. Frade JM, Barde YA. Microglia-derived nerve growth factor causes cell death in the developing retina. *Neuron* 1998; **20**: 35–42.

44. Miyata Y, Kashihara Y, Homma S, Kuno M. Effects of nerve growth factor on the survival and synaptic function of Ia sensory neurons axotomized in neonatal rats. *J Neurosci* 1986; **6**: 2012–2018.

45. Sendtner M, Holtmann B, Kolbeck R et al. Brain-derived neurotrophic factor prevents the death of motoneurons in newborn rats after nerve section. *Nature* 1992; **360**: 757–758.

46. Henderson CE, Camu W, Mettling C et al. Neurotrophins promote motor neuron survival and are present in embryonic limb bud. *Nature* 1993; **363**: 266–270.

47. Griesbeck O, Parsadanian AS, Sendtner M, Thoenen H. Expression of neurotrophins in skeletal muscle: quantitative comparison and significance for motoneuron survival and maintenance of function. *J Neurosci Res* 1995; **42**: 21–33.

48. Yan Q, Elliott J, Snider WD. Brain-derived neurotrophic factor rescues spinal motor neurons from axotomy-induced cell death. *Nature* 1992; **360**: 753–755.

49. Oppenheim RW, Qin-Wei Y, Prevette D, Yan Q. Brain-derived neurotrophic factor rescues developing avian motoneurons from cell death. *Nature* 1992; **360**: 755–757.

50. Kucera J, Ernfors P, Jaenisch R. Reduction in the number of spinal motor neurons in neurotrophin-3-deficient mice. *Neuroscience* 1995; **69**: 312–330.

51. Ernfors P, Kucera J, Lee KF et al. Studies on the physiological role of brain-derived neurotrophic factor and neurotrophin-3 in knock-out mice. *Int J Dev Biol* 1995; **39**: 799–807.

52. Ernfors P, Persson H. Developmentally regulated expression of NDNF/NT-3 mRNA in rat spinal cord motoneurons and expression of BDNF mRNA in embryonic dorsal root ganglion. *Eur J Neurosci* 1991; **3**: 953–961.

53. Acheson A, Conover JC, Fandl JP et al. A BDNF autocrine loop in adult sensory neurons prevents cell death. *Nature* 1995; **374**: 450–453.

54. Snider WD. Functions of the neurotrophins during nervous system development: what the knockouts are teaching us. *Cell* 1994; **77**: 627–638.

55. Hallböök F, Ibanez CF, Ebendahl T, Persson H. Cellular localization of brain-derived neurotrophic factor and neurotrophin-3 mRNA in the early chicken embryo. *Eur J Neurosci* 1993; **5**: 1–14.

56. Funakoshi H, Belluasdo N, Arenas E et al. Muscle-derived neurotrophin-4 as an activity-dependent trophic signal for adult motor neurons. *Science* 1995; **268**: 1495–1499.

57. Lohof AM, Ip NY, Poo M. Potentiation of developing neuromuscular synapses by the neurotrophins NT-3 and BDNF. *Nature* 1993; **363**: 350–353.

58. Lin LFH, Doherty DH, Lile JD et al. GDNF: A glial cell line-derived neurotrophic factor for midbrain dopaminergic neurons. *Science*

1993; **260**: 1130–1132.

59. Henderson CE, Phillips HS, Pollock RA et al. GDNF: a potent survival factor for motoneurons present in peripheral nerve and muscle. *Science* 1994; **266**: 1062–1064.

60. Trupp M, Ryden M, Jornvall H et al. Peripheral expression and biological activities of GDNF, a new neurotrophic factor for avian and mammalian peripheral neurons. *J Cell Biol* 1995; **130**: 137–148.

61. Treanor JJ, Goodman L, de Sauvage F et al. Characterization of a multicomponent receptor for GDNF. *Nature* 1996; **328**: 80–83.

62. Jing S, Wen D, Yu Y et al. GDNF-induced activation of the ret protein tyrosine kinase is mediated by GDNFR-alpha, a novel receptor for GDNF. *Cell* 1996; **85**: 1113–1124.

63. Durbec P, Marcos Gutierrez CV, Kilkenny C et al. GDNF signalling through the Ret receptor tyrosine kinase. *Nature* 1996; **381**: 789–793.

64. Moore MW, Klein RD, Farinas I et al. Renal and neuronal abnormalities in mice lacing GDNF. *Nature* 1996; **382**: 76–79.

65. Kotzbauer PT, Lampe PA, Heukeroth RO et al. Neurturin, a relative of glial-cell-line-derived neurotrophic factor. *Nature* 1996; **384**: 467–470.

66. Milbrandt J, de Sauvage FJ, Fahrner TJ et al. Persephin, a novel neurotrophic factor related to GDNF and neurturin. *Neuron* 1998; **20**: 245–253.

67. Baloh RH, Gorodinsky A, Golden JP et al. GFRalpha3 is an orphan member of the GDNF/neurturin/persephin receptor family. *Proc Natl Acad Sci USA* 1998; **95**: 5801–5806.

68. Duberley RM, Johnson IP, Martin JE, Anand P. RET-like immunostaining of spinal motoneurons in amyotrophic lateral sclerosis. *Brain Res* 1998; **789**: 351–354.

69. Matsumoto K, Kagoshima M, Nakamura T. Hepatocyte growth factor as a potent survival factor for rat pheochromocytoma PC12 cells. *Exp Cell Res* 1995; **220**: 71–78.

70. Ebens A, Brose K, Leonardo ED et al. Hepatocyte growth factor/scatter factor is an axonal chemoattractant and a neurotrophic factor for spinal motor neurons. *Neuron* 1996; **17**: 1157–1172.

71. Bladt F, Riethmacher D, Isenmann S et al. Essential role for the c-met receptor in the migration of myogenic precursor cells into the limb bud. *Nature* 1995; **376**: 768–771.

72. Wong V, Glass DJ, Arriga R et al. Hepatocyte growth factor promotes motor neuron survival and synergizes with ciliary neurotrophic factor. *J Biol Chem* 1997; **272**: 5187–5191.

73. Yamamoto Y, Livet J, Polock R et al. Hepatocyte growth factor (HGF/SF) is a muscle-derived survival factor for a subpopulation of embryonic motoneurons. *Development* 1997; **124 (Suppl)**: 2903–2913.

74. LeRoith D, Roberts CT Jr. Insulin-like growth factors. *Ann N Y Acad Sci* 1993; **692**: 1–9.

75. Cheng HL, Randolph A, Yee D et al. Characterization of insulin-like growth factor-I and its receptor and binding proteins in transected nerves and cultured Schwann cells. *J Neurochem* 1996; **66**: 525–536.

76. Liu JP, Baker J, Perkins AS et al. Mice carrying null mutations of the genes encoding insulin-like growth factor I (Igf-1) and type 1 IGF receptor (Igf1r). *Cell* 1993; **75**: 59–72.

77. Beck KD, Powell Braxton L, Widmer HR et al. Igf1 gene disruption results in reduced brain size, CNS hypomyelination, and loss of hippocampal granule and striatal parvalbumin-containing neurons. *Neuron* 1995; **14**: 717–730.

78. De Chiara TM, Robertson EJ, Efstratiadis A. Parental imprinting of the mouse insulin-like growth factor II gene. *Cell* 1991; **64**: 849–859.

79. Hughes RA, Sendtner M, Thoenen H. Members of several gene families influence survival of rat motoneurons in vitro and in vivo. *J Neurosci Res* 1993; **36**: 663–671.

80. Caroni P, Grandes P. Nerve sprouting in innervated skeletal muscle induced by exposure to elevated levels of insulin-like growth factors. *J Cell Biol* 1990; **110**: 1307–1317.

81. Caroni P, Schneider C. Signalling by insulin-like growth factors in paralyzed skeletal muscle: rapid induction of IGF1 expression in muscle fibers and prevention of interstitial cell proliferation by IGF-BP5 and IGF-BP4. *J Neurosci* 1994; **14**: 3378–3388.

82. Caroni P, Schneider C, Kiefer MC, Zapf J. Role of muscle insulin-like growth factors in

nerve sprouting: suppression of terminal sprouting in paralyzed muscle by IGF-binding protein 4. *J Cell Biol* 1994; **125**: 893–902.

83. Troost D, Aten J, Morsink F, de Jong JM. Apopotosis in amyotrophic lateral sclerosis is not restricted to motor neurons. Bcl-2 expression is increased in unaffected post-central gyrus. *Neuropathol Appl Neurobiol* 1995; **21**: 498–504.

84. Haase G, Kennel P, Pettmann B et al. Gene therapy of murine motor neuron disease using adenoviral vectors for neurotrophic factors. *Nature Med* 1997; **3**: 429–436.

85. Gravel C, Götz R, Lorrain A, Sendtner M. Adenoviral gene transfer of ciliary neurotrophic factor and brain-derived neurotrophic factor leads to longterm survival of axotomized motoneurons. *Nature Med* 1997; **3**: 765–770.

86. Eriksson NP, Lindsay RM, Aldskogius H. BDNF and NT-3 rescue sensory but not motoneurones following axotomy in the neonate. *NeuroReport* 1994; **5**: 1445–1448.

87. Vejsada R, Sagot Y, Kato AC. BDNF-mediated rescue of axotomized motor neurones decreases with increasing dose. *NeuroReport* 1994; **5**: 1889–1892.

88. Vejsada R, Sagot Y, Kato AC. Quantitative comparison of the transient rescue effects of neurotrophic factors on axotomized motoneurons in vivo. *Eur J Neurosci* 1995; **7**: 108–115.

89. Dittrich F, Ochs G, Grosse-Wilde A et al. Pharmacokinetics of intrathecally applied BDNF and effects on spinal motoneurons. *Exp Neurol* 1996; **141**: 225–239.

90. Aebischer P, Schluep M, Deglon N et al. Intrathecal delivery of CNTF using encapsulated genetically modified xenogeneic cells in amyotrophic lateral sclerosis patients. *Nature Med* 1996; **2**: 696–699.

91. Reinhardt RR, Bondy CA. Insulin-like growth factors cross the blood-brain barrier. *Endocrinology* 1994; **135**: 1753–1761.

92. Dittrich F, Thoenen H, Sendtner M. Ciliary neurotrophic factor: pharmacokinetics and acute phase response. *Ann Neurol* 1994; **35**: 151–163.

93. Arakawa Y, Sendtner M, Thoenen H. Survival effect of ciliary neurotrophic factor (CNTF) on chick embryonic motoneurons in culture: comparison with other neurotrophic factors and cytokines. *J Neurosci* 1990; **10**: 3507–3515.

94. ALS CNTF Treatment Study (ACTS) Phase I–II Study Group. A phase I study of recombinant human ciliary neurotrophic factor (rhCNTF) in patients with amyotrophic lateral sclerosis. *Clin Neuropharmacol* 1995; **18**: 515–532.

95. Brooks BR, Sanjak M, Mitsumoto H et al. Recombinant human ciliary neurotrophic factor (rhCNTF) in amyotrophic lateral sclerosis (ALS) patients: dose selection strategy in phase I-II safety, tolerability and pharmakokinetic studies. *Can J Neurol Sci* 1993; **20 (suppl 4)**: 83.

96. Miller RG, Bryan WW, Dietz M et al. Safety, tolerability and pharmakokinetics of recombinant human ciliary neurotrophic factor (rhCNTF) in patients with amyotrophic lateral sclerosis. *Ann Neurol* 1993; **34**: 304.

97. The ALS CNTF Study Group. A double-blind placebo-controlled clinical trial of subcutaneous recombinant human ciliary neurotrophic factor (rHCNTF) in amyotrophic lateral sclerosis. ALS CNFT Treatment Study Group. *Neurology* 1996; **46**: 1244–1249.

98. Miller RG, Bryan WW, Dietz MA et al. Toxicity and tolerability of recombinant human ciliary neurotrophic factor in patients with amyotrophic lateral sclerosis. *Neurology* 1996; **47**: 1329–1331.

99. Miller RG, Petajan JH, Bryan WW et al. A placebo-controlled trial of recombinant human ciliary neurotrophic (rhCNTF) factor in amyotrophic lateral sclerosis. *Ann Neurol* 1996; **39**: 256–260.

100. Penn RD, Kroin JS, York MM, Cedarbaum JM. Intrathecal ciliary neurotrophic factor delivery for treatment of amyotrophic lateral sclerosis. *Neurosurgery* 1997; **40**: 94–100.

101. The BDNF Study Group, Bradley WE. A phase I/II study of recombinant brain-derived neurotrophic factor (r-metHuBDNF) in patients with amyotrophic lateral sclerosis (abstract). 120th Annual Meeting of the American Neurological Association, Washington, 1995.

102. Lai EC, Felice BW, Festoff BW et al. A double-blind, placebo-controlled study of recombinant human insulin-like growth factor in the treatment of amyotrophic lateral sclerosis. *Ann Neurol* 1995; 38: 971.

17

Involvement of immune factors in motor neuron cell injury in amyotrophic lateral sclerosis

Stanley H Appel, Maria Alexianu, József I Engelhardt, Lászlós Siklós, R Glenn Smith, Dennis Mosier and Mohamed Habib

Introduction

Our understanding of the mechanisms of motor neuron injury and cell loss in sporadic amyotrophic lateral sclerosis (ASL) is limited. Studies from the authors' own laboratory suggest a prominent role for increased intracellular calcium in motor neuron degeneration.[1-4] Other studies emphasize the importance of excitotoxic[5-7] and free radical[8,9] mechanisms in mediating cell death in ALS. However, none of these explanations is mutually exclusive, and altered calcium homeostasis, free radicals, and glutamate excitotoxicity may all participate in the cell injury cascade that leads to motor neuron death. In fact, alterations in one parameter can lead to alterations in other parameters, and each can enhance and propagate the injury cascade. Increased intracellular calcium can enhance free radical production[10] and glutamate release,[11-14] which in turn can further increase intracellular calcium.[15] Increased free radicals can also increase glutamate, which in turn can increase intracellular calcium or free radicals, or both. Free radicals can enhance lipid peroxidation, leading to increased intracellular calcium.[16]

These changes of increased intracellular calcium, increased production of free radicals, and enhanced glutamate excitotoxicity are likely to represent a (self-)propagating stage in motor neuron injury. The pertinent question is whether any of these factors are the initial event or whether they are only a late consequence of other processes in the pathogenesis of sporadic ALS. In familial ALS, at least in those cases that are due to mutations in the copper-zinc superoxide dismutase (SOD1) gene, free radical damage is possibly an early event.[17,18] However, there is presently no evidence that genetic defects in the homeostasis of free radicals, calcium, or glutamate can explain the majority of cases of sporadic ALS.

The authors' hypothesis was originally based on several clinical facets of sporadic ALS as well as on circumstantial evidence supporting the presence of an immune–inflammatory process, such as the presence of other immune disorders, paraproteinemias, and lymphomas. In addition, inflammatory cells are clearly present in ALS spinal cord[19,20] and provide a possible explanation for the spread of clinical manifestations from a focal onset in one extremity to the involvement of a contralateral extremity, and then in a rostral direction to involve other extremities and bulbar musculature. This clinical progression has no simple explanation, but certainly suggests the involvement of a pool of motor neurons with diffusion across the spinal cord to involve contralateral motor neurons followed by rostral diffusion of factors, such as cytokines released from inflammatory cells, to involve more rostral motor neurons. Evidence for

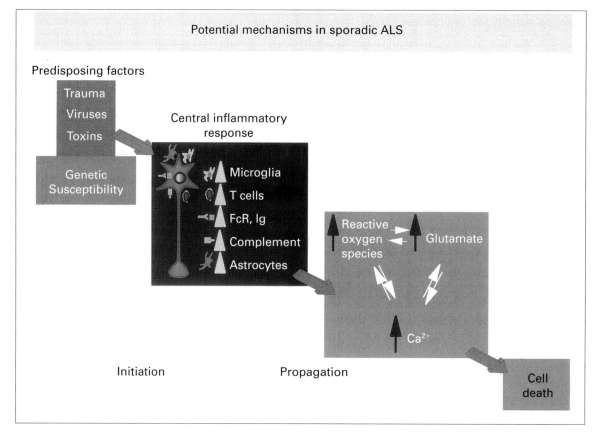

Figure 17.1
Potential mechanisms in sporadic ALS.

increased free radicals and lipid peroxidation is also present in sporadic ALS spinal cord, and products such as 4-hydroxynonenal within the cerebrospinal fluid (CSF) are also potent diffusible toxins.[21,22] Whether the inflammatory reaction represents an attempt to repair altered motor neurons or contributes to motor neuron injury is presently unclear. Nevertheless it is of interest that peripheral trauma, which is cited as a risk factor in ALS,[23] can injure motor axons and, in turn, initiate central microglial[24] and lymphocytic[25]

responses, which could contribute to motor neuron injury through contact or through diffusible cytokines.

In the discussion that follows, evidence is provided for calcium influx and increased intracellular calcium as an early change in ALS, and for immune–inflammatory reactions as a possible triggering or initiating cause. The selective vulnerability of motor neurons is attributed to their relative absence of calcium-binding proteins (especially calbindin D28K and parvalbumin), and their resulting sensitivity is attributed to an increased calcium load resulting from immune–inflammatory processes or enhanced glutamate excitotoxicity or both. The immune–inflammatory reaction in the central nervous system (CNS) is largely characterized by activation and then proliferation of microglia and infiltration of T cells and IgG. It may have three possible roles:

(a) an attempt to repair;
(b) participation in the injury process; and
(c) phagocytosis of injured motor neurons.

Which of these roles are being carried out and the mechanism by which they are mediated are presently undefined in ALS. *Figure 17.1* provides a model of how potential mechanisms could lead to motor neuron injury in sporadic ALS.

CNS inflammation in ALS

Although early studies of ALS tissue did not describe the presence of inflammatory cells in ALS, reports beginning in 1988 suggested that inflammatory cell infiltration may be more common than previously suspected.[26–29] Further studies by Lampson and colleagues[30] demonstrated activated microglia and small numbers of T cells in degenerating white matter of ALS cords. The authors' own studies[31] documented the presence of lymphocytes in the spinal cord in 18 of 27 consecutive ALS autopsies. Lymphocytes were predominantly CD4+ in the vicinity of degenerating cortical spinal tracts. However, more significantly, CD4+ and CD8+ cells were found in ventral horns. Activated microglia were also prominent in the ventral horn of spinal cords from ALS patients. Kawamata and colleagues[32] demonstrated the presence of significant numbers of CD8-reactive T cells and, to a lesser extent, CD4+ cells marginating along capillaries in the parenchyma of spinal cord and

brains of 13 ALS patients. Cells, including lymphocytes and activated microglia expressing major histocompatability complex (MHC) class I and class II, leukocyte common antigen, $Fc_\gamma RI$, and β-2 integrins were present in ALS tissue. Recent studies on peripheral blood lymphocytes of ALS patients have also shown that two rare subsets expressing Fc_γ RIII (CD16) — CD8 with or without CD57 — are significantly increased in the blood of ALS patients with upper motor neuron and bulbar signs.[33]

The diversity of T cells in ALS spinal cord has also been examined employing the reverse transcriptase polymerase chain reaction (PCR) with variable region sequence-specific oligonucleotide primers to amplify Vβ T cell receptor transcripts.[34] A greater expression of $V\beta_2$ transcripts was detected in ALS specimens, independent of the human leukocyte antigen (HLA) genotype of the individual. As additional confirmation, cells were assayed from the CSF of 22 consecutive ALS patients for the presence of $V\beta_2$ transcripts. This specific T cell receptor was demonstrated in the CSF of 17 of 22 ALS patients, whereas only 4 of 19 disease control patients had similar expression. It is of interest that $V\beta_2$ is a T cell receptor that is known to respond to superantigens. Whether superantigen stimulation of lymphocytes with $V\beta_2$ receptors are a primary factor in motor neuron injury or the consequence of motor neuron injury resulting from other causes is not known, but the presence of T lymphocyte restriction does suggest the involvement of immune mechanisms.

Microglia: mediator of immune–inflammatory reactions in the CNS

Microglia comprise about 10% of the brain parenchyma and are distributed throughout the CNS, where they play important roles as mediators of immune inflammatory responses.[35,36] CNS microglia can proliferate and become activated after inflammatory, mechanical, or neurotoxic insults to the peripheral nerve.[37] This suggests that different kinds of tissue damage can trigger anatomically limited microglial responses within the anterior horn of relevant spinal cord levels. Following peripheral axonal injury, changes in microglia appear first, followed by the appearance of components of complement, infiltration of IgG, astroglial proliferation, and T cell recruitment.[38] These reactions then gradually subside. The specific signals from motor neurons that activate microglia after peripheral injury are far from clear, although γ-interferon has been implicated. Activated microglia are fully competent antigen-presenting cells[39] and may play a role in the recognition, uptake, processing, and presentation of foreign antigens in the CNS. These microglia have been described as having both positive and negative effects associated with cell injury (i.e. they may facilitate repair or enhance injury).[38,40] The negative effects involve the production of cytotoxic mediators such as free radicals,[41–44] tumor necrosis factor-α, quinolinic acid, and other factors. The signals that trigger these negative responses have not been well delineated in any of the neurodegenerative diseases, including ALS, although in Alzheimer's disease the β-amyloid in senile plaques has been demonstrated to activate microglia and trigger neuronal injury.[45] Activated microglia have been well delineated as participating in the pathogenesis of demyelination in multiple sclerosis;[46] and the peripheral counterpart, the macrophage, has been documented as contributing to the pathogenesis of demyelination in inflammatory neuropathies.[47,48]

The fact that an immune–inflammatory reaction is present in ALS spinal cord and that it can occur in the setting of distal (peripheral) trauma provides a novel rationale for the immune–inflammatory reaction in ALS. Peripheral trauma is a well known risk factor in ALS[33] and could initiate a central response. However, since trauma is a common occurrence and ALS is relatively uncommon,[49,50] trauma alone might not be sufficient to produce a sustained response without implicating prior genetic or environmental sensitizing factors.

Circumstantial evidence for immune–inflammatory reactions in ALS

Associated autoimmune diseases, paraproteinemias, lymphomas

In the past decade, circumstantial evidence for immune mechanisms has included a higher incidence of immune disorders in patients with ALS, the presence of paraproteinemias and lymphomas, the presence of lymphocytes and activated macrophages in ALS spinal cord, and the presence of IgG within ALS motor neurons. In the authors' recent series of more than 1,200 patients, 21% had thyroid disease, as determined either by history or by laboratory investigations.[46] With respect to paraproteinemias, Shy and colleagues[51] reported that 5.6% of 202 patients with motor neuron disease had paraproteinemia, compared to only 1% of control subjects. Subsequently, paraproteins were demonstrated in 9% of patients by using immunofixation electrophoresis, compared to 3% of patients by using cellulose acetate electrophoresis.[52] Employing more sensitive techniques, Duarte and colleagues[53] demonstrated that 60% of ALS patients had serum monoclonal immunoglobulins, while only 13% of control subjects had such abnormalities. In nine patients, lymphoma was associated with motor neuron disease,[54] and a similar association was present in 25 additional cases from the literature.

Although the presence of lymphoma is most commonly associated with lower motor neuron disease, six of the first 25 published cases of lymphoma and motor neuron disease had both upper and lower motor neuron signs. In none of the cases could direct lymphomatous infiltration of the meninges, nerve roots, or nerves be demonstrated. The presence of paraproteinemias raises the possibility that the paraproteins may directly cause motor neuron injury.[54] However, no passive transfer experiments document that such paraproteins directly lead to motor neuron injury. A more plausible explanation is that paraproteins as well as lymphoma reflect alterations in the immune system, and that these alterations give rise to motor neuron injury by diverse humoral and/or cell-mediated mechanisms.

Cellular immunity

No studies have demonstrated a consistent difference in cellular immunity in ALS. Studies of histocompatability antigen subgroups in ALS have not demonstrated the predominance of any single subtype. In the authors' own laboratory, in more than 1,200 patients studied, no single or predominant HLA subtype was noted.[50] In fact, in recent studies of T cell receptors in the spinal cord and spinal fluid of ALS patients, a number of different MHC class II subtypes were noted.[26] The lack of unique HLA association does not rule out an autoimmune mechanism, since a number of well-defined autoimmune disorder do not have a single or predominant association.

IgG in ALS motor neurons

The demonstration of IgG in ALS motor neurons provides additional circumstantial evidence for immune mechanisms. In 13 of 15 consecutive ALS autopsies, IgG was present in spinal motor neurons in a patchy and coarse granular cytoplasmic localization.[19] In the motor cortices of 11 ALS patients, IgG was demonstrated in pyramidal motor neurons in six patients. Minimal IgG reactivity was found in spinal motor neurons and pyramidal motor neurons in 10 disease control patients. Although limited uptake of IgG can be demonstrated in motor neurons following intraperitoneal injection,[56] the intraperitoneal injection of ALS IgG results in much greater uptake of IgG in motor neurons than the injection of disease control IgG does. In addition, following ALS IgG injection, IgG is found in proximity to microtubules, the endoplasmic reticulum, and the Golgi apparatus, whereas disease control IgG is primarily lysosomal.[57] However, both ALS IgG and disease control IgG can be detected in motor neuron lysosomes. In human spinal cord, IgG can be detected in association with microtubules in ALS specimens but not in disease control specimens.

Despite this localization, the significance of IgG reactivity within motor neurons is unclear, and there is no specific correlation of IgG reactivity in ALS specimens with the rate of progression or stage of the disease, nor is there any indication that the IgG within the motor neuron contributes to cell degeneration. Recent studies from the authors' laboratory using in situ hybridization and immunohistochemistry suggest the possible dependence of ALS IgG uptake on interaction with FcRI at the neuromuscular junction (Habib M, unpublished data). As noted previously, IgG accumulates in spinal cord ventral horn after peripheral trauma to motor axons, and the association of IgG with motor neurons in ALS could be a reflection of motor axon injury. However, IgG could possibly contribute to motor neuron injury.

Clearly, any or all of these immune–inflammatory changes (i.e. microglial activation, the presence of IgG, T cell infiltration) could be functioning to repair rather than injure motor neurons. Thus, cellular infiltrates within ALS spinal cord ventral horns could be secondary to motor neuron destruction rather than its cause. Furthermore, the increased incidence of paraproteinemias and lymphomas could be due to a common factor that may also compromise motor neurons independently.

Animal models of immune-mediated motor neuron disease

Experimental autoimmune motor neuron disease and experimental autoimmune gray matter disease

Two distinct models of immune-mediated motor neuron destruction provide evidence that immune–inflammatory reactions do have the capacity to mediate motor neuron injury in ALS. Experimental autoimmune motor neuron disease (EAMND) is a lower motor neuron syndrome induced in guinea pigs by the inoculation of purified bovine motor neurons in Freund's adjuvant.[58] In EAMND, the affected animals demonstrated gradual onset of hind limb weakness associated with electromyographic and morphologic evidence of denervation, spinal motor neuron injury, and cell death. Experimental autoimmune gray matter disease (EAGMD) is a more acute disorder involving lower and upper motor neurons. It is induced in guinea pigs by the inoculation of spinal cord ventral horn homogenates.[57] EAGMD is clinically characterized by the relatively rapid onset of extremity weakness, with bulbar signs in approximately 25–30% of cases. There is evidence of denervation by both EMG and morphologic criteria. Scattered foci of perivascular inflammation are present within the CNS, as well as injury and loss of spinal cord motor neurons in large pyramidal cells in the motor cortex. Early in the course of both disorders there is an increased resting frequency of spontaneous miniature end-late potentials (MEPP) whereas the muscle membrane resting potential and MEPP amplitude and time course are normal.[59] Such data suggest enhanced release of acetylcholine from motor nerve terminals, possibly owing to increased intracellular calcium.

The animal models of motor neuron destruction, especially EAGMD, resemble human ALS with respect to the loss of upper and lower motor neurons; the presence of inflammatory foci, including activated microglia within the spinal cord; the presence of IgG within upper and lower motor neurons; and the presence of physiologic changes at the neuromuscular junction.[60]

The animal models clearly suggest the potential relevance of immune–inflammatory mechanisms in the pathogenesis of ALS, but in no sense do they suggest that the specific antigens involved in immune–mediated models of motor neuron injury are necessarily involved in human ALS.

Passive transfer experiments

To provide more evidence for the importance of immune mechanisms, the authors developed an immune-mediated passive transfer experimental model in which animals exhibit both systemic weakness and altered morphology in motor neurons.[2] Antimotor neuronal antibodies were produced by immunization of goats with ventral horn homogenates of bovine spinal cord, and these IgG were passively transferred to mice to induce motor neuron dysfunction. Twelve hours after intraperitoneal injection, the mice manifested muscle stiffness but no clinical weakness. Intracellular calcium was increased, and synaptic vesicles were increased in axon terminals at the neuromuscular junction and synaptic boutons residing on spinal motor neurons. The earliest clinical signs in animals injected with anti-motor neuronal IgG suggested cholinergic hyperactivity at the neuromuscular junction (muscle stiffness) and in the autonomic nervous system (increased sweating, slight diarrhea, mucous discharge in the eyes). These signs are the opposite of those found in Lambert–Eaton myasthenic syndrome, which is mediated by calcium channel antibodies and which results in decreased calcium influx.[61,62] By 20–24 hours, injected mice became more sluggish and developed a generalized hypotonia that involved the respiratory muscles and led to death. Administration of the same amount of pre-immune IgG caused no signs. Electron microscopic cytochemistry within 12 hours demonstrated significantly increased density of synaptic vesicles and calcium both in axon terminals of neuromuscular junctions and synaptic boutons on spinal motor neurons. After 24 hours, the number of synaptic vesicles was still larger than normal, but calcium was depleted from axon terminals and synaptic boutons. The motor neuron perikarya demonstrated dilatation of the Golgi system and the rough endoplasmic reticulum with an increased amount of calcium. The NMDA receptor antagonist, MK-801, and the dihydropyridine calcium channel antagonist, diltiazem, prevented the appearance of clinical signs and some of the morphologic alterations.

Mice injected with IgG from ALS patients did not manifest weakness, but they did have similar ultrastructural features, with increased intracellular calcium and altered synaptic vesicles in motor axon terminals and an increased amount of calcium in rough endoplasmic reticulum, mitochondria, and the Golgi complex of motor neuron cell bodies.[1] A total depletion of intracellular calcium was less commonly observed. In parallel experiments, IgG from ALS patients injected intraperitoneally into mice increased the frequency of miniature end plate potentials at the neuromuscular junction, with no effect on MEPP amplitude or the resting membrane potential of the muscle.

Thus, the morphologic and the electrophysiologic data were in accord with increased intracellular calcium, which could alter the resting acetylcholine release from axon terminals. The injection of control guinea pig or goat IgG or human disease control IgG produced no effects on MEPP frequency or acetylcholine release.[63]

In vitro studies with ALS IgG in passive transfer experiments

Effects on L-type channel-mediated calcium current

Since acetylcholine release at the neuromuscular junction is dependent on increasing intracellular calcium, which may enter through voltage-gated calcium channels (VGCC), it was postulated that the increased intracellular calcium might have been triggered by immunoglobulins enhancing the VGCC. Since muscle contains the highest concentrations of VGCC in mammalian cells, we used single mammalian skeletal muscle fibers in vitro to test this hypothesis. The addition of 1–3 mg/ml of ALS IgG resulted in L-type calcium currents as well as charge movement without any effect on sodium-dependent action potentials.[64] F_{AB} fragments from ALS IgG also altered calcium currents, similar to the effects of whole ALS IgG.[65] In artificial phospholipid bilayers, ALS IgG also altered L-type VGCCs. In each preparation there was a decrease in the calcium current produced by ALS IgG, as well as a change in the channel open time.[65]

Effects on neuronal calcium currents

The significance of ALS IgG effects on L-type calcium current was unclear, primarily because there is no evidence of L-type calcium current modulating acetylcholine release at mammalian neuromuscular junctions. In fact, recent studies suggest that P-type calcium currents modulate acetylcholine release at mammalian neuromuscular junctions.[66] By testing ALS IgG on neuronal calcium currents, the authors were able to resolve the potential discrepancy. By employing P-type channels in Purkinje cells and lipid bilayers, enhancement rather than inhibition of calcium current was documented with ALS IgG but not with disease control IgG.[67] In the motor neuron cell line ((ventral spinal cord) VSC4.1) with neuronal calcium currents, ALS but not disease control IgGs enhanced calcium current and mean open time.[68,69] Thus, ALS IgGs were found to enhance calcium currents in several systems that are known to have the same type of neuronal type VGCC in motor nerve terminals and to modulate acetylcholine release.

Increased intracellular calcium in ALS motor terminals

These data suggest that motor nerve terminals can be a site of immune attack and that increased intracellular calcium may be an early event leading to neuronal injury. However, no data were available to determine the similarity of ultrastructural changes induced by passive transfer of ALS IgG and the pathologic alterations in human ALS. To accomplish this goal, the authors employed ultrastructural techniques with oxalate–pyroantimonate fixation to characterize morphometric alterations in intracellular calcium in motor nerve terminals from patients with ALS and with different neurological disorders.[3] Muscle biopsy specimens from seven patients with ALS, 10 non-denervating control subjects, and five patients with denervating neuropathies were analysed. Motor nerve terminals from ALS specimens contained significantly increased calcium, increased mitochondrial volume, and increased numbers of synaptic vesicles compared to any of the disease controls, without exhibiting excess Schwann cell envelopment specific to denervating terminals.

These results parallel the effects produced when ALS IgG is passively transferred to mice, and they provide the first demonstration that neuronal calcium is, in fact, increased in ALS in vivo. A comparison of the ultrastructural changes induced by the passive transfer of sporadic ALS IgG to mice with the changes observed in patients with sporadic ALS are given in *Table 17.1*.

Effects of ALS IgG on a motor neuron cell line

To model the alteration in calcium channel current in vitro, we employed our motor neuron-neuroblastoma hybrid cell line. This VSC4.1 motor neuron cell line was produced by fusion of murine N18TG2 neuroblastoma cells with dissociated embryonic rat ventral spinal cord, employing techniques that had previously yielded a substantia nigra cell line.[69] The VSC4.1 cell line contains specific antagonist binding sites for L-type VGCCs, N-type VGCCs, and P-type VGCCs. In addition, VSC4.1 cells possess neuron-specific enolase, immunoreactive 200 kDa neurofilament pro-

Sporadic ALS IgG in mice	Human sporadic ALS
Increased synaptic vesicle number and pre-terminal density at neuromuscular junctions	Increased synaptic vesicle number and pre-terminal density at neuromuscular junctions
Increased synaptic mitochondrial volume at neuromuscular junctions	Increased synaptic mitochondrial volume at neuromuscular junctions
Swelling and occasional fragmentation of somal Golgi apparatus outer leaflet	Extensive fragmentation of somal Golgi apparatus
Increased calcium ion concentration in synaptic mitochondria at neuromuscular junctions	Increased calcium ion concentration at neuromuscular junctions
Increased calcium ion concentration in axons, somal mitochondria, Golgi apparatus, endoplasmic reticulum	Not tested
Increased calcium ion concentration and vesicle density in terminals contacting lower motor neurons	Not tested

Table 17.1
Comparison of ultrastructural changes in motor neurons and at neuromuscular junctions induced by passive transfer of sporadic ALS IgG to mice with changes observed in patients with sporadic ALS.

tein, synaptophysin, and cAMP-inducible choline acetyl transferase. ALS IgG was found to kill 40–70% of such cells differentiated with cAMP within several days.[70] The cytotoxicity was dependent on calcium entry from the extracellular fluid, and was prevented by antagonists of N-type or P-type VGCCs but not by dihydropyridine inhibitors of L-type VGCCs. Pre-incubating the ALS IgG with either purified intact calcium channels or isolated α-1-subunits (but not the α-2- or β-subunits or unrelated proteins) also removed IgG-mediated cytotoxicity. Following the addition of ALS IgG, the VSC4.1 cells underwent apoptotic cell death, with DNA fragmentation observed within 12 hours and cell blebbing and fragmentation beginning shortly thereafter.[71] Cell death and nuclear changes were prevented by prior incubation of cells with the inhibitor, aurintricarboxylic acid, or with the protein synthesis inhibitor, cyclohex-imide, but not with antagonists of glutamate receptors or nitric oxide scavengers. Additional experiments have documented that the cell death mediated by ALS IgG is triggered by a transitory increase of intracellular calcium within the first several minutes, followed by cell death within 2 days.[72]

Potential mechanisms of enhanced calcium entry

These studies confirm the importance of calcium entry through calcium channels in mediating the cytotoxic effects of ALS IgG, at least in vitro. The key question in these experiments is whether the ALS IgG interacts directly with the calcium channel to mediate the effects or whether the effects on the calcium channel are indirect. At the present time there is no definitive answer to this question. The authors have purified L-type VGCCs from skeletal muscle and employed the complexes in enzyme-linked immunoabsorbant assays (ELISA).[73] With this assay, sera from 75% of ALS patients reacted with the calcium channels. Antibody titers correlated with the rate of ALS disease progression rather than with the stage of disease, and calcium channel antibodies were not present in patients with familial ALS or with spinal muscular atrophy. None of the patients studied had antibodies to gangliosides and none had paraproteinemias. However, the presence of antibodies to L-type specific calcium channels was not completely specific for ALS, since antibodies were also noted in 20% of patients with Guillain–Barré syndrome and in the majority of patients with the Lambert–Eaton myasthenic syndrome (a condition in which antibodies to calcium channels have been previously described).[61,62] The authors have not been able to detect antibodies to N-type channels using radioactive antagonists in immunoprecipitation assays, and other groups have also failed to identify antibodies to N-type channels.[74] Antibodies to P–Q type calcium channels have been found in 23% of sporadic ALS patients using immunoprecipitation assays.[75] But more than 70% of ALS sera and IgG enhance calcium currents in vitro and in vivo. Thus, a clear discrepancy exists between the ability of ALS IgG to interact directly with calcium channels in vitro in ELISA assays and to enhance calcium current and calcium entry into motor neurons in vitro and motor nerve endings in vivo. This difficulty may be related either to technical problems in the calcium channel assays or to the possibility that alterations in calcium homeostasis mediated by

ALS IgG require interactions with non-calcium channel surface membrane constituents, which can still alter calcium currents through calcium channels. Our recent studies of the in vivo reactivity of ALS IgG in mice suggests that interaction with FcRI may serve this function (Habib M, unpublished data).

The failure of immunosuppression in ALS

Immunosuppression with corticosteroids, cyclophosphamides, plasmapheresis, and total lymphoid irradiation have been ineffective in halting the progression of ALS.[76,77] The authors' study with cyclosporine suggested a possible slowing of the course of ALS in a subpopulation of patients with no effect on the overall population.[78] However, a follow-up study failed to demonstrate any effect of immunosuppression with cyclosporine on the rate of progression of ALS in the subgroup of men with recent-onset ALS. The fact that immunosuppressant therapy has not been proven to halt progression remains a major stumbling block for an immune-mediated etiology. However, several explanations for this lack of efficacy may exist. Firstly immunosuppression may be too little and too late. By the time symptoms and signs appear, extensive CNS damage may already have occurred owing to increased calcium and free radicals and it may be difficult to stop the process that the immune–inflammatory reactions initiated. Furthermore, it is not clear that the immunosuppression therapies can adequately access and suppress the CNS-selective inflammatory reactions, especially microglial responses. Immunosuppression has similarly failed to ameliorate type 1 diabetes mellitus or other endocrinopathies without invalidating the important role of immune mechanisms in initiating those disorders. In addition, in the chronic progressive stage of multiple sclerosis, with its marked CNS inflammatory lesions, immunosuppression is of limited value. The levels of immunosuppression employed have also been limited by toxic side effects. It is also possible that what initiates the disease may be different from what propagates the disease (increased calcium, free radicals, and glutamate) or administers the final cellular *coup de grâce* (the presence of T cells and activated microglia releasing cytokines). The death of neurons may no longer require the initial immune-initiated cell injury, but rather may result from alterations in intracellular calcium and free radicals through a number of processes. The destructive effects of oxidative stress and 4-hydroxynonenal may play a role, as may increased glutamate and the presence of reactive microglia releasing destructive cytokines. Thus the failure of immunosuppression does not, per se, invalidate the possible participation of immune–inflammatory mechanisms in the pathogenesis of motor neuron injury and death in ALS.

Selective vulnerability of motor neurons

Our understanding of the factors dictating selective vulnerability of motor neurons is incomplete. It is unlikely to be explained by the interaction of ALS IgG with unique calcium channels in motor neurons, since such channels are present in the plasma membrane of most neurons and antibodies to VGCC should therefore affect most neurons. Purkinje cells, for example, have an abundance of P-type calcium channels and ALS IgG can be documented to enhance currents through P-type calcium channels.[67] However, Purkinje cells are not compromised in ALS. Furthermore, in the authors' passive transfer experiments, increased calcium could not be detected

within Purkinje cells, suggesting that regulation of calcium homeostasis may be more active or more finely adjusted in Purkinje cells than in motor neurons.[1] Thus, a susceptible type of calcium channel, per se, cannot explain the pattern of selective vulnerability, and other factors may also influence the ability of neurons to cope with an increased calcium load.

In addition, despite extensive investigations of SOD1 mutations in familial ALS and excitotoxicity in sporadic ALS, neither mechanism provides a definitive explanation for motor neuron selective vulnerability in ALS. The SOD1 mutations are present in all motor neurons, yet oculomotor neurons are spared in the SOD1 mutant transgenic mouse.[2] In the motor cortex and spinal cord of patients with ALS, Rothstein and colleagues[79] have documented a loss of high-affinity glutamate transporters, with the major transporter most significantly decreased being the GLT-1 (glutamate transporter) glial transporter excitatory amino acid transporter (EAAT2). No quantitative change in mRNA for GLT-1 in ALS motor cortex has been found even with large loss of GLT-1 (EAAT2) protein and decreased tissue glutamate transporters.[80] Further studies have demonstrated changes in RNA splicing of the EAAT2 protein, with both elongated introns and exon elimination.[7] However, there is no evidence that the loss of the glial glutamate transporter is a primary event in ALS, and other injuries have also been reported to down-regulate the glutamate transporter.

Specific glutamate receptors have also been proposed as an explanation for selective vulnerability. However, a recent paper by Morrison and colleagues,[81] demonstrated no changes in the distribution of the GluR2 subunit of the AMPA receptor in motor neurons that are affected in ALS and those that are resistant. Thus there is presently no cogent evidence to support specific glutamate receptor or transporter localization as major determinants of selective vulnerability.

Calcium-binding proteins

Another potential approach to selective vulnerability involves the calcium-binding proteins calbindin D28K and parvalbumin, which clearly influence calcium homeostasis.[82,83] Calcium-binding proteins are normally elevated in Purkinje cells and physiologically absent from adult motor neurons. In fact, the lack of calbindin D28K and parvalbumin immunohistochemical reactivity in motor neurons parallels the known selective vulnerability of motor neurons in ALS. Motor neurons that are affected early in the disease (spinal motor neurons and the twelfth cranial nerve) lack immunoreactivity for these calcium-binding proteins, while motor neurons that control the eye muscles (the third, fourth, and sixth cranial nerves) as well as Onuf's nucleus motor neurons, which control bladder muscles, are relatively spared and have high levels of calcium-binding proteins.[84] In the authors' motor neuron cell line, VSC4.1, only differential cells are injured by ALS IgG; and such differentiated cells lack calbindin D28K and parvalbumin. Undifferentiated VSC4.1 cells possess ample calbindin D28K and parvalbumin and are relatively resistant to cytotoxic effects of ALS IgG. Transfection of VSC4.1 cells with calbindin cDNA with a phosphoglycerate kinase promoter yielded cells that, when differentiated, still maintained high levels of calbindin. These differentiated transfected cells were resistant to ALS IgG mediated cytotoxicity.[85] Furthermore, in the SOD1 mutant mouse, spinal motor neurons (which lack calbindin and parvalbumin) undergo degenerative changes with vacuoles filled with calcium, and oculomotor neurons that possess ample parvalbumin undergo no degenerative changes and have normal calcium homeostasis.[3]

The function of calbindin D28K and parvalbumin is still unclear, but these calcium-binding proteins appear to enhance calcium homeostasis not only by their ability to bind calcium but also possibly by altering calcium entry through VGCCs, as well as by promoting calcium extrusion and compartmentalization.[86] Thus, regardless of whether the damage to motor neurons is mediated by oxidant stress,[8,9] immune mechanisms, or excitotoxic mechanisms,[5,87] the regulatory effects of calbindin D28K and parvalbumin may influence the selective resistance and vulnerability in motor neurons to cell death in ALS.

Interaction of immune-mediated excitotoxic mechanisms in motor neuron cell death

Although excitotoxic mechanisms are clearly involved in motor neuron injury, whether it is induced by SOD1 mutation or by other toxins, it is not clear what factors are responsible for initiating the excitotoxic process. In sporadic ALS cases, there is no evidence for a genetic defect in glutamate release, uptake, or receptors that could lead to motor neuron injury. Thus, glutamate excitotoxicity must be triggered by some other process. To determine whether immune mechanisms could lead to increased glutamate, the authors injected rats with ALS IgG and disease control IgG and monitored CSF amino acids. After 24 and 72 hours, ALS IgG-injected rats demonstrated a statistically significant increase in CSF glutamate compared to basal levels of glutamate and compared to levels of glutamate in disease-control-injected rats.[88] There was no increase in glutamine or glutathione. With repeated injections of ALS IgG, evidence of motor neuron injury was present by light microscopic and ultrastructural techniques,[89] just as earlier studies with a single injection of low-dose IgG had documented motor nerve terminal changes.[2] Further work is required to determine whether the increased CSF glutamate has been released from nerve terminals. Nevertheless, the fact that immune mechanisms can initiate an increase in CSF glutamate suggests that both processes may participate in a cell death cascade. Since ALS IgG can be documented to increase intracellular calcium as well as CSF glutamate, and since increased intracellular calcium can give rise to increased free radical formation, the authors suggest that all three constituents (calcium, free radicals, and glutamate) are interrelated, with the final common pathway leading to cell injury in sporadic ALS being increased intracellular calcium. After traumatic spinal cord injury, 4-hydroxynonenal, a lipid peroxidation product, increases dramatically and leads to a marked decrease in glutamate uptake.[90] The authors have recently demonstrated a relatively specific increase in CSF 4-hydroxynonenal in ALS patients.[21] Furthermore, it is possible that the elevated 4-hydroxynonenal could contribute to the down-regulation of the glial glutamate transporter in ALS spinal cord, stimulating effects noted in vitro.[91]

Triggering of increased calcium in motor neurons

Although motor neurons may be selectively vulnerable to an increased calcium load in ALS because of the physiologic absence of the calcium-binding proteins, calbindin D28K and parvalbumin, it is still not clear what triggers the increase in motor neuron calcium. The authors' data suggest a prominent role for immune mechanisms in initiating the increase

in motor neuron calcium and subsequent free radical formation. Alterations in glutamate transport, perhaps initiated by the immune mechanisms and mediated by 4-hydroxynonenal, could aggravate the initial motor neuron injury. However, even with repeated intraperitoneal injections of ALS IgG, significant motor neuron cell death does not occur despite changes in motor neuron calcium and early changes of motor neuron injury. An additional factor, which is presently unknown, appears to be required, possibly mediated by the inflammatory cells known to be present in ALS spinal cord or mediated by a breakdown of the blood–brain barrier permitting higher concentrations of IgG to enter the CNS.

An instructive model may well be experimental allergic encephalomyelitis produced in marmosets.[92] In this model, inflammation and demyelination occur following immunization with myelin oligodendrocyte glycoprotein (MOG). If myelin basic protein (MBP) is employed, a central inflammatory process occurs but minimal demyelination is noted. If animals are immunized with MBP followed by the intravenous administration of antibodies to MOG, then marked demyelination occurs. The explanation for these events is that the antibodies, per se, cannot penetrate the blood–brain barrier in sufficient quantities to contribute to demyelination unless the barrier has been broken by a prior inflammatory response. A similar process may be occurring in immune-mediated motor neuron injury. The immunoglobulins that lead to increased intracellular calcium and enhanced acetylcholine release by action at the motor nerve terminal are clearly not sufficient to trigger motor neuron cell death. However, the increasing changes in the motor neurons that occur with chronic immune attack may lead to central inflammatory processes, as noted following axotomy of cranial nerves.[93] Subsequently, down-regulation of the glial glutamate transporter, in addition to the presence of an inflammatory response of T cells and microglia, may enhance the oxidant stress and free radicals and increase the access of immune–inflammatory components to the CNS. Certainly, this hypothesis merits testing, and it may lead to new therapeutic approaches.

Acknowledgments

This work was supported by grants from the Muscular Dystrophy Association, Cephalon, Inc, the Fogarty International Research Collaboration Award (FIRCA), the US–Hungarian Science and Technology Joint Fund, the Hungarian Academy of Science (AKP), the Hungarian Ministry of Welfare, and the National Scientific Research Fund of Hungary (OTKA).

References

1. Engelhardt JI, Siklos L, Komuves L et al. Antibodies to calcium channels from ALS patients passively transferred to mice selectively increase intracellular calcium and induce ultrastructural changes in motor neurons. *Synapse* 1995; 20: 185–199.

2. Engelhardt JI, Siklos L, Appel SH. Altered calcium homeostasis and ultrastructure in motoneurons of mice caused by passively transferred anti-motoneuronal IgG. *J Neuropathol Exp Neurol* 1997; 56: 21–39.

3. Siklos L, Engelhardt JI, Harati Y et al. Ultrastructural evidence for altered calcium in motor nerve terminals in amyotrophic lateral sclerosis. *Ann Neurol* 1996; 39: 203–216.

4. Siklos L, Engelhardt JI, Alexianu ME et al. Intracellular calcium parallels motoneuron degeneration in SOD-1 mutant mice. *J Neuropathol Exp Neurol* 1998; 57: 571–587.

5. Rothstein JD, Tsai G, Kuncl RW et al. Abnormal excitatory amino acid metabolism in amyotrophic lateral sclerosis. *Ann Neurol* 1990;

28: 18–25.

6. Rothstein JD, Martin LJ, Kuncl RW. Decreased glutamate transport by the brain and spinal cord in amyotrophic lateral sclerosis. *N Engl J Med* 1992; 326: 1464–1468.

7. Lin CL, Bristol LA, Jin L et al. Aberrant RNA processing in a neurodegenerative disease: the cause for absent EAAT2, a glutamate transporter, in amyotrophic lateral sclerosis. *Neuron* 1998; 20: 589–602.

8. Bowling AC, Schulz JB, Brown RH Jr, Beal MF. Superoxide dismutase activity, oxidative damage, and mitochondrial energy metabolism in familial and sporadic amyotrophic lateral sclerosis. *J Neurochem* 1993; 61: 2322–2325.

9. Yim MB, Kang JH, Kwak HS et al. A gain-of-function of an amyotrophic lateral sclerosis-associated Cu, Zn superoxide dismutase mutant: an enhancement of free radical formation due to a decrease in Km for hydrogen peroxide. *Proc Natl Acad Sci USA* 1996; 93: 5709–5714.

10. Dykens JA. Isolated cerebral and cerebellar mitochondria produce free radicals when exposed to elevated Ca^{2+} and Na^+: implications for neurodegeneration. *J Neurochem* 1994; 63: 584–591.

11. Coyle JT, Putterfarcken P. Oxidative stress, glutamate and neurodegenerative disorders. *Science* 1993; 262: 689–696.

12. Tymianski M, Charlton MP, Carlen PL, Tator CH. Source specificity of early calcium neurotoxicity in cultured embryonic spinal neurons. *J Neurosci* 1993; 13: 2085–2104.

13. Dugan LL, Sensi S, Canzoniero LMT et al. Mitochondrial production of reactive oxygen species in cortical neurons following exposure to N-methyl-D-aspartate. *J Neurosci* 1995; 15: 6377–6388.

14. Carriedo SG, Yin HZ, Sensi S, Weiss JH. Rapid Ca^{2+} entry through Ca^{2+}-permeable AMPA/Kainate channels triggers marked intracellular Ca^{2+} rises and consequent oxygen radical production. *J Neurosci* 1998; 18: 7727–7738.

15. Sheen VL, Dryer EB, Macklis JD. Calcium-mediated neuronal degeneration following singlet oxygen production. *NeuroReport* 1992; 3: 705–708.

16. Kakkar P, Mehrota S, Viaswanathan PN.

Interrelation of active oxygen species, membrane damage and altered calcium functions. *Mol Cell Biochem* 1992; **111:** 11–15.

17. Siddique T, Figlewicz D, Pericak-Vance MA et al. Linkage of a gene causing familial amyotrophic lateral sclerosis to chromosome 21, and evidence of genetic locus heterogeneity. *N Engl J Med* 1991; **324:** 1381–1384.

18. Rosen DR, Siddique T, Patterson D et al. Mutations in Cu/ZN superoxide dismutase genes are associated with familial amyotrophic lateral sclerosis. *Nature* 1993; **362:** 59–62.

19. Engelhardt JI, Appel SH. IgG reactivity in the spinal cord and motor cortex in amyotrophic lateral sclerosis. *Arch Neurol* 1990; **47:** 1210–1216.

20. Engelhardt JI, Tajti J, Appel SH. Lymphocytic infiltrates in the spinal cord in amyotrophic lateral sclerosis. *Arch Neurol* 1993; **50:** 30–36.

21. Smith RG, Henry KY, Mattson MP, Appel SH. Presence of 4-hydroxynonenal in the cerebrospinal fluid of patients with sporadic amyotrophic lateral sclerosis. Ann Neurol 1998; **44:** 696–699.

22. Keller JN, Mattson MP. Roles of lipid peroxidation in modulation of cellular signaling pathways, cell dysfunction, and death in the nervous system. *Rev Neurosci* 1998; **9:** 105–116.

23. Kurtzke JF, Kurland LT. The epidemiology of neurologic disease. In: Joint RJ, ed. *Clinical Neurology* vol 4. Philadelphia: JB Lippincott, 1983,1–43.

24. Streit WJ, Graeber MB, Kreutzberg GW. Expression of Ia antigen on perivascular and microglial cells after sublethal and ethal motor neuron injury. *Exp Neurol* 1989; **105:** 115–126.

25. Raivich G, Jones LL, Kloss CUA et al. Immune surveillance in the injured nervous system: T-lymphocytes invade the axotomized mouse facial motor nucleus and aggregate around sites of neuronal degeneration. *J Neurosci* 1998; **18:** 5804–5816.

26. Troost D, Van den Oord JJ, de Jong JMBV. Analysis of the inflammatory infiltrate in amyotrophic lateral sclerosis. *J Neuropathol Appl Neurobiol* 1988; **14:** 255–256.

27. Troost D, Van den Oord JJ, de Jong JMBV, Swaab DF. Lymphocytic infiltration in the spinal cord of patients with amyotrophic lateral sclerosis. *Clin Neuropathol* 1989; **8:** 289–294.

28. Lampson LA, Kushner PD, Sobel RA. Strong expression of class II major histocompatibility complex (MHC) antigens in the absence of detectable T-cell infiltration in amyotrophic lateral sclerosis. *J Neuropathol Exp Neurol* 1988; **47:** 353.

29. McGeer PL, Itagaki S, McGeer EG. Expression of histocompatibility glycoprotein HLA-DR in neurologic disease. *Acta Neuropathol (Berl)* 1988; **76:** 550–557.

30. Lampson LA, Kushner PD, Sobel RA. Major histocompatibility complex antigen expression in the affected tissue in amyotrophic lateral sclerosis. *Ann Neurol* 1990; **28:** 365–372.

31. Englehardt JI, Tajti J, Appel SH. Lymphocytic infiltrates in the spinal cord in amyotrophic lateral sclerosis. *Arch Neurol* 1993; **50:** 30–36.

32. Kawamata T, Akiyama H, Yamada T, McGeer PL. Immunologic reactions in amyotrophic lateral sclerosis, brain and spinal cord. *Am J Pathol* 1992; **140:** 691–707.

33. Schubert W, Schwann H. Detection by 4-parameter microscopic imaging and increase of rare mononuclear blood leukocyte types expressing FcγR III receptor (CD16) for immunoglobulin G in human sporadic amyotrophic lateral sclerosis. *Neurosci Lett* 1995; **198:** 29–32.

34. Panzara MA, Gussoni E, Begovich AB et al. T-cell receptor V_β gene rearrangements in the spinal cords and cerebrospinal fluids of patients with amyotrophic lateral sclerosis. *Neurobiology* 1999; in press.

35. Fedoroff S. Development of microglia. In: Kettenmann H, Ransom BR, eds. *Neuroglia*. New York: Oxford University Press, 1995, 162–181.

36. Streit WJ. Microglia-neuronal interactions. *J Chem Neuroanat* 1993; **6:** 261–266.

37. Zielasek J, Hartung HP. Molecular mechanisms of microglial activation. *Adv Neuroimmunol* 1996; **6:** 191–222.

38. Kreutzberg GW. Microglia: a sensor for pathological events in the CNS. *Trends Neurosci* 1996; **19:** 312–318.

39. Matsumoto Y, Ohmori K, Fujiwara M. Immune regulation by brain cells in the central nervous system: microglia but not

astrocytes present myelin basic protein to encephalitogenic T cells under in vivo-mimicking conditions. *Immunology* 1992; **76**: 209–216.

40. Merrill JE, Benveniste EN. Cytokines in inflammatory brain lesions: helpful and harmful. *Trends Neurosci* 1996; **19**: 331–338.

41. Banati RB, Schubert P, Rothe G et al. Modulation of intracellular formation of reactive oxygen intermediates in peritoneal macrophages and microglia/brain macrophages by propentofylline. *J Cereb Blood Flow Metab* 1994; **14**: 145–149.

42. Gehrmann J, Banati R, Wiessner C et al. Reactive microglia in cerebral ischemia: an early mediator of tissue damage? *Neuropathol Appl Neurobiol* 1995; **21**: 277–289.

43. Hu S, Sheng WS, Peterson PK, Chao C. Cytokine modulation of murine microglial cell superoxide production. *Glia* 1995; **13**: 45–50.

44. Hu S, Chao CC, Khanna KV et al. Cytokine and free radical production by porcine microglia. *Clin Immunol Immunopathol* 1996; **78**: 93–96.

45. Banati RB, Gehrmann J, Czech C et al. Early and rapid de novo synthesis of Alzheimer beta A4-amyloid precursor protein (APP) in activated microglia. *Glia* 1993; **9**: 199–210.

46. Sriram S, Rodriguez M. Indictment of the microglia as the villain in multiple sclerosis. *Neurology* 1997; **48**: 464–470.

47. Hall SM, Hughes RA, Atkinson PF et al. Motor nerve biopsy in severe Guillain–Barré syndrome. *Ann Neurol* 1992; **31**: 441–444.

48. Hartung HP, Pollard JD, Harvey GK, Toyka KV. Immunopathogenesis and treatment of the Guillain–Barré syndrome. *Muscle Nerve* 1995; **18**: 137–153.

49. Annegers JF, Appel S, Lee JR, Perkins P. Incidence and prevalence of amyotrophic lateral sclerosis in Harris County, Texas, 1985–1988. *Arch Neurol* 1991; **48**: 589–593.

50. Haverkamp LJ, Appel V, Appel SH. Natural history of amyotrophic lateral sclerosis in a database population: validation of a scoring system and a model for survival prediction. *Brain* 1995; **118**: 707–719.

51. Shy ME. Rowland LP, Smith T et al. Motoneuron disease and plasma cell dyscrasia. *Neurology* 1986; **36**: 1429–1436.

52. Younger DS, Rowland LP, Latov N et al. Motoneuron disease and amyotrophic lateral sclerosis: relation of high CSF protein content to paraproteinemia in clinical syndromes. *Neurology* 1990; **40**: 595–599.

53. Duarte F, Binet S, Lacomblex L et al. Quantitative analysis of monoclonal immunoglobulins in serum of patients with amyotrophic lateral sclerosis. *J Neurol Sci* 1991; **104**: 88–91.

54. Younger DS, Rowland LP, Latov N et al. Lymphoma, motoneuron diseases, and amyotrophic lateral sclerosis. *Ann Neurol* 1991; **29**: 78–86.

55. Hays AP, Roxas A, Siddiq S et al. A monoclonal IgA in a patient with amyotrophic lateral sclerosis reacts with neurofilaments and surface antigen on neuroblastoma cells. *J Neuropath Exp Neurol* 1990; **49**: 383–398.

56. Fabian R. Uptake of plasma IgG by CNS motor neurons: comparison of anti-neuronal and normal IgG. *Neurology* 1988; **38**: 1775–1780.

57. Engelhardt JI, Appel SH, Killian JM. Motor neuron destruction in guinea pigs immunized with bovine spinal cord ventral horn homogenate: experimental autoimmune gray matter disease. *J Neuroimmunol* 1990; **27**: 21–31.

58. Engelhardt JI, Appel SH, Killian JM. Experimental autoimmune motor neuron disease. *Ann Neurol* 1989; **26**: 368–376.

59. Garcia J, Engelhardt JI, Appel SH, Stefani E. Increased mepp frequency as an early sign of experimental immune-mediated motor neuron disease. *Ann Neurol* 1990; **28**: 329–334.

60. Maselli R, Wollman R, Leung C et al. Neuromuscular transmission in amyotrophic lateral sclerosis. *Muscle Nerve* 1993; **16**: 1193–1203.

61. Lang B, Newsom-Davis J, Wray D, Vincent A. Autoimmune etiology for myasthenic (Eaton–Lambert) syndrome. *Lancet* 1981; **2**: 224–226.

62. Kim YJ, Neher E. IgG from patients with Lambert–Eaton syndrome blocks voltage-dependent calcium channels. *Science* 1988; **239**: 405–408.

63. Appel SH, Engelhardt JI, Garcia J, Stefani E. Immunoglobulins from animal models of motor neuron disease and from human amyotrophic lateral sclerosis patients passively

transfer physiological abnormalities to the neuromuscular junction. *Proc Natl Acad Sci USA* 1991; **88**: 647–651.

64. Delbono O, Garcia J, Appel SH, Stefani E. Calcium current and charge movement of mammalian muscle: action of amyotrophic lateral sclerosis immunoglobulins. *J Physiol* 1991; **444**: 723–742.

65. Delbono O, Magnelli V, Sawanda T et al. F$_{ab}$ fragments from amyotrophic lateral sclerosis IgG affect calcium channels of skeletal muscle. *Am J Physiol* 1993; **265**: C537–C543.

66. Uchitel OD, Protti DA, Sanchez V et al. P-voltage-dependent calcium channel mediates presynaptic calcium influx and transmitter release in mammalian synapsis. *Proc Natl Acad Sci USA* 1992; **89**: 3330–3333.

67. Llinas R, Sugimori M, Cherksey BD et al. IgG from amyotrophic lateral sclerosis patients increases current through P-type calcium channels in mammalian cerebellar Purkinje cells and in isolated channel protein in lipid bilayers. *Proc Natl Acad Sci USA* 1993; **90**: 11743–11747.

68. Mosier DR, Baldelli P, Delbono O et al. Amyotrophic lateral sclerosis immunoglobulins increase Ca^{2+} currents in a motor neuron cell line. *Ann Neurol* 1995; **37**: 102–109.

69. Crawford G, Le WD, Smith RG et al. A novel N18TG2X mesencephalon cell hybrid expresses property that suggests a dopaminergic cell line of substantia nigra origin. *J Neurosci* 1992; **12**: 3392–3398.

70. Smith RG, Alexianu M, Crawford G et al. Cytotoxicity of immunoglobulins from amyotrophic lateral sclerosis patients on a hybrid motor neuron cell line. *Proc Natl Acad Sci USA* 1994; **91**: 3393–3397.

71. Alexianu ME, Mohamed AH, Smith RG et al. Apoptotic cell death of a hybrid motor neuron cell line induced by immunoglobulin from patients with ALS. *J Neurochem* 1994; **63**: 2365–2368.

72. Colom LV, Alexianu ME, Mosier DR et al. Amyotrophic lateral sclerosis immunoglobulins increase intracellular calcium in a motoneuron cell line. *Exp Neurol* 1997; **146**: 354–360.

73. Smith RG, Hamilton S, Hoffman F et al. Serum antibodies to L-type calcium channels in patients with amyotrophic lateral sclerosis. *N Engl J Med* 1992; **327**: 1721–1728.

74. Arsac C, Raymond C, Martin-Moutot N et al. Amino assays fail to detect antibodies against neuronal calcium channels in amyotrophic lateral sclerosis serum. *Ann Neurol* 1996; **40**: 695–700.

75. Lennon VA, Kryzert J, Griessmann GE et al. Calcium channel antibodies in the Lambert–Eaton syndrome and other paraneoplastic syndromes. *N Engl J Med* 1995; **332**: 1467–1474.

76. Brown RH, Hauser SL, Harrington H, Weiner HL. Failure of immunosuppression with a 10- to 14-day course of high-dose intravenous cyclophosphamide to alter the progression of amyotrophic lateral sclerosis. *Arch Neurol* 1986; **43**: 383–384.

77. Drachman DB, Chaudhry V, Cornblath D et al. Trial of immunosuppression in amyotrophic lateral sclerosis using total lymphoid irradiation. *Ann Neurol* 1994; **35**: 142–150.

78. Appel SH, Steward SS, Appel V et al. A double-blind study of the effectiveness of cyclosporine in amyotrophic lateral sclerosis. *Arch Neurol* 1988; **45**: 381–386.

79. Rothstein JD, Van Kammen M, Levy AI et al. Selective loss of glial glutamate transporter (GLT-1) in amyotrophic lateral sclerosis. *Ann Neurol* 1995; **38**: 73–84.

80. Bristol LA, Rothstein JD. Glutamate transporter gene expression in amyotrophic lateral sclerosis motor cortex. *Ann Neurol* 1996; **39**: 676–679.

81. Morrison BM, Janssen WGM, Gordon JW, Morrison JH. Light and electron microscopic distribution of the AMPA receptor subunit, Glu R2, in the spinal cord of control and G68R mutant superoxide dismutase transgenic mice. *J Comp Neurol* 1998; **395**: 523–534.

82. Celio MR, Baier W, Scharer L et al. Monoclonal antibodies directed against the calcium-binding protein parvalbumin. *Cell Calcium* 1988; **9**: 81–86.

83. Cellio MR, Baier W, Scharer L et al. Monoclonal antibodies directed against the calcium-binding protein calbindin-D$_{28K}$. *Cell Calcium* 1990; **11**: 599–602.

84. Alexianu ME, Ho BK, Mohamed AH et al. The role of calcium-binding proteins in selective motor neuron vulnerability in amyotrophic

lateral sclerosis. *Ann Neurol* 1994; **36:** 846–858.

85. Ho BK, Alexianu ME, Colom LV et al. Expression of calbindin-D_{28K} in motoneuron-hybrid cells following retroviral infection with calbindin-D_{28k} cDNA prevents amyotrophic lateral sclerosis IgG-mediated cytotoxicity. *Proc Natl Acad Sci USA* 1996; **93:** 6796–6801.

86. Lledo PM, Somasundaram B, Morton AJ et al. Stable transfection of calbindin-D_{28K} into GH_3 cell line alters calcium currents and intracellular calcium in homeostasis. *Neuron* 1992; **9:** 943–954.

87. Appel SH. Excitotoxic neuronal cell death in amyotrophic lateral sclerosis. *Trends Neurosci* 1993; **16:** 3–4.

88. La Bella V, Goodman JC, Appel SH. Increased CSF glutamate following injection of ALS immunoglobulins. *Neurology* 1997; **48:** 1270–1272.

89. Alexianu ME, La Bella V, Manole E et al. The interaction of immune and excitotoxic mechanisms leading to altered intracellular calcium and ultrastructure in rat motoneurons. *Soc Neurosci* 1997; **23:** 832.

90. Springer JE, Azbill RD, Mark RJ et al. 4-hydroxynonenal, a lipid peroxidation product, rapidly accumulates following traumatic spinal cord injury and inhibits glutamate uptake. *J Neurochem* 1997; **68:** 2469–2476.

91. Blanc EM, Keller JN, Fernandez S, Mattson MP. 4-hydroxynonenal, a lipid peroxidation product, impairs glutamate transport in cortical astrocytes. *Glia* 1998; **22:** 149–160.

92. Genain CP, Nguyen MH, Letvin NL et al. Antibody facilitation of multiple sclerosis-like lesions in a nonhuman primate. *J Clin Invest* 1995; **96:** 2966–2974.

93. Kristensson K, Aldskogius H, Peng ZC et al. Co-induction of neuronal interferon-gamma and nitric oxide synthase in rat motor neurons after axotomy: a role for nerve cell repair or death? *J Neurocytol* 1994; **23:** 453–459.

18

Does autoimmunity play a role in amyotrophic lateral sclerosis?

Daniel B Drachman

Introduction

The possibility that autoimmune mechanisms may be involved in the pathogenesis of amyotrophic lateral sclerosis (ALS) has been considered and debated for more than 30 years. About 10 years ago the author reviewed the evidence for and against this hypothesis[1] and proposed a set of criteria by which to evaluate the evidence for a suspected autoimmune disorder.[2] Since then, concepts of the pathogenesis of ALS have evolved in important ways, changing the questions that are now being asked. It is now generally accepted that ALS is not a single disease entity, autoimmune or otherwise; instead, it is most likely that the rather stereotyped clinicopathological picture of ALS results from the peculiar vulnerability of motor neurons to a variety of different insults, any of which can trigger the cascades of events that lead to their death.

Thus, the questions now being asked deal less with primary causes and more with mechanisms involved in the neuron-damaging cascades. In this context, this chapter examines the evidence that autoimmune mechanisms may play a significant pathogenic role in some or all forms of ALS. This issue is of fundamental importance because the answer could substantially influence therapeutic efforts to interrupt or slow the otherwise inevitable progression of ALS. On balance, there are still doubts as to whether the tantalizing clues suggesting autoimmune phenomena in at least some cases of ALS play a significant role in the disease process, or whether they represent epiphenomena.

Experimental disease models of autoimmune processes that may produce an ALS syndrome

There is persuasive evidence from the development of experimental animal models of motor neuron disease by Engelhardt and colleagues[3–5] that an autoimmune attack *can* reproduce features of ALS. Immunization of guinea pigs with preparations enriched for motor neurons from spinal cords of swine or cattle have resulted in loss of motor neurons in the spinal cord and in muscle weakness and atrophy.[3,4] Immunization with a cruder ventral spinal cord homogenate has produced damage both to cortical motor neurons and to spinal motor neurons.[5]

These models provide convincing evidence that immune responses evoked by immunization with one or more components of the spinal cord preparations can potentially induce damage to motor neurons. The specific antigens responsible for the pathologic immune response have not been elucidated, but their precise identification might allow further investigation of the role of autoimmunity in spontaneous ALS.

Role of antibodies directed against motor neuron targets in ALS

This hoary and controversial area may be divided into several topics:

(a) cytotoxic antibodies;
(b) physiologic effects of antibodies;
(c) antibodies to calcium channels;
(d) autoantibodies to other neuronal components; and
(e) intraneuronal IgG.

Antibodies that are cytotoxic to motor neurons

More than 30 years ago, various investigators first reported that neurons cultured in the presence of serum from ALS patients were damaged or killed.[6–10] Although others were unable to reproduce their findings,[11–13] the blinded studies of Wolfgram[9] and Roisen and colleagues[10] (using cultured mouse motor neurons) suggested a neurotoxic humoral factor. More recently, Smith and colleagues[14] reported that IgG from ALS patients was lethal to hybrid rat motor neurons and neuroblastoma cells in culture. The exposure time required for killing was remarkably brief: incubation of the cells for only 30 minutes in medium containing as little as 200 µg/ml of ALS IgG produced a maximal toxic effect, with the eventual death of more than 50% of the IgG-exposed cells. This effect was calcium-dependent. It was prevented by omission of calcium from the medium, or by blockade of N-type calcium channels with ω-conotoxin, or by blockade of P-type calcium channels with agatoxin IVa (please see below for brief definition of calcium channels). The

concept that IgG-mediated influx of calcium could lead to motor neuron death is particularly attractive because of independent evidence for a role of calcium in the ALS cascade. However, as with previous studies that demonstrated cytotoxic effects of ALS sera, this investigation involved isolated cells in culture, a condition that can accentuate their vulnerability.

In order to relate this intriguing finding to the pathogenesis of ALS, it is important to determine whether IgG from ALS patients induces loss of motor neurons in the intact spinal cord. To examine the effect of IgG from ALS patients on spinal motor neurons in situ, studies were performed that made use of an organotypic spinal cord culture system.[15,16] Transverse slices of spinal cords from 8-day-old rats were maintained in culture on permeable membranes with excellent viability of motor neurons for up to several months.[16] This system has the advantage of allowing direct application of the putative pathogenic IgG to motor neurons in the more physiologic environment of the spinal cord for long periods of time. Moreover, anterior horn cells in these cultures have been shown to undergo subacute or chronic cell death when subjected to conditions thought to contribute to their loss in ALS, including the presence of agents that enhance glutamate excitotoxicity or inhibit superoxide dismutase, or both.[16,17] In these experiments, IgG that had been purified from sera of 20 patients with classic sporadic ALS and 13 controls was added to the culture medium. A relatively high concentration of IgG (600 µg/ml) was used, and the culture medium was changed twice a week for the 2-week duration of the experiment. Triplicate culture wells, each containing five spinal cord preparations, were used for each subject's IgG. At the end of the 2-week experimental period, choline acetyltransferase (ChAT) was measured. In the lumbar spinal cord, ChAT is present exclusively in motor neurons,[18] and it is decreased in spinal cords cultured with agents that enhance excitotoxicity or decrease superoxide dismutase activity.[16,17] Contrary to expectations, there was no significant difference in ChAT activity in any of the spinal cord preparations cultured with IgG from ALS patients compared with the controls.[19] This disappointing result, observed in two separate sets of experiments, suggested that IgG from ALS patients does not lead to the death or dysfunction of mammalian anterior horn cells in the context of the spinal cord environment.

Physiologic effects of antibodies

It is well known that fatiguability and abnormalities of neuromuscular transmission occur in patients with ALS.[20–22] Microelectrode studies of neuromuscular preparations from ALS patients have shown several changes, including variability of miniature end-plate potential (MEPP) frequency (but not a significant *increase* in frequency), as well as a reduction in MEPP amplitudes and a decrease in quantal stores and quantal content of endplate potentials.[23] Guinea pigs with experimentally-induced autoimmune motor neuron disease have also shown abnormalities of neuromuscular transmission, consisting of *increased* MEPP frequency,[24] which differed somewhat from the features described in ALS. To determine whether antibodies from ALS patients could induce similar changes in neuromuscular transmission, immunoglobulin preparations from patients or controls were added acutely to mouse nerve–muscle preparations in vitro[25] or passively transferred in vivo.[26] The results showed an increase in MEPP frequency induced by immunoglobulins from a majority of ALS patients. A more recent study of passive transfer of serum from ALS patients to mice[27] has confirmed these observations, showing increased frequencies of MEPPs induced by just over half the sera.

These findings, which indicate that humoral factors from ALS patients — presumably antibodies — can alter neuromuscular transmission, raise two key questions. First, what is the mechanism of this physiologic phenomenon? Secondly, and more importantly, does it contribute to the ultimate death of motor neurons and, if so, how?

Antibodies to calcium channels

Calcium channels are a family of related proteins that have different localization and susceptibility to various blocking agents.[28] L-type calcium channels are found in skeletal muscle membranes, while channels at motor nerve terminals are thought to be of the N, P, or P–Q types. Increases in MEPP frequency are usually associated with opening of calcium channels at motor nerve terminals. The resultant increase in calcium influx triggers the release of acetylcholine from the nerve terminals. Therefore, an explanation of the ALS antibody-mediated increase in MEPP frequency would be expected to relate to increased calcium flux through these channels. Somewhat paradoxically, immunoglobulin from ALS patients was first shown to *decrease* calcium currents in L-type calcium channels of skeletal muscle fibers.[29] Moreover, it was reported[30] that:

(a) ALS patients had abnormally high levels of antibodies to L-type calcium channels;
(b) the antibodies bound selectively to the α-1 subunits of the channels; and
(c) the serum antibody levels correlated with the rapidity of disease progression.

These findings — binding to L-type calcium channels and inhibition of calcium currents — seemed inconsistent with the reported effects on motor nerve terminals. In the first place, inhibition of calcium entry would be expected to result in a decrease rather than an increase in MEPP frequency. Furthermore, the relevant calcium channels at the motor nerve terminal are not L-type but N-type, P-type, and P–Q-type. In addition, the cytotoxic effect of ALS immunoglobulins on cultured hybrid motor neurons[14] also suggested an increase in calcium entry, via N-type or P-type channels. These apparently contradictory findings raised certain questions, both about the type of channels to which the ALS patients' antibodies bound and about whether these antibodies blocked or enhanced calcium translocation.

More consistent with the physiologic evidence were reports that immunoglobulin preparations from ALS patients increased calcium currents through P-type channels of cerebellar Purkinje cells and increased the open times of purified P-type channels in lipid bilayers.[31] A similar increase in calcium currents was also reported when the hybrid motor neuron cells were exposed to ALS immunoglobulins, although the effects were rather weak and variable and the pattern of blockade by calcium channel toxins was inconsistent with previously reported protection of these cells from cytotoxic cell death.[32] In any case, an effect on P-type channels could theoretically explain the apparent paradox: the antibodies might produce an increase in calcium flux through P-type channels, but they could have an opposite effect on calcium flux through L-type channels and they could bind to all three types of channels (P-type, N-type, and L-type). Since the *increase* in calcium flux occurred through P-type channels, and since they are known to be present on motor neurons, perhaps the P-type channels represent the main site of ALS IgG-induced calcium entry into the motor neurons.

Antibodies to calcium channels can also be measured by immunoprecipitation of ^{125}I-neurotoxin-labeled channels, as has been successfully demonstrated in Lambert–Eaton myasthenic syndrome.[33,34] Lennon and colleagues[34] found that nearly one-quarter of ALS patients had antibodies to P–Q-type channels and that 13% had antibodies to N-type channels, using specific ^{125}I-ω-conotoxin-labeled channel preparations to measure the antibodies. At that point one might have accepted the presence of the antibodies, at least in some patients, even if their pathogenic relevance was not yet clear. However, we examined the binding of serum IgG from 26 patients with classic ALS to these calcium channels, using ^{125}I-ω-conotoxin GVIA to label N-type channels, and ^{125}I-ω-conotoxin MVIIC to label P-type channels.[19] Only one of the 26 ALS sera gave a weakly positive result in the radioimmunoassay for binding to either the N-type or the P-type channel (a different serum was positive in each assay). By contrast, 44% of Lambert–Eaton myasthenic syndrome sera were positive in the N-type assay and 95% were positive in the P-type assay.[19] Other investigators have also attempted to demonstrate antibodies to L-type or N-type calcium channels by immunoprecipitation assays or enzyme-linked immunosorbent assays, with negative results.[35] The reasons for these conflicting results and others concerning antibodies to calcium channels[36,37] remain unresolved at present. It is obviously extremely important to have an assay that could identify any patients with a putative autoimmune form of ALS, in whom early and vigorous immunosuppressive therapy could be attempted (see below).

Regardless of the presence or absence of antibodies to calcium channels, mechanisms that could increase intraneuronal calcium concentrations should be taken seriously. An increase in intracellular calcium can result in cell death by activating cytosolic proteases or other cytoplasmic cascades. Such calcium-mediated mechanisms, which are triggered by excitotoxicity or other processes, are thought to have an important role in ALS as well as in other 'neurodegenerative' disorders.[38–40] Indeed, Appel and colleagues have reported an increase in intracellular calcium, predominantly in synaptic vesicles or mitochondria, in motor nerve terminals of ALS patients.[41] Passive transfer of relatively large amounts of selected cytotoxic IgG from ALS patients to mice has also been shown to induce an increase in intracellular calcium in nerve terminals, although 'high-dose' IgG had a curiously opposite, depleting effect on vesicle calcium content.[42] If IgG-induced calcium influx into motor neurons can be shown to reproduce cell damage like that seen in ALS, this would provide a further argument in favor of autoimmunity.

Other antibodies in ALS and paraproteins

The concept that various other types of antibodies might be related to ALS probably acquired its original support from a series of clinical observations of patients with ALS-like syndromes who also had serum paraproteins.[43–54] The incidence of monoclonal paraproteins in patients with ALS is uncertain. An early report[48] gave a figure of nearly 5% but later studies[54] using the more sensitive immunofixation method noted an incidence of nearly 10%. However, another study[55] found no increase in paraproteins compared with controls. Although the clinical manifestations generally involved lower motor neurons or motor neuropathy, some patients with classic clinical features of upper and lower motor neuron involvement were also described.[45,46,48] In a retrospective analysis of 21 cases, Rowland[54] reported that 10 had classic ALS and another seven had probable upper motor neuron signs as well as lower motor neuron involvement.

Immunologic studies of paraproteins from some of these cases revealed that they reacted with the gangliosides GM1 or GD1b, or both.[52,53] It is now well established that some patients with motor neuropathies have high levels of antibodies to glycolipids, chiefly GM1.[56] Early reports of antibodies to GM1 overestimated the prevalence of elevated levels of antibodies to glycolipids in classic ALS,[57] mainly because moderately elevated levels of antiglycolipid antibodies are not specific to ALS but also occur in a variety of other disorders, including multiple sclerosis, myasthenia gravis, and lupus erythematosus.[57,58] More recent results indicate that relatively few patients with ALS have truly high levels of antibodies to gangliosides.[59,60] In our own series only 29% of patients with definite ALS had levels of antibodies to GM1 or GD1a that were more than 2 standard deviations above the mean for normal control subjects, and only three of 61 ALS patients had more highly elevated serum levels of antiganglioside antibodies, that were comparable to the levels seen in multifocal motor neuropathy or Guillain–Barré syndrome. Thus, the role of antiganglioside antibodies in the pathogenesis of ALS now seems doubtful at best.

A variety of other humoral changes have also been reported in ALS. An increase in immune complexes in serum and kidney biopsies of ALS patients was found in one study,[61] which is possibly consistent with an alteration of immunoglobulin isotype patterns,[62] but another investigation failed to detect increased immune complexes.[63] IgM antibodies to sulfoglucuronyl paragloboside (SGPG), a glycolipid component of motor nerves, have been reported to be elevated in more than one-third of 72 ALS patients, with high titers in 22%.[64] Autoantibodies to diverse antigens, including various neuronal components,[65] acetylcholinesterase,[66] fetal muscle proteins,[67] and vascular antigens[68] have been detected in ALS.

What do these deviations in humoral factors mean? At present, most of the findings remain unexplained curiosities. The very diversity of these autoantibodies suggests that no single one of them plays a key role in the pathogenesis of ALS. The fact that so many immune peculiarities have been unearthed could mean that there is some underlying generalized disturbance in immune regulation, or alternatively it could merely reflect the intensity of the search, which predisposes to the 'discoveries'.

Intraneuronal IgG: specific or non-specific?

IgG has been found within anterior horn cells of guinea pigs with experimental autoimmune motor neuron disease and in animals that had been passively injected with immunoglobulins from the affected animals.[3,69] This suggested that antibodies could enter the neurons via retrograde transport and damage them from within the cytoplasm. These observations prompted an examination of spinal cords of human ALS patients, and 13 of 15 spinal cord specimens also showed immunocytochemical staining for IgG.[70] In order to distinguish whether the IgG was internalized by selective or non-selective mechanisms, we undertook a detailed study of intraneuronal proteins in ALS, using immunocytochemistry to detect not only the immunoglobulins IgG and IgM, but also the non-immune serum protein α-2 macroglobulin (α-2Mac) in spinal cords from nine ALS patients.[71] α-2Mac is a particularly useful control, since it is present in the serum at a concentration close to that of IgG but has a much higher molecular weight (800 kDa), which is similar to that of IgM.[72,73] The findings showed that both IgG and α-2Mac were present in motor neurons from all nine ALS spinal cords. More importantly, there was a close concordance between the distribution and intensity of staining of IgG and α-2Mac in motor neurons. In contrast, staining for IgM was weak or absent in motor neurons, apparently reflecting the lower serum concentration of this protein. It was concluded that, although IgG can be detected in the cytoplasm of motor neurons in ALS, it does not appear to be internalized on an immune-specific basis. The presence of α-2Mac in motor neurons in a similar distribution and with an intensity similar to that of IgG implies that motor neurons in patients with ALS may internalize plasma proteins, including IgG, by non-selective endocytosis. These findings cast doubt on the concept that internalization of IgG into the cytoplasm of motor neurons in ALS is mediated by a selective immune mechanism.

Autoimmune ALS-like syndromes

Perhaps the most compelling clue in favor of an autoimmune mechanism in at least some ALS patients is the occurrence of disorders that mimic ALS in settings of immune abnormalities plausibly directed against neurons.

Multifocal motor neuropathy

Multifocal motor neuropathy (MMN) is the best characterized of these conditions. Clinically, it is manifested by slowly progressive asymmetrical weakness that preferentially involves distal muscles. It affects males 1.5–2 times more commonly than females.[56] Upper motor neuron signs are not present in these patients. The diagnosis is based on the finding of motor nerve conduction block or increased levels of antibodies to GM1. Although the lesions primarily affect myelin of peripheral nerves, axons may also be involved. Antibodies to GM1 have been convincingly shown to induce focal physiologic changes typical of MMN.[74,75] The motor neuropathies often respond to immunotherapy with either cyclophosphamide or intravenous immuno-globulin, but not to corticosteroids. Some MMN patients were originally thought to have lower motor neuron forms of ALS, and the similarity of these conditions provides support for the idea that damage to the motor system may occur naturally as a result of autoimmune mechanisms.

Malignancy-related syndromes

The association of neoplasms with motor neuron diseases has attracted interest since the papers by Brain and colleagues[76] and by Norris and Engel.[77] Epidemiologic studies of the incidence of cancer in patients with motor neuron diseases gave mixed results, with conclusions varying from an association that was no greater than chance to a figure of more than 7%.[78] However, case reports of the co-occurrence of lymphoproliferative disorders and motor neuropathy or classic ALS were particularly striking.[79–81]

Most recently, Posner's group at Sloan-Kettering Memorial Hospital, New York, USA, has described three groups of patients with motor neuron syndromes and cancer.[82] The first group of three patients was distinguished by antineuronal antibodies. All three patients had evidence of widespread denervation, and two had clinical signs of upper motor neuron involvement, but there were additional neurological features that are not part of ALS in all three. The two autopsies showed anterior horn cell depletion, but no abnormalities of the corticospinal tracts. The second group consisted of five women with a rather special syndrome of primary lateral sclerosis in association with breast cancer. The cancer was detected from 5 years before the neurological disorder to 6.5 years after it. In addition to spasticity, signs of

lower motor neuron involvement were definite in one and possible in two of these patients. The third group consisted of six patients who had classic ALS and a variety of different neoplasms.

The rationales for linking the motor neuron syndromes and the malignancies in these 14 patients are plausible but as yet not proven. In the first group, the presence of antineuronal antibodies that have established relationships to paraneoplastic neurological disorders provides support for a pathogenic, although rare, mechanism of immune damage to motor neurons. In the second group, the uniqueness of the syndrome is a tantalizing clue, although the temporal relationship is rather loose. The third group may well represent a coincidental association of two conditions that are not rare in the older age group.

Finally, there are scattered reports in the literature of remission of motor neuron syndromes following treatment of malignancy.[80]

In summary, these presumptive paraneoplastic motor neuron syndromes suggest a reasonable relationship based on autoimmune processes.

Effects of immunosuppression

Perhaps the most important goal in the search for the pathogenesis of ALS is to develop rational treatment for this disease. If autoimmunity plays a role in the pathogenesis of ALS, then immune suppression, if adequate, should alter the course of the disease process. To date, immunosuppression has failed to influence the relentlessly progressive course of ALS in several uncontrolled trials using adrenal corticosteroids, plasmapheresis, azathioprine, cyclophosphamide, or various combinations of these agents.[83–86] A controlled trial of cyclosporin A had no significant beneficial effect.[87] In an effort to achieve highly potent suppression of the immune system, we carried out a randomized, double-blind, controlled trial of total lymphoid irradiation in 61 patients with ALS.[88] The findings showed that total lymphoid irradiation suppressed all measured aspects of humoral, cellular, and delayed-type immunity, yet failed to influence the course of ALS. Based on the idea that even more powerful immunosuppression might be needed, a third group of patients was added; these patients were treated with high-dose intravenous cyclophosphamide followed by continued oral cyclophosphamide (D Drachman and colleagues, unpublished work). This study was limited by the drop-out of patients as a result of adverse effects of cyclophosphamide, but again no beneficial effect was shown.

An important focus of these studies was to examine the results in light of the autoimmune hypothesis of ALS. If these powerful treatments failed to influence the course of ALS, was their ineffectiveness due to an erroneous hypothesis or to inadequacy of immunosuppression? It is well known that even profound immunosuppression may be selective and does not necessarily inhibit all immune responses.[89] It is possible that the methods used to date have merely failed to suppress the appropriate immune mechanisms and have thereby missed the mark. Finally, it remains possible that once the pathologic process is set in motion, or has reached a certain point, it cannot be halted even if the pathogenic mechanism is suppressed.

Conclusions

The concept that an autoimmune attack can be directed against motor neurons is a priori logical and is supported by experimental and clinical findings. Autoimmune response to virtually all organs, most tissues, and an enormous variety of self-molecules either occur spontaneously or can be provoked by immunization. Motor neurons are no exception, as demonstrated by the models of experimental motor neuron disease induced by immunization with preparations of cells derived from the spinal cord. There is no doubt that distal parts of motor neurons — axons, myelin, and nerve terminals — are subject to autoimmune attack, both clinically and experimentally. Moreover, there are hints that cell bodies of motor neurons may be damaged in patients with cancer-associated antineuronal antibodies, and possibly in patients with paraproteins.

If autoimmune damage to motor neurons can occur, the first question we must ask is whether it does occur as part or all of the pathogenic process in most, or even some, patients with classic ALS. Secondly, what is the relationship between any of the antibodies that have been reported to occur and the disease process? Are they pathogenic? Are they indicators of generalized immune autoreactivity? Do they result from a secondary response to damage to motor neurons? Thirdly, and most importantly, can immunotherapy intervene in the pathologic process and halt or slow the disease progression? These questions become all the more complex in view of the generally accepted concept that the clinical syndrome of ALS can result from a wide variety of different causes.[90]

As a framework for the evaluation of the role of autoimmunity in ALS, I have used a set of the following five 'criteria' proposed for the assessment of antibody-mediated autoimmune diseases.[2]

1. **Antibodies are present in patients with the disease:** The importance of identifying putative pathogenic antibodies in ALS cannot be overemphasized. If such antibodies exist, their early detection could lead to prompt

treatment long before clinical criteria for ALS are satisfied and before the disease process has become irreversible. The search for such antibodies is detailed above. In brief, antibodies to L-type calcium channels have been reported in 75% of patients by one group, but have not been found in another study. Antibodies to N-type or P-type calcium channels have been identified in ALS sera by certain physiologic effects, but they have not been detected by sensitive radioimmunoassays. Contrary to early hopes, antibodies to gangliosides have not proven to be markedly elevated in ALS, except in a very few patients. Paraprotein antibodies are present in a small minority of ALS patients, and their relationship to the disease process remains uncertain. Antineuronal antibodies are found only in rare patients with associated cancer and atypical clinical features. Thus, the evidence for plausibly pathogenic antibodies in ALS is scattered and controversial. Whether this uncertainty reflects the multifactorial pathogenesis of ALS, indicates that we have not yet learned to identify the important antibodies, or means that antibody-mediated mechanisms are not relevant to ALS, is not yet clear.

2. **Antibodies interact with the target antigen:** The target antigen is uncertain in ALS. Antibodies damage hybrid motoneuron and neuroblastoma cells in culture and produce physiologic effects on different calcium channels but do not affect anterior horn cells in organotypic spinal cord cultures.

3. **Passive transfer of the antibody reproduces features of the disease:** Passive transfer induces an increase in MEPP frequency and changes in intracellular calcium, but the hallmark of ALS — loss of motor neurons — has not been demonstrated.

4. **Immunization with the antigen produces a model disease:** The experimental models of motor neuron disease induced by immunization with xenogeneic spinal cord cells show intriguing similarities to motor neuron disease or ALS.

5. **Reduction of the antibodies ameliorates the disease:** Potent immunosuppression has failed to influence the course of ALS. However, the ability of the suppressive methods to reduce the putative pathogenic antibodies cannot be evaluated until more is known about the particular antibodies involved. As discussed above, the effects of immunosuppressive treatment on different immune responses varies and does not guarantee suppression of the potentially relevant response.

Summary

Thus, we remain uncertain at best about the role of autoimmunity in ALS. Although negative results cannot prove the null hypothesis, the findings summarized here do not provide convincing support for autoimmunity as a major pathogenetic mechanism in ALS. On balance, it is doubtful that autoimmune mechanisms have a major role in the pathogenesis of classic ALS.

Acknowledgments

I am grateful to Ms Lori Clawson RN, Dr P Fishman, Dr R Kuncl, Dr ED Mellits, Dr A Pestronk, Dr J Rothstein, and Dr A Vincent for their role in the original work described here.

The work carried out in the author's laboratory was supported in part by grants from the Muscular Dystrophy Association, the National Institutes of Health, the C Walder Parke Family Foundation, the Eleanor Denmead Ingram Fund, and the Baltimore Relief Foundation.

References

1. Drachman DB, Kuncl RW. Amyotrophic lateral sclerosis: an unconventional autoimmune disease? *Ann Neurol* 1989; **26**: 269–274.

2. Drachman DB. How to recognize an antibody-mediated autoimmune disease: criteria. In: Waksman BH, ed. *Immunologic Mechanisms in Neurologic and Psychiatric Disease.* New York: Raven, 1990, 183–186.

3. Engelhardt JI, Joo F. An immune-mediated guinea pig model for lower motor neuron disease. *J Neuroimmunol* 1986; **12**: 279–290.

4. Engelhardt JI, Appel SH, Killian JM. Experimental autoimmune motoneuron disease. *Ann Neurol* 1989; **26**: 368–376.

5. Engelhardt JL, Appel SH, Killian JM. Motor neuron destruction in guinea pigs immunized with bovine spinal cord ventral horn homogenate: experimental autoimmune gray matter disease. *J Neuroimmunol* 1990; **47**: 21–31.

6. Field EJ, Hughes D. Toxicity of motor neurone disease serum for myelin in tissue culture. *Br Med J* 1965; **2**: 1399–1401.

7. Bornstein MB, Appel SH. Tissue culture studies of demyelination. *Ann N Y Acad Sci* 1965; **122**: 280–286.

8. Wolfgram F, Myers L. Amyotrophic lateral sclerosis: effect of serum on anterior horn cells in tissue culture. *Science* 1973; **179**: 579–580.

9. Wolfgram F. Blind studies on the effect of amyotrophic lateral sclerosis sera on motor neurons in vitro. In: Andrews JM, Johnson RT, Brazier MAB, eds. *Amyotrophic Lateral Sclerosis: Recent Research Trends.* New York: Academic Press, 1976, 145–151.

10. Roisen FJ, Bartfeld H, Donnenfeld H, Baxter J. *Muscle Nerve* 1982; **5**: 48–53.

11. Horwich MS, Engel WK, Chauvin PB. Amyotrophic lateral sclerosis sera applied to cultured motor neurons. *Arch Neurol* 1974; **30**: 332–333.

12. Liveson J, Frey H, Bornstein MB. The effect of serum from ALS patients on organotypic nerve and muscle tissue cultures. *Acta Neuropathol* 1975; **32**: 127–131.

13. Ecob MS, Brown AE, Young C et al. Is there a circulating neurotoxic factor in motor neurone disease? In: Clifford-Rose F, ed. *Research Progress in Motor Neurone Disease.* London: Pitman, 1984, 249–254.

14. Smith RG, Alexianu ME, Crawford G et al. Cytotoxicity of immunoglobulins from amyotrophic lateral sclerosis patients on a hybrid motoneuron cell line. *Proc Natl Acad Sci U S A* 1994; **91**: 3393–3397.

15. Stoppini L, Buchs PA, Muller DJ. A simple method for organotypic cultures of nervous tissue. *Neurosci Methods* 1991; **37**: 173.

16. Rothstein JD, Dykes-Hoberg M, Kuncl RW. Chronic glutamate uptake inhibition produces a model of slow neurotoxicity. *Proc Natl Acad Sci U S A* 1993; **90**: 6591–6595.

17. Rothstein JD, Bristol LA, Hosler B et al. Chronic inhibition of superoxide dismutase produces apoptotic death of spinal neurons. *Proc Natl Acad Sci U S A* 1994; **91**: 4155–4159.

18. Phelps PE, Baraber RP, Houser CR et al. Postnatal development of neurons containing choline acetyl transferase in rat spinal cord: an immunohistochemical study. *J Comp Neurol* 1984; **229**: 347–361.

19. Drachman DB, Fishman PS, Rothstein JD et al. Amyotrophic lateral sclerosis: an autoimmune disease? In: Serratrice G, Munsat T, eds. *Advances in Neurology.* Philadelphia: Lippincott–Raven, 1995, 59–65.

20. Mulder DW, Lambert EH, Eaton LM. Myasthenic syndrome in patients with amyotrophic lateral sclerosis. *Neurology* 1959; **9**: 627–631.

21. Denys EH, Norris FH. Amyotrophic lateral sclerosis: impairment of neuromuscular transmission. *Arch Neurol* 1979; **36**: 202–205.

22. Bernstein LP, Antel JP. Motor neuron disease: decremental responses to repetitive nerve stimulation. *Neurology* 1981; **31**: 204–207.

23. Maselli RA, Wollman RL, Leung C et al. Neuromuscular transmission in amyotrophic lateral sclerosis. *Muscle Nerve* 1993; **16**: 1193–1203.

24. Garcia J, Engelhardt JI, Appel SH et al. Increased MEPP frequency as an early sign of experimental immune mediated motor neuron disease. *Ann Neurol* 1990; **28**: 329–334.

25. Uchitel OD, Appel SH, Crawford F et al. Immunoglobulins from amyotrophic lateral sclerosis patients enhance spontaneous transmitter release from motor-nerve terminals. *Proc Natl Acad Sci U S A* 1998; **85**:

7371–7374.

26. Appel SH, Engelhardt JI, Garcia J et al. Immunoglobulins from animal models of motor neuron disease and from human amyotrophic lateral sclerosis patients passively transfer physiological abnormalities to the neuromuscular junction. *Proc Natl Acad Sci U S A* 1991; **88**: 647–651.

27. O'Shaughnessy TJ, Yan H, Kim J et al. Amyotrophic lateral sclerosis: serum factors enhance spontaneous and evoked transmitter release at the neuromuscular junction. *Muscle Nerve* 1998; **21**: 81–90.

28. Birnbaumer L, Campbell KP, Catterall WA et al. The naming of voltage-gated calcium channels. *Neuron* 1994; **13**: 505–506.

29. Delbono O, Garcia J, Appel SH et al. Calcium current and charge movement of mammalian muscle: action of amyotrophic lateral sclerosis immunoglobulins. *J Physiol* 1991; **444**: 723–742.

30. Smith RG, Hamilton S, Hofmann F et al. Serum antibodies to L-type calcium channels in patients with amyotrophic lateral sclerosis. *N Engl J Med* 1992; **327**: 1721–1728.

31. Llinas R, Sugimore M, Cherksey BD et al. IgG from amyotrophic lateral sclerosis patients increases current through P-type calcium channels in mammalian cerebellar Purkinje cells and in isolated channel protein in lipid bilayer. *Proc Natl Acad Sci U S A* 1993; **90**: 11743–11747.

32. Mosier DR, Baldelli P, Delbono O et al. Amyotrophic lateral sclerosis immunoglobulins increase Ca^{2+} currents in a motoneuron cell line. *Ann Neurol* 1995; **37**: 102–109.

33. Motomura M, Johnston I, Lang B et al. An improved diagnostic assay for Lambert–Eaton myasthenic syndrome. *J Neurol Neurosurg Psychiatry* 1995; **58**: 85–87.

34. Lennon VA, Kryzer TJ, Griesmann GE et al. Calcium channel antibodies in the Lambert–Eaton myasthenic syndrome and other paraneoplastic syndromes. *N Engl J Med* 1995; **332**: 1467–1474.

35. Arsac C, Raymond C, Martin-Moutot N et al. Immunoassays fail to detect antibodies against neuronal calcium channels in amyotrophic lateral sclerosis serum. *Ann Neurol* 1996; **40**: 695–700.

36. Vincent A, Drachman DB. Amyotrophic lateral sclerosis and antibodies to voltage-gated calcium channels: new doubts. *Ann Neurol* 1996; **40**: 691–693.

37. Zhainazarov AB, Annunziata P, Toneatto S et al. Serum fractions from amyotrophic lateral sclerosis patients depress voltage-activated Ca^{2+} currents of rat cerebellar granule cells in culture. *Neurosci Lett* 1994; **172**: 111–114.

38. Schanne FAX, Kane AB, Young EE et al. Calcium dependence of toxic cell death: a final common pathway. *Science* 1979; **206**: 700–702.

39. Choi DW. Calcium-mediated neurotoxicity: relationship to specific channel types and role in ischemic damage. *Trends Neurosci* 1988; **11**: 465–467.

40. Rothstein JD. Excitotoxic mechanisms in the pathogenesis of amyotrophic lateral sclerosis. *Adv Neurol* 1995; **68**: 7–20.

41. Siklos L, Engelhardt J, Harati Y et al. Ultrastructural evidence for altered calcium in motor nerve terminals in amyotrophic lateral sclerosis. *Ann Neurol* 1996; **39**: 203–216.

42. Engelhardt JI, Siklos L, Komuves L et al. Antibodies to calcium channels from ALS patients passively transferred to mice selectively increase intracellular calcium and induce ultrastructural changes in motoneurons. *Synapse* 1995; **20**: 185–199.

43. Peters HA, Clotanoff DV. Spinal muscular atrophy secondary to macroglobulinemia: reversal with chlorambucil therapy. *Neurology* 1968; **18**: 101–108.

44. Bauer M, Bergstrom R, Ritter B et al. Macroglobulinemia Waldenstrom and motor neuron syndrome. *Acta Neurol Scand* 1977; **55**: 245–250.

45. Latov N. Plasma cell dyscrasia and motor neuron disease. In: Rowland LP, ed. *Human Motor Neuron Diseases*. New York: Raven, 1982, 273–279.

46. Krieger C, Melmed C. Amyotrophic lateral sclerosis and paraproteinemia. *Neurology* 1982; **32**: 896–898.

47. Patten BM. Neuropathy and motor neuron syndromes associated with plasma cell disease. *Acta Neurol Scand* 1984; **70**: 47–61.

48. Shy ME, Rowland LP, Smith T et al. Motor neuron disease and plasma cell dyscrasia. *Neu-*

rology 1986; **36**: 1429–1436.

49. Parry GJ, Holtz SJ, Ben Zeev D et al. Gammopathy with proximal motor axonopathy simulating motor neuron disease. *Neurology* 1986; **36**: 273–276.

50. Rudnicki S, Chad DA, Drachman DA et al. Motor neuron disease and paraproteinemia. *Neurology* 1987; **37**: 335–337.

51. Rowland LP, Defendini R, Sherman W et al. Macroglobulinemia with peripheral neuropathy simulating motor neuron disease. *Ann Neurol* 1981; **11**: 532–536.

52. Latov N, Hays AP, Donofrio PE et al. Monoclonal IgM with unique specificity to gangliosides GM1 and GD1b and to lacto-*N*-tetraose associated with human motor neuron disease. *Neurology* 1998; **38**: 763–768.

53. Freddo L, Yu RK, Latov N et al. Gangliosides GM1 and GD1b are antigens for IgM M-protein in a patient with motor neuron disease. *Neurology* 1986; **36**: 454–458.

54. Rowland LP. Amyotrophic lateral sclerosis with paraproteins and autoantibodies. In: Serratrice G, Munsat T, eds. *Advances in Neurology*. Philadelphia: Lippincott–Raven, 1995, 93–105.

55. Willison HJ, Chancellor AM, Patterson G et al. Anti-glycolipid antibodies, immunoglobulins, and paraproteins in motor neuron disease: a population-based case-control study. *J Neurol Sci* 1993; **114**: 209–215.

56. Kornberg AJ, Pestronk A. Chronic motor neuropathies: diagnosis, therapy, and pathogenesis. *Ann Neurol* 1995; **37** (**suppl 1**): S43–S50.

57. Pestronk A, Adams RN, Cornblath D et al. Patterns of serum antibodies to GM1 and GD1a gangliosides in ALS. *Ann Neurol* 1989; **25**: 98–102.

58. Endo T, Scott DD, Stewart SS et al. Antibodies to glycosphingolipids in patients with multiple sclerosis and SLE. *J Immunol* 1994; **132**: 1793–1797.

59. Drachman DB, Chaudhry V, Cornblath D et al. Trial of immunosuppression in amyotrophic lateral sclerosis using total lymphoid irradiation. *Ann Neurol* 1994; **35**: 142–150.

60. Kinsella LJ, Lange DJ, Trojaborg W et al. Clinical and electrophysiological correlates of elevated anti-GM1 antibody titers. *Neurology* 1994; **44**: 1278–1282.

61. Oldstone MBA, Perrin LH, Wilson CB et al. Evidence for immune-complex formation in patients with amyotrophic lateral sclerosis. *Lancet* 1976; **2**: 269–272.

62. Westarp ME, Bartmann P, Kornhuber HH. Immunoglobulin-G isotype changes in human sporadic amyotrophic lateral sclerosis (ALS). *Neurosci Lett* 1994; **173**: 124–126.

63. Behan PO, Behan WMH. Are immune factors involved in motor neurone disease? In: Clifford-Rose F, ed. *Research Progress in Motor Neurone Disease*. London: Pitman, 1984, 405–411.

64. Ben Younes-Chennoufi A, Rozier A, Dib M et al. Anti-sulfoglucuronyl paragloboside IgM antibodies in amyotrophic lateral sclerosis. *J Neuroimmunol* 1995; **57**: 111–115.

65. Sakoda S, Azuma T, Mizumo R et al. A novel antineuronal antibody in serum and CSF of a patient with motor neuron disease. *Eur Neurol* 1991; **31**: 430–433.

66. Conradi S, Ronnevi LO. Selective vulnerability of alpha motor neurons in ALS: relation to antibodies towards acetylcholinesterase (AChE) in ALS patients. *Brain Res Bull* 1993; **30**: 369–371.

67. Ordonez G, Sotelo J. Antibodies against fetal muscle proteins in serum from patients with amyotrophic lateral sclerosis. *Neurology* 1989; **39**: 683–686.

68. Greiner A, Marx A, Muller-Hermelink HK et al. Vascular autoantibodies in amyotrophic lateral sclerosis. *Lancet* 1992; **340**: 378–379.

69. Engelhardt JI, Appel SH. Motor neuron reactivity of sera from animals with autoimmune models of motor neuron destruction. *J Neurol Sci* 1990; **96**: 333–352.

70. Engelhardt JI, Appel SH. IgG reactivity in the spinal cord and motor cortex in amyotrophic lateral sclerosis. *Arch Neurol* 1990; **47**: 1210–1216.

71. Fishman PS, Drachman DB. Internalization of IgG in motoneurons of patients with ALS: selective or nonselective? *Neurology* 1995; **45**: 1551–1554.

72. Fishman PS, Farrand DA, Kristt DA. Penetration and internalization of plasma proteins in the human spinal cord. *J Neurol Sci* 1991; **104**: 166–175.

73. Keyser JW. *Human Plasma Proteins: Their*

Investigation in Pathological Conditions 2nd edn. New York: Wiley, 1987, 426–428.

74. Roberts M, Willison HJ, Vincent A, Newsom-Davis J. Multifocal motor neuropathy human sera block distal motor nerve conduction in mice. *Ann Neurol* 1995; **38**: 111–118.

75. Newsom-Davis J. Effects of human mono-clonal anti-GM1 ganglioside antibodies derived from multifocal motor neuropathy patients block distal motor nerve conduction. *Proceedings of the VIII International Congress on Neuromuscular Disease.* World Federation of Neurology, Research Group on Neuromuscular Disease. Kyoto, Japan, 10–15 July 1994.

76. Brain WR, Croft PB, Wilkinson M. Motor neurone disease as a manifestation of neoplasm (with a note on the course of classical motor neurone disease). *Brain* 1965; **88**: 479–500.

77. Norris FH Jr, Engel WK. Carcinomatous amy-otrophic lateral sclerosis. In: Brain WR, Norris FH Jr, eds. *The Remote Effects of Cancer on the Nervous System.* New York: Grune and Stratton, 1965, 24–34.

78. Rowland LP. Paraneoplastic primary lateral sclerosis and amyotrophic lateral sclerosis. *Ann Neurol* 1977; **41**: 703–705.

79. Rowland LP, Schneck SA. Neuromuscular dis-orders associated with malignant neoplastic disorders. *J Chron Dis* 1963; **16**: 777–795.

80. Schold SC, Cho ES, Sonasundaram M et al. Subacute motor neuronopathy: a remote effect of lymphoma. *Ann Neurol* 1979; **5**: 271–287.

81. Louis ED, Hanley AE, Brannagan TH et al. Motor neuron disease, lymphoproliferative dis-ease and bone marrow biopsy. *Muscle Nerve* 1996; **19**: 1334–1337.

82. Forsyth PA, Dalmau J, Graus F et al. Motor neuron syndromes in cancer patients. *Ann Neurol* 1997; **41**: 722–730.

83. Norris FH, Denys EH, Mielke CH. Plasma-pheresis in amyotrophic lateral sclerosis. In: Dau PC, ed. *Plasmapheresis and the Immuno-biology of Myasthenia Gravis.* Boston, Massa-chussets: Houghton–Mifflin, 1979, 258–264.

84. Kelemen J, Hedlund W, Orlin JB et al. Plasma-pheresis with immunosuppression in amy-otrophic lateral sclerosis. *Arch Neurol* 1986; **40**: 752–753.

85. Brown RH, Hauser SL, Harrington H et al. Failure of immunosuppression with a 10–14 day course of high-dose intravenous cyclophos-phamide to alter the progression of amy-otrophic lateral sclerosis. *Arch Neurol* 1986; **43**: 383–384.

86. Tan E, Lynn DJ, Amato AA et al. Immunosup-pressive treatment of motor neuron syndromes. Attempts to distinguish a treatable disorder. *Arch Neurol* 1994; **52**: 230–231.

87. Appel SH, Stewart SS, Appel V et al. A double blind study of the effectiveness of cyclosporine in amyotrophic lateral sclerosis. *Arch Neurol* 1988; **45**: 381–386.

88. Drachman DB, Chaudhry V, Cornblath D et al. Trial of immunosuppression in amyotrophic lateral sclerosis using total lymphoid irradia-tion. *Ann Neurol* 1994; **35**: 142–150.

89. Pestronk A, Adams RN, Kuncl RW et al. Dif-ferential effects of prednisone and cyclophos-phamideon autoantibodies in human neuromuscular disorders. *Neurology* 1989; **39**: 628–633.

90. Eisen A. Amyotrophic lateral sclerosis: a multi-factorial disease. In: Serratrice GT, Munsat TL, eds. *Advances in Neurology.* Philadelphia: Lip-pincott–Raven, 1995, 121–134.

19

Neurofilament and familial amyotrophic lateral sclerosis-linked mutant copper–zinc superoxide dismutase-mediated motor neuron degeneration: insights from transgenic mouse models

Lucie I Bruijn, Toni L Williamson, Mark W Becher, Donald L Price and Don W Cleveland

Introduction

Amyotrophic lateral sclerosis (ALS), the most common form of adult motor neuron disease in humans, is a progressive neurodegenerative disorder resulting from the selective dysfunction and loss of large motor neurons in the motor cortex, brainstem, and spinal cord, which in turn causes atrophy of the skeletal muscles, ultimately culminating in paralysis and death.[1,2] Between 5 and 10% of ALS cases are familial, inherited in an autosomal-dominant manner. The mechanisms leading to degeneration of motor neurons in familial and sporadic ALS are not clearly understood. One of the most frequently described pathological findings in ALS is the presence of aberrant neurofilament accumulations in the perikarya and proximal axons of motor neurons.[3–5] The only known cause to date, accounting for 20% of familial ALS cases, is the presence of mis-sense mutations[6] in the metalloenzyme copper–zinc superoxide dismutase (SOD1). How these mutations lead to motor neuron death is still unknown. This chapter focuses on recent studies that have examined possible mechanisms involved in motor neuron degeneration through the use of transgenic mouse models, with specific emphasis on the role

that neurofilaments and familial ALS-linked mutants in SOD1 play in disease progression.

Clinical pathology

ALS typically afflicts adults in mid-life and usually begins asymmetrically. The disease is characterized by selective failure, degeneration, and death of the lower motor neurons in the brainstem and spinal cord, which leads to generalized weakness, muscle atrophy, and loss of upper motor neurons in the cortex, which in turn leads to spasticity and hyper-reflexia. In contrast, Onuf's nuclei in the sacral cord and motor neurons that control eye movements are relatively spared. Motor neuron loss is accompanied by reactive gliosis;[7] intracytoplasmic neurofilament abnormalities and axonal spheroids;[3,5,89] ubiquitin-positive inclusions;[10] and apparent fragmentation of the Golgi apparatus.[11] In end-stage disease there is a significant loss of large myelinated fibers in corticospinal tracts and ventral roots, as well as evidence of Wallerian degeneration and atrophy of axonal myelinated fibers.[1] Although non-motor neuron systems, including dorsal root ganglia and sensory nerves, are relatively spared, ALS patients maintained on respirators for long periods of time show multi-system degeneration of Clarke's dorsal nuclei, the spinocerebellar tracts, the posterior column, and the substantia nigra.[12,13]

Neurofilaments and motor neuron degeneration

The molecular basis for the selective vulnerability of subsets of neurons to disease remains one of the most puzzling aspects of ALS. A possible explanation focuses on the cytoarchitecture of these highly asymmetric neurons (*Fig. 19.1a*), which have cell body sizes typical for an animal cell (about 50 μm in diameter) but whose axons may extend to more than 1 m in length (e.g. in the human sciatic nerve). The most abundant structural proteins in the neurons are neurofilaments, the major intermediate (10 nm) filaments in many types of

mature neurons (see *Fig. 19.1b*). These filaments are assembled from three polypeptide subunits, neurofilament (NF)-L (68 kDa), NF-M (95 kDa) and NF-H (115 kDa). NF-L is required for filament assembly under physiological conditions both in vitro[14,15] and in vivo.[16,17] NF-M and NF-H have long tail domains that extend from the surface of the filament and establish the interactions that neurofilaments have with each other and with other axonal components. A filament–filament spacing of approximately 50 nm is found in the myelinated portion of axons (the internodes), where NF-M and NF-H are fully phosphorylated, whereas spacing drops to 30 nm in the unmyelinated portions (both in the initial segment and at nodes) (see *Fig. 19.1a*).

Since the initial visualization of neurofilaments by silver staining in the late 19th century, mounting evidence has pointed to the importance of neurofilaments in specifying the

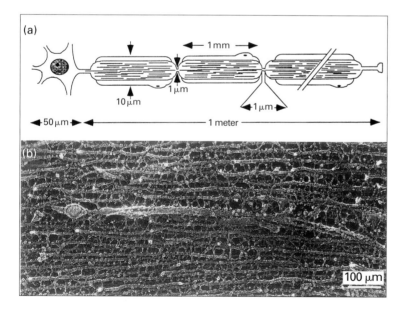

Figure 19.1
Structure of axoplasm. (a) Schematic representation of the structural features and asymmetry of a human motor neuron. The enlarged portion shows neurofilament arrays in the 10 μm diameter internodes (myelinated by single Schwann cells) and in the 1 μm diameter nodes (unmyelinated). Phosphorylation of tail domains of NF-M and NF-H is restricted to myelinated segments. (b) Quick-freeze, deep-etch view of the cytoplasm of a myelinated axon from a rat sciatic nerve. A single (25 nm) microtubule is seen in the center; all the remaining filaments (10 nm) are neurofilaments. (Micrograph kindly provided by N Hirokawa.)

diameter (caliber) of large myelinated axons,[18–23] itself a crucial determinant of conduction velocity through axons.[22] Early correlative studies showed a linear relationship between neurofilament number and the cross-sectional area throughout normal radial growth and during regrowth after axonal injury. The fact that neurofilaments are a primary influence, and not a consequence, of axonal caliber has been proven unequivocally with the identification of a recessive point mutant (named quiver or Quv) in a Japanese quail that accumulates no neurofilaments in axons. The one nucleotide mutation causes premature translation termination in NF-L,[24] resulting in no detectable NF-L protein, total absence of neurofilaments, and axons that almost completely fail to grow radially.[21] This has also been demonstrated in mice, either by disruption of the NF-L gene[23] or by expressing a NF-H β-galactosidase fusion polypeptide[18] that blocks transport of all neurofilaments into axons.

A functional role for NF-M is uncertain, although raising its concentration in transgenic mouse models has led to the proposal that it contributes to setting nearest neighbor spacing between filaments.[25] For NF-H, much interest has been focused on the 610 amino acid-long tail domain that projects from the central core of the filaments.[26–28] In humans, the tail contains 43[29] or 44[30] lysine–serine–proline (KSP) repeats that are heavily phosphorylated on serine.[31] This phosphorylation is found almost exclusively in myelinated axonal segments and correlates with wider filament spacing.[32–34]

The idea that aberrant accumulation of neurofilaments may play a role in disease progression was first suggested by the discovery that accumulation and abnormal assembly of neurofilaments are common pathological hallmarks in several types of neurodegenerative diseases, including sporadic ALS[3,8,35] and familial ALS[5] (*Fig. 19.2a*), infantine spinal muscular atrophy[37] and hereditary sensory–motor neuropathy. A central question has been whether aberrant accumulations of neurofilaments are merely byproducts of the pathogenic process or whether they contribute to the process of motor neuron degeneration. Direct evidence that neurofilamentous accumulations can cause motor neuron disease emerged from the expression in transgenic mice of three or four times the normal level of NF-L[37] or wild-type human NF-H. Both sets of mice have large accumulations of perikaryal neurofilaments, which leads to swollen cell bodies with eccentrically located nuclei (see *Fig. 19.2b*), similar to aberrant neurofilament accumulations seen in humans (see *Fig. 19.2a*). Neurofilament accumulations are accompanied by proximal axon swellings, motor neuron dysfunction, and atrophy of skeletal muscle. However, unlike in human ALS, these mice do not exhibit extensive motor neuron death.[37,38]

To examine directly whether aberrant neurofilament subunits could be a direct cause of motor neuron disease, several lines of transgenic mice were constructed to express a point mutation at the end of the rod domain of NF-L.[39] Since mutations in keratins, the intermediate filament proteins of skin, were known to cause dominantly inherited skin blistering diseases,[40–42] a mutation analogous to one of the frequently occurring keratin mutations was engineered into the end of the conserved helical region of the mouse NF-L subunit. Expression of the mutant protein at levels appropriate for a dominantly inherited disease does yield selective motor neuron death (and progressive disease) that is reminiscent of ALS.[39] Transgenic mice showed abnormal gait, reduced activity, and weakness in both upper and lower limbs as early as 18 days after birth. These abnormalities progressively increased in

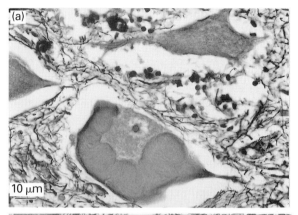

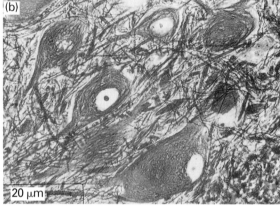

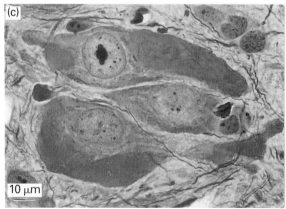

Figure 19.2
Misaccumulation of neurofilaments in motor neurons in motor neuron disease. Silver-stained, high-power view of motor neurons in the anterior horn in (a) a case of rapidly progressing ALS, (b) a transgenic mouse model that develops a rapidly progression neuronopathy from expressing wild-type NF-L at four times the normal level, and (c) a transgenic mouse that expresses a level of an NF-L mutant appropriate for a dominantly inherited disease. ((a) kindly provided by A Hirano.[97] (b) is reproduced with permission from Xu et al.[37])

severity and, in most lines, progressed to death. Prominent neurofilament-rich swellings could be seen by silver staining in motor neuron cell bodies and proximal axons (see *Fig. 19.2c*).

Since these findings proved that neurofilament mutants can cause motor neuron degeneration in mice, it was plausible that neurofilament mutations might be responsible for some ALS cases. Early efforts focused on the 80% of familial ALS not arising from SOD1 mutation, but did not identify neurofilament mutants. Subsequent efforts examining the repetitive tail domain of the large neurofilament subunit NF-H[43–45] have now identified a set of small in-frame deletions or insertions in ~1% of more than 1300 ALS patients, almost all of which appear in 'sporadic' cases. Excluding family members not yet affected, no similar mutants have been seen in a comparable number of control DNAs. Search of this one domain alone has thus yielded mutations in the overall patient population about half as frequent as SOD1 mutants. It should be realized that variation in timing of disease onset and incomplete penetrance can befuddle identifying an underlying genetic component. While the neurofilament sequence variants are surely not by themselves capable of provoking disease with high penetrance, the collective evidence now strongly hints that variants in neurofilaments are, at the least, important risk factors for apparently sporadic disease. It should be borne in mind that these apparent mutations add further weight to the possibility that indirect damage to neurofilaments can be involved.

SOD1 mutations in ALS

The only proven primary cause of ALS is the presence of missense mutations in the ubiquitously expressed, intracellular enzyme SOD1, which is now known to underlie about 20% of familial ALS. More than 45 such mutations have been reported.[46,47] SOD1 consists of 153 amino acids and is encoded by a 15 kb gene comprising five exons on chromosome 21. It is a homodimer with a β-barrel structure containing a central copper ion (*Fig. 19.3a*) that is essential for enzymatic activity through its alternating reduction and oxidation by superoxide. The superoxide dismutases (copper–zinc cytosolic SOD1, manganese-dependent mitochondrial SOD2, and copper–zinc extracellular SOD3) form part of a free radical scavenger system, catalysing the dismutation of superoxide anions into hydrogen peroxide and oxygen.[48,49] Superoxide, generally thought to arise predominantly from mitochondrial errors in oxidative phosphorylation, has itself been proposed to cause oxidative degradation of DNA, lipids, and proteins. SOD1 is very abundant in nervous tissue and immunolocalization studies have demonstrated that SOD1 is present in many populations of neurons, especially motor neurons.[50,51]

A toxic property, not increased or decreased activity, of familial ALS-linked SOD1 mutants causes disease

A long series of earlier studies indicating that SOD1 possesses neuroprotective activities fueled the initial hypothesis[52,53] that SOD1-linked familial ALS results from free radical damage caused by diminished superoxide scavenging activity. Diminished SOD1 activity is associated with increased neuronal death in several culture systems.[54,55] Moreover, initial measurements of SOD1 activity levels in patients who had familial ALS with SOD1 mutations showed reductions of dismutase activity in a variety of cells and tissues, including red blood cells,[52,53] lymphocytes, and brain.[52,53,56]

Despite this early focus on loss of activity as the mechanism underlying human disease, subsequent in vitro studies demonstrated that familial ALS mutations vary in their effects on enzymatic activity and that, at least in some instances (such as the substitution of arginine for glycine at position 37 — SOD1[G37R]), the

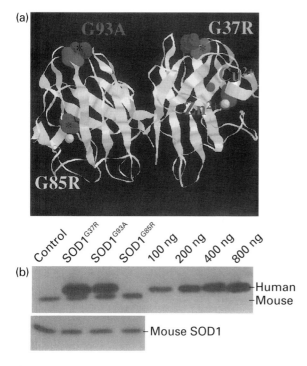

(a)

(b)

Figure 19.3

SOD1 mutations and ALS. (a) Schematic representation of the homodimeric enzyme SOD1 showing the positions of the catalytic copper, the bound zinc atom, and the human mutations SOD1[G37R], SOD1[G93A], and SOD1[G85R], which have been proven to produce ALS-like motor neuron disease when expressed in mice. (b) Immunoblot analysis showing mutant SOD1 (upper panel) and the unaltered endogenous mouse SOD1 levels (lower panel) in spinal cord extracts of transgenic mice SOD1[G37R]-, SOD1[G93A]-, and SOD1[G85R]-expressing familial ALS-linked SOD1 mutants.

transgenic mouse models that express human SOD1 with familial ALS-linked mutations, SOD1[G93A], SOD1[G37R], and SOD1[G85R] (*Fig. 18.3a*), as well as one transgenic mouse model expressing mutant mouse SOD1[G86R] (corresponding to human SOD1[G85R]). All of these mice develop severe hind limb weakness despite normal or highly elevated SOD1 activity levels. Accumulated protein levels of mutant human SOD1[G37R] vary from five-fold (in the lowest expressing SOD1[G37R] line) to 12-fold endogenous mouse SOD1 (see *Fig. 19.3b*) in the highest expressing line. Similarly, mutant SOD1 protein levels in the SOD1[G93A] line[59] are six-fold that of endogenous mouse SOD1 (see *Fig. 19.3b*), whereas much lower levels of accumulated mutant can provoke progressive motor neuron disease in mice expressing SOD1[G85R] (varying from 0.2 times to equal to endogenous mouse SOD1; see *Fig. 19.3b*). (Note that unlike SOD1[G93A] and SOD1[G85R], which migrate with lower electrophoretic mobilities than mouse SOD1, SOD1[G85R] co-migrates under these conditions with mouse SOD1.) Levels of RNA in the various transgenic lines are similar for the three different mutations, supporting in vitro evidence that mutants vary in their protein stability.[59]

Using antibodies and activity gels that distinguish the mouse SOD1 from human SOD1, it can be seen that disease in all of these mice arises despite a normal level of the wild-type mouse SOD1 (see *Fig. 19.3c*). Reducing or eliminating wild-type SOD1 by disrupting one or both of the alleles that encode SOD1 indicates that copper–zinc SOD1 is not required for normal development of mice and does not result in motor neuron disease,[60] a finding that is inconsistent with familial ALS arising from a loss of SOD1 activity. Furthermore, since multiple lines of mice expressing wild-type SOD1 at up to 10 times the level of endoge-

mutant enzyme retains full specific activity.[57] Moreover, only a modest reduction in the abundance of the SOD1[G37R] polypeptide is observed in lymphocytes from patients, and the mutant polypeptide in the human sample is fully active.[57]

The most compelling evidence for the gain of a toxic property comes from a series of nous SOD1 in spinal cord do not develop any detectable phenotype, the collective data prove that neither loss nor increase in SOD1 activity mediates disease in familial ALS-linked SOD1 mutant mice. Rather, disease in these mice must derive from one or more aberrant (toxic) properties of the mutant subunits. Indeed, since neither age at disease onset nor duration of disease correlates with SOD1 activity in patient samples,[61] this is almost certainly also the situation in human disease.

Prominent vacuolar pathology seen in SOD1^{G93A} and SOD1^{G37R} transgenic mice

To examine how familial ALS-linked mutants are toxic to motor neurons, the progression of pathologic abnormalities was followed in affected mice of different ages. In 2-month-old transgenic mice expressing the SOD1^{G93A} mutation, a striking and unexpected finding was the presence of prominent membrane-bounded structures, referred to as vacuoles, primarily in the perikarya of motor neurons.[62] As disease progresses, motor neurons decrease in number and pathological alterations, including grossly distended axonal swellings, spread into the neurophil, which becomes crowded with axonal and dendritic vacuoles of various dimensions (*Fig. 19.4a*). Similar membrane-bound vacuolar inclusions are also prominent in axons of transgenic mice that express SOD1^{G37R} mutant protein[63] and are apparent as early as 5 weeks of age (see *Fig. 19.4b*). As disease progresses, vacuoles in SOD1^{G37R} mice become more prominent in both dendrites and axons, with multiple vacuoles often occupying almost the entirety of the axoplasm (see *Fig. 19.4c*). In contrast to the perikarya of SOD1^{G93A} mice, the perikarya

of SOD1^{G37R} are relatively spared throughout disease.

Examination of vacuoles of all three neuronal compartments at the electron microscopic level reveals that many vacuoles in both SOD1^{G93A} and SOD1^{G37R} mice (see *Fig. 19.4c*) appear to derive from mitochondria in varying stages of degeneration (see *Fig. 19.4d*). Mitochondria in the processes of the majority of non-motor neurons and in adjacent non-neuronal cells (i.e. glia) are uniformly unaffected. Indeed, careful analysis of the disease stages in SOD1^{G93A} mice shows a correlation between decline in muscle strength and an increase in vacuoles derived from degenerating mitochondria.[64] At end-stage disease in both SOD1^{G93A} and SOD1^{G937R} mice, there is a marked reduction in the number of motor neurons in the lumbar spinal cord, extensive wallerian degeneration of large myelinated axons at the level of the ventral root exit zone and the motor nerve roots, and denervation atrophy of muscle.[63,65]

Lewy body-like inclusions in both astrocytes and neurons in transgenic mice expressing SOD1^{G85R}

Unlike the situation for the SOD^{G37R} and SOD^{G93A} mice, the most striking finding in transgenic mice that express human SOD1^{G85R} is the presence of numerous inclusions[66] with a dense central core and a clear peripheral halo that is observable by conventional staining with hematoxylin and eosin (*Figs 19.5a* and *19.5b*). These Lewy body-like inclusions are present in both astrocytes (as determined by the presence of glial fibrillary acidic protein (GFAP); see *Fig. 19.5a*) and neurons (see *Fig. 19.5c*) and are highly immunoreactive for SOD1 (see *Figs 19.5b* and *19.5d*). The periphery of inclusions (see *Fig. 19.5e*) is also

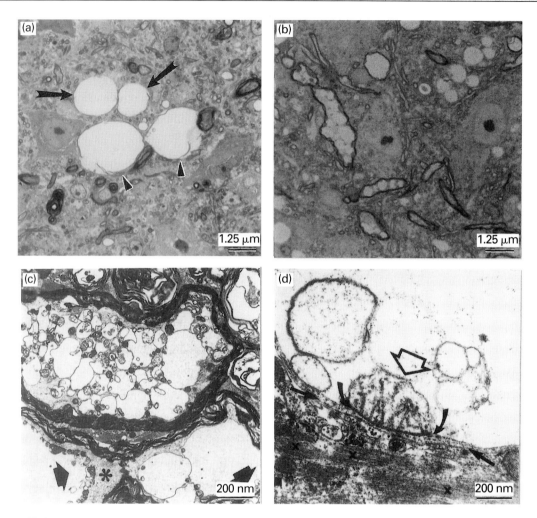

Figure 19.4

Vacuolar accumulations in the spinal cords of transgenic mice expressing familial ALS-linked SOD1 mutants. Ventral horn region of the lumbar spinal cord of end-stage mice expressing (a) the SOD1[G93A] mutation[58] or (b) the SOD1[G37R] mutation. The arrows in (a) point to dendritic vacuoles, as judged by the absence of obvious myelin. The arrowheads in (a) point to large axonal vacuoles with visible remnants of myelin. (c) Swollen axons, some with axoplasmic vesicles (as indicated by the arrows) in the anterior horn and anterior root of a transgenic mouse expressing the SOD1[G37R] mutation.[63] (d) Higher magnification of axons from (c) showing that vacuoles apparently originate from degenerating mitochondria. (Reproduced with permission from Wong et al.[63])

immunoreactive for ubiquitin (see *Fig. 19.5f*). Although no autopsy material is available for familial cases with the SOD1[G85R] mutation (T Siddique and T Siddique, personal commu-

nication), neuronal SOD1-positive inclusions have been described in some familial ALS patients with mutation SOD1[A4V],[67] and inclusions with similar SOD1 immunoreactivity in

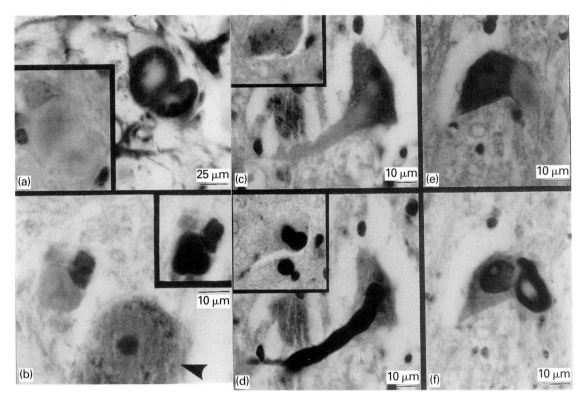

Figure 19.5

Striking presence of astroglial and neuronal inclusions in transgenic mice expressing mutant SOD1^{G85R}. (a) Lewy body-like cytoplasmic inclusions in astrocytes (inset), consisting of a pale periphery and dense central core, seen with hematoxylin and eosin staining as one of the earliest pathological findings in a 6-month-old transgenic mouse that expresses SOD1^{G85R}. The astrocytic nature of the cells that contain these inclusions is demonstrated (main figure) by the peripheral, halo-like staining with antibodies to GFAP. (b) Hematoxylin and eosin staining reveals an astrocytic inclusion and (arrowhead) a normal motor neuron in a spinal cord section from a SOD1^{G85R} animal after clinical onset. In the inset, the same astrocyte after destaining and restaining with an antibody recognizing human and mouse SOD1 is shown. (c–f) Neurons from SOD1^{G85R} transgenic animals following clinical onset reveal intracellular inclusions distinguishable by hematoxylin and eosin staining (c) both in cell bodies (c, inset and e) and in processes (c). Destaining and restaining of the same neurons with antibodies to SOD1 (d) or ubiquitin (f) demonstrate that the core of the inclusions are intensely reactive with SOD1 antibodies, whereas only the periphery is reactive with antibodies to ubiquitin (f). (Reproduced with permission from Bruijn et al.[66])

astrocytes have also been reported in a familial ALS patient with a two base pair deletion in the 126th codon of SOD1 leading to a frame shift and truncation of the final 27 amino acids.[68] As seen by electron microscopy, the core consists of a heterogeneous mass of short

(200–300 nm in length), disorganized filaments covered with small granules (about 20 nm in diameter) in which organelles are entrapped, with a less dense and, in some cases, a linear array of filaments (about 10 nm in diameter) at the periphery of the inclusion.[66] Vacuoles such as those in cell bodies, dendrites, and axons of previously reported transgenic mice that express the SOD1[G93A] mutant[62] or the SOD1[G37R] mutant[63] are not seen in transgenic mice that express SOD1[G85R], and mitochondria appear morphologically normal at all stages of disease.

Transgenic mice that express mutant SOD1 as models for motor neuron degeneration in ALS

At first glance, the pathology seen in the transgenic mice that express the SOD1[G85R] mutant appears very different to that in the SOD1[G93A] and SOD1[G37R] mice. This underscores the fact that the striking vacuolar degeneration seen in the latter transgenic mice is not a recognized component of familial or sporadic ALS. A plausible explanation for these differences in pathology could be the overall acceleration of the pathogenic process in mice as a result of highly elevated levels of SOD1[G37R] and SOD1[G93A] mutant protein, which in turn increases the rate of mutant enzyme-mediated damage. Indeed, consistent with this, in the transgenic lines expressing lower levels of the SOD1[G93A] mutant[69] and the SOD1[G37R] mutant (M Becher and DL Price, unpublished data), vacuoles are less conspicuous and inclusions are seen in neurons. Furthermore, although this was not evident from earlier reports,[62,65,70] astrocytic inclusions (*Fig. 19.6a*), as determined by GFAP immunoreactivity (see *Fig. 19.6b*) (similar to those seen in SOD1[G85R]

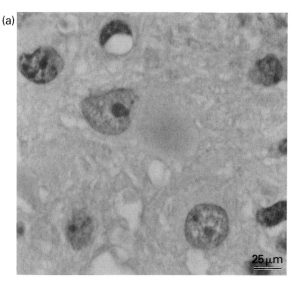

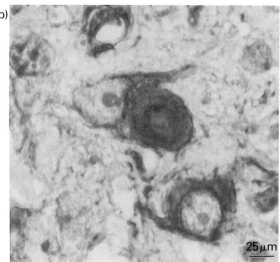

Figure 19.6
Inclusions in astrocytes observed in SOD1[G93A] mice. (a) Lewy body-like cytoplasmic inclusions consisting of a pale periphery and dense central core seen by hematoxylin and eosin staining in an end-stage animal that expresses SOD1[G93A]. (b) The astrocytic nature of the cells that contain these inclusions is demonstrated by the peripheral, halo-like staining with antibodies to glial fibrillary acidic protein.

transgenic mice) are present in both the higher expressing SOD1^{G93A} mice (see *Figs 19.6a* and *19.6b*) as well as in lower expressing lines.[69]

Neurofilament accumulations, a hallmark of the human disease (see *Fig. 19.3a*), are prominent features only of SOD1^{G93A}-mediated disease in mice.[70,71] Silver staining of spinal cord sections reveals intensely staining accumulations in axonal spheroids (*Fig. 19.7a*), which at the electron microscopic level are seen to be masses of filaments[71] similar to those reported in human disease.[9] In SOD1^{G37R} mice (see *Fig. 19.7b*), numerous axonal swellings in the root exit zone are found, but these are composed of clusters of vacuoles around which the neurofilaments are marginated. Neurofilamentous aggregates are only very rarely observed. In SOD1^{G85R} transgenic mice (see *Fig. 19.7c*), axonal swellings are themselves very rare, although the strong staining of these swellings with silver suggests a neurofilamentous character.

At a minimum, it must be concluded that both the overall character of the pathology and the degree of neurofilamentous involvement arising from these three familial ALS-linked SOD1 mutants is surprisingly heterogeneous. Perhaps of most relevance is the finding that it is the large-caliber motor axons (less than 4 μm in diameter) — those that are most enriched in neurofilaments — that are lost during disease in humans (see *Fig. 19.7e*), in mice with a mutation in NF-L (see *Fig. 19.7f*), and in SOD1^{G85R} mice (see *Fig. 19.7d*). In all these cases, the small-diameter, relatively neurofilament-deficient axons, are spared. Indeed, although this has not been reported for the SOD1^{G93A} and SOD1^{G37R} animals, for the SOD1^{G85R} animals, the involvement of large, neurofilament-rich axons is absolute: about 70% of the large-caliber axons are lost during disease progression, but exhaustive examination[66] of ventral roots reveals no degeneration of axons less than 4 μm in diameter (see *Fig. 19.7d*).

Mechanisms of disease
Mutant SOD1-mediated nitration of proteins

Central to understanding the mechanism of mutant SOD1-mediated familial ALS is the identity of the toxic property or properties that lead to motor neuron degeneration. One hypothesis put forward by Beckman and colleagues[72] is that improper folding of the mutant subunits fails to shield the copper co-factor of the enzyme, allowing inappropriate substrates to contact the catalytic copper. Indeed, retention of at least partial copper binding catalysed by the specific copper chaperone for SOD1[73] has been found to be a common feature of several classes of familial ALS-linked SOD1 mutations.[74] The aberrant substrate initially proposed[72] is peroxynitrite ($^-$ONOO) (formed spontaneously from nitric oxide and superoxide anion), which, in the presence of the mutant enzyme, may nitrate tyrosine residues on proteins. Evidence in vivo for accelerated production of nitrotyrosine by the mutant enzymes comes from measurements of elevated free nitrotyrosine in two lines of transgenic mice that express the SOD1^{G37R} mutant[75] (*Fig. 19.8*) and the SOD1^{G93A} mutant.[76] In addition, an antibody to nitrotyrosine has been reported to show a focal increase in reactivity in patients with familial ALS[77,78] and sporadic ALS.[78,79]

However, it must be recognized that direct search for such nitration has produced no in vivo evidence to support neurofilaments (or any other protein target, for that matter) as targets for this aberrant chemistry at any stage of disease in mice.[75]

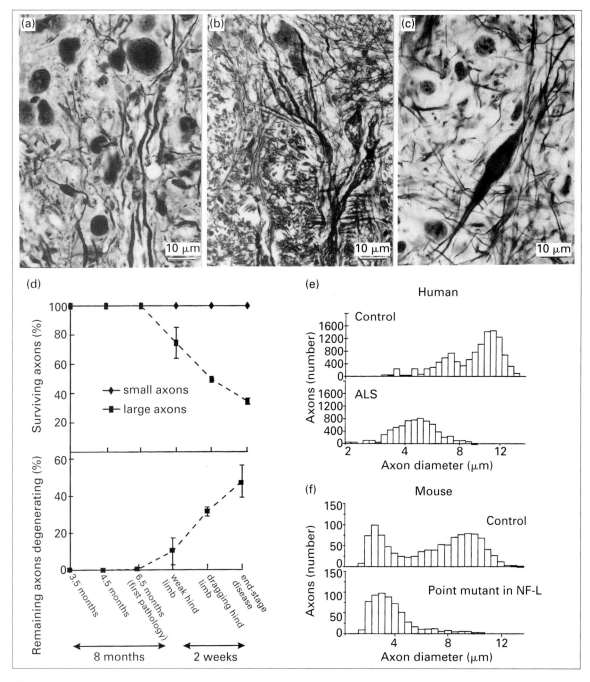

Figure 19.7
Variable incidence of neurofilamentous accumulations caused by mutants SOD1^{G37R}, SOD1^{G93A}, and SOD1^{G85R}. Sections of ventral root exit zones from mice with motor neuron disease caused by expression of mutants (a) SOD1^{G93A}, (b) SOD1^{G37R}, and (c) SOD1^{G85R} stained with silver to highlight neurofilamentous accumulations. Prominent, neurofilament-rich spheroids are seen in (a) SOD1^{G93A}

Moreover, use of genetics to manipulate SOD1 activity levels in mice that develop disease from expression of an SOD1 mutant has demonstrated that the nitration hypothesis is very unlikely to play a central role. In mice that develop disease from expressing a mutant (SOD1^{G85R}) that confers only a ~10% increase in the activity of the endogenous, wild type SOD1, neither elimination nor elevation (by ~6 fold) of wild type SOD1 affected disease onset, progression or pathology.[80] The insensitivity of toxicity to SOD1 activity levels is inconsistent with damage arising from superoxide or any spontaneous reaction product of it (such as $^-$ONOO), since absence of the wild type protein would accelerate toxicity by raising superoxide levels and/or forcing all catalysis through the mutant, while elevating it would do the opposite. This was clearly not the case, at least for the SOD1^{G85R} mutant.

Increased use of hydrogen peroxide by mutant SOD1 leading to production of highly toxic hydroxyl radicals

A second proposal for the nature of the toxic property is that the mutants catalyse the formation of hydroxyl radicals from hydrogen peroxide via the Fenton reaction. Hydroxyl radicals have been proposed to damage a variety of cellular targets, including SOD1, mitochondrial membranes (via lipid peroxidation), and glutamate transporters (via oxidation).[81] In vitro, at least two mutations can increase the rate of hydroxyl radical formation, probably because of increased availability of the active copper site to hydrogen peroxide.[82] Although this is plausible, it is important to realize that only two of the more than 45 mutants (SOD1^{A4V} and SOD1^{G93A}) have been tested for accelerated use of hydrogen peroxide as an aberrant substrate, and both these mutants display only modest increased use relative to wild-type SOD1. Indeed, if, as seems likely, many mutants accumulate to lower in vivo levels than wild-type SOD1, the combination of a modestly elevated rate of usage of hydrogen peroxide and a more significantly reduced level of mutant protein would *reduce* overall SOD1-mediated damage through this pathway. Moreover, no in vivo support for the predicted damage that should accumulate through usage of hydrogen peroxide has yet emerged either in human examples or in the spinal cords of transgenic mice expressing the SOD1^{G37R} mutant[75] or the SOD1^{G93A} mutant[76] using an established hydroxyl spin trap assay.

---

mice, whereas distended axoplasm full of membrane bounded vacuoles are abundantly seen in (b) SOD1^{G37R} mediated disease. (c) Only a rare silver stained axonal swelling is detectable in exhaustive searches through spinal cord sections from SOD1^{G85R} mice. (d, top) Percentage of surviving (both healthy and degenerating) large-caliber (>5 μm) and small-caliber axons in fourth lumbar ventral roots from SOD1^{G85R} transgenic mice, measured at ages before the onset of clinical symptoms (3.5, 4.5, and 6.5 months), at the onset of clinical signs, and at end-stage. A dramatic loss of large-caliber axons is seen, beginning with disease onset; small-caliber axons are unaffected at all ages. (d, bottom) Percentage of remaining large axons actively degenerating. No degeneration was observed in small axons. (e) The selective loss of large-caliber motor neurons in human ALS and (f) in mice that express a point mutant in NF-L. The human data are from Kawamura et al.,39[98] The mouse data are from Lee et al.[40] ((d) reproduced with permission from Bruijn et al.[66])

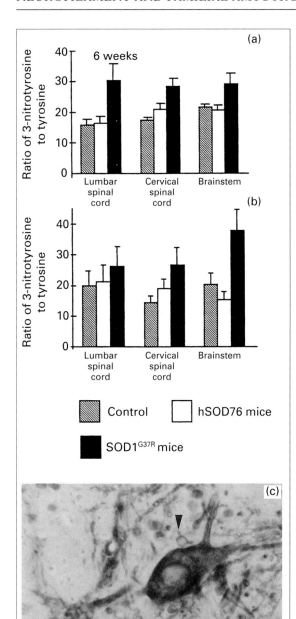

Figure 19.8

Elevated levels of free nitrotyrosine in two lines of mice expressing SOD1^{G37R}. Ratios of 3-nitrotyrosine to tyrosine ($\times 10^{-2}$) were measured in cervical and lumbar spinal cord and the brainstem of control mice, transgenic mice that overexpress wild-type human SOD1 (hSOD76), and transgenic mice that express human mutant SOD1^{G37R} at (a) 6 weeks of age and (b) 20 weeks of age. (c) Early pathology in transgenic mice expressing mutant SOD1^{G37R}.

Immunocytochemistry on a spinal cord section of a 6-week-old SOD1^{G37R} transgenic mouse using antibodies against a phosphorylated determinant on neurofilament proteins. Numerous small vacuoles are evident in processes (marked with arrows) in the spinal cord. (Data and photograph reproduced with permission from Bruijn et al.[75])

Neurofilaments as targets for SOD1-mediated damage

The frequent neurofilamentous misaccumulations found in human disease,[9] including disease caused by SOD1^{A4V} mutants[5,67] and polypeptide sequence variants in the NF-H subunit in a few sporadic ALS patients,[44–46] coupled with neurofilament aggregates in one mouse model of SOD1^{G93A}-mediated disease[70,71] and proof that primary mutation in a neurofilament subunit can cause motor neuron disease in mice,[39] have implicated neurofilaments in ALS pathogenesis, including that mediated by SOD1 mutants. To test more directly how the absence of neurofilaments affects SOD1 mutant-mediated disease, onset and progression, mice deleted for the NF-L gene (the major neurofilament subunit required for filament assembly) were bred with mice that express the SOD1^{G85R} mutant.[83] The absence of neurofilaments slowed disease onset (*Fig. 19.9a*) and produced a significantly increased life span (see *Fig. 19.9b*), with the

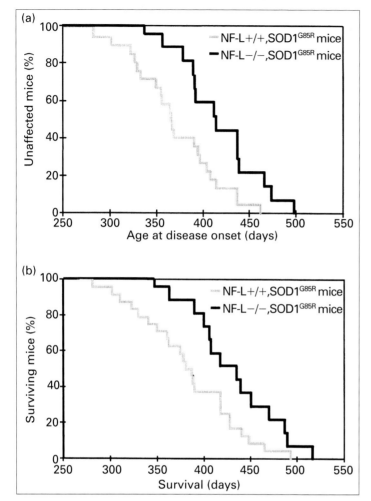

Figure 19.9

Delayed disease onset and extended survival in SOD1^{G85R} mice that lack neurofilaments. Kaplan–Meier curves showing (a) age at onset and (b) survival of SOD1^{G85R} mice in the presence or absence of neurofilaments. (Reproduced with permission from Williamson et al.[83])

average survival of 388 ± 11 days for SOD1^{G85R} mice with a normal level of neurofilaments ($n = 24$) compared with 433 ± 14 days for SOD1^{G85R} mice that lacked neurofilaments ($n = 14$). This slowing of disease onset and lengthening of survival occurred despite the loss, early in life, of about 13% of the normal number of motor neurons as a consequence of chronic absence of neurofilaments. Moreover, absence of neurofilaments also reduced the selectivity of the SOD1 mutant-mediated toxicity for motor neurons.

Although these findings prove that neither axonal or perikaryal neurofilaments are necessary for SOD1-mutant mediated disease, the absence of neurofilaments does slow the onset and progression of motor neuron disease onset even from an SOD1 mutant that does not produce detectable neurofilament misaccumulation.

As to what mechanism underlies the toxicity of the SOD1 mutants and how neurofilaments contribute to it, the findings of two additional mutating experiments are relevant.

First, the SOD1[G37R] mutant can promote disease in the absence of axonal neurofilaments in the NF-H β-galactosidase mice in which neurofilaments are trapped in the neuron cell bodies.[32] However, compared to mice with normal neurofilament levels, the NF-H β-galactosidase mice are at a significant disadvantage: chronic neurofilamentous aggregates in their perikarya and a 25% loss of motor axons occurs during the first 14 months of life.[31] Thus, comparing the life spans of mice that express the SOD1[G37R] mutant alone and mice that express both SOD1[G37R] and NF-H β-galactosidase[32] firmly supports a conclusion that the absence of axonal neurofilaments retards motor neuron loss from the SOD1[G37R] mutant, similar to the situation reported here for SOD1[G85R] mice.

Secondly, an additional mating experiment has tested how elevating the synthesis of NF-H affects disease mediated by the familial ALS SOD1[G37R] mutant.[85] Despite the prior finding that mice that express high levels of human NF-H develop a late-onset motor neuronopathy,[22] expression of human NF-H at lower levels reduced SOD1[G37R] toxicity very significantly and increased the mean life span of SOD1[G37R] mice by up to 65% (i.e. 6 months). The increased synthesis of NF-H traps an increased proportion of neurofilaments in the perikarya of motor neurons, with a corresponding reduction in axonal neurofilaments, so that maximal slowing of disease onset was achieved with marked reduction in axonal neurofilaments and increased perikaryal levels of both neurofilaments and all three subunits.

Taken together, amelioration of SOD1 mutant toxicity in each of these mating experiments correlates with reduction in axonal neurofilaments and increased perikaryal neurofilament subunits, especially NF-H. A portion of the protective effect may arise from the enhancement axonal transport by the removal of a major cargo whose incorporation is known to correlate with the slowing of slow axonal transport.[85]

Another proposed protective effect of NF-H overexpression is based on previous reports that indicated that neurofilament proteins have multiple calcium binding sites, including high-affinity sites.[86] It is therefore conceivable that increasing NF-H protein levels might confer protection in perikarya against rises in intracellular calcium that result from SOD1 mutant-mediated damage, particularly as reflected in the mitochondrial damage reported in some mutant SOD1 transgenic mice.[66,88] Direct support for involvement of calcium in SOD1-mediated disease has also come from overexpression of the calcium-binding protein, calbindin-D28K. This was recently reported to confer protection against mutant SOD1-mediated death of cultured motor neurons[88] that express mutant SOD1[G93A]. A calcium involvement in ALS has also been supported by the selective vulnerability of motor neurons that lack the typical calcium-binding proteins, parvalbumin and calbindin, as has been shown in ALS patients and monkeys[89–92] and in a line of SOD1 transgenic mice.[93]

Astrocytes as targets for mutant SOD1-mediated damage

The presence of SOD1-immunoreactive inclusions in astrocytes, initially reported for transgenic mice expressing familial ALS-linked mutant SOD1[G85R] (see *Fig. 19.5a*)[66] and more recently shown in SOD1[G93A] mice (see *Fig. 19.6*) and SOD1[G37R] mice,[81] supports the idea that there are molecular targets within astrocytes that can be damaged by mutant SOD1. Dysfunction of astrocytes could have significant consequences, since these cells are essential for neuronal viability, in part because they contain glutamate transporters that

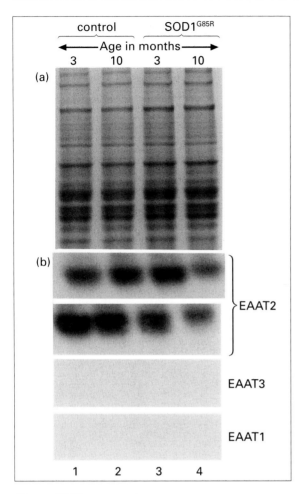

control   SOD1[G85R]

←—Age in months—→

3   10   3   10

(a)

(b)

}EAAT2

EAAT3

EAAT1

1   2   3   4

Figure 19.10
Levels of EAAT2 (GLT-1), the most abundant glial transporter in the spinal cord, are decreased in transgenic mice expressing SOD1[G85R]. (a) Coomassie blue-stained gel of total spinal cord extracts from 3- and 10-month-old control or SOD1[G85R] transgenic mice. (b) Immunoblots of the same spinal cord extracts as in (a), probed for the glial glutamate transporters EAAT2 and EAAT1 or for the neuronal transporter EAAT3. (Reproduced with permission from Bruijn et al.[66])

recover extracellular, synaptic glutamate, thereby limiting excitotoxic neuronal firing. Moreover, 60–70% of sporadic ALS patients[94] show a significant loss of the astroglial glutamate transporter (excitatory amino acid transporter (EAAT)2, originally named GLT-1) that is concomitant with the appearance in affected tissue regions of aberrantly spliced EAAT2 mRNA.[95] Four transporters have been cloned and sequenced from mice, but immunoblotting of whole mouse spinal cord extracts with antibodies against EAAT2, EAAC1 (now renamed EAAT3), and GLAST (now renamed EAAT1) has demonstrated that EAAT2 is the most abundant glutamate transporter in the spinal cord (*Fig. 19.10*).[66] Moreoever, similar analyses comparing levels of EAAT2 in control and transgenic SOD1[G85R] mice have demonstrated an approximately 50% decrease at end-stage disease (see *Fig. 19.10b*), proving that one consequence of this SOD1 mutation is a selective loss of this glial cell-specific transporter. Since this mimics the reduction seen in human disease,[94] it seems highly likely that glutamate-mediated excitoxicity represents at least one important secondary factor common to familial and sporadic ALS.

Moreover, using DNA microinjection into Xenopus oocytes, ALS-linked SOD1 mutants, but not wild type SOD1, were found to catalyze inactivation of EAAT2 in the presence of high levels of hydrogen peroxide[96]. This supports a unifying hypothesis that damage within astrocytes initiated either by SOD1 mutation *per se* or by other (yet unidentified) initiators yields diminished defense from synaptic glutamate as a key aspect of the cascade of toxicity. If so, this would, at last, offer a direct mechanistic link between sporadic and SOD1-mediated disease.

Conclusion

Studies of transgenic mice have not only conclusively proven that mutations in SOD1 lead to a gain of a toxic property, they have also provided a means to begin to address how these mutations actually cause selective degeneration and death of motor neurons. Two most likely hypotheses for toxic properties remain. In the first hypothesis, the mutant enzymes, by way of copper, catalyze damage to proteins or membranes through action on aberrant substrates. In the second hypothesis, intracytoplasmic aggregates composed at least in part of mutant SOD1, may choke an essential process or sequester (by precipitation) an essential component.

References

1. Delisle MB, Carpenter S. Neurofibrillary axonal swellings and amyotropic lateral sclerosis. *J Neurol Sci* 1984; **63**: 241–250
2. Banker BQ. The pathology of the motor neuron diseases. In: Engel AG, Banker BQ, eds. *Myology*. New York: McGraw-Hill, 1986, 2031–2066.
3. Carpenter S. Proximal axonal enlargement in motor neuron disease. *Neurology* 1968; **18**: 841–851.
4. Chou SM. Pathology of intraneuronal inclusions in ALS. In: Tsubaki T, Toyokura Y, eds. *Amyotrophic Lateral Sclerosis: Proceedings of the International Symposium on ALS*. Baltimore: University Park Press, 1979, 135–176.
5. Hirano A, Nakano I, Kurland LT et al. Fine structural study of neurofibrillary changes in a family with amyotrophic lateral sclerosis. *J Neuropathol Exp Neurol* 1984; **43**: 471–480.
6. Rosen DR, Siddique T, Patterson D et al. Mutations in Cu/Zn superoxide dismutase gene are associated with familial amyotropic lateral sclerosis. *Nature* 1993; **362**: 59–62.
7. Leigh PN, Swash M. Cytoskeletal pathology in motor neuron diseases. *Adv Neurol* 1991; **56**: 115–124.
8. Chou SM, Fakadej AV. Ultrastructure of chromatolytic motoneurons and anterior spinal roots in a case of Werdnig–Hoffmann disease. *J Neuropathol Exp Neurol* 1971; **30**: 368–379.
9. Hirano A, Donnenfeld H, Sasaki S, Nakano I. Fine structural observations of neurofilamentous changes in amyotrophic lateral sclerosis. *J Neuropathol Exp Neurol* 1984; **43**: 461–470.
10. Leigh PN, Whitwell H, Garofalo O et al. Ubiquitin-immunoreactive intraneuronal inclusions in amyotrophic lateral sclerosis. Morphology, distribution, and specificity. *Brain* 1991; **114**: 775–788.
11. Gonatas NK, Stieber A, Mourelatos Z et al. Fragmentation of the Golgi apparatus of motor neurons in amyotrophic lateral sclerosis. *Am J Pathol* 1992; **140**: 731–737.
12. Kato S, Oda M, Tanabe H. Diminution of dopaminergic neurons in the substantia nigra of sporadic amyotrophic lateral sclerosis. *Neuropathol Appl Neurobiol* 1993; **19**: 300–304.
13. Mizutani T, Sakamaki S, Tsuchiya N. Amyotrophic lateral sclerosis with opthalmoplegia and multisystem degeneration in patients on long-term use of respirators. *Acta Neuropathol* 1992; **84**: 372–377.
14. Geisler N, Weber K. Self-assembly in vitro of the 68,000 molecular weight component of the mammalian neurofilament triplet proteins into intermediate-sized filaments. *J Mol Biol* 1981; **151**: 565–571.
15. Liem RK, Hutchison SB. Purification of individual components of the neurofilament triplet: filament assembly from the 70 000-dalton subunit. *Biochemistry* 1982; **21**: 3221–3226.
16. Ching GY, Liem RK. Assembly of type IV neuronal intermediate filaments in nonneuronal cells in the absence of preexisting cytoplasmic intermediate filaments. *J Cell Biol* 1993; **122**: 1323–1335.
17. Lee MK, Xu Z, Wong PC, Cleveland DW. Neurofilaments are obligate heteropolymers in vivo. *J Cell Biol* 1993; **122**: 1337–1350.
18. Eyer J, Peterson A. Neurofilament-deficient axons and perikaryal aggregates in viable transgenic mice expressing a neurofilament-beta-galactosidase fusion protein. *Neuron* 1994; **12**: 389–405.
19. Friede RL, Samorajski T. Axon caliber related to neurofilaments and microtubules in sciatic nerve fibers of rats and mice. *Anat Rec* 1970;

167: 379–387.

20. Hoffman PN, Cleveland DW, Griffin JW et al. Neurofilament gene expression: a major determinant of axonal caliber. *Proc Natl Acad Sci U S A* 1987; **84:** 3472–3476.

21. Sakaguchi T, Okada M, Kitamura T, Kawasaki K. Reduced diameter and conduction velocity of myelinated fibers in the sciatic nerve of a neurofilament-deficient mutant quail. *Neurosci Lett* 1993; **153:** 65–68.

22. Yamasaki H, Bennett GS, Itakura C, Mizutani M. Defective expression of neurofilament protein subunits in hereditary hypotrophic axonopathy of quail. *Lab Invest* 1992; **66:** 734–743.

23. Zhu Q, Couillard-Despres S, Julien JP. Delayed maturation of regenerating myelinated axons in mice lacking neurofilaments. *Exp Neurol* 1997; **148:** 299–316.

24. Ohara O, Gahara Y, Miyake T et al. Neurofilament deficiency in quail caused by nonsense mutation in neurofilament-L gene. *J Cell Biol* 1993; **121:** 387–395.

25. Wong PC, Marszalek J, Crawford TO et al. Increasing neurofilament subunit NF-M expression reduces axonal NF-H, inhibits radial growth, and results in neurofilamentous accumulation in motor neurons. *J Cell Biol* 1995; **130:** 1413–1422.

26. Hirokawa N, Glicksman MA, Willard MB. Organization of mammalian neurofilament polypeptides within the neuronal cytoskeleton. *J Cell Biol* 1984; **98:** 1523–1536.

27. Hisanaga S, Hirokawa N. Structure of the peripheral domains of neurofilaments revealed by low angle rotary shadowing. *J Mol Biol* 1988; **202:** 297–305.

28. Mulligan L, Balin BJ, Lee VM, Ip W. Antibody labeling of bovine neurofilaments: implications on the structure of neurofilament sidearms. *J Struct Biol* 1991; **106:** 145–160.

29. Lees JF, Shneidman PS, Skuntz SF et al. The structure and organization of the human heavy neurofilament subunit (NF-H) and the gene encoding it. *EMBO J* 1988; **7:** 1947–1955.

30. Figlewicz DA, Rouleau GA, Krizus A, Julien JP. Polymorphism in the multi-phosphorylation domain of the human neurofilament heavy-subunit-encoding gene. *Gene* 1993; **132:** 297–300.

31. Elhanany E, Jaffe H, Link WT et al. Identification of endogenously phosphorylated KSP sites in the high-molecular-weight rat neurofilament protein. *J Neurochem* 1994; **63:** 2324–2335.

32. de Waegh SM, Lee VM, Brady ST. Local modulation of neurofilament phosphorylation, axonal caliber, and slow axonal transport by myelinating Schwann cells. *Cell* 1992; **68:** 451–463.

33. Hsieh ST, Kidd GJ, Crawford TO et al. Regional modulation of neurofilament organization by myelination in normal axons. *J Neurosci* 1994; **14:** 6392–6401.

34. Nixon RA, Paskevich PA, Sihag RK, Thayer CY. Phosphorylation on carboxyl terminus domains of neurofilament proteins in retinal ganglion cell neurons in vivo: influences on regional neurofilament accumulation, interneurofilament spacing, and axon caliber. *J Cell Biol* 1994; **126:** 1031–1046.

35. Hirano A. Cytopathology of amyotrophic lateral sclerosis. *Adv Neurol* 1991; **56:** 91–101.

36. Wiley CA, Love S, Skoglund RR, Lampert PW. Infantile neurodegenerative disease with neuronal accumulation of phosphorylated neurofilaments. *Acta Neuropathol (Berl)* 1987; **72:** 369–376.

37. Xu Z, Cork LC, Griffin JW, Cleveland DW. Increased expression of neurofilament subunit NF-L produces morphological alterations that resemble the pathology of human motor neuron disease. *Cell* 1993; **73:** 23–33.

38. Cote F, Collard JF, Julien JP. Progressive neuronopathy in transgenic mice expressing the human neurofilament heavy gene: a mouse model of amyotrophic lateral sclerosis. *Cell* 1993: **73:** 35–46.

39. Lee MK, Marszalek JR, Cleveland DW. A mutant neurofilament subunit causes massive, selective motor neuron death: Implications for the pathogenesis of human motor neuron disease. *Neuron* 1994; **13:** 975–988.

40. Coulombe PA, Hutton ME, Letai A et al. Point mutations in human keratin 14 genes of epidermolysis bullosa simplex patients: genetic and functional analyses. *Cell* 1991; **66:** 1301–1311.

41. Ishida-Yamamoto A, McGrath JA, Chapman SJ et al. Epidermolysis bullosa simplex (Dowling–Meara type) is a genetic disease character-

ized by an abnormal keratin-filament network involving keratins K5 and K14. *J Invest Dermatol* 1991; **97**: 959–968.

42. Chipev CC, Yang JM, DiGiovanna JJ et al. Preferential sites in keratin 10 that are mutated in epidermolytic hyperkeratosis. *Am J Hum Genet* 1994; **54**: 179–190.

43. Figlewicz DA, Krizus A, Martinoli MG et al. Variants of the heavy neurofilament subunit are associated with the development of amyotrophic lateral sclerosis. *Hum Mol Genet* 1994; **3**: 1757–1761.

44. al-Chalabi A, Andersen PM, Nilsson P et al. Deletions of the heavy neurofilament subunit tail in amyotrophic lateral sclerosis. *Hum Mol Genet* 1999; **8**: 157–164.

45. Tomkins J, Usher P, Slade JY et al. Novel Insertion in the KSP regin of the neurofilament heavy gene in amyhotrophic lateral sclerosis (ALS). *Neuroport* 1998; **9**: 3967–3970.

46. Siddique T, Nijhawan D, Hentati A. Molecular genetic basis of familial ALS. *Neurology* 1996; **47**: S27–S34.

47. Radunovic A, Leigh PN. Cu/Zn superoxide dismutase gene mutations in amyotrophic lateral sclerosis: correlation between genotype and clinical features. *J Neurol Neurosurg Psychiatry* 1996; **61**: 565–572.

48. Imlay JA, Linn S. DNA damage and oxygen radical toxicity. *Science* 1988; **240**: 1302–1309.

49. Stadtman ER. Protein oxidation and aging. *Science* 1992; **257**: 1220–1224.

50. Pardo CA, Xu Z, Borchelt DR et al. Superoxide dismutase is an abundant component in cell bodies, dendrites, and axons of motor neurons and in a subset of other neurons. *Proc Natl Acad Sci U S A* 1995; **92**: 954–958.

51. Tsuda T, Muthasser S, Fraser PE et al. Analysis of the functional effects of a mutation in SOD1 associated with familial amyotrophic lateral sclerosis. *Neuron* 1994; **13**: 727–736.

52. Bowling AC, Schulz JB, Brown RH Jr, Beal MF. Superoxide dismutase activity, oxidative damage, and mitochondrial energy metabolism in familial and sporadic amyotrophic lateral sclerosis. *J Neurochem* 1993; **61**: 2322–2325.

53. Deng H-X, Hentati A, Tainer JA et al. Amyotrophic lateral sclerosis and structural defects in Cu,Zn superoxide dismutase. *Science* 1993; **261**: 1047–1051.

54. Silos-Santiago I, Greenlund LJ, Johnson EM Jr, Snider WD. Molecular genetics of neuronal survival. *Curr Opin Neurobiol* 1995; **5**: 42–49.

55. Rothstein JD, Bristol LA, Hosler B et al. Chronic inhibition of superoxide dismutase produces apoptotic death of spinal neurons. *Proc Natl Acad Sci U S A* 1994; **91**: 4155–4159.

56. Robberecht W, Sapp P, Viaene MK et al. Cu/Zn superoxide dismutase activity in familial and sporadic amyotrophic lateral sclerosis. *J Neurochem* 1994; **62**: 384–387.

57. Borchelt DR, Lee MK, Slunt HS et al. Superoxide dismutase 1 with mutations linked to familial amyotrophic lateral sclerosis possesses significant activity. *Proc Natl Acad Sci U S A* 1994; **91**: 8292–8296.

58. Gurney ME, Pu H, Chiu AY et al. Motor neuron degeneration in mice that express a human Cu,Zn superoxide dismutase mutation. *Science* 1994; **264**: 1772–1775.

59. Borchelt DR, Guarnieri M, Wong PC et al. Superoxide dismutase 1 subunits with mutations linked to familial amyotrophic lateral sclerosis do not affect wild-type subunit function. *J Biol Chem* 1995; **270**: 3234–3238.

60. Reaume AG, Elliott JL, Hoffman EK et al. Motor neurons in Cu/Zn superoxide dismutase-deficient mice develop normally but exhibit enhanced cell death after axonal injury. *Nat Genet* 1996; **13**: 43–47.

61. Cleveland DW, Laing N, Hurse PV, Brown RH. Toxic mutants in Charcot's sclerosis. *Nature* 1995; **378**: 342–343.

62. Dal Canto MC, Gurney ME. Development of central nervous system pathology in a murine transgenic model of human amyotrophic lateral sclerosis. *Am J Pathol* 1994; **145**: 1271–1279.

63. Wong PC, Pardo CA, Borchelt DR et al. An adverse property of a familial ALS-linked SOD1 mutation causes motor neuron disease characterized by vacuolar degeneration of mitochondria. *Neuron* 1995; **14**: 1105–1116.

64. Kong J, Xu Z. Massive mitochondrial degeneration in motor neurons triggers the onset of amyotrophic lateral sclerosis in mice expressing a mutant SOD1. *J Neurosci* 1998; **18**: 3241–3250.

65. Gurney ME, Pu H, Chiu AY et al. Motor neuron degeneration in mice that express a human Cu,Zn superoxide dismutase mutation. *Science* 1994; **164**: 1772–1775.

66. Bruijn LI, Becher MW, Lee MK et al. ALS-linked SOD1 mutant G85R mediates damage to astrocytes and promotes rapidly progressive disease with SOD1-containing inclusions. *Neuron* 1997; **18**: 327–338.

67. Shibata N, Hirano A, Kobayashi M et al. Intense superoxide dismutase-1 immunoreactivity in intracytoplasmic hyaline inclusions of familial amyotrophic lateral sclerosis with posterior column involvement. *J Neuropathol Exp Neurol* 1996; **55**: 481–490.

68. Kato S, Shimoda M, Watanabe Y et al. Familial amyotrophic lateral sclerosis with a two base pair deletion in superoxide dismutase 1 gene: multisystem degeneration with intracytoplasmic hyaline inclusions in astrocytes. *J Neuropath Exp Neurol* 1996; **55**: 1089–1101.

69. Dal Canto MC, Gurney ME. A low expressor line of transgenic mice carrying a mutant human Cu,Zn superoxide dismutase (SOD1) gene develops pathological changes that most closely resemble those in human amyotrophic lateral sclerosis. *Acta Neuropathol* 1997; **93**: 537–550.

70. Tu PH, Raju P, Robinson KA et al. Transgenic mice carrying a human mutant superoxide dismutase transgene develop neuronal cytoskeletal pathology resembling human amyotrophic lateral sclerosis lesions. *Proc Natl Acad Sci U S A* 1996; **93**: 3155–3160.

71. Zhang B, Tu P, Abtahian F et al. Neurofilaments and orthograde transport are reduced in ventral root axons of transgenic mice that express human SOD1 with a G93A mutation. *J Cell Biol* 1997; **139**: 1307–1315.

72. Beckman JS, Carson M, Smith CD, Koppenol WH. ALS, SOD and peroxynitrite. *Nature* 1993; **364**: 584.

73. Culotta VC, Klomp LWJ, Strain J et al. The copper chaperone for superoxide dismutase. *J Biol Chem* 1997; **272**: 23469–23472.

74. Corson LB, Strain J, Culotta VC, Cleveland DW. Chaperone-facilitated loading of copper is a common in vivo property of familial ALS-linked SOD1 mutants. *Proc Natl Acad Sci U S A* 1998; **95**: 6361–6366.

75. Bruijn LI, Beal MF, Becher MW et al. Elevated free nitrotyrosine levels, but not protein-bound nitrotyrosine or hydroxyl radicals, throughout amyotrophic lateral sclerosis (ALS)-like disease implicate tyrosine nitration as an aberrant in vivo property of one familial ALS-linked superoxide dismutase 1 mutant. *Proc Natl Acad Sci U S A* 1997; **94**: 7606–7611.

76. Ferrante RJ, Shinobu LA, Schulz JB et al. Increased 3-nitrotyrosine and oxidative damage in mice with a human copper/zinc superoxide dismutase mutation. *Ann Neurol* 1997; **42**: 326–334.

77. Chou SM, Wang HS, Komai K. Colocalization of NOS and SOD1 in neurofilament accumulation within motor neurons of amyotrophic lateral sclerosis: an immunocytochemical study. *J Chem Neuroanat* 1996; **10**: 249–258.

78. Beal MF, Ferrante RJ, Browne SE et al. Increased 3-nitrotyrosine in both sporadic and familial amyotrophic lateral sclerosis. *Ann Neurol* 1997; **42**: 644–654.

79. Abe K, Pan LH, Watanabe M et al. Upregulation of protein-tyrosine nitration in the anterior horn cells of amyotrophic lateral sclerosis. *Neurol Res* 1997; **19**: 124–128.

80. Burijn LI, Beal MF, Becher MW et al. Elevated free nitrotyrosine levels, but not protein-bound nitrotyrosine or hydroxyl radicals, throughout amyotrophic lateral sclerosis (ALS)-like disease implicate tyrosine nitration as an aberrant in vivo property of one familial ALS-linked superoxide dismutase 1 mutant. *Proc Natl Acad Sci USA.* 1997; **94**: 7606–7611.

81. Pogun S, Dawson V, Kuhar MJ. Nitric oxide inhibits L-glutamate transport in synaptosomes. *Synapse* 1994; **18**: 21–26.

82. Wiedau-Pazos M, Goto JJ, Rabizadeh S et al. Altered reactivity of superoxide dismutase in familial amyotrophic lateral sclerosis. *Science* 1996; **271**: 515–518.

83. Williamson TL, Bruijn LI, Zhu Q et al. Absence of neurofilaments reduces the selective vulnerability of motor neurons and slows disease caused by familial amyotrophic lateral sclerosis-linked superoxide dismutase 1 mutant. *Proc Natl Acad Sci USA* 1998; **95**: 9631–9636.

84. Couillard-Despres S, Zhu Q, Wong P, Price DL, Cleveland DW, Julien F-P. Protective

effect of neurofilament NF-H overexpression in motor neuron disease induced by mutant superoxide dismutase. *Proc Natl Acad Sci USA.* 1998; **95**: 9626-9630.

85. Hoffman PN, Lasek RJ, Griffin JW, Price DL. Slowing of the axonal transport of neurofilament proteins during development. *J Neurosci* 1983; **3**: 1694–1700.

86. Lefebvre S, Mushynski WE. Calcium binding to untreated and dephosphorylated porcine neurofilaments. *Biochem Biophys Res Commun* 1987; **145**: 1006–1011.

87. Dal Canto MC, Gurney ME. Neuropathological changes in two lines of mice carrying a transgene for mutant human Cu,Zn SOD, and in mice overexpressing wild type human SOD: a model of familial amyotrophic lateral sclerosis (FALS). *Brain Res* 1995; **676**: 25–40.

88. Roy J, Minotti S, Dong L, Figlewicx DA, Durham HD. Glutamate potentiates the toxicity of mutant Cu/Zn-superoxide dismutase in motor neurons by postsynaptic calcium-dependent mechanisms. *J Neurosci* 1998; **18**: 9673–9684.

89. Reiner A, Medina L, Figueredo-Cardenas G, Anfinson S. Brainstem motoneuron pools that are selectively resistant in amyotrophic lateral sclerosis are preferentially enriched in parvalbumin: evidence from monkey brainstem for a calcium-mediated mechanism in sporadic ALS. *Exp Neurol* 1995; **131**: 239–250.

90. Elliott JL, Snider WD. Paralbumin is a marker of ALS-resistant motor neurons. *NeuroReport* 1995; **6**: 449–452.

91. Ince P, Stout N, Shaw P et al. Parvalbumin and calbindin D28K in the human motor system and in motor neuron disease. *Neuropathol Appl Neurobiol* 1993; **19**: 291–299.

92. Ho BK, Alexianu ME, Colom LV et al. Expression of calbindin-D28K in motoneuron hybrid cells after retroviral infection with calbindin-D28K cDNA prevents amyotrophic lateral sclerosis IgG-mediated cytotoxicity. *Proc Natl Acad Sci U S A* 1996; **93**: 6796–6801.

93. Morrison BM, Gordon JW, Ripps ME, Morrison JH. Quantitative immunocytochemical analysis of the spinal cord in G86R superoxide dismutase transgenic mice: neurochemical correlates of selective vulnerability. *J Comp Neurol* 1996; **373**: 619–631.

94. Rothstein JD, Van Kammen M, Levey AI et al. Selective loss of glial glutamate transporter GLT-1 in amyotrophic lateral sclerosis. *Ann Neurol* 1995; **38**: 73–84.

95. Lin CL, Bristol LA, Jin L et al. Aberrant RNA processing in a neurodegenerative disease: the cause for absent EAAT2, a glutamate transporter, in amyotrophic lateral sclerosis. *Neuron* 1998; **20**: 589–602.

96. Trotti D, Rolfs A, Danbolt NC, Brown RH Jr, Hediger MA. SOD1 mutants linked to amyotrophic lateral sclerosis selectively inactivate a glial glutamate transporter. *Nat Neurosci* 1999; **2**: 427–433.

97. Hirano A. *Color Atlas of Pathology of the Nervous System* 2nd edn. New York: Igaku-shoin, 1988.

98. Kawamura Y, Dyck PJ, Shimono M et al. Morphometric comparison of the vulnerability of peripheral motor and sensory neurons in amyotrophic lateral sclerosis. *J Neuropathol Exp Neurol* 1981; **40**: 667–675.

20

Apoptosis in amyotrophic lateral sclerosis: a review

Piera Pasinelli and Robert H Brown Jr

Overview of apoptosis

Apoptosis is a mode of cell death in which the cell actively participates in its own destruction by activating pre-programmed intracellular suicide machinery. For this reason, apoptosis is also known as programmed cell death. Morphological criteria still represent the best basis for the identification of an apoptotic death process[1], since genetic and biochemical markers of apoptotic cell death often differ between cell types. Primary morphologic features of apoptosis include chromatin condensation, cytoplasmic vacuolization, cell shrinkage, and plasma membrane blebbing followed by formation of membrane-enclosed apoptotic bodies that contain intracellular material.[1] In vivo, these apoptotic bodies are rapidly phagocytosed by neighbouring cells[2,3] whereas, in the absence of phagocytosis (e.g. in vitro cell culture systems), secondary necrosis may occur, which leads to cell lysis and loss of plasma membrane.[4] In contrast to necrosis, apoptosis is characterized by early preservation of intracellular organelles as well as of nuclear and plasma membranes, and it does not induce inflammatory responses.

At the biochemical level, apoptosis is often associated with internucleosomal DNA fragmentation,[5] producing integral multiples of 180 base pair 'ladders' as seen in the electrophoresis of DNA from apoptotic cells.

Whether DNA cleavage always correlates with apoptosis is controversial; in some cells, apoptosis can occur in the absence of DNA fragmentation.[6]

The transduction of apoptosis involves both positive and negative regulatory elements such as the Bcl-2–Bax family of proteins,[7–12] the p53 tumor suppressor gene,[13] members of the tumor necrosis factor receptors[14,15] superfamily, and several cell cycle-related genes.[16] The relative expression patterns of these genes in the cells determines the threshold for apoptosis and may explain the selective vulnerability of some cells to apoptotic stimuli. The central components of the cell death machinery are the interleukin-1-β converting enzyme (ICE)-like cysteine proteases, which are also known as caspases. The caspase family consists of 11 members that can be divided into three subfamilies. These proteases are translated as inactive proenzymes that are activated after cleavage at specific aspartate residues. Processing and activation of a protease can induce additional processing of molecules of the same protease family or of other protease families, which leads to an amplified death cascade. Once activated, caspases cleave their substrates after aspartate residues. It is the cleavage of selected key proteins that appears to direct destruction and packing of the cell for clearance.[17–19] Only a few of these selected targets have been identified so far, and their contribution to the apoptotic process remains largely hypothetical. Assuming that a relevant substrate is expressed in a tissue-specific manner, it would be expected that some of the effects mediated by its cleavage will also be tissue-specific or cell type-specific, influencing the likelihood that the tissue or cell will undergo apoptosis.

Apoptosis plays an important role in neuronal cell death. For years it has been recognized as the physiological process by which developing neurons are destroyed.[20] It is now clear that it can occur in pathological conditions. In neurons in vitro, apoptosis can be induced by diverse pathological stimuli such as exposure to β-amyloid,[21,22] viral infections,[8] mitochondrial toxins,[23] and oxidative stress.[24–27] Moreover, there is increasing evidence that apoptosis contributes to neuronal loss in many acute and chronic neurological diseases[28,29] including stroke, Alzheimer's disease, Parkinson's disease, Huntington's disease, and possibly amyotrophic lateral sclerosis (ALS). For several reasons, the role of apoptosis in these diseases and the precise signals that are involved are far from clear. First, it may be difficult to detect cells that exhibit morphological criteria of apoptosis because apoptotic cells are rapidly phagocytosed. Secondly, during apoptosis only a few cells die at any given time and those that die may be widely scattered among viable cells. Moreover, the rate of the death process is low. Thus, although cell death might involve a significant number of cells, at a precise moment dying cells might represent less than 1% of the total cellular population. This complicates biochemical analysis, since molecular signals generated by the infrequent apoptotic cells may be undetectable against the background of normal cells. For this reason, in situ techniques must be used to identify single apoptotic cells in vivo with confidence. This may pose difficul-

ties if the monitored signals are also potentially characteristic of necrotic cells.[30]

Apoptosis in ALS tissues

Several reports have described evidence for apoptosis in tissues of patients with ALS. An early study identified the expression of an apoptosis-related antigen and DNA breaks in cervical spinal cord sections of ALS patients. Immunostaining with an antibody to Le(Y), a difucosylated type 2 chain determinant that is characteristic of cells undergoing apoptosis, showed positive immunostaining in seven out of the 10 ALS cases analysed. In the same seven cases, apoptosis was confirmed by double staining with TdT mediate biotin-dUTP nick end labelling (TUNEL).[31] Another report detected DNA fragmentation in situ in brain and spinal cord tissues from 12 ALS cases, together with cell shrinkage and small Nissl-positive bodies. None of the six non-neurological controls used in the study showed the apoptotic features seen in the ALS cases.[32] However, the significance of the findings is unclear since apoptosis was not restricted to the motor system but was also detected in other neuronal and non-neuronal cells. In addition, immunostaining showed identical distribution of bcl-2 between ALS and non-neurological controls. In a more recent paper, Mu and colleagues,[33] used in situ hybridization to analyse bcl-2 and bax mRNA levels in control sections and ALS lumbar spinal cord sections. Compared with controls, bcl-2 mRNA levels were significantly lower (4.7-fold) in ALS, whereas bax mRNA hybridization signal was significantly higher (2.8-fold). Interestingly, bax expression was selectively increased in ALS motor neurons. At the protein level, strong expression of bax and ICE-promoting apoptosis was also found in muscle fibers of two ALS patients. Activation of these proapoptic genes was followed by DNA proapoptotic as determined by TUNEL method. However, high expression of the anti-apoptotic product bcl-2 was also found.[34] A recent report indicated that neuronal death in ALS has all the characteristics of apoptosis as revealed by signs of typical chromatolysis in spinal cords of ALS patients as well as increased bax and decreased bcl-2 expression in the mitochondria-enriched membrane compartment of vulnerable regions.[35]

Few data exist that correlate the neurochemical pathology of ALS with the signal transduction pathways associated with apoptosis. An immunohistochemical analysis showed that the c-Jun-JNK–SAPK kinase pathway is dramatically overexpressed in ALS spinal cords. However, the strongest activation was found in astrocytes, whereas motor neurons showed an unusually low expression of the pathway.[36] While motor neurons appeared to be apoptotic, as assessed by in situ end-labeling, this was not the case in astrocytes, in which JNK–SAPK overexpression was related not to apoptosis but to activation of the nuclear factor κB. This nuclear transcription factor mediates resistance of neuronal cells to oxidative stress.[37] Because oxidative stress has been implicated in the pathogenesis of ALS, these findings were therefore interpreted to support the view that astrocytes are involved in ALS via activation of an apoptotic pathway that is mediated by stress-activated kinases, and that motor neurons are selectively killed because of their lack of antioxidant defenses. Cyclin-dependent kinase-5 (cdk-5) has recently been associated with neuronal apoptosis.[38] Intense cdk-5 immunoreactivity has been detected in degenerating motor neurons of ALS cases,[39,40] although the exact role of cdk-5 in ALS remains a matter of conjecture. Since cdk-5 phosphorylates neurofilament protein (NF), it has been implicated as a candidate kinase to explain the heightened NF phosphorylation that is characteristic of ALS.[39,41] However, one study[40] reported that cdk-5 co-localizes with lipofuscin and not with accumulated NF proteins in motor neurons. As is the case with cdk-5, lipofuscin plays a role in apoptosis. The biogenesis of lipofuscin is presumed to be linked to oxidative stress and oxidative stress-related apoptosis. Therefore, the authors of this study argue that, in ALS patients, high levels of cdk-5 that co-localizes with lipofuscin are more likely to be linked to lipofuscin-related apoptosis than to NF phosphorylation.[40]

Another possible correlation between ALS and apoptosis has been suggested by Migheli and co-workers,[42] who found that dying motor neurons are ubiquitin-positive. Since activation of polyubiquitin gene has been observed in developmental apoptosis,[43] the authors suggested that in addition to its protective role, ubiquitin could be directly implicated in the mechanism (or mechanisms) of apoptotic cell death in ALS.

The evidence that apoptosis actually occurs in motor neurons in ALS is therefore still less than fully compelling. Although most of the above reports demonstrated DNA fragmentation, the corresponding morphology was not clearly apoptotic and, in some cases, was not confined selectively to motor neurons. Moreover, although expression of the pro- and anti-apoptotic genes correlates with apoptosis at the mRNA level, this has not been consistently demonstrated at the protein level.

Mutant SODI apoptosis

Intriguing data relating ALS to apoptosis have been generated in studies that examine the role of Cu–Zn superoxide dismutase (SOD1) in neuronal cell death. The genetic finding that a subset of cases with familial ALS is associated with mutations in the gene that encodes for SOD1[44] has provided a useful molecular basis for the study of the mechanism of neurodegeneration in ALS. The primary function of SOD1 is to detoxify or dismutate the superoxide anion, which is generated during normal metabolism in the cell, to form hydrogen peroxide. In turn, hydrogen peroxide is detoxified by glutathione peroxidase or catalase to form water. Thus, SOD1 represents an important line of defense against free radicals and oxidative stress.

Evidence from several laboratories indicates that reactive oxygen species (ROS) play an important role in neuronal apoptosis.[45–48] Given its role in dismutating superoxide, it is not entirely surprising that overexpression of the wild-type SOD1 protein in cultured neuronal cells inhibits ROS-mediated apoptosis that has been induced by insults such as nerve growth factor deprivation or calcium ionophores.[49–51] Moreover, increased SOD1 activity results in a greater resistance to a variety of neurotoxic insults both in vivo and in vitro.[52–55] This enzyme also promotes the development and survival of cultured postnatal midbrain neurons[56] and is a determinant of lifespan in *Drosophila*.[57]

In striking contrast, mutations associated with familial ALS transform SOD1 into a proapoptotic gene. The hypothesis that the mutant SOD1 protein might promote apoptosis was first prompted by the observation that overexpression of the A4V mutant in a rat nigral neural cell line enhances apoptosis induced by serum and growth factor deprivation.[51] Expression of two familial ALS-related mutants using a replication-deficient adenovirus caused cell death of differentiated PC12 cells, hippocampal pyramidal neurons, and superior cervical ganglion neurons. Death could be prevented by caspase inhibitors, bcl-

2, glutathione, and vitamin E, which clearly indicates an apoptotic cell death mechanism that is possibly associated with disturbed free-radical homeostasis.[58] In primary cultures of spinal motor neurons, forced expression of high levels of mutant but not wild-type SOD1 protein results in cytoplasmic aggregation of SOD1. Neurons that develop the SOD1 aggregates subsequently undergo apoptotic cell death.[59] The proapoptotic influence of mutant SOD1 protein is not confined to motor neurons in culture. Primary midbrain cultures of 1-week-old transgenic mice that express the G93A mutation have significantly fewer midbrain neurons and more apoptotic and necrotic cells than non-transgenic cultures. The opposite was observed in cultured neurons from transgenic mice that express the wild-type enzyme. These cultures had significantly more midbrain neurons and fewer necrotic and apoptotic cells than non-transgenic cultures. Interestingly, midbrain neurons from G93A mice were more sensitive to oxidative stress induced by L-dihydroxyphenyl alanine (L-DOPA) than neurons from non-transgenic mice. L-DOPA had no effect on wild-type transgenic cultures.[60]

These findings in neuronal cultures are supported by genetic analyses of motor neuron cell death in the G93A familial ALS mice. Overexpression of bcl-2 delays the onset of motor neuron disease and prolongs survival in transgenic mice that express the G93A mutation. However, it does not prolong the duration of the disease once it has been initiated.[61] Bcl-2 overexpression protects from mutant SOD1-induced cytotoxicity as well. The G93A mice that overexpress bcl-2 have significantly fewer c-Jun or ubiquitin-positive motor neurons than the G93A mice. Another study showed that inhibition of caspase-1 (or ICE), via a dominant negative ICE-derived protein slows disease progression in the same G93A mouse model without affecting the timing of onset.[62] We recently found that caspase-1 is activated in two other lines of transgenic mice that carry the G37R or G85R mutations and also in differentiated mouse neuroblastoma (line N2a) cells.[63] In the N2a cells, this activation of caspase-1 is enhanced by oxidative challenge, which triggers cleavage and secretion of pro-interleukin-1-β (the ICE substrate) and induces apoptosis. Consistent with an apoptotic cell death pathway, caspase inhibitors prevent oxidative stress-induced cell death, caspase-1 activation, and mature interleukin-1-β secretion in these N2a cells in vitro.

Mechanism of apoptosis in ALS

The mechanism by which mutant SOD1 promotes apoptosis is unclear. Studies in neuronal cultures have demonstrated that reductions in the levels of wild-type SOD1 protein and activity can precipitate apoptotic neuronal death.[64–66] It is clear in many experimental paradigms that the mutant SOD1 molecule is apoptotic not through subnormal levels of SOD1 activity but through an acquired, adverse function. Thus, although many mutations associated with familial ALS do reduce total cellular activity of SOD1,[67,68] many retain normal catalytic activity.[69,70] Moreover, the dominant inheritance pattern favors an acquired toxic property; available data indicate that the mutant SOD1 protein does not act through a dominant negative mechanism.[71] Yeast that lacks the SOD1 gene are rescued as efficiently from paraquat-induced toxicity by the mutated SOD1 molecule as by the wild-type SOD1 molecule.[51] Finally, particularly convincing are two observations in genetically altered mice. While mice that are devoid of SOD1 activity develop normally and survive into mature adulthood with normal motor function,[72] transgenic mice that express high levels of the mutant protein without loss of enzymatic activity develop a paralytic disease similar to ALS.[73–75] Thus, although it remains possible that the loss of dismutase function observed in some ALS patients contributes to the pathogenesis of the motor neuron death process, one or more alternative, adverse mechanisms must be active.

Two broad categories of hypotheses have been proposed for the putative gain of function of the mutant SOD1 protein. Both are predicted on the observation that the mutant molecule is unstable and subject to conformational modifications.[69,76] One category invokes a novel enzymatic activity. Thus, it is proposed that the mutant SOD1 molecule has an enhanced ability to accept hydrogen peroxide or peroxynitrite as substrates, leading to increased intracellular concentrations of hydroxyl radicals or nitronium ions, respectively. These models predict increased oxidation or nitration, or both, of target proteins.[77–79] A parallel suggestion is that improperly folded mutant SOD1 protein may release either copper or zinc, thereby initiating catalytic metal toxicity.

A second set of hypotheses invokes aberrant protein chemistry without necessitating aberrant catalytic properties. It is proposed that conformational alterations induce the mutant molecule to precipitate and form toxic aggregates in motor neurons. At least three reports describe aggregated SOD1 protein in motor neurons in both sporadic and familial ALS.[80–82] Moreover, two recent reports imply that both in vitro and in vivo the mutant protein forms toxic cytoplasmic aggregates in motor neurons.[59,83] A second protein-based toxic function supposes that the mutant SOD1 molecule has an abnormally enhanced affinity for one or more cellular protein binding partners.[84]

Whether the ability of the mutant protein to cause apoptosis operates through one of the above mechanisms is still under debate. Remarkably, data from different laboratories indicate that whatever the precipitating factors are (e.g. reduced enzymatic activity, altered intracellular levels of hydrogen peroxide, or SOD1 aggregates) the mode of cell death has features characteristic of apoptosis. This observation may have important therapeutic implications.

If apoptotic cell death itself, as opposed to events further upstream in the apoptotic pathway, is crucial for the manifestation of ALS, one might expect that blocking one or more of the final events of the pathway would be useful therapeutically. Caspases are attractive potential targets as they represent one of the final steps in the execution of apoptosis.[85] In view of this possibility, some important questions have to be considered. First, do we have any direct in vivo evidence that caspase inhibition may be beneficial to ALS? Secondly, among the different caspases, what are the best targets? To date, only one report has suggested that blockade of caspase is activated in neuronal cell death;[85] similarly, many caspases are likely to be activated in motor neuron cell death. It may be very informative to investigate the expression and activation pattern of the caspases in brain and spinal cord of ALS patients (and ALS mice). The development of drugs that are non-selective caspase inhibitors or the use of cocktails of different inhibitors may offer advantages relative to those currently being developed for single caspases.

It is also possible that more than one mechanism of neuronal degeneration occurs in ALS and that antiapoptotic therapy may be beneficial only to those patients who can be treated early in the course of the disease, even possibly before the onset of overt clinical symptoms.

Finally, knowing whether there is any direct link between one of the proteins that are caspase targets and ALS may provide new insight into the selective vulnerability of motor neurons and new possibilities in the treatment of the disease.

Conclusions

The hypothesis that apoptosis or an abnormal activation of a specific death program contributes to motor neuron degeneration in ALS is provocative but must be viewed as speculative at present. As outlined above, there are compelling data favoring the view that the mutant SOD1 protein can be proapoptotic in vitro. By contrast, in ALS mice that express mutant transgenic SOD1, it is by no means clear that neuronal death is apoptotic. Moreover, in ALS patients (of whom fewer than 5% have SOD1 mutations), the evidence that neuronal death is apoptotic is still limited and indirect.

What data then are required to test the hypothesis conclusively? Ultimately, a definitive proof of the hypothesis would be a demonstration that specific, antiapoptotic compounds significantly ameliorate the course of ALS in patients. Until such a demonstration is forthcoming, two types of evidence would bear on this question. First, it would be helpful to see systematic morphological studies of apoptosis in ALS tissues (both murine and human). Strikingly absent in the present literature are any reports that motor neuron cell death in ALS fulfils the morphological criteria for apoptosis. Is this because there is no apoptosis or is it because most human neuropathological studies in ALS are necessarily conducted late in the course of the disease? The latter cannot be the only explanation: in many cases of ALS at autopsy, motor neurons deteriorate at different rates in different regions. One would anticipate that within those segments of the spinal cord at the earlier stages of the disease, it might be possible to detect morphological evidence of apoptosis.

Secondly, in determining whether neuronal cell death in human ALS is apoptotic, it would also be useful to see a systematic search for well-defined biochemical markers of apoptotic cell death. Presumably, these might be detected in several ways, including immuno-histochemical analyses of specific cell types at the single cell level or analyses of whole cord and brain preparations using sensitive methods such as reverse transcriptase polymerase chain reaction, radioimmunoassays, or activity assays. It would be extremely useful to detect profiles of such markers in the cerebrospinal fluid. The cerebrospinal fluid analyses can be performed over time in the same patient and thus might provide a temporal profile of the markers in the death process. Such markers would have considerable utility as monitors of the efficacy of therapy as well. If, indeed, specific biomarkers are defined in ALS, cellular studies may then be critical in defining the signal transduction pathways and effector molecules that these biomarkers implicate. This will have immediate significance for understanding the full sequence of molecular events that trigger cell death, discerning new disease biomarkers, and defining new ALS therapeutic targets.

Acknowledgments

Robert H Brown Jr is supported by grants from the Amyotrophic Lateral Sclerosis Association, the Muscular Dystrophy Association, the National Institute of Health (the National Institute of Neurological Disorders and Stroke and the National Institute on Aging), the Pierre L de Bourgknecht ALS Research, and the Myrtle May MacLellan Fund. Piera Pasinelli is the recipient of a fellowship from Telethon Italia.

References

1. Kerr JFR, Wyllie AH, Currie AR. Apoptosis: a basic biological phenomenon with wide-ranging implications in tissue kinetics. *Br J Cancer* 1972; **26**: 239–257.
2. Duvall E, Wyllie AH, Morris RG et al. Macrophage recognition of cells undergoing programmed cell death (apoptosis). *Immunology* 1985: **56**: 351–358.
3. Savill J, Fadok V, Henson P, Haslett C. Phagocyte recognition of cells undergoing apoptosis. *Immunol Today* 1993; **14**: 131–136.
4. Leist M, Gantner F, Bohlinger I et al. Tumor necrosis factor-induced hepatocyte apoptosis precedes liver failure in experimental murine shock models. *Am J Pathol* 1995; **146**: 1220–1234.
5. Wyllie AH. Glucocorticoid-induced thymocyte apoptosis is associated with endogenous endonuclease activation. *Nature* 1980; **284**: 555–556.
6. Tomei LD, Shapiro JP, Cope FO. Apoptosis in C3H/10T1/2 mouse embryonic cells: evidence for internucleosomal DNA modification in the absence of double-strand cleavage. *Proc Acad Natl Sci U S A* 1993; **90**: 853–857.
7. Bredesen DE, Widedau-Pazos M, Goto JJ et al. Cell death mechanisms in ALS. *Neurology* 1996; **47**(Suppl 2): S36–S39.
8. Adams MJ, Cory S. The bcl-2 protein family: arbiters of cell survival. *Science* 1998; **281**: 1322–1326.
9. Oh JH, O'Malley KL, Krajewski S et al. Bax accelerates staurosporine-induced but suppresses nigericin-induced neuronal cell death. *NeuroReport* 1997; **8**: 1851–1856.
10. Pinon LG, Middleton G, Davies AM. Bcl-2 is required for cranial sensory neuron survival at defined stages of embryonic development. *Development* 1997; **124**: 4173–4178.
11. Martinou JC, Dubois-Dauphin M, Staple JK et al. Overexpression of BCL-2 in transgenic mice protects neurons from naturally occurring cell death and experimental ischemia. *Neuron* 1994; **13**: 1017–1030.

12. Zanjani HS, Vogel MW, Delhaye-Bouchaud N et al. Increased cerebellar Purkinje cell numbers in mice overexpressing a human bcl-2 transgen. *J Comp Neurol* 1996; **374**: 332–341.

13. Wood KA, Youle RJ. The role of free radicals and p53 in neurone apoptosis in vivo. *J Neurosci* 1995; **15**: 5851–5857.

14. Rabizadeh S, Oh J, Zhong LT et al. Induction of apoptosis by the low affinity NGF receptor. *Science* 1993; **261**: 345–348.

15. Yeo TC, Chua-Couzens J, Larry L et al. Absence of p75NTR causes increased basal forebrain cholinergic neuron size, choline acetyltransferase activity, and target innervation. *J Neurosci* 1997; **17**: 7594–7605.

16. Freeman RS, Estus S, Johnson EM. Analysis of cell cycle related gene expression in postmitotic neurons: selective induction of Cyclin D1 during programmed cell death. *Neuron* 1994; **12**: 343–355.

17. Casciola-Rosen L, Nicholson DW, Chong T et al. Apopain/CPP32 cleaves proteins that are essential for cellular repair: a fundamental principle of apoptotic death. *J Exp Med* 1996; **183**: 1957–1964.

18. Nicholson DW, Thornberry NA. Caspases: killer proteases. *Trends Biochem Sci* 1997; **22**: 299–306.

19. Green DR. Apoptotic pathways: the roads to ruin. *Cell* 1998; **94**: 695–698.

20. Golstein P. Cell death in us and others. *Science* 1998; **281**: 1283.

21. Loo DT, Copani A, Pike CJ et al. Apoptosis is induced by beta-amyloid in cultured central nervous system neurons. *Proc Natl Acad Sci USA* 1993; **90**: 7951–7955.

22. Pappolla MA, Sos M, Omar RA et al. Melatonin prevents death of neuroblastoma cells exposed to the Alzheimer amyloid peptide. *J Neurosci* 1997; **17**: 1683–1690.

23. Beherns MI, Koh J, Canzoniero LM et al. 3-Nitropropionic acid induces apoptosis in cultured striatal and cortical neurons. *NeuroReport* 1995; **6**: 545–548.

24. Ratan RR, Murphy TH, Baraban JM. Oxidative stress induces apoptosis in embryonic cortical neurons. *J Neurochem* 1994; **62**: 376–379.

25. Bonfoco E, Krainc D, Ankarcrona M et al. Apoptosis and necrosis: two distinct events induced, respectively, by mild and intense insults with N-methyl-D-aspartate or nitric oxide/superoxide in cortical cell cultures. *Proc Natl Acad Sci USA* 1995; **92**: 7162–7166.

26. Green DR, Reed JC. Mitochondria and apoptosis. *Science* 1998; **281**: 1309–1312.

27. Murphy AN, Bredesen D. In: *Mitochondria and Free Radicals in Neurodegenerative Diseases* 1997, 159–182.

28. Bredesen DE. Neural apoptosis. *Ann Neurol* 1995; **38**: 839–851.

29. Pettmann B, Henderson CE. Neuronal cell death. *Neuron* 1998; **20**: 633–647.

30. Grasl-Kraupp B. In situ detection of fragmented DNA (TUNEL assay) fails to discriminate among apoptosis, necrosis, and autolytic cell death: a cautionary note. *Hepatology* 1995; **21**: 1465–1468.

31. Yoshiyama Y, Yamada T, Asanuma K, Asahi T. Apoptosis related antigen, Le(Y) and nick-end labeling are positive in spinal motor neurons in amyotrophic lateral sclerosis. *Acta Neuropathol (Berl)* 1994; **88**: 207–211.

32. Troost D, Aten J, Morsink F, de Jong JM. Apoptosis in amyotrophic lateral sclerosis is not restricted to motor neurons. Bcl-2 expression is increased in unaffected post-central gyrus. *Neuropathol Appl Neurobiol* 1995; **21**: 498–504.

33. Mu X, Anderson DW, Trojanowski JQ et al. Altered bcl-2 and bax mRNA in amyotrophic lateral sclerosis spinal cord motor neurons. *Ann Neurol* 1996; **40**: 379–386.

34. Tews DS, Goebel HH, Meinck HM. DNA-fragmentation and apoptosis-related proteins of muscle cells in motor neuron disorders. *Acta Neurol Scand* 1997; **96**: 380–386.

35. Martin LJ. Neuronal death in amyotrophic lateral sclerosis is apoptosis: possible contribution of a programmed cell death mechanism. *J Neuropathol Exp Neurol* 1999; **58**: 459–471.

36. Migheli A, Piva R, Atzori C et al. c-Jun, JNK-SAPK Kinases and transcription factor NF-Kappa B are selectively activated in astrocytes, but not motor neurons, in amyotrophic lateral sclerosis. *J Neurophatol Exp Neurol* 1997; **56**: 1314–1322.

37. Lezoualc'h F, Sagara Y, Holsboer F, Behl C. High constitutive NF-kappaB activity mediates resistance to oxidative stress in neuronal cells. *J Neurosci* 1998; **18**: 3224–3232.

38. Henchcliffe C, Burke RE. Increased expression of cyclin-dependent kinase 5 in induced apoptotic neuron death in rat substantial nigra. *Neurosci Lett* 1997; **230**: 41–44.

39. Nakamura S, Kawamoto T, Nakano S et al. Cyclin-dependent kinase 5 in lewy body-like inclusions in anterior horn cells of a patient with sporadic amyotrophic lateral sclerosis. *Neurology* 1997; **48**: 267–270.

40. Bajaj NP, Al-Sarraj ST, Anderson V et al. Cyclin-dependent kinase-5 is associated with lipofuscin in motor neurones in amyotrophic lateral sclerosis. *Neurosci Lett* 1998; **245**: 45–48.

41. Toyoshima I, Yamamoto A, Masamune O, Satake M. Phosphorylation of neurofilament proteins and localization of axonal swellings in motor neuron disease. *J Neurol Sci* 1989; **89**: 269–277.

42. Migheli A, Attanasio A, Schiffer D. Ubiquitin and neurofilament expression in anterior horn cells in amyotrophic lateral sclerosis: possible clues to the pathogenesis. *Neuropathol Appl Neurobiol* 1994; **20**: 282–289.

43. Schwartz LM, Myer A, Kosz L et al. Activation of polyubiquitin gene expression during developmentally programmed cell death. *Neuron* 1990; **5**: 411–419.

44. Rosen DR, Siddique T, Patterson D et al. Mutations in Cu/Zn superoxide dismutase gene are associated with familial amyotrophic lateral sclerosis. *Nature* 1993; **362**: 59–62.

45. Halliwell B, Gutteridge JMC. Oxygen radicals and the nervous system. *Trends Neurol Sci* 1993; **16**: 439–444.

46. Buttke MT, Sandstrom PA. Oxidative stress as a mediator of apoptosis. *Immunol Today* 1994; **15**: 7–10.

47. Cookson MR, Shaw PJ. Oxidative stress and motor neurone disease. *Brain Pathol* 1999; **9**: 165–186.

48. Facchinetti F, Dawson VL, Dawson TM. Free radicals as mediators of neuronal injury. *Cell Mol Neurobiol* 1998; **18**: 667–682.

49. Greenlund LJ, Deckwerth TL, Johnson EM Jr. Superoxide dismutase delays neuronal apoptosis: a role for reactive oxygen species in programmed neuronal death. *Neuron* 1995; **14**: 303–315.

50. Jordan J, Ghadge GD, Prehn JH et al. Expression of human copper/zinc-superoxide dismutase inhibits the death of rat sympathetic neurons caused by withdrawal of nerve growth factor. *Mol Pharmacol* 1995; **47**: 1095–1110.

51. Rabizadeh S, Gralla EB, Borchelt DR et al. Mutations associated with amyotrophic lateral sclerosis convert superoxide dismutase from an antiapoptotic gene to a proapoptotic gene: studies in yeast and neural cells. *Proc Natl Acad Sci USA* 1995; **92**: 3024–3028.

52. Elroy-Stein O, Bernstein Y, Groner Y. Overproduction of human Cu/Zn-superoxide dismutase in transfected cells: extenuation of paraquat-mediated cytotoxicity and enhancement of lipid peroxidation. *EMBO J* 1986; **5**: 615–622.

53. Chan PH, Yang GY, Chen SF et al. Cold-induced brain edema and infarction are reduced in transgenic mice overexpressing CuZN-superoxide dismutase. *Ann Neurol* 1991; **29**: 482–486.

54. Huang TT, Carlson EJ, Leadon SA, Epstein CJ. Relationship of resistance to oxygen free radicals to CuZN-superoxide dismutase activity in transgenic, transfected, and trisomic cells. *FASEB J* 1992; **6**: 903–910.

55. Przedborski S, Kostic V, Jackson-Lewis V et al. Transgenic mice with increased Cu/Zn-superoxide dismutase activity are resistant to N-methyl-4-phenyl-1,2,3,6-tetrahydropyridine-induced neurotoxicity. *J Neurosci* 1992; **12**: 1658–1667.

56. Przedborski S, Kahn U, Kostic V et al. Increased superoxide dismutase activity improves survival of cultured postnatal midbrain neurons. *J Neurochem* 1996; **67**: 1383–1392.

57. Parkes TL, Elia AJ, Dickinson D et al. Extension of *Drosophila* lifespan by overexpression of human SOD1 in motor neurons. *Nat Genet* 1998; **19**: 171–174.

58. Ghadge GD, Lee JP, Bindokas VP et al. Mutant superoxide dismutase-1-linked familial amyotrophic lateral sclerosis: molecular mechanisms of neuronal death and protection. *J Neurosci* 1997; **17**: 8756–8766.

59. Durham HD, Roy J, Dong L, Figlewicz DA. Aggregation of mutant Cu/Zn superoxide dismutase proteins in a culture model of ALS. *J Neuropathol Exp Neurol* 1997; **56**: 523–530.

60. Mena MA, Khan U, Togasaki DM et al. Effects of wild-type and mutated copper/zinc superoxide dismutase on neuronal survival and

L-DOPA-induced toxicity in postnatal midbrain culture. *J Neurochem* 1997; **69**: 21–33.

61. Kostic V, Jackson-Lewis V, de Bilbao F et al. Bcl-2: prolonging life in a transgenic mouse model of familial amyotrophic lateral sclerosis. *Science* 1997; **277**: 559–562.

62. Friedlander RM, Brown RH. Gagliardini V et al. Inhibition of ICE slows ALS in mice. *Nature* 1997; **388**: 31.

63. Pasinelli P, Borchelt DR, Houseweart M et al. Caspase-1 is activated in neural cells and tissue with amyotrophic lateral sclerosis-associated mutations in copper-zinc superoxide dismutase. *Proc Natl Acad Sci USA* 1998; **95**: 15763–15768.

64. Rothstein J, Bristol LA, Hosler B et al. Chronic inhibition of superoxide dismutase produces apoptotic death of spinal neurons. *Proc Natl Acad Sci USA* 1994; **91**: 4155–4159.

65. Troy C, Stefanis L, Prochiantz A et al. The contrasting roles of ICE family proteases and interleukin-1beta in apoptosis induced by trophic factor withdrawal and by copper/zinc superoxide dismutase down-regulation. *Proc Natl Acad Sci USA* 1994; **91**: 6384–6387.

66. Troy C, Derossi D, Prochiantz A et al. Downregulation of Cu/Zn superoxide dismutase leads to cell death via the nitric oxide-peroxynitrite pathway. *J Neurosci* 1996; **16**: 253–261.

67. Deng HX, Hentati A, Tainer JA et al. Amyotrophic lateral sclerosis and structural defects in Cu,Zn superoxide dismutase. *Science* 1993; **261**: 1046–1051.

68. Bowling AC, Schulz JB, Brown RH Jr et al. Superoxide dismutase activity, oxidative damage, and mitochondrial energy metabolism in familial and sporadic amyotrophic lateral sclerosis. *J Neurochem* 1993; **61**: 2322–2325.

69. Borchelt DR, Lee MK, Slunt HS et al. Superoxide dismutase 1 with mutations linked to familial amyotrophic lateral sclerosis possesses significant activity. *Proc Natl Acad Sci USA* 1994; **91**: 8292–8296.

70. Marklund SL, Andersen PM, Forsgren L et al. Normal binding and reactivity of copper in mutant superoxide dismutase isolated from amyotrophic lateral sclerosis patients. *J Neurochem* 1997; **69**: 675–681.

71. Borchelt DR, Guarnieri M, Wong PC et al. Superoxide dismutase 1 subunits with mutations linked to familial amyotrophic lateral scle-

rosis do not affect wild-type subunit function. *J Biol Chem* 1995; **270**: 3234–3238.

72. Reaume AG, Elliott JL, Hoffman EK et al. Motor neurons in Cu/Zn superoxide dismutase-deficient mice develop normally but exhibit enhanced cell death after axonal injury. *Nat Genet* 1996; **13**: 43–47.

73. Gurney ME, Pu H, Chiu AY et al. Motor neuron degeneration in mice that express a human Cu,Zn superoxide dismutase mutation. *Science* 1994; **264**: 1772–1775.

74. Ripps ME, Huntley GW, Hof PR et al. Transgenic mice expressing an altered murine superoxide dismutase gene provide an animal model of amyotrophic lateral sclerosis. *Proc Natl Acad Sci USA* 1995; **92**: 689–693.

75. Wong PC, Pardo CA, Borchelt DR et al. An adverse property of a familial ALS-linked SOD1 mutation causes motor neuron disease characterized by vacuolar degeneration of mitochondria. *Neuron* 1995; **14**: 1105–116.

76. Lyons TJ, Liu H, Goto JJ et al. Mutations in copper-zinc superoxide dismutase that cause amyotrophic lateral sclerosis alter the zinc binding site and the redox behaviour of the protein. *Proc Natl Acad Sci USA* 1996; **93**: 12240–12244.

77. Wiedau-Pazos M, Goto JJ, Rabizadeh S et al. Altered reactivity of superoxide dismutase in familial amyotrophic lateral sclerosis. *Science* 1996; **271**: 515–518.

78. Yim MB, Kang JH, Yim HS et al. A gain-of-function of an amyotrophic lateral sclerosis-associated Cu,Zn-superoxide dismutase mutant: an enhancement of free radical formation due to a decrease in K_m for hydrogen peroxide. *Proc Natl Acad Sci USA* 1996; **93**: 5709–5714.

79. Beckman J, Carson M, Smith CD, Koppenol WH. ALS, SOD and peroxynitrite. *Nature* 1993; **364**: 584.

80. Shibata NA, Hirano A, Kobayashi M et al. Cu/Zn superoxide dismutase-like immunoreactivity in Lewy body-like inclusions of sporadic amyotrophic lateral sclerosis. *Neurosci Lett* 1994; **79**: 149–152.

81. Chou SM, Wang HS, Taniguchi A, Bucala R. Advanced glycation endproducts in neurofilament conglomeration of motoneurons in familial and sporadic amyotrophic lateral sclerosis. *Mol Med* 1998; **4**: 324–332.

82. Kato S, Hayashi H, Nakashima K et al. Pathological characterization of astrocytic hyaline inclusions in familial amyotrophic lateral sclerosis. *Am J Pathol* 1995; **151**: 611–620.

83. Bruijn LI, Houseweart MK, Kato S et al. Aggregation and motor neuron toxicity of an ALS-linked SOD1 mutant independent from wild-type SOD1. *Science* 1998; **281**: 1851–1854.

84. Kunst CB, Mezey E, Brownstein MJ, Patterson D. Mutations in SOD1 associated with amyotrophic lateral sclerosis cause novel protein interactions. *Nat Genet* 1997; **15**: 91–94.

85. Thornberry NA, Lazebnik Y. Caspases: enemies within. *Science* 1998; **281**: 1312–1316.

SECTION V

THERAPEUTIC APPROACHES

21

Health outcome measures

Crispin Jenkinson and Michael Swash

Introduction

The purpose of the vast majority of medical interventions is to maintain or improve function and well-being, and consequently to have a positive impact upon quality of life. Indeed, even in those instances in which the primary purpose of a treatment regime is to prevent death it is desirable that there should be positive effects on subjective health status. There are, after all, health states that many believe are worse than death.[1] Despite the obvious centrality of the patient's perspective to the assessment of health, the medical profession has not traditionally undertaken systematic evaluation of subjective, patient-based reports.[2] Undeniably, doctors have often asked patients how they are feeling or to describe symptoms, but the attempt to build this into a standardized measure that could take its place beside laboratory and radiological data or beside morbidity and mortality statistics is a relatively recent phenomenon. However, epidemiologists, clinicians, and medical researchers are now only too well aware that quality of life must in some way be measured.[3] With growing concern as to the efficacy of treatments, patients are increasingly being asked to report on their own health status in a way that can be analysed quantitatively and in a way that will inform medical practice. In a relatively short period of time, questionnaires designed to measure subjective health status measures have become an increasingly valued aspect of medical evaluation. Health outcomes are no longer narrowly conceived within the traditional biomedical model but now also incorporate the personal and social aspects of illness and its treatment.[4] The purpose of this chapter is to outline the potential uses of subjective health outcomes measures and the variety of types of measures that are available.

The move to quality of life outcomes

Amyotrophic lateral sclerosis (ALS) is a progressive, fatal disorder with an incidence of about 2/100,000 per year and a prevalence of about 6/100,000.[5] It is characterized by increasing weakness of limb, trunk, ventilatory, and bulbar muscles, usually without impairment of sphincters or of intellectual faculties. As a result, there is increasing dependency on family and other carers.[6] In the longer term this leads to a state of physical dependency and immobility. Despite the substantial impact this disease has on subjective health status and quality of life, there has been little attempt to measure these aspects of the illness. In part this may be because the data are seen as difficult to collect and interpret. However, one recent study found subjective health status to be strongly associated with measures of muscle strength and pulmonary function.[7]

This result suggests that the application of health status questionnaires to ALS patients is both feasible and informative. Future studies should seek to apply such measures when evaluating treatment regimes. The development of disease-specific measures will probably provide important additional information. It is fair to say, however, that neurology has been slower than many other areas of clinical medicine to utilize subjective health outcome measures, although this attitude is now changing. One area that has seen substantial growth in the application of health outcome measures to research and treatment in recent years is Parkinson's disease. In this disorder, generic measures have been applied and disease-specific measures have been developed.[8–12] It is likely that research in ALS will follow this move to the inclusion of patient-based reports in evaluation.

The centrality of quality of life as an outcome measure is heightened by developments in the pharmaceutical industry that suggest for the first time a feasible treatment for the disease. Until the advent of the antiglutamate drug, riluzole, there was no recognized, effective treatment. Riluzole slows progression of the disease, but it does not offer a cure.[13,14] Furthermore, its impact on quality of life remains uncertain. The clinical benefits of such new therapies should be assessed not only in terms of the quantity of life gained but in terms of the assessment of the experiences of individual patients and their families. In future, it would seem essential to assess new therapies in ALS by such means during the process of evaluation of biological efficacy, since the latter does not necessarily equate with perceived health status.[15,16]

Measurement properties

It is essential that any measure, whether assessing quality of life or, indeed, any other phenomenon, is both meaningful and accurate. The design of questionnaires is sometimes seen as a straightforward undertaking that anyone with a word processor and a competent grasp of language could master in a few moments. However, the design of questionnaires is a rigorous discipline. There are numerous examples of questionnaires that have produced meaningless or limited data owing to ignorance of some of the principles of questionnaire design.[17] The measures employed in assessing health outcomes and quality of life must be valid, reliable, and sensitive to change.

Validity

The term 'validity' refers to whether a questionnaire actually measures what it claims to measure. At one level this can be assessed by simply reading a questionnaire and determining whether it appears to make sense. This is the face validity of the questionnaire and is perhaps the first check that an investigator should undertake when testing a questionnaire. Asking members of the target group to assess the face validity of a measure is a simple but often illuminating undertaking.

Content validity refers to the questions themselves: in particular, whether they cover the range of topics that are under investigation. Measures that pass these requirements can then be assessed for criterion and construct validity.

Criterion validity is a concept that describes a given measure in relation to its correlate with some form of 'gold standard'. Given that health status measures are distinct from clinical assessment (traditionally the 'gold standard' in medical evaluations), then one would expect only modest levels of association between the two. Consequently, the search for a 'gold standard' is problematic. In most cases, therefore, new health outcome measures are compared to similar questionnaires. Short form measures, which are currently popular in response to a realization that many of the measures introduced into research are too long and burdensome for ordinary clinical use or even for use in clinical trials, are usually compared to the longer parent measure.

Finally, measures are tested for construct validity, in which certain hypotheses are constructed and the measure tested against them. Clearly, the essential variable in construct validity testing is the hypothesis itself.

Reliability

Reliability is an important aspect of assessing a questionnaire. A questionnaire that produced unreliable results would be of little value in the assessment of treatment regimes. Questionnaires should provide the same data when used repeatedly under the same conditions. Reliability is assessed by, for example, internal consistency and test–retest reliability.

Internal reliability refers to the correlation of items within a scale. One would assume that if a scale is measuring a single phenomenon (e.g. emotional distress) the questions should be related to one another and, therefore, correlated. The internal consistency of measures is often assessed by Cronbach's α-statistic.[18]

Test–retest reliability refers to the administration of a questionnaire at two separate times, usually only a few days apart. Those respondents who claim that their health has not changed between the two administrations would be expected to achieve identical, or at least very similar, scores.

Finally, if a study aims to assess outcome or change, it is imperative that questionnaires

used are sensitive to a change that is itself important to the respondents. These issues are considered in greater depth by Streiner and Norman[2] and Jenkinson.[19]

The applications of quality of life measures

There are a number of potential applications of subjective health assessment measures in the evaluation of health care (*Table 21.1*). Perhaps the most obvious use for standardized health assessment profiles is as outcome measures in randomized controlled trials and cohort studies.[20] For example, in a randomized control trial of transdermal glyceryl trinitrate against placebo in the treatment of angina, a health assessment questionnaire (the Sickness Impact Profile) showed a significant adverse effect of active drug treatment, suggesting that the continuous use of this drug in the relief of chest pain might have adverse implications for the quality of life of patients with this condition.[21] Quality of life measures have yet to play a major role in clinical trials of new therapies for ALS. It seems essential that any pharmaceutical trials to be run in the future should

Clinical trials
Regular monitoring of patient care
Screening
Improving doctor–patient interactions
Monitoring the health of populations
Economic evaluation of health care

Table 21.1
Some potential applications of health status measures.

include reliable, valid and appropriate measures of subjective health status.

On a more day-to-day level, the regular completion of health assessment questionnaires by patients has been advocated as a routine procedure that should be put in place to assess the impact of medical care. This approach is advocated by the Health Outcomes Institute in the USA, which suggests that groups of patients should be followed through treatment and beyond. This philosophy underlines the Outcomes Management System approach to health care, which suggests that quality of life data should be routinely collected and patient outcomes then assessed from this information.[22] Bardsley and colleagues used such a system to evaluate short-term outcomes of cholecystectomy with the Nottingham Health Profile.[23] They found that patients were willing to complete the questionnaires and that valuable additional data on the health of patients was collected using subjective measures of health.

It has also been found that measures of health status that can be easily and quickly completed and then scored by the physician can lead to improved doctor–patient communication. It has been found that health status data can act as adjuncts to the standard clinical interview and can appropriately inform medical practitioners of the well-being of individual patients in their care. A series of studies run in the USA suggest that both patients and clinicians believe that the use of the such simple measures of health status has led to improved interaction, better communication, and, consequently, better treatment.[24]

Related to the use of health status measures in the clinicians office is the idea that health status measures may be used to screen patients. Although the use of psychiatric screening questionnaires can be useful in increasing doctors' awareness of psychological problems in their patients,[24] to date there has not been a great rush by physicians to adopt health status measures for screening purposes, in part because quality of life measures are not designed to detect specific treatable conditions. In this context it may be remembered that general health questionnaires were extensively used in certain clinics in the 1950s and 1960s. Typically, patients were asked to complete a series of questions related to health status classified by body systems, with a number of additional general questions, and the answers were made available to the doctor and nurse when they came to evaluate the patient in consultation. This approach was particularly popular in stratified clinical evaluations such as in colorectal practice, where it is still used in some centres. It has the advantage that it allows information to be collected in a non-threatening way.

Health assessment questionnaires have been advocated as useful in the monitoring of the health of the general population, which cannot be well understood by analyses of treatment survival rates or from population mortality statistics. Population mortality statistics tell us little about the health of general populations in developed countries, and standardized health assessment measures may be used for monitoring the health of whole towns, regions, or countries.[26] Furthermore, data gathered from general population samples can be used as a yardstick by which data from clinical samples can be interpreted.[27] Thus, population data constitute normative values giving an indication as to what extent any subsample differs from the whole population. This method of interpreting generic questionnaires has been advocated as a way of making health status data more meaningful.[28]

Perhaps the most controversial application of health status data is in the prioritization of health-care resources, or what is perhaps more accurately called rationing. Health economists attempt to answer two related questions:

(a) What proportion of a society's resources should be spent on health care?

(b) How should this sum be distributed between different individuals and different types of health care?

This approach is not intended to be used to deny the importance of clinical evaluation of alternative therapies, which can identify the range of effective treatments from which a choice must be made. The task of an economic evaluation is to compare the costs and consequences of alternative procedures under consideration and so to determine the most effective allocation of resources.[29]

The use of subjective health measures is central to utility measurement. Utility refers to a subjective assessment of the well-being gained from an intervention. This measure therefore takes account of qualitative as well as quantitative medical outcomes. The most common approach is to adjust the number of life years estimated as gained from an intervention by the quality of life enjoyed by those treated. This procedure can produce a statistic known as the quality-adjusted life year (QALY) and it is possible to determine the cost per QALY gained per treatment applied. The trick here is to be able to create a single figure that measures the complex phenomena of quality of life. Most health status measures produce a profile of scores that are of little use to the health economist.

In order to generate a single unit index of life quality three issues must be addressed:[30]

(a) the relevant dimensions of life quality need to be determined;

(b) utility must be measured for each dimension; and

(c) valuations of utility for each dimension need to be aggregated.

This is a complex undertaking in itself, and potential pitfalls exist at almost every turn.

Perhaps, however, more worrying for clinicians and patients is that QALYs are potentially ageist,[31] since the multiplier in the calculation is the number of life years gained or remaining. Thus, those with only a short number of years remaining in their lives are unlikely to come top of any prioritized list even if their quality of life could be improved. Some people suggest that the elderly have had a 'fair innings',[32] but this rather trite assessment of the value of life is untenable in those patients who, in mid-life, develop illnesses that swiftly bring disability and consequently death; it is equally ill-thought out in the elderly, many of whom are capable of a high quality of life on any standard measure, even if the special attributes of the elderly are not considered in the assessment.

Finally, quality of life measures can play an important role in the assessment of the impact of a disease such as ALS on carers. The impact of taking care of someone with such a serious, progressive, and disabling condition places considerable burdens on family members. Although generic measures of health status may give some indication of carers' quality of life, it is also important that measures are developed to assess the specific aspects of the burden of care giving. Issues such as financial problems, social limitations, and emotional distress need to be explored in a systematic manner, and they will require the development of carer-specific questionnaires. This is an area that has received only scant attention to date.

Measurement instruments applicable to ALS

Neurology has at its disposal a large number of clinical measures of health state. The ALS Functional Rating Scale (ALS-FRS) was devised to assess functional status in the disease, and it has been found to be sensitive and reliable.[33] It is a physician-administered scale and as such is not suitable for wide application in large outpatient populations, in which it would be more appropriate to use a patient-administered scale. Nonetheless, this scale consists of subsections relevant to ALS — including speech, salivation, swallowing, handwriting, cutting food, dressing and hygiene, turning in bed, walking, climbing stairs, and breathing — that could be answered as easily by a patient as by a physician. Previously used measures, such as the Norris scale[34] and the Appel scale[35] consisted of a number of medical measures and clinical examination results, together with data concerning a patient's functioning and well-being. These scales are therefore composite measures, rather than quality of life measures. Indeed, most of the categories in these assessments required the physician to complete the data collection.

A number of generic measures are potentially valuable in the self-reported assessment of health status in ALS patients and have been successfully used across a wide range of illnesses. The most frequently reported generic health measures have been the Sickness Impact Profile,[36] the Functional Limitations Profile,[37] the Nottingham Health Profile,[38] and, more recently, the COOP Charts,[39] the Short-Form 36 (SF-36),[40] and the Short-Form 12.[41,42] These measures cover a wide variety of dimensions of health status and are not primarily designed to give a single index of health status but rather to provide a profile of scores. However, for most of these measures, methods of data reduction have been suggested. *Table 21.2* presents some of the attributes of these questionnaires.

The measures have all undergone extensive testing for validity (to ensure that they measure what they claim to measure) and reliability (to ensure that the same results are gained

under the same conditions at different times). All the measures are fixed-format questionnaires in which respondents indicate the frequency or extent of health problems, and they are applicable to all conditions and populations. However, many questionnaires have been designed for use in specific illnesses. Such disease-specific measures exist for a variety of different conditions and address questions that are of particular concern to patients with specific illnesses. For example, questionnaires exist for use with patients with cancer, rheumatoid arthritis, and Parkinson's disease.[43]

Generally, these questionnaires are developed by asking patients to describe in their own words the demands of their illness, and what impact it has had upon their daily lives. Content analysis is then undertaken on the material gained from these interviews to determine the most frequently discussed areas. Questions are then developed from the areas selected, matching the terminology of the patients as closely as possible. The resulting questionnaire is then tested with patients for face validity (i.e. does it make sense and appear to cover salient areas) and then, by statistical procedures, items are removed, because they appear to get the same responses as related questions or seem to be actually asking the same question. An example of this procedure can be seen in a manual documenting a Parkinson's disease questionnaire.[44] At the time of writing, an ALS-specific measure is not available, but one is at present under development and should be available in late 1999.[45]

Disease-specific questionnaires have the advantage over generic measures in that they reflect areas of concern of direct relevance to the illness and are therefore likely to be more sensitive to changes in health.[46] However, a number of researchers have begun to address the possibility of both asking individual

Functional Limitations Profile (FLP)/Sickness Impact Profile (SIP)	Nottingham Health Profile (NHP)	Short Form 36 (SF-36) Health Survey	Short Form 12 (SF-12) Health Survey	COOP Charts
Number of items: 136 **Number of dimensions:** 12	**Number of items:** 38 **Number of dimensions:** 6	**Number of items:** 36 **Number of dimensions:** 8	**Number of items:** 12 **Number of dimensions:** 2 Summary scores	**Number of items:** 9 **Number of dimensions:** 9
Dimensions Ambulation Body care and movement Mobility Household management Recreation and pastimes Social interaction Emotion Alertness Sleep and rest Eating Communication Work	**Dimensions** Energy Pain Emotional reactions Sleep Social isolation Physical mobility	**Dimensions** Physical functioning Role limitations caused by physical problems Role limitations caused by emotional problems Social functioning Mental health Energy Pain Health perception	**Dimensions** Designed to provide the PCS and MCS (see SF-36 column), but can provide eight dimensions of SF-36	**Dimensions** Physical fitness Feelings Daily activities Social activities Change in health Overall health Social support Quality of life Pain
Notes The FLP is the Anglicized version of the SIP. An overall single index score can be derived from the FLP/SIP, as can a psychosocial dimension score and a physical dimension score. Note scoring rules differ slightly for the FLP and SIP.	**Notes** The original NHP contained a second section but the developers no longer recommend its use. A single index (the NHP distress index) can be created from a subset of the items.	**Notes** Two summary scores can be derived from the SF-36: the physical component summary (PCS) and mental component summary (MCS).	**Notes** The developers do not recommend the SF-12 for use when the eight dimensions are required, but in instances when only the PCS and MCS scores are required (see SF-36 column). The SF-12 was designed to provide these scores yet in a shorter form instrument.	**Notes** There is only one item for each dimension. The charts were intended for use in the clinical interview.

Adapted from Jenkinson and McGee.[54]

Table 21.2
Properties of some commonly used generic health status measures.

patients to nominate areas of their life that have been adversely affected by their health status, and to then assess the extent of this impact. The results from each of the items selected is then aggregated to form a single index figure. A variety of methodologies for this approach exist, but in essence they all permit each individual patient to select and weight his or her own chosen areas.[47] Such a procedure has the advantage of not imposing pre-existing definitions of health status on respondents.[48] Research in this area has been undertaken in a number of groups, including patients undergoing orthopaedic surgery, human immunodeficiency virus-positive patients, patients with arthritis, and patients reporting low back pain.[49–52]

Finally, measures such as the EuroQol,[53] which is a generic measure, provide a single index and are intended to reflect the utility of given health states. In this instance, the questions in the measure are not chosen by patients but are intended to reflect the most important areas of health-related quality of life. The EuroQol contains five questions covering the areas of mobility, self-care, pain and discomfort, and anxiety–depression. Each question has three response categories (1: no problems; 2: some problems; 3: inability or extreme problems). Proponents of the measure claim that a score for overall health state can be calculated from responses to these simple questions. For example the response set '11111' indicates perfect health. There are 243 (i.e. 3^5) possible health states, each of which is weighted by values gained from the general population indicating the relative severity of the various combinations. Such single-index utility measures are used by health economists in the calculations of QALYs, the use of which remains controversial.

Conclusion

Patient-based outcome and quality of life research takes a wider perspective than the purely medical model of disease that has hitherto dominated clinical trials and other assessments of the value of treatments. It is striking to think that neurology is only now moving towards patient-based assessment. The reliance on clinical scales of health status has been dominant for so long and the apparent difficulties in measuring quality of life have been so daunting, that the move to subjective health status has been relatively slow in coming. However, it should be stressed that these measures are complementary to the traditional methods of medical evaluation of the effectiveness of any treatment and are not to be regarded as alternatives; they add an important dimension to evaluation, which has placed such a great reliance on technical and supposedly 'objective' end-points.

The future of treatment for ALS is beginning to show promise. However, assessing functional ability or length of life will not give a full insight into the impact of new treatment regimes. Subjective reports of patients will provide a far more comprehensive understanding of the effects of treatment. Furthermore, a very strong case can be made for measuring carer burden and quality of life. The full potential of quality of life measurements will only begin to be realized when the full social and economic effects are understood. After the development of new disease-specific measures for ALS, the next important task will be the creation of measures to be completed by those who care for those with the disease.

Finally, it is argued that in studies of future treatments for ALS, research should systematically measure quality of life and health status. Given the limited impact that medicine can have at present on the prognosis of this disease, it is essential that treatment at the very least improves well-being and quality of life. Further validation and experience with generic measures will increase their use and their value to the neurological community, and the development of ALS-specific outcome measures and carer questionnaires will provide important end-point measures for future trials and cohort studies.

Indeed, quality of life and health outcome measures may be used to assess personal benefit from new treatments shown to have biological effects on ALS as part of Phase III clinical trials. These data may also be used, perhaps, to assess the likely economic impact of new treatments.

References

1. Rosser R. A health index and output measure. In Walker SR, Rosser R, eds. *Quality of Life Assessment: Key Issues in the 1990s*. London: Kluwer, 1993. 151–178.
2. Streiner D, Norman G. *Health Measurement Scales: A Guide to their Development and Use* 2nd edn. Oxford: Oxford University Press, 1995.
3. Patrick DL, Erickson P. Assessing health-related quality of life for clinical decision making. In Walker SR, Rosser R, eds. *Quality of Life Assessment: Key Issues in the 1990s*. London: Kluwer, 1993. 11–64.
4. Testa MA, Simonson DC. Assessment of quality-of-life outcomes. *N Engl J Med* 1996; **334**: 835–840.
5. Brooks BR. Clinical epidemiology of amyotrophic lateral sclerosis. *Neurol Clin* 1966; **14**: 399–420.
6. Leigh PN, Swash M. *Motor Neuron Disease: Biology and Management*. London: Springer-Verlag, 1995.
7. McGuire D, Garrison L, Arman C et al. Relationship of the Tufts Quantitative Neuromuscular Exam and the Sickness Impact Profile in measuring disease progression in ALS. *Neurology* 1996; **46**: 1442–1444.
8. Shindler JS, Brown R, Welburn P, Parkes JD. Measuring the quality of life of patients with Parkinson's disease. In Walker SR, Rosser R, eds. *Quality of Life Assessment. Key Issues in the 1990s*. London: Kluwer, 1993. 289–300.
9. Peto V, Jenkinson C, Fitzpatrick R, Greenhall R. The development and validation of a short measure of functioning and well-being for individuals with Parkinson's disease. *Qual Life Res* 1995; **4**: 241–248.
10. Jenkinson C, Fitzpatrick R, Peto V et al. The Parkinson's Disease Questionnaire (PDQ-39): development and validation of a Parkinson's disease summary index score. *Age Ageing* 1997; **26**: 353–357.
11. Jenkinson C, Peto V, Fitzpatrick R et al. Self reported functioning and well-being in patients with Parkinson's disease: comparison of the SF-36 and the PDQ-39. *Age Ageing* 1995; **24**: 505–509.
12. de Boer AGEM, Wijker W, Speelman JD, de Haes JCJM. Quality of life in patients with Parkinson's disease: development of a questionnaire. *J Neurol Neurosurg Psychiatry* 1996; **61**: 70–74.
13. Lacomblez L, Bensimon G, Leigh PN et al for the Amyotrophic Lateral Sclerosis Study Group II. Dose-ranging study of riluzole in amyotrophic lateral sclerosis. *Lancet* 1996; **347**: 1425–1431.
14. Wokke J. Riluzole. *Lancet* 1996; **348**: 795–799.
15. Jenkinson C. Measuring health and medical outcomes: an overview. In: Jenkinson C, ed. *Measuring Health and Medical Outcomes*. London: UCL Press, 1994. 1–6.
16. MacIntye S. Health and illness. In: Burgess RG, ed. *Key Variables in Social Investigation*. London: Routledge and Kegan Paul, 1986.
17. Oppenheim AN. *Questionnaire Design, Interviewing and Attitude Measurement*. London: Pinter, 1992.
18. Cronbach LJ. Coefficient alpha and the internal structure of tests. *Psychometrica* 1951; **22**: 293–296.
19. Jenkinson C, ed. *Measuring Health and Medical Outcomes*. London: UCL Press, 1994.
20. Spilker B. Introduction. In: Spilker B, ed. *Quality of Life and Pharmacoeconomics in Clinical Trials*. Philadelphia: Lippincott–Raven, 1996. 1–11.

21. Fletcher A, McLoone P, Bulpitt C. Quality of life in angina therapy: a randomised controlled trial of transdermal glyceryl trinitrate against placebo. *Lancet* 1988; **2**: 4–8.

22. Anon. *The SF-36 User's Manual.* Minneapolis: Quality Quest, 1988.

23. Bardsley MJ, Venables CW, Watson J, Goodfellow J, Wright PD. Evidence for the validity of a health status measure in assessing short term outcomes in cholecystectomy. *Qual Health Care* 1992; **1**: 10–14.

24. Nelson EC, Landgraf JM, Hays RD et al. The functional status of patients: how can it be measured in patients offices? *Med Care* 1990; **28**: 1111–1126.

25. Johnstone A, Goldberg D. Psychiatric screening in general practice. *Lancet* 1976; **1**: 605–608.

26. Ware JE. Measures for a new era of health assessment. In: Stewart A, Ware JE, eds. *Measuring Functioning and Well Being.* Durham: Duke, 1992. 3–11.

27. Jenkinson C. The SF-36 physical and mental summary measures: an example of how to interpret scores. *Journal of Health Services Research and Policy,* 1998; **3**: 92–96.

28. Ware JE. Measuring patients views: the optimum outcome measure. *Br Med J* 1993; **306**: 1429–1430.

29. Mooney G. *Economics, Medicine and Health Care* 2nd edn. London: Harvester Wheatsheaf, 1992.

30. Brookes R. *Health Status Measurement: a Perspective on Change.* London: MacMillan, 1995.

31. Evans JG. Rationing health care by age: the case against. *Br Med J* 1997; **314**: 822–825.

32. Williams A. Intergenerational equity: an exploration of the 'fair innings' argument. *Health Econ* 1997; **6**: 117–132.

33. ALS CNTF Treatment Study (ACTS) Phase I-II Study Group. The amyotrophic lateral sclerosis functional rating scale; assessment of activities of daily living in patients with amyotrophic lateral sclerosis. *Arch Neurol* 1996; **53**: 141–147.

34. Norris F, Shepherd R, Denys E et al. Onset, natural history and outcome in idiopathic motor neuron disease. *J Neurol Sci* 1993; **118**: 48–55.

35. Haverkamp LJ, Appel V, Appel SH. Natural history of amyotrophic lateral sclerosis in a database population. *Brain* 1995; **118**: 707–719.

36. Bergner JL, Bobbitt RA, Pollard W et al. The Sickness Impact Profile; validation of a health status measure. *Med Care* 1976; **14**: 57–67.

37. Patrick D, Peach H, eds. *Disablement in the Community.* Oxford: Oxford University Press, 1989.

38. Hunt S, McEwan J, McKenna S. *Measuring Health Status.* Dover, UK: Croom Helm, 1986.

39. Wasson J, Keller A, Rubenstein L et al and the Dartmouth Primary Care COOP Project. Benefits and obstacles of health status assessment in ambulatory settings: the clinicians point of view. *Med Care* 1992; **30** (**suppl**): MS42–MS49.

40. Ware J, Sherbourne C. The MOS 36 item short-form survey: conceptual framework and item selection. *Med Care* 1992; **30**: 473–483.

41. Ware J, Kosinski M, Keller S. A 12-item short-form health survey. Construction of scales and preliminary tests of reliability and validity. *Med Care* 1995; **33** (**suppl**): AS264–AS279.

42. Jenkinson C, Layte R. Development and testing of the UK SF-12. *J Health Serv Res Policy* 1997; **2**: 14–18.

43. Bowling A. *Measuring Disease.* Buckingham, UK: Open University Press, 1995.

44. Jenkinson C, Fitzpatrick R, Peto V. *Manual for The Parkinsons Disease Questionnaire: User Manual for the PDQ-39, PDQ-8 and PDQ Summary Index.* Oxford: Health Services Research Unit, University of Oxford, 1998.

45. Jenkinson C, Fitzpatrick R, Swash M. *Development and Validation of the ALS-QLS (the ALS Quality of Life Scales).* Grant proposal to the Motor Neurone Disease Society, UK, 1996.

46. Jenkinson C, Stradling J, Petersen S. Comparison of three measures of quality of life outcome in the evaluation of continuous positive airways pressure therapy for sleep apnoea. *J Sleep Res* 1997; **6**: 199–204.

47. Ruta D, Garratt A. Health status to quality of life measurement. In: Jenkinson C, ed. *Measuring Health and Medical Outcomes.* London: UCL Press, 1994.

48. Ruta D, Garratt A, Leng M et al. A new approach to the measurement of quality of life: the Patient Generated Index. *Med Care* 1994;

32: 1109–1123.

49. Hickey A, Bury G, O'Boyle C et al. A new short form quality of life measure (SEIQoL-DW) application in a cohort of individuals with HIV/AIDS. *Br Med J* 1996; **313:** 29–33.

50. McGee H, O'Boyle C, Hickey A et al. Assessing the quality of life of the individual: the SEIQoL with a healthy and gastroenterology population. *Psychol Med* 1991; **21:** 749–759.

51. Garratt A, Ruta D. Taking a patient centred approach to outcome measurement. In: Hutchinson A, McColl E, Christie M, Riccalton C, eds. *Health Outcome Measures in Primary and Out-Patient Care.* Amsterdam: Harwood Academic, 1996.

52. Tugwell C, Bombardier C, Buchanan W et al. Methotrexate in rheumatoid arthritis: impact on quality of life assessed by traditional standard item and individualized patient preference health status questionnaires. *Arch Intern Med* 1990; **150:** 59–62.

53. EuroQol Group. EuroQol — a new facility for the measurement of health related quality of life. *Health Policy* 1990; **16:** 199–208.

54. Jenkinson C, McGee H. Patient assessed outcomes: measuring health status and quality of life. In: Jenkinson C, ed. *Assessment and Evaluation of Health and Medical Care: A Methods Text.* Buckingham, UK: Open University Press, 1997.

22

Review of clinical trials

Vincent Meininger and François Salachas

A wide variety of pharmaceutical agents has been tested to try to modify the course of amyotrophic lateral sclerosis (ALS). The results of almost all these trials have been considered to be negative. In consequence, not only the compounds but also the putative pathogenic mechanisms were discarded. This chapter summarizes most of the therapeutic trials undertaken since the early 1980s. The rationale for these trials is reviewed elsewhere in the book. This chapter therefore focuses on the main characteristics of the trials, namely the number of patients, the study design, evaluation criteria, data, statistical analysis, and results.

Thyrotropin-releasing hormone

The publication by Engel and colleagues[1] of a clinical functional improvement in ALS patients receiving thyrotropin-releasing hormone (TRH) triggered a number of trials. The aim was not to intervene in the mechanism of the degenerating process, but to improve the symptoms related to the motor neuron insult. Three groups of patients were studied: the first group (n = 5) received intravenous (iv) TRH 200 mg/day for four days and a placebo at day five; the second group (n = 3) received iv TRH 320–500 mg/day for two days and no placebo; and the third group (n = 9) received iv TRH

500 mg/day for 2 days and no placebo. The evaluation criteria for spasticity and motor function were not described. A transient benefit was reported in the second and third groups of patients.

In 1984, Imoto and colleagues[2] performed a double-blind, crossover trial with two treatment periods of 2 weeks each, using intramuscular (im) TRH 4 mg or placebo daily, followed by 3 weeks of observation without treatment. The seven patients were evaluated weekly over a 12-week period. Evaluation criteria were bulbar function and function of upper and lower limbs, most items involving an analysis of the time taken to perform a given task. Statistical analysis was based on the regression slope calculated with the minimal square method for each item and a t-test comparison of the TRH versus placebo period. The results were negative. Data are provided for mean and standard deviation (SD) of the grip power of the upper extremities.

Engel and Spiel[3] reported in abstract form the results of an open trial in which patients self-administered TRH at various doses (25–60 mg/day) for a period of 12–32 weeks. Sixteen patients were included: 11 had ALS, two had primary lateral sclerosis, one had progressive muscular atrophy, and two had spinal muscular atrophy. No evaluation criteria and no statistical plans are reported. Symptomatic improvement was considered to be excellent in five patients, good in five, fair in four, and poor in two.

Strober and colleagues[4] used an open trial to evaluate the efficacy of intrathecal injection of TRH at doses ranging from 10.6 to 43.2 mg over 2–4 months in six ALS patients. Evaluation criteria were measurement of atrophy, Norris score, and manual muscle testing (MMT) (but details on muscles and grades are missing). Statistical analysis was not provided, the results were negative, and no data were given.

Caroscio and colleagues[5] included 12 patients in a double-blind, placebo-controlled trial using a subcutaneous (sc) injection of TRH 150 mg or placebo and an iv infusion of TRH 500 mg or placebo over 72 hours. Evaluation criteria were bulbar score, spinal score (MMT: eight grades, 26 muscles), and upper motor neuron score (modified Ashworth scale), a voice recording, vital capacity measurement, a dynamometric recording of four or five muscles, a grip score, and time taken to perform a walking task. Statistical analysis was based on a t-test comparison of each item at 1, 3, and 8 hours. Results were negative. No values were provided. Plots of individual patients were shown.

Brooke and colleagues[6] performed a double-blind, placebo-controlled trial with 30 patients, stratified by sex and by use of a wheelchair, who received im TRH 150 mg/day or placebo for 2 months. Evaluation criteria were MMT (10 grades, 34 muscles), timed functional tests, respiratory measures (including vital capacity), quantitative forearm muscle testing for strength and fatigue, and EMG measures. Evaluation was done weekly for 2 months and then at weeks 9, 11, 14, and 16, except for EMG measures. The authors reported a partial unblinding owing to side effects. Results were negative. No data were provided. Plots of means were shown.

Serratrice and colleagues[7] included nine patients (seven with ALS) in an open trial using a sequential iv infusion of TRH 120 mg at day 1 and 240 mg at days 2, 7, 15, 30, 45, 60, and 75. Evaluation criteria were MMT (five grades, 30 muscles) at times 0 hours and 24 hours for each infusion. Statistical analysis was the analysis of variance (ANOVA) of the mean MMT score at 0 hours and 24 hours. Improvement was obtained at each period of evaluation. Means were provided without SD.

Mitsumoto and colleagues[8] examined the effects of a short-term administration of iv TRH 500 mg or placebo or a long-term administration of sc TRH 25 mg or placebo (over 3 months) in a double-blind, crossover trial. There were 41 patients in the trial. Evaluation criteria were respiratory variables, time-dependent items, MMT (five grades, 28 muscles), muscle stretch reflexes, manual grip strength, EMG variables, and isometric strength (four muscles). Statistical analysis was non-parametric for short-term treatment and parametric for quantitative variables for long-term treatment. Results were negative. Slopes of means without SD were given.

Brooks and colleagues[9] reported the results in 14 patients, previously selected as good responders, of an iv infusion of TRH 10 mg/kg or placebo on alternate days over a 10-week period. Evaluation criteria were a quantitative assessment of bulbar and limb muscles, pulmonary function tests, and timed motor tests. Items were compared using a t-test. Positive results were obtained for some variables (jaw movements, vital capacity, and lower limb functions). Histograms of means were shown.

The report of the National TRH Group[10] is in abstract form. Their double-blind, placebo-controlled trial included 108 patients who received sc TRH 5 mg/kg or placebo. The evaluation criterion was MMT (16 muscles). The results were not statistically significant. No demographic data and no detailed results were reported.

Munsat and colleagues[11] performed a double-blind, crossover trial in 36 patients. TRH 3 mg/day was delivered intrathecally for 6 months followed by 1 month wash-out. Patients had previously been selected as fast or slow decliners. Evaluation criteria were based on the Tufts Quantitative Neuromuscular Exam (TQNE) every 3 weeks. Twenty-five patients completed the trial, and the results were not statistically significant. Data were provided, with means.

Treatments for immune abnormalities in ALS

Various agents have been used to try to modify the immunological status of ALS patients.

Cyclophosphamide

Cyclophosphamide has been tested in two open trials. Brown and colleagues[12] reported the effects of 10–14 days of cyclophosphamide at a dose sufficient to obtain a white blood cell count of less than 2000/mm³. Six patients were enrolled. No evaluation criteria are given. Results were negative and no data are provided.

Smith and colleagues[13] analysed the efficacy of a total loading dose of 3 g/m² (five doses given over 8 days) followed by 6-monthly injections of 750–1000 mg/m² in 18 patients. Evaluation criteria were vital capacity, isometric strength (four muscle groups), and timed bulbar and hand function assessed every month. t-tests were used to compare the slopes of deterioration of patients to a matched control group provided by historical database. Results were negative. No data were given.

Cyclosporine

Cyclosporine was tested by Appel and colleagues[14] in a double-blind, placebo-controlled trial at 10 mg/kg per day over 48 weeks; the dose was adjusted by an unblinded investigator. Seventy patients stratified by disease duration were enrolled. The evaluation criterion was the Appel amyotrophic lateral sclerosis scale (AALS) every 4 weeks. A stopping rule was applied for an AALS score over 130 or a vital capacity less than 1000 ml. Statistics are one sided with a progression of deterioration analysed with Kaplan–Meier curves and Cox regression analysis. Results were not significant, except in men with a disease duration of less than 18 months. Means of deterioration and SD were provided.

Azathioprine

Azathioprine has been used in combination with other agents. Werdelin and colleagues[15] associated this compound (2 mg/kg per day) with prednisolone in an open trial in 21 patients (seven with ALS, five with progressive bulbar palsy, and nine with progressive muscular atrophy). Evaluation criteria were based on MMT (grades are missing, 38 muscles) every month for 3 months and then every 2 months. Results were negative. No data and no statistics were given.

Kelemen and colleagues[16] used azathioprine (2 mg/kg per day for 3 weeks) before plasmapheresis (three times a week for 2 weeks, then once a week for 3 months) in five patients (four with ALS, one with progressive muscular atrophy) in an open trial. A control group matched for age, sex, clinical course, and disease duration was used for statistical comparison. Evaluation criteria were isometric strength (eight muscles) and vital capacity. Results were not statistically significant. No data were given.

Total lymphoid irradiation

Drachman and colleagues[17] reported the results of a total lymphoid irradiation (30.6 Gr) in a double-blind placebo-controlled trial in 61 patients. Evaluation criteria were quantitative dynamometry (18 muscles), MMT (five grades, 18 muscles), timed functional variables, vital capacity, and Kurtzke scale. Assessment was done at 1 month and then every 3 months from month 6 to year 2. The expected difference was 25% between placebo and treatment. Statistical analysis was performed using a t-test comparison of each item and survival (death or respirator) with Kaplan–Meier curves. No data were given. Kaplan–Meier curves and plotting of means for dynamometry and MMT were shown.

Antiviral agents

Guanidine

Guanidine was used by Norris.[18] Two open trials were carried out: one uncontrolled trial with 175 patients (84 treated; 91 untreated, matched for sex and age); one controlled trial with 24 patients. The uncontrolled trial used a natural history control group for statistical comparison. The controlled trial used two doses (a low dose: 2 mg/kg per day and a high dose: 25 mg/kg per day) over 6 months. Evaluation criteria were the Norris scale, pulmonary function including vital capacity, and MMT (grades and muscles were not reported) every 3 months. The statistical study comprised a comparison of the Norris score, vital capacity, and maximal voluntary ventilation at entry and at 6 months. In the second study, the results were considered as significant for MMT and vital capacity. Data at entry were provided with mean and standard error (SE).

Amantadine and guanidine

Amantadine and guanidine were tried in 20 patients by Munsat and colleagues[19] in a 6-month double-blind, placebo-controlled trial. Randomization was by treatment group (amantadine or guanidine) and within strata by treatment groups (amantadine 300 mg/day, guanidine 25 mg/kg/day or placebo). Evaluation criteria consisted of a 68-item score (not defined), which was able to quantify functional performance and strength. Assessment was every month for 1 year. Statistics were not detailed and no data were reported. Results were negative.

Inosiplex (Isoprinosine)

Inosiplex was used in two trials. Brody and colleagues[20] performed a double-blind, trial that included 33 selected patients from Guam: eight paired patients were randomly allocated to treatment (inosiplex 4 g/day) or placebo, five were allocated to treatment, and 12 were not allocated (reasons not stated). Duration of treatment was 2 years. Evaluation criteria was a composite score (not detailed) that was assessed weekly for the first month, monthly for 6 months, and every other month for the remainder of the trial. Data provided were means at entry without SD or SE.

Fareed and Tyler[21] included 25 patients in a 3-month double-blind, placebo-controlled trial that used inosiplex 3–6 g/day. Evaluation criteria were clinical status, pulmonary function, EMG, and speech recording (no details provided). Statistics were not detailed. Results were negative. No data were provided.

α-interferon

α-interferon was tested by Mora and colleagues[22] in an open trial that included 10 patients who received intrathecal α-interferon weekly for a mean period of 18.4 weeks. Evaluation criteria were based on TQNE and were assessed monthly. Statistical analysis consisted of a t-test comparison of the slope of progression. No change was observed. No data were provided.

Tilorone

Tilorone 1 g once a week was used in 16 patients in a 48-week double-blind, placebo-controlled trial.[23] Evaluation criteria were pulmonary function (including vital capacity), MMT (grade and muscles missing) and speech, all assessed monthly. Statistics and data were not provided. Results were negative.

Agents that disturb cholinergic function
Physostigmine

In an open trial, Aquilonius and colleagues[24] included seven patients, who received physostigmine 1 mg/day and neostigmine 1.5 mg/day, both iv (bolus), then, in a crossover trial after a wash-out period of 2 days, physostigmine 10 mg/day for 3 days, neostigmine 45 mg/day for 3 days, and a placebo, all orally. Evaluation criteria were quantitative myometry (different muscles were used, depending on the patient) and quantitative EMG. Assessment was made during the infusion (at 0, 10, 30, and 60 minutes) and after 3 days of oral treatment. Statistical analysis included a comparison (paired and unpaired t-tests) of values at baseline and during treatment per patient and within the whole group. Results were negative. No data were provided. Plotting of individual patients was shown.

Tetrahydroaminoacridine

Ashmark and colleagues[25] included eight patients in an open trial to analyse the efficacy of tetrahydroaminoacridine 30 mg by iv infusion and oral treatment (dose increased in increments from 25 mg/day to 200 mg/day). Evaluation criteria were the Hillel scale and isometric strength (muscles not specified), which were assessed before treatment, during infusion (at 5, 15, 30, 60, and 90 minutes) and after 1, 3, and 7 weeks of oral treatment. EMG parameters were also recorded but at a lower frequency of assessment. Statistical analysis included an ANOVA comparison of parameters and t-tests for paired observations. Results were negative. Data were not provided. Slopes of deterioration were shown.

3-4 Diaminopyridine

3-4 Diaminopyridine was tested by Aisen and colleagues[26] in a double-blind, crossover trial with two evaluation periods. The starting dose was 10 mg, given orally, which was increased up to the maximum tolerated dose (mean period of time: 44.4 days for drug, and 46.1 for placebo). Nine patients were evaluated 30 minutes after the maximum dose had been administered, using EMG parameters, pulmonary function (maximal pressure), functional scale, motor function (not detailed), muscle strength (muscles not specified, five grades) and the Ashworth scale. Statistics were not detailed. No differences were observed. Data (mean, SD) were provided for functional score and muscle strength at entry.

Antioxidant drugs

Vyth and colleagues[27] reported the efficacy of an 'array of antioxidants' tested in 36 selected ALS patients (selection criteria not detailed) from a group of patients with various degenerative diseases. This open trial tested various compounds (N-acetylcysteine, Dithiothreitol (DTT), Dithioerythritol (DTE), vitamin C, vitamin E, N acetylmethionine (NAM), 2,3 dimercaptosuccinic acid (DMSA)). Evaluation criteria were the Norris score and survival. Statistics were a comparison with a historical control group (107 patients out of 307, matched for age and site of onset). No differences were observed in terms of survival. Data were not provided. Kaplan–Meier curves were shown.

Acetylcysteine

Acetylcysteine sc 50 mg/kg per day was used for 12 months by Louwerse and colleagues[28] in 111 patients in a double-blind, placebo-controlled trial. Randomization was balanced for prognostic factors (age, disease duration, bulbar symptoms, vital capacity, and disability). Evaluation criteria were MMT (20 muscles, grades missing), hand myometry, pulmonary functions (vital capacity), assessment of disability and handicap (Barthel Index, Rankin Scale), and bulbar function (Frenchay). Assessment was made monthly for MMT and pulmonary function and at irregular intervals for the other items. The primary end-point was survival at 1 year. Statistics were survival analysis unadjusted (log rank) and proportional hazard regression. Secondary analyses were rate of progression in the various parameters using the least square estimates and F statistics. Power was estimated. Despite a favorable trend, the primary end-point was not achieved. No differences in the rate of progression were observed. Data were provided with means and SE at entry.

Deprenyl

Deprenyl 10 mg/day was tested in two trials. In an open randomization (sequential entry, blinded randomization) 6-month double-blind, placebo-controlled trial, Mazzini and colleagues[29] evaluated 111 patients. Evaluation criteria were MMT (18 muscles, five grades), Norris score, bulbar score, and vital capacity, assessed every 3 months. There were three end-points: survival, mean disability score (not defined), and treatment withdrawal for adverse reaction. Statistics were a t-test comparison of the parameters at 3 and 6 months. Results were not significant. No data were provided. Plots of means and SE were shown.

Jossan and colleagues[30] designed a double-blind, crossover trial with 10 patients. Evaluation criteria were Norris score, bulbar score, and limb score (according to Plaitakis and colleagues[31]), assessed every 6 weeks. Statistical analysis was based on a t-test comparison of parameters. Results were negative. No data were provided. Plots of means and SE were shown.

Excitotoxicity
Branched-chain amino acids

The initial attempts to intervene in the mechanism of excitotoxicity were made in 1988 by Plaitakis and colleagues,[31] who used an association of three branched-chain amino acids (BCAA) — leucine, isoleucine, and valine — in 22 patients in a 12-month double-blind, placebo-controlled trial. Evaluation criteria were spinal score (MMT, 26 muscles, eight grades), bulbar score (four grades, five items), and a timed ability to walk; these were assessed every 3 months. Primary end-points were rate of decline in scores and ability to walk. Statistics comprised a t-test comparison of mean clinical scores, differences in baseline compared with an unpaired t-test, and an analysis of complete data with ANOVA for repeated measures. The primary end-point was not achieved, but the rate of decline of spinal scores showed a significant difference between the two treatment groups. No data were provided. Mean and SE were plotted.

In 1992, Plaitakis and colleagues[32] reported in abstract form the result of a confirmatory double-blind, placebo-controlled trial that included 90 patients who were studied for 9 months. Evaluation criteria were identical to those defined in the earlier trial by the same group.[31] Statistics and end-points were not reported. Results were negative. Means without SD or SE at entry were reported.

In 1993, the Italian Subgroup of the European Study Group[33] analysed the efficacy of BCAA and reported a possible increase in the risk of death in the treated group, based on a double-blind, placebo-controlled trial. Criteria for evaluation were MMT (28 muscles, five grades), modified Norris and Appel scales, and vital capacity. A sequential analysis of death rate was decided after the initial 65 patients, owing to a high death rate. The Italian Subgroup decided to abandon the trial after 126 patients because of a higher death rate in the BCAA group, both in unadjusted and adjusted analysis.

Tandan and colleagues[34] designed a three-arm, 6-month trial with BCAA, L-threonine 4 g/day and placebo in 95 patients. One investigator was unblinded for adverse events. Stratification was by treatment group, center, age, and Norris score. Assessment was made every 2 months on Norris score, MMT (21 muscles, grades missing), bulbar score (not detailed), daily activity (not detailed), forced vital capacity, timed activities, maximal voluntary isometric contraction (MVIC) (Z score, eight muscles) and EMG parameters. The primary end-point was the slope of regression of MMT and MVIC (Z score); secondary end-points were the other items. The results were not significant. Data were given, with means and SD at entry.

L-threonine

L-threonine has been tested in two trials. Testa and colleagues[35] used this compound in 30 patients in a double-blind trial. Patients received either oral L-threonine 4 g/day or an association of L-carnitine (dose not specified) and vitamin B (dose not specified) for 1 year. Evaluation criteria were based on the Norris scale, which was assessed every 3 months. Statistics were not detailed. Results were not significant. Data were given, with means at entry.

Blin and colleagues[36] conducted a 1-year double-blind, placebo-controlled trial in which they gave L-threonine 2 g/day or placebo to 23 patients. Evaluation criteria were a modified Norris score, MMT (10 muscles, grades missing), grip strength, and visual analogic scales (cramps and fasciculations). The primary end-point was the rate of decline in the Norris score with non-parametric tests at each stage. Results were not significant. Data were given for MMT (mean and SD) at entry.

Dextromethorphan

Owing to its known action on N-methyl-d-aspartate (NMDA) receptors, dextromethorphan (DMP) has been tested in four trials. Appelbaum and colleagues[37] reported the results of a 6-month double-blind, crossover trial in which patients received DMP 120 mg/day or a placebo. Eighteen patients were enrolled. Evaluation criteria and statistics were not given. Results were negative.

Ashmark and colleagues[38] tested DMP 150 mg/day in a 12-week double-blind, crossover trial with a 4-week wash-out period. Fourteen patients were enrolled. Evaluation criteria were the Plaitakis spinal and bulbar scores,[31] Norris score, myometry (different muscles in each patient), and EMG parameters assessed at the beginning and end of each period of treatment. Statistical analysis was based on an ANOVA for crossover design. Results were not significant. No data were given. Plots of means with SE were shown.

Blin and colleagues[39] tested DMP 1.5 mg/kg

per day in a 1-year double-blind, placebo-controlled trial in 49 patients. Evaluation criteria were the modified Norris scores for limbs and bulbar regions.[40] Statistics were an intention-to-treat analysis of survival and the rate of deterioration of Norris scores. Results were not significant. No data were given.

Gredal and colleagues[41] used DMP 150 mg/day in a 1-year double-blind, placebo-controlled trial. Randomization was balanced for age, site of onset, and vital capacity. Evaluation criteria were the Hillel scale and vital capacity, which were assessed every 3 months. Primary end-point was death at 1 year (log rank and Cox); secondary end-points were vital capacity and slope of deterioration of Hillel score. Analysis was based on an intention-to-treat analysis with stratification by site of onset. Results were not significant. Data at entry were given with means and SD.

Calcium channel blockers

Verapamil

Verapamil was used in an open trial[42] in 72 patients matched for age and time since diagnosis with a natural history control group. The evaluation criterion was Tufts Quantitive Neuromuscular Exam (TQNE) assessed monthly from 3 months before treatment to month 6 of treatment. A statistical comparison was made with the control group. Results were not significant. Data at entry were given.

Niomodipine

Nimodipine was tested in two trials. Miller and colleagues[43] designed a double-blind, crossover trial with nimodipine 60 mg/day or placebo in 87 patients during a 3-month treatment period with a 1-month wash-out period. The evaluation criterion was TQNE, which was assessed monthly. The end-point was the slope of deterioration of vital capacity and arm megascore of TQNE during the first 4

months. Statistical analysis was based on a one-tailed t-test for comparison of means and individuals. Results were not significant. Data were given.

Ziv and colleagues,[44] in an open trial with two patients, considered their results to be not significant.

Lamotrigine

Eisen and colleagues[45] used lamotrigine 100 mg/day in 67 patients in a double-blind, placebo-controlled trial. The duration of treatment was determined by interim analysis. Evaluation criteria comprised a composite score with bulbar, walking, age, and daily parameters, which were assessed every 3 months, and EMG parameters. The primary end-point was survival. Secondary end-points were rate of decline of the various scores. Statistical analysis consisted of a sequential analysis for the primary end-point and a t-test comparison for secondary end-points. After 18 months, results were not significant and the trial was stopped.

Gabapentin

Gabapentin was tested in a double-blind, placebo-controlled trial[46] in 152 patients at increasing doses from 800 mg/day to 2000 or 2400 mg/day (adjusted according to adverse reactions). Evaluation criteria were MVIC (eight arm muscles) and vital capacity, which were assessed every 4 weeks. The primary end-point was the mean slope of arm megascore of the intention-to-treat population (excluding patients with only one measure). Secondary end-points were the rate of decline of vital capacity and arm megascore of completers. The trial was completed by 117 patients. The primary end-point was not achieved, but a trend was observed at 0.06, with a 24% difference in slope. Secondary end-point results were not significant and the trend was not observed in the completers. No data were given.

Riluzole

Two trials were conducted with riluzole.[40,47] Both trials were double-blind and placebo-controlled. Randomization was stratified by center and according to the site of disease onset: bulbar or spinal. Criteria for evaluation were modified Norris spinal and bulbar scores, MMT (five grades, 22 muscles), vital capacity, and visual analogic scales (fatigue, fasciculations, cramps, and stiffness). Assessment was every 2 months except for vital capacity, which was assessed every 6 months. In the first trial,[40] 155 patients were included and riluzole was administered at 100 mg/day for 12 months after the enrollment of the final patient. Primary end-points were survival (tracheostomy-free) and the rate of decline of the functional status (spinal and bulbar scores). Secondary end-points were the other parameters.

In the second trial,[47] 959 patients were treated with riluzole 50, 100, 200 mg/day or placebo during 18 months. The primary end-point was survival (tracheostomy-free). Secondary end-points were the other parameters. Statistical analysis was identical in each trial: for survival, unadjusted analysis (Kaplan–Meier and log rank) and adjusted analysis (Cox regression model); for rate of change, the unweighted least-squares method.

In both trials, the primary end-point was achieved and the death rate was decreased in the treated group compared to the placebo. Data at entry and risk factors were provided. Slopes of deterioration (mean and SE) were shown.

Neurotrophic factors and axonal spouting
Gangliosides

Gangliosides suspected of having neurotrophic properties and of enhancing axonal sprouting have been tested in three double-blind, placebo-controlled trials, each of which included 40 patients.

Bradley and colleagues[48] used im gangliosides 40 mg/day for 6 months. Evaluation criteria were vital capacity, isometric strength (18 muscles), timed activities, and bulbar function. Statistical analysis was a comparison of variables using a t-test (120 comparisons). Results were not significant. Data were not provided.

Harrington and colleagues[49] used the same dosage of gangliosides. Criteria for evaluation were MMT (22 muscles, grades missing), strain gauge dynamometer and vital capacity, which were assessed every 2 months for 6 months. Results were not significant. Results at entry were provided.

Lacomblez and colleagues[50] used im gangliosides 300 mg/day or placebo for 3 months. Evaluation criteria were a modified Norris scale and MMT (28 muscles, five grades), which were assessed every month. Statistics were ANOVA for continuous data and chi square comparison for categorical data. Results were not significant. Data at entry were provided.

Growth hormone

Growth hormone was used im at 0.1 mg/kg three times a week and compared to placebo for up to 18 months in 75 patients in a double-blind, placebo-controlled trial.[51] Evaluation criteria were TQNE and MMT (20 muscles, four grades) assessed every 2 months.

End-points and statistics were not given. Results were not significant. Data were not given, but slopes of decline of TQNE were shown.

Neurotrophic factors

Brain-derived neurotrophic factor

Brain-derived neurotrophic factor was tested in two trials, one exploratory and the other pivotal. Neither trial was published.

Ciliary neurotrophic factor

Subcutaneous injections of ciliary neurotrophic factor (CNTF) have been tested in two double-blind, placebo-controlled trials. In the first trial,[52] CNTF was administered at 30 or 15 μg/kg/day and compared to placebo for 9 months in 730 patients. Evaluation criteria were isometric muscle strength (muscles not specified), pulmonary function (including vital capacity), the Amyotrophic Lateral Sclerosis Functional Rating Scale (ALSFRS) and the Schwab scale. The primary end-point was the rate of decline in muscle strength; secondary end-points were the other parameters. Statistical analysis compared the 30 μg group versus placebo and all the CNTF patients versus placebo. Results were not significant. The death rate was identical in the various groups. Data (means and SE) were provided for arm megascore and vital capacity. Slopes of means and SE were shown for muscle strength and vital capacity.

The second trial[53] analysed 570 patients who received CNTF 0.5, 2 or 5 μg/kg per day or placebo for 6 months. Evaluation criteria were MVIC (18 muscles, Z megascore), vital capacity and Sickness Impact Profile (SIP) assessed every 4 weeks. The primary end-point was a change in megascore from the baseline. Secondary end-points were the other parame-

ters and survival in two populations: the intention-to-treat group and completers. Results were not significant. Death rate was doubled in the 5 μg group. Data (means and SD) were provided for arm megascore and vital capacity. Plots of arm megascore and vital capacity slopes were shown (means and SD).

Insulin growth factor

Insulin growth factor (IGF)-I was tested in 266 patients in a double-blind, placebo-controlled trial[54] with three arms (placebo, IGF-I 0.05 mg/kg per day, and 0.1 mg/kg per day). Evaluation criteria were Appel scale and SIP, which were assessed every month. Treatment failure was determined as an Appel scale >115, vital capacity <39% of the predicted value, or both. The primary end-point was the slope of Appel scale after the randomization period. Secondary end-points were a change in the score from the baseline, time to failure, and a change in SIP or vital capacity. Statistical analysis for the primary end-point was a co-variate adjusted ANOVA. The primary end-point was not achieved. A significant result was obtained in a subgroup (high rate decliners) of the group of patients who received IGF-I 0.1 mg/kg per day. Data were provided.

Conclusions

If the design of the trials conducted over the past 10 years in ALS is considered, in approximately half of the 51 long-term trials, the number of patients per treatment arm was 18 or fewer and the mean duration was 24 weeks or less. The evaluation criteria used in the trials varied considerably. Among the most commonly used end-parameters were vital capacity in 45% of the trials, MMT in 41%, bulbar function in 35%, isometric strength (including trials with only a grip strength evaluation) in 33%, the Norris scale in 31%, and survival in 25%. Some scales are used very infrequently: timed activities were used in 15%, TQNE in 13%, the Appel scale in 6%, and the Hillel scale in 4%. The end-points were defined clearly at entry in 47% of the trials, and data were provided in 43%. For most of the trials, the data provided were the demographic characteristics of the patients at entry. However, the most useful data, namely the means and SD of the end-points, such as the slopes of deterioration, were provided clearly in fewer than 5% of the trials. Only six trials defined the expected difference between placebo and treatment as stated in the study design.

These results raise some important issues.

(a) It is often impossible to obtain sufficient information on the characteristics of the patients. This information is essential to be able to compare the data. Even a negative trial can provide very useful information on the ALS population.

(b) It is very difficult to compare the results of the various trials, owing to the great differences between the end-points that were used. Despite the extreme diversity of evaluation criteria, two criteria — vital capacity and MMT — are used frequently. However, there is clearly considerable uncertainty over which procedures were used to assess these parameters.

(c) Most of the trials were double-blind and placebo-controlled. Fewer than 10% used natural history control groups.

(d) The most puzzling results concern the information on the drugs and on the disease mechanisms that can be ascertained from the published trials. With the exception of the riluzole trials,[40,47] all trials have been considered to be negative. These negative results have had important repercus-sions since they have led to the tested compound being discarded and frequently to potential candidate mechanisms of the disease being rejected. However, very few of the trials stated the degree of improvement in symptomatology that would have allowed the investigators to conclude that the drug could be considered as active. In this respect, two parameters are essential: the SD and the number of patients. The SD of the slopes of deterioration for most parameters tested (including isometric strength) were 0.7 and 1.5 of the mean. As stated above, the number of patients in the majority of trials was 18 or fewer. Using an SD of 1 and 18 patients and calculating the expected difference between a placebo and an active compound for vital capacity or MMT gives approximately an 80–90% difference. It follows, therefore, that for most of the trials the answer is not that the compound was not active, but rather that the compound did not achieve an expected 80–90% difference compared to the placebo. Since such a huge difference seems totally unrealistic in ALS, it is also reasonable to conclude that none of the published trials was able to eliminate a possible activity of the compounds that were tested and thus discard the associated putative etiopathogenic mechanism of ALS.

References

1. Engel WK, Siddique T, Nicoloff JT. Effect on weakness and spasticity in amyotrophic lateral sclerosis of thyrotropin-releasing hormone. *Lancet* 1983; **1**: 73–75.
2. Imoto K, Saida K, Iwamura K et al. Amyotrophic lateral sclerosis: a double-blind crossover trial of thyrotropin-releasing hormone. *J Neurol Neurosurg Psychiatry* 1984; **47**: 1332–1334.

3. Engel WK, Spiel RH. Prolonged at-home treatment of motor neuron disorders with self-administered subcutaneous (sq) high-dose TRH. *Neurology* 1985; **35** (suppl 1): 106–107.

4. Strober T, Shimrigk K, Dietzsch S, Thielen T. Intrathecal thyrotropin-releasing hormone therapy of amyotrophic lateral sclerosis. *J Neurol* 1985; **232**: 13–14.

5. Caroscio JT, Cohen JA, Zawodniak J et al. A double-blind, placebo-controlled trial of TRH in amyotrophic lateral sclerosis. *Neurology* 1986; **36**: 141–145.

6. Brooke MH, Florence JM, Heller SL et al. Controlled trial of thyrotropin releasing hormone in amyotrophic lateral sclerosis. *Neurology* 1986; **36**: 146–151.

7. Serratrice G, Desnuelles C, Crevat A et al. Traitement de la sclérose latérale amyotrophique par le facteur de libération de l'hormone thyréotrope (TRH). *Rev Neurol* 1986; **142**: 133–139.

8. Mitsumoto H, Salgado ED, Negroski D et al. Amyotrophic lateral sclerosis: effects of acute intravenous and chronic subcutaneous administration of tyrotropin-releasing hormone in controlled trials. *Neurology* 1986; **36**: 152–159.

9. Brooks BR, Sufit RL, Montgomery GK et al. Intravenous thyrotropin-releasing hormone in patients with amyotrophic lateral sclerosis. Dose-response and randomized concurrent placebo-controlled pilot studies. *Neurol Clin* 1987; **5**: 143–158.

10. National TRH Study Group. Multicenter controlled trial: no effect of alternate-day 5 mg/kg subcutaneous thyrotropin-releasing hormone (TRH) on isometric-strength decrease in amyotrophic lateral sclerosis. *Neurology* 1989; **39** (suppl 1): 322.

11. Munsat TL, Taft J, Jackson IM et al. Intrathecal thyrotropin-releasing hormone does not alter the progressive course of ALS: experience with an intrathecal drug delivery system. *Neurology* 1992; **42**: 1049–1053.

12. Brown RH Jr, Hauser SL, Harrington H, Weiner HL. Failure of immunosuppression with a Ten- to 14-Day course of high-dose intravenous cyclophosphamide to alter the progression of amyotrophic lateral sclerosis. *Arch Neurol* 1986; **43**: 383–384.

13. Smith SA, Miller RG, Murphy JR, Ringel SP. Treatment of ALS with high dose pulse cyclophosphamide. *J Neurol Sci* 1994; **124** (suppl): 84–87.

14. Appel SH, Stewart SS, Appel V et al. A double-blind study of the effectiveness of cyclosporine in amyotrophic lateral sclerosis. *Arch Neurol* 1988; **45**: 381–386.

15. Werdelin L, Boysen G, Jensen TS, Mogensen P. Immunosuppressive treatment of patients with amyotrophic lateral sclerosis. *Acta Neurol Scand* 1990; **82**: 132–134.

16. Kelemen J, Hedlund W, Orlin JB et al. Plasmapheresis with immunosuppression in amyotrophic lateral sclerosis. *Arch Neurol* 1983; **40**: 752–753.

17. Drachman DB, Chaudhry V, Cornblath D et al. Trial of immunosuppression in amyotrophic lateral sclerosis using total lymphoid irradiation. *Ann Neurol* 1994; **35**: 142–150.

18. Norris FH, Calanchini PR, Fallat RJ et al. The administration of guanidine in amyotrophic lateral sclerosis. *Neurology* 1974; **24**: 721–728.

19. Munsat TL, Easterday CS, Levy S et al. Amantadine and guanidine are ineffective in ALS. *Neurology* 1981; **31**: 1054–1055.

20. Brody JA, Chen KM, Yase Y et al. Inosiplex and amyotrophic lateral sclerosis. Therapeutic trial in patients on Guam. *Arch Neurol* 1974; **30**: 322–323.

21. Fareed GC, Tyler HR. The use of isoprinosine in patients with amyotrophic lateral sclerosis. *Neurology* 1971; **21**: 937–940.

22. Mora JS, Munsat TL, Kao KP et al. Intrathecal administration of natural human interferon alpha in amyotrophic lateral sclerosis. *Neurology* 1986; **36**: 1137–1140.

23. Olson WH, Simons JA, Halaas GW. Therapeutic trial of tilorone in ALS: lack of benefit in a double-blind, placebo-controlled study. *Neurology* 1978; **28**: 1293–1295.

24. Aquilonius SM, Ashmark H, Eckernas SA et al. Cholinesterase inhibitors lack therapeutic effect in amyotrophic lateral sclerosis. A controlled study of physostigmine versus neostigmine. *Acta Neurol Scand* 1986; **73**: 628–632.

25. Askmark H, Aquilonius SM, Gillberg PG et al. Functional and pharmacokinetic studies of tetrahydroaminoacridine in patients with amy-

otrophic lateral sclerosis. *Acta Neurol Scand* 1990; **82**: 253–258.

26. Aisen ML, Sevilla D, Edelstein L, Blass J. A double-blind placebo-controlled study of 3,4-diaminopyridine in amytrophic lateral sclerosis patients on a rehabilitation unit. *J Neurol Sci* 1996; **138**: 93–96.

27. Vyth A, Timmer JG, Bossuyt PM et al. Survival in patients with amyotrophic lateral sclerosis, treated with an array of antioxidants. *J Neurol Sci* 1996; **139** (suppl): 99–103.

28. Louwerse ES, Weverling GJ, Bossuyt PM et al. Randomized, double-blind, controlled trial of acetylcysteine in amyotrophic lateral sclerosis. *Arch Neurol* 1995; **52**: 559–564.

29. Mazzini L, Testa D, Balzarini C, Mora G. An open-randomized clinical trial of selegiline in amyotrophic lateral sclerosis. *J Neurol* 1994; **241**: 223–227.

30. Jossan SS, Ekblom J, Gudjonsson O et al. Double blind cross over trial with deprenyl in amyotrophic lateral sclerosis. *J Neural Transm Suppl* 1994; **41**: 237–241.

31. Plaitakis A, Smith J, Mandeli J, Yahr MD. Pilot trial of branched-chain aminoacids in amyotrophic lateral sclerosis. *Lancet* 1988; **1**: 1015–1018.

32. Plaitakis A, Sivak M, Fesdjian CO, Mandeli J. Treatment of amyotrophic lateral sclerosis with branched chain amino acids (BCAA): results of the secondary study. *Neurology* 1992; **42** (suppl 3): 454.

33. The Italian ALS Study Group. Branched-chain amino acids and amyotrophic lateral sclerosis: a treatment failure? *Neurology* 1993; **43**: 2466–2470.

34. Tandan R, Bromberg MB, Forshew D et al. A controlled trial of amino acid therapy in amyotrophic lateral sclerosis: I. Clinical, functional, and maximum isometric torque data. *Neurology* 1996; **47**: 1220–1226.

35. Testa D, Caraceni T, Fetoni V, Girotti F. Chronic treatment with L-threonine in amyotrophic lateral sclerosis: a pilot study. *Clin Neurol Neurosurg* 1992; **94**: 7–9.

36. Blin O, Pouget J, Aubrespy G et al. A double-blind placebo-controlled trial of L-threonine in amyotrophic lateral sclerosis. *J Neurol* 1992; **239**: 79–81.

37. Appelbaum JS, Salazar-Grueso EF, Richman JG et al. Dextromethorphan in the treatment of ALS: a pilot study. *Neurology* 1991; **41** (suppl 1): 393.

38. Askmark H, Aquilonius SM, Gillberg PG et al. A pilot trial of dextromethorphan in amyotrophic lateral sclerosis. *J Neurol Neurosurg Psychiatry* 1993; **56**: 197–200.

39. Blin O, Azulay JP, Desnuelle C et al. A controlled one-year trial of dextromethorphan in amyotrophic lateral sclerosis. *Clin Neuropharmacol* 1996; **19**: 189–192.

40. Bensimon G, Lacomblez L, Meininger V, the ALS/riluzole study group. A controlled trial of riluzole in amyotrophic lateral sclerosis. *N Eng J Med* 1994; **330**: 585–589.

41. Gredal O, Werdelin L, Bak S et al. A clinical trial of dextromethorphan in amyotrophic lateral sclerosis. *Acta Neurol Scand* 1997; **96**: 8–13.

42. Miller RG, Smith SA, Murphy JR et al. A clinical trial of verapamil in amyotrophic lateral sclerosis. *Muscle Nerve* 1996; **19**: 511–515.

43. Miller RG, Shepherd R, Dao H et al. Controlled trial of nimodipine in amyotrophic lateral sclerosis. *Neuromuscul Disord* 1996; **6**: 101–104.

44. Ziv I, Achiron A, Djaldetti R et al. Can nimodipine affect progression of motor neuron disease? A double blind pilot study. *Clin Neuropharmacol* 1994; **17**: 423–428.

45. Eisen A, Stewart H, Schulzer M, Cameron D. Anti-glutamate therapy in amyotrophic lateral sclerosis: a trial using lamotrigine. *Can J Neurol Sci* 1993; **20**: 297–301.

46. Miller RG, Moore D, Young LA et al. Placebo-controlled trial of gabapentin in patients with amyotrophic lateral sclerosis. WALS Study Group. Western Amyotrophic Lateral Sclerosis Study Group. *Neurology* 1996; **47**: 1383–1388.

47. Lacomblez L, Bensimon G, Leigh PN et al for the amyotrophic lateral sclerosis/riluzole study group II. Dose-ranging study of riluzole in amyotrophic lateral sclerosis. *Lancet* 1996; **347**: 1425–1431.

48. Bradley WG, Hedlund W, Cooper C. A double-blind controlled trial of bovine brain gangliosides in amyotrophic lateral sclerosis. *Neurology* 1984; **34**: 1079–1082.

49. Harrington H, Hallett M, Tyler HR. Ganglio-

sides therapy for amyotrophic lateral sclerosis: a double blind controlled trial. *Neurology* 1984; **34**: 1083–1085.

50. Lacomblez L, Bouche P, Bensimon G, Meininger V. A double-blind placebo controlled trial of high doses of gangliosides in amyotrophic lateral sclerosis. *Neurology* 1989; **39**: 1635–1637.

51. Smith RA, Melmed S, Sherman B et al. Recombinant growth hormone treatment of amyotrophic lateral sclerosis. *Muscle Nerve* 1993; **16**: 624–633.

52. ALS CNTF Treatment Study Group. A double-blind placebo-controlled clinical trial of subcutaneous recombinant human ciliary neurotrophic factor (rHCNTF) in amyotrophic lateral sclerosis. *Neurology* 1996; **46**: 1244–1249.

53. Miller RG, Petajan JH, Bryan WW et al. A placebo-controlled trial of recombinant human ciliary neurotrophic (rhCNTF) factor in amyotrophic lateral sclerosis. rhCNTF ALS Study Group. *Ann Neurol* 1996; **39**: 256–260.

54. Lai EC, Felice KJ, Festoff BW et al. Effect of recombinant human insulin-like growth factor-I on progression of ALS. *Neurology* 1997; **49**: 1621–1630.

SECTION VI

PATIENT CARE

23

A treatable disease: a guide to the management of amyotrophic lateral sclerosis

Deborah F Gelinas and Robert G Miller

Introduction

Amyotrophic lateral sclerosis (ALS), also known as Lou Gehrig's disease, is a frightening disease to patient, family, and friends. In addition to the ongoing deterioration of the muscles, ALS can cause the loss of the ability to speak and to swallow. This can have obvious negative effects on the quality of life of the patient. This chapter stresses informed management decision making for patients as well as empowerment for caregivers. This chapter introduces strategies for coping with decreasing physical abilities, various stages of disability, and patient bereavement over lost health.

Perhaps the best way to begin a chapter on the management of ALS is to review the disease itself. ALS is an uncommon disease that affects both men and women in middle adulthood and results in paralysis of voluntary muscles. For the most part, the patient's intellect and personality remain intact. ALS inexorably progresses with increasing physical disability accompanied by consequent emotional and almost inevitable financial hardship. The diagnosis of ALS challenges a person to unlearn mastery of the body, to unlearn personal control and independence, and to return to a state of almost complete dependence. The diagnosis of ALS forces a person to become slowly and increasingly dependent on others for the smallest want or desire. Know-

ing the inevitability of what disability lies ahead for their patient, it is not surprising that many physicians feel powerless to give patients adequate assistance in managing ALS. The task appears overwhelming. Furthermore, the definition of managing is 'to bring about or succeed in accomplishing'. Managing ALS may therefore seem to be an oxymoron — how can a physician succeed with a disease that defies cure or containment? What is there to oversee besides progressive loss?

Before discussing management, it is useful to try to conceptualize the goal. The over-riding objective is for the patient to live as fully as possible. The man or woman with a diagnosis of ALS must struggle to live each day well while being forced to let go of many capabilities that in the past have made life worth living. The physician must assist patients in cherishing their lives regardless of the difficulties; by befriending, advising, educating, and preparing them for the next challenge. From birth, a child is prepared by a good parent to face the challenges of growth and development. From diagnosis, a patient is prepared by a good physician to face the escalating challenges imposed by ALS. Until the time of that diagnosis, the patient may not have acquired many of the necessary skills that will be required to live fully while suffering from ALS. The physician must therefore oversee this entire educational process. The physician alone is familiar both with the disease and the grieving over lost vitality that is brought about by the very nature of this progressive illness.

ALS patients frequently complain that their physicians do not want to see them, do not want to talk to them, and do not know how to comfort them. The physician has no ability to comfort a patient until the physician accepts the fact that ALS cannot be cured. Once the physician accepts this limitation, he or she can then lend strength and solace to those who suffer by making a commitment of time and availability. Although sometimes undeserving of respect, physicians are in fact greatly respected by patients. Time with the physician is therefore highly valued. Even if no specific therapeutic intervention occurs, a patient begins to feel comforted when spending time with his or her physician. Patients do not necessarily expect their physician to be experts but they do expect them to take the time to become informed about their specific problems with ALS. At each patient encounter, the physicians must learn more about ALS from the patient and share information about ALS with the patient. This can not be accomplished in a hurry.

Diagnosis

Initially, diagnosis will entail a careful review of the patient's history and tests to ascertain that ALS is the correct diagnosis. The El Escorial Criteria[1] serve as a helpful guide. A history of progressive weakness is essential for the diagnosis.

The term ALS should be avoided until there is diagnostic confidence and the patient has been offered a second opinion. The possibility of error must always be entertained and a more 'treatable' disease must always be sought. The variability of the disease should be stressed, as should the variability in disease progression.[2] The patients should always be left with hope. Offering hope is not lying; it is allowing life.

Every patient should be seen as exceptional and as having the potential to face and rise above the challenges that lie ahead while retaining personal dignity and joy in living.

General management principles

Periodic evaluations with forced vital capacity and vital signs should take place every 2–3 months, depending on disease progression.[3] At each visit, the physician should reassess the patient's understanding of the disease and the patient's desire for more or less active disease management. The patient is autonomous and ultimately decides the course of disease — whether to be aggressive or passive. The physician serves as an advisor, informing the patient of various options and the consequences of those options.

This entails an ongoing discussion and ongoing re-evaluation of the desires of the patient. Too often, physicians seek to resolve these issues in one session, exhorting patients to write their wishes regarding invasive life support and resuscitation. A statement of patient autonomy — advance directives — that clearly states the patient's desires is a very important document and helps physicians in managing the ALS patient. However, this 'living will', as with all wills, must be revisited periodically and revised as the circumstances dictate. Patients change during the course of ALS and sometimes life becomes so precious that conditions that would have once been considered intolerable are not so any longer.

For this reason periodic re-evaluations of the patient's physical status as well as emotional and psychologic outlook are essential. An excellent tool to evaluate patient function is the ALS Function Rating Scale (ALSFRS), which identifies key issues in the progression of ALS (*Table 23.1*).[4] Below-normal scores on

ALS FUNCTIONAL RATING SCALE (ALSFRS)

Date Performed: ☐☐ day ☐☐☐ month ☐☐ year

1. SPEECH
- 4 ☐ Normal speech processes
- 3 ☐ Detectable speech disturbance
- 2 ☐ Intelligible with repeating
- 1 ☐ Speech combined with non-vocal communication
- 0 ☐ Loss of useful speech

2. SALIVATION
- 4 ☐ Normal
- 3 ☐ Slight but definite excess of saliva in mouth; may have night-time drooling
- 2 ☐ Moderately excessive saliva; may have minimal drooling
- 1 ☐ Marked excessive of saliva with some drooling
- 0 ☐ Marked drooling; requires constant tissue or handkerchief

3. SWALLOWING
- 4 ☐ Normal eating habits
- 3 ☐ Early eating problems; occasional choking
- 2 ☐ Dietary consistency changes
- 1 ☐ Needs supplemental tube feeding (subject must be excluded from the study)
- 0 ☐ Nil by mouth (exclusively parenteral or enteral feeding) (subject must be excluded from the study)

4. HANDWRITING (with dominant hand prior to ALS onset)
- 4 ☐ Normal
- 3 ☐ Slow or sloppy; all words are legible
- 2 ☐ Not all words are legible
- 1 ☐ Able to grip pen but unable to write
- 0 ☐ Unable to grip pen

5a. CUTTING FOOD AND HANDLING UTENSILS (Subjects without gastrotomy)
- 4 ☐ Normal
- 3 ☐ Somewhat slow and clumsy, but no help needed
- 2 ☐ Can cut most foods, although clumsy and slow, some help needed
- 1 ☐ Food must be cut by someone, but can still feed slowly
- 0 ☐ Needs to be fed

Total Score _____

5b. CUTTING FOOD AND HANDLING UTENSILS (Subjects with gastrotomy)
- 4 ☐ Normal
- 3 ☐ Clumsy but able to perform all manipulations independently
- 2 ☐ Some help needed with closures and fasteners
- 1 ☐ Provides minimal assistance to caregiver
- 0 ☐ Unable to perform any aspect of task

6. DRESSING AND HYGIENE
- 4 ☐ Normal function
- 3 ☐ Independent and complete self-care with effort or decrease in efficiency
- 2 ☐ Intermittent assistance or substitute methods
- 1 ☐ Need attendant for self-care
- 0 ☐ Total dependence

7. TURNING IN BED/ADJUSTING BEDCLOTHES
- 4 ☐ Normal
- 3 ☐ Somewhat slow and clumsy, but no help needed
- 2 ☐ Can turn alone or adjust sheets, but with great difficulty
- 1 ☐ Can initiate, but not turn or adjust sheets alone
- 0 ☐ Helpless

8. WALKING
- 4 ☐ Normal
- 3 ☐ Early ambulation difficulties
- 2 ☐ Walks with assistance (any assistive device, including ankle–foot orthoses)
- 1 ☐ Non-ambulatory functional movement only
- 0 ☐ No purposeful leg movement

9. CLIMBING STAIRS
- 4 ☐ Normal
- 3 ☐ Slow
- 2 ☐ Mild unsteadiness or fatigue
- 1 ☐ Needs assistance (including handrail)
- 0 ☐ Cannot do

10. BREATHING
- 4 ☐ Normal
- 3 ☐ Shortness of breath with minimal exertion (e.g., walking, talking)
- 2 ☐ Shortness of breath at rest
- 1 ☐ Intermittent (e.g. nocturnal) ventilatory assistance
- 0 ☐ Ventilator-dependent

Table 23.1
The ALS functional rating scale.

1. Do you have difficulty sleeping?
2. Do you wake up frequently during the night?
3. Do you snore?
4. Does your spouse say that you snore?
5. Are you sleepy during the daytime?
6. Are you more tired than you used to be?
7. Do you fall asleep frequently during the day?
8. Have you ever fallen asleep during a meal?
9. Has anyone noticed that you stop breathing during sleep?

Table 23.2
Sleep symptom questionnaire administered to patients with amyotrophic lateral sclerosis. From Gay et al.[5]

the ALSFRS naturally lead to further questions and allow the physicians to evaluate symptoms in a comprehensive manner. Since adequate sleep is a major component of daytime well-being, questions relating to the quality of the patient's sleep should also be addressed routinely (*Table 23.2*).[5] Even minor sleep disturbances can cause a major disruption in a patient's well-being, and therapeutic options should be offered accordingly (see below).

Disease-specific treatment

Once the diagnosis is established, patients will be interested in pursuing treatment. The only disease-specific treatment for ALS that is approved in the USA by the Food and Drug Administration at this time is riluzole, a glutamate inhibitor. Two placebo-controlled, double-blind trials demonstrated that riluzole modestly extends survival for patients with ALS (by an average of 2–3 months).[6,7] The advantages and disadvantages of treatment with riluzole should be discussed, and riluzole should be offered (where it is available) in the hope of slowing the progress of the disease.

Patients will usually also be interested in pursuing investigational treatment possibili-ties. Thus, patients should be informed of ongoing clinical trials, especially if they live near an ALS center and are interested in participating. Patients cope better with ALS when they are not merely passive victims of the disease but partners in a search for the optimum treatment. The ALS Association as well as the Muscular Dystrophy Association publishes periodic newsletters announcing research trials in ALS. This information is also available unofficially through various Internet locations such as the ALS Digest (www.brunel.ack.uk~hssrsdn/alsig/alsig.htm) or (http://www.flash.net/~gnichola).

Alternative treatment

ALS patients are often dissatisfied (as are their physicians) with the disease specific treatment offered by conventional medicine. Many patients therefore seek other, alternative, solutions to their disease. These holistic approaches may benefit the patient greatly in affording a sense of mastery over the disease. Nutritional regimens that stress the role of antioxidant vitamins in postponing symptom manifestation have some experimental basis, but are still not of proven value to patients, yet these and other approaches (such as therapeutic massage, visual imagery etc) may offer support, encouragement, and hope.[8]

Patients cannot live without hope and should not be disabused of their hope. Instead, patients should be encouraged to share their exploration into alternative treatments with their physicians. The physician should serve as an advisor steering patients away from exploitative and harmful therapies and towards those in which the provider is doing no harm and seeking to do good. For patients who desire a holistic approach, it is important for the physician to listen with an open mind, to seek to understand, and to ask to be kept informed. In this way, the patient will feel free to ask for more conventional therapies when the need arises. It is not necessary to be encouraging of alternative therapies, but neither is it prudent to be condemning. Ultimately, it is the trust between patient and physician that must be preserved.

Symptom-specific treatment

Commonly used medications for specific clinical features in ALS are listed in *Table 23.3*.

Weakness

Although physicians cannot reverse the inexorable muscle weakness of ALS, there are alternative means of compensating for weakness. ALS patients should be evaluated by specialists in rehabilitation in order to maximize their function at all stages of disease. Occupational therapists can provide hundreds of assistive devices to maintain independence with activities of daily living, such as feeding, dressing, and maintaining hygiene. Physical therapists can teach stretching exercises to maintain range of motion and minimize joint pain, and they can provide ankle–foot orthoses to compensate for foot drop, knee

sleeves for buckling of the legs, and abdominal binders for paraspinal weakness. Physical and occupational therapists are also invaluable in assessing and teaching patient transfer techniques that maximize safety for both the patient and the caregiver. Wheeled walkers can compensate for weakened trunks and leg muscles and permit continued ambulation. Various lifts are available to assist with patient transfers, as is adaptive equipment for the bathroom.

When ambulation is no longer an option, manual and motorized wheelchairs continue to permit patient mobility. When prescribing durable medical equipment such as wheelchairs, it is important to consider the progressive nature of this disease. When possible, equipment should be rented, since patient needs may change quickly. Lightweight portable wheelchairs are ideal in the early stages of ALS as energy saving devices. Later, as the disease progresses, a more appropriate wheelchair would be one with a head support, reclining back, removable adjustable-height arm rests, lap table, removable and elevating leg rests, and a gel or air cushion for seating.[9]

It is preferable to order equipment before it is actually necessary so that the patient's needs can be anticipated.[9] However, some patients are simply not ready to see themselves as disabled and refuse canes, walkers, and wheelchairs until very late in the course of the disease. The stigma associated with adaptive equipment can be overcome through education and continued exposure. Modeling equipment in the clinic setting has proven to be an effective means of desensitizing patients. The myriad of insurance plans available today pose serious challenges to obtaining the correct equipment to meet patient needs. Advocating for the patient can be a time-consuming project that requires skilled case management.

Symptoms	Treatment
Cramps, spasms, myalgias	Lioresal 10–20 mg qid prn Zanaflex slow increase to 8 mg tid Intrathecal lioresal
Excessive crying or laughter	Amitriptyline 10–75 mg every day Fluroextine 10–40 mg every day Paroxetine 10–40 mg every day
Urinary urgency or frequency	Oxybutynin 5 mg every day or tid prn
Sialorrhea	Amitriptyline 10–25 mg tid prn Glycopyrrolate 1–2 mg qid prn Scopolamine 0.125 mg tid prn
Thick phlegm or post-nasal drip	Guaifenesin 300 mg q4h prn Propranolol 10–40 mg tid prn Nebulized acetylcysteine 10% solution 2 ml tid prn
Jaw quivering or jaw clenching	Clonazepam 0.5 mg tid prn Diazepam 2.5–5 mg bid–qid prn Lorazepam 0.5–1.0 mg q8h prn
Laryngospasm	Clonazapam 0.5 mg Diazepam 2.5–5 mg q8h prn Lorazepam 0.5–1.0 mg prn
Gastroesophagel reflux disease	Omeprazole 20 mg every day Famotidine 20 mg bid at bedtime Ranitidine 150 mg bid Cimetidine 400 mg at bedtime Cisapride 10–20 mg before meals and at bedtime prn Metoclopramide 10–15 mg before meals and at bedtime prn
Nasal congestion	Over-the-counter nasal sprays Beclomethasone dipropionate nasal spray 42 mg (1–2 puffs) Diphenhydramine 25-5 mg q8h prn Pseudoephedrine sulfate 30–60 mg q8h prn
Sleep disturbance	Amitriptyline 25–75 mg at bedtime Trazodone 50 mg at bedtime Zolpidem 5–10 mg at bedtime Temazepam 7.5–30 mg at bedtime Sertraline 50–100 mg at bedtime Bupropion 100–150 mg bid
Depression or anxiety	Fluoxetine 10–40 mg each morning Paroxetine 10–40 mg at bedtime Sertraline 50–100 mg at bedtime Bupropion 100–150 mg bid
Dyspnea	Morphine sulfate elixir 20 mg/ml, 0.5–2.0 mg dose
Pain or pressure sores	Ibuprofen 200–800 mg Morphine sulfate elixir 20 mg/ml, 0.5–2.0 mg dose
Terminal management	Lorazepam 1–3 mg tid, Morphine sulphate elixir 20 mg/ml, 0.5–2.0 mg dose Morphine by subcutaneous pump 1–5 mg/hour. May bolus with 0.5–2.5 mg q 15 minutes as needed.
Nausea	Prochloperazine 5–10 mg tid prn
Agitation or anxiety	Lorazepam 0.5–3 mg tid prn Diazepam 2.5–10 mg tid

Table 23.3
Commonly used medications for symptomatic ALS treatment.

Cramps, spasms, myalgias, and spasticity

A muscle cramp is a sudden involuntary muscle contraction that may be triggered by voluntary exertion of any muscle group in the arms, legs, chest, back, abdomen, jaw, or throat. Cramps are caused by a brief contraction of a weakened muscle as a result of an explosive overactivity of motor nerves. These contractions may be extremely painful and prolonged and can actively interfere with waking as well as sleep. Patients may notice visible knotting in the muscle and abnormal posture until the cramp passes.

Cramps can be effectively managed through several strategies, including proper hydration and diet as well as avoiding overexertion of weakened muscles. Manual stretching of a muscle cramp is universally effective. When cramps and muscle spasms are particularly frequent and severe, medications such as quinine sulfate, lioresal, dantrolene, clonazepam, lorazepam, diphenylhydantoin, and gabapentin can be prescribed.[10]

Intrathecal administration of lioresal via subcutaneous pump is effective when spasticity is not adequately controlled by oral medication.[11] Certain musculoskeletal problems are particularly problematic in ALS. In patients with shoulder weakness, adhesive capsulitis (also known as frozen shoulder) can develop and cause a limitation in range of motion and excruciating pain. Neck weakness may result in painful myalgias and stiffness. The best treatment is prevention with joint stabilization and a daily home exercise program consisting of stretching and range-of-motion exercises. Manuals on appropriate therapeutic exercise for ALS patients are available and should be recommended to patients.

Fatigue

General muscle fatigue and exhaustion are common features in ALS. As neurons die, remaining ones send signals to activate the otherwise unused muscle and a single surviving neuron may be doing a hundred times its normal workload. This may result in temporary exhaustion of overburdened neurons. Thus, there may be times when a patient is able to perform a certain task (such as climbing stairs) only after resting beforehand. Patients should be instructed to pace themselves judiciously in terms of energy expenditure throughout the day and the week.

Various medications have been tried for fatigue with limited success.[12] These medications include pyridostigmine, amantadine, and stimulants such as methylphenidate and pemoline. The authors have not experienced success with medical regimens for fatigue and do not advocate their use. When the patient has persistent overwhelming fatigue, the quality of sleep should be evaluated with a polysomnogram (see below) or, as a more cost effective measure, nocturnal oximetry.[13]

Sleep disturbance

Sleep disturbance can lead to many quality of life consequences, such as depression and fatigue (as mentioned above).[14] Many factors can contribute to insomnia. Sleep disorders in ALS include central and obstructive apneas, hypopneas, and increased airway resistance.[5] Other factors include periodic movements of sleep as well as depression and anxiety.[15]

A polysomnogram is the best method to investigate sleep difficulties. However, a nocturnal oximetry is a simpler and less expensive way to monitor the heart rate and oxygen saturation throughout the night.[13] Desaturations of more than 3% from baseline are indicative of hypopneas.

Obstructive apneas may be difficult to diagnose in ALS patients, even with a polysomnogram, since ALS patients may be unable to generate an inspiratory pressure greater than the upper airway critical closing pressure.[16] Often repeated microarousals occur, owing to hypoventilation, excess secretions or periodic upper airway obstruction. These microarousals fragment sleep and may result in daytime fatigue.[17–19]

Hypopneas, whether central or obstructive, may respond to non-invasive ventilatory support with positive-pressure devices such as pressure ventilators or volume ventilators.[17–19] Success in using non-invasive ventilatory support depends on patient motivation and the control of upper airway secretions.[20]

Simpler measures for helping a patient with nocturnal hypopneas are elevation of the head of the bed and the use of the lateral decubitus position instead of the supine position in bed. Protriptyline hydrochloride, a tricyclic antidepressant, has been used with some success, owing to its ability to increase the tone of the nasopharynx.[18] Both tricyclic antidepressants and SSRI antidepressants decrease time spent in rapid eye movement (REM) sleep, the period of greatest breathing disturbance, and thus may be used with some positive result.[21] Periodic leg movements caused by spasticity or muscle spasms can be alleviated through the use of medications such as L-dopa, lioresal, and codeine. Anxiety and depression respond well to SSRI or tricyclic antidepressants. Sleep disturbances occur more frequently during the REM stage of sleep and can sometimes be effectively treated by use of amitriptyline, trazodone, or certain SSRI antidepressants. Respiratory muscle fatigue has been reported to respond favorably to theophylline.[22] Sedatives should be avoided. If other options have failed and care and comfort are the main concern, short-acting sedatives may be effective.

Pseudobulbar affect

Patients with ALS may develop difficulty controlling emotion and may sometimes cry or laugh inappropriately or excessively. Emotional incontinence, or pseudobulbar affect, is thought to be caused by the loss of frontal inhibition over the bulbar nuclei that are involved in laughing and crying. SSRI antidepressants, as well as tricyclic antidepressants and lithium, are often effective in treating these unwanted emotional displays.[12,23,24]

Dementia

Dementia is infrequently reported in ALS; it occurs in only 5–10% of cases,[25] although subtle cognitive dysfunction relating to mental flexibility may be present in as many as 25% of ALS patients. It is more prevalent in patients who present with bulbar and pseudobulbar symptoms, and it may include frontal features such as apathy, altered social skills, and personality changes. In those rare patients in whom frank dementia is present, it is important to encourage the family to pursue conservatorship early in the course of disease so that appropriate medical decisions regarding life support can be made.

Urinary urgency and frequency

Although ALS is not thought to involve the autonomic nervous system, patients with ALS can frequently develop spastic bladder, urinary urgency, and urinary frequency. This may be due to the lack of frontal inhibition over micturition centers. Superimposed urinary tract infections will also increase bladder spasms and polyuria can arise. Therefore, in the presence of frequency or urgency, a urinalysis should be checked and, if the urine is infected, the patient should be treated with antibiotics. If there is no infection, oxybutynin may be helpful in relaxing the bladder and helping the patient to regain continence.

Dependent edema of the hands and feet

Dependent edema frequently occurs in a very weak limb, owing to the failure of muscle pumping action to increase venous return. Passive range-of-motion exercises, elevation of paralysed limbs, and compression hose are helpful. When swelling is painful or if it fails to decrease after overnight elevation, a deep vein thrombosis (DVT) should be ruled out immediately because of the risk of a pulmonary embolism. Consideration should be given to DVT prophylaxis before prolonged periods of inactivity.

Sialorrhea

Excess saliva is a common feature of ALS, resulting in increased drooling, choking, or coughing. The problem is not believed to be due to overproduction but to decreased clearance.[26] In ALS, saliva is not swallowed automatically and repetitive volitional swallowing is needed to compensate for this. Sialorrhea may be further increased by anxiety, hunger, and gastroesophageal reflux disease.[27]

Medications that can decrease saliva production include glycopyrrolate, amitriptyline, diphenhydramine, oxybutynin, scopolamine, and other anticholinergics such as artane.[12,28,29] Surgery and radiation therapy have both been tried in the past for excess secretions but they often result in excessively thickened secretions and are therefore not recommended.[30]

Thick phlegm and post-nasal drip

ALS patients may develop a habit of mouth breathing, owing to fatigue of jaw muscles or nasal congestion. Mouth breathing causes saliva to dry out and thicken. Furthermore, medications taken to reduce drooling can cause excessive dryness and tenacious secretions. This can result in a bothersome sensation of post-nasal drip, chronic cough, or a need to clear the throat.

β-Antagonists such as metoprolol or propanolol have been reported to thin secretions when added to antisialorrhea regimens.[29] Expectorant medications such as guaifenesin, or even homeopathic treatments such as papaya juice, may be helpful in thinning secretions. Over-the-counter expectorants, hot tea, and the use of room humidifiers and nebulized breathing treatments with acetylcysteine solutions can also help. When allergies contribute to post-nasal drip, antihistamines and corticosteroid nasal inhalers may be useful. A mechanical insufflation–exsufflation cofflator is an excellent way of clearing thick upper airway secretions.[31]

Jaw quivering and jaw clenching

Patients with pseudobulbar involvement may experience uncomfortable release of bulbar reflexes to noxious stimuli such as cold, anxiety, or pain. Benzodiazepines such as clonazepam, diazepam, and lorazepam may be helpful in relieving these symptoms.

Laryngospasm

Laryngospasm is an abrupt and prolonged closure of the vocal cords resulting in sudden gasping for breath and an expiratory wheeze. This phenomenon can cause panic as a result of airway constriction and fear of suffocation.[32] Laryngospasm can occur when patients are exposed to increased emotion, smoke, strong smells, alcohol, cold or rapid bursts of air, and even spicy foods. It can also occur with aspirated liquids or saliva as well as gastroesophageal reflux disease.[33]

Laryngospasm normally resolves spontaneously in a few seconds but it can be more immediately relieved by having the patient breathe through the nose and repetitively swallow. Possible precipitants of laryngospasm should be eliminated and a trial of antacids instituted.

Gastroesophageal reflux

Gastroesophageal reflux disease (GERD) is a common condition in patients with ALS, owing to weakness of the diaphragmatic muscle fibers that form the lower esophageal sphincter. The signs and symptoms may include heartburn, acid taste, throat irritation, chest pain, hoarseness, shortness of breath, nausea, and insomnia.[32] These symptoms are thought to be caused by the reflux of stomach acid into the distal esophagus.[34] Caffeine, spicy foods, overeating, and diaphragm weakness all increase acid reflux into the esophagus.

Particular care in managing GERD must be maintained when instituting a feeding tube because the stomach may be easily overfed after weeks of starvation. Peristaltic agents, such as metoclopramide and cisapride, and antacids, such as ranitidine hydrochloride, cimetidine, and famotidine omeprazole, are reasonably effective.[34]

Nasal congestion

If there is bulbar involvement, the tone of the muscles in the nasopharynx may be weakened, resulting in a failure to elevate and open the nostrils, upper airways, and eustachian tubes. The nasal bridge may be effectively elevated with nasal tape. In addition, antihistamines and topical decongestants may be used to decrease mucosal edema and bring relief.

Constipation

Constipation is very common in ALS and can be difficult to manage. Constipation can result in hours spent on the commode with abdominal pain and bloating. The causes include decreased fluid intake, inadequate diet, lack of exercise, and reduced ability to bear down with the abdominal muscles.

Proper management is essential since hospitalization can occur for bowel obstruction if this condition persists. Medications taken to control excessive saliva and pain can contribute to constipation and should be decreased if possible or discontinued if necessary. An excellent dietary adjunct to normalize bowel movement is 'power pudding': equal parts of prunes, prune juice, apple sauce, and bran. Two tablespoons with each meal and at bed time, along with adequate fluid intake and fruits and vegetables in the diet, is helpful in maintaining a bowel regimen. When necessary, stool softeners, laxatives, and periodic enemas should be used liberally.

Depression and anxiety

Depression is very common in patients with increasing physical disability and should be aggressively treated.[35] Depression is dramatically underdiagnosed in patients presenting with medical disease and it has a negative impact on the quality of life both of patients and of their families.[36] SSRI antidepressants such as fluoxetine, sertraline, and paroxetine are preferable to older monomine oxidase inhibitors and tricyclic antidepressants such as amitriptyline because of their lesser incidence of side effects and their greater efficacy. When effective, antidepressants should be continued for at least 6–12 months and then slowly tapered as indicated.[15] When anxiety is the problem, buspirone and benzodiazepines can be used on an as-needed basis. Buspirone is a preferable first agent, owing to its lack of respiratory depression.

Dysphagia

Weakness and disco-ordination of pharyngeal muscles can result in dysphagia. A swallowing evaluation by a speech therapist can be invaluable in determining which foods cause the greatest difficulty. A video esophagram or a modified barium swallow may sometimes be indicated to detect silent aspiration, since some patients are unaware of swallowing difficulties and are at great risk of aspiration pneumonia.[37] These patients should be fed by alternative routes such as percutaneous gastrostomy. For milder dysphagia patients should be instructed to:[38]

1. tuck their chin down while swallowing;
2. swallow two to three times per mouthful of food;
3. avoid foods that cause the greatest difficulty; and
4. perform a clearing cough after each swallow.

When dysphagia results in weight loss or when a patient becomes fatigued from attempts to consume a meal, a percutaneous gastrostomy (PEG) should be considered. Ideally the procedure should be performed while a patient still has an adequate forced vital capacity (FVC) (i.e. more than 50% of the predicted value), since risks of the procedure increase as FVC decreases below 50%.[39] Although a PEG does not prevent aspiration it does increase patient comfort and provide a route for adequate nutrition. The PEG should be placed by an experienced gastroenterologist, and general anesthesia should be avoided. Patients should be educated to increase PEG feedings only as tolerated and to avoid overfeeding, which may lead to stomach distension, nausea, and even pulmonary aspiration. Patients should only be fed in an upright position and should avoid bending or lying flat for at least 1 hour after feeding. In many instances, peristaltic agents such as metoclopramide or cisapride should be added.[35] Most patients prefer bolus feedings three or four times a day to leave many hours for other activities. Various feeding formulas are available. In general, formulas with high osmolarity and high sugar content are harder to digest and may result in cramping and diarrhea. Iso-osmolar solutions are preferable and these may be specifically selected to meet a patient's individual needs (e.g. high-fiber formulas for constipation, high-protein, high-lipid, low-carbohydrate formulas for patient with carbon dioxide retention).[40]

Cricopharyngeal myotomy has been tried for ALS patients with dysphagia but it is not recommended. Mortality is high and benefits are small and transient.[41]

Dysarthria

Slurred, slow, or strangulated speech is caused by inco-ordination and weakness of the lips, tongue, and pharyngeal muscles. Patients with dysarthria should be evaluated by a speech therapist and augmentative communication methods should be offered. Strengthening exercises will not improve dysarthria and should not be encouraged. Pen and paper or keyboard devices may be used if hand function is adequate. Scanning computer programs with a single switch device may be used by patients even with severely limited movements. An eye-gaze alphabet board is helpful if any reliable eye movement remains. Some form of communication can usually be established and must be sought.[37] It is important for the physician to allot sufficient time for the patient since augmentative communication can be extremely slow. In a busy office practice it can be frustrating and tedious to have patients spell out a word using eye movements but it is essential that the patient's need to communicate is respected.

Dyspnea

Dyspnea may have many etiologies in ALS. For this reason, breathing difficulties should be evaluated by a physician who is familiar with pulmonary problems and with ALS. Some respiratory physicians have little experience in managing patients with neuromuscular disease and may not be familiar with the many non-invasive devices that are now available.

Reversible causes of dyspnea must always be sought and treated where appropriate. These include intercurrent infections, excess secretions, and pulmonary emboli. When dyspnea is due to progression of ALS and chronic hypoventilation, it typically presents initially during sleep, especially REM sleep.[14,15] Patients may complain of frequent arousals, bad dreams, attacks of anxiety, and daytime somnolence.[18] Later they may complain of headaches, confusion, and frank hallucinations.

Chronic hypoventilation can be treated successfully in many patients, and non-invasive ventilatory support may increase patient well-being and possibly also survival.[22] When patients are unable to tolerate non-invasive support as a result of failure to manage upper airway secretions or other factors, invasive ventilation should be discussed. Although the financial and emotional costs of tracheostomy ventilation are high, the majority of ALS patients who choose this option report a satisfactory quality of life.[42,43]

Modes of mechanical ventilation

Ventilators may be either:

(a) invasive (administered via a tracheostomy or endotracheal tube); or
(b) non-invasive (applied directly to the face or body).

Invasive ventilators offer the advantage of bypassing the upper airway and thus can be used in patients with upper airway obstruction resulting from bulbar involvement or heavy secretions. Tidal volume and positive end-expiratory pressure can be selected to reduce dead space and prevent the collapse of peripheral airways and subsequent atelectasis. Patient survival can thus be extended indefinitely, although the disease course will progress unabated with the eventual loss of all patient communication and independence.

Invasive ventilation has a number of major drawbacks, including the exorbitant costs involved, the need for 24-hour nursing care and its significant detrimental impact on the quality of life of both the patient and caregiver. Indeed, in many countries invasive ventilation is not available to patients with ALS, owing to the progressive, incurable nature of the illness, and even in countries where it is available it is seldom used.[42]

Non-invasive mechanical ventilators can be categorized as either negative- or positive-pressure devices. Negative-pressure devices passively expand the chest, thereby increasing the inspiratory volume. The best-known historical example of this type of ventilator is the 'iron lung', in which patients are placed in an airtight cylinder with their head protruding. Air is then pumped out of the cylinder, causing the chest wall to expand, thus simulating the action of the diaphragm. However, this type of ventilator is large and confining, and does not afford ease of movement or hygiene for the patient. Thus, they tend to be unpopular and are not widely used.

Other more patient-friendly negative-pressure devices are the chest shell, also known as the cuirass, and the pulmo-wrap. The cuirass is a rigid shell that is applied to the chest from the neck down to the bottom of the rib cage, and that adheres to the thorax by negative pressure suction. A seal around the edge of the cuirass allows air to be pumped out from under the shell, creating negative pressure and expanding the lungs like a smaller, more mobile version of the iron lung. Since the patient's limbs are outside the cuirass, greater mobility is possible. The pulmo-wrap is an air-tight body suit that covers the chest and is sealed at the neck, shoulder, and hips. It tends to be more comfortable than the cuirass, but it is much more difficult to apply.

A disadvantage with all negative-pressure ventilators is the possibility of exacerbating upper airway obstruction by creating negative pressure in the glottis and further narrowing the upper airway. However, even patients with severe bulbar involvement have occasionally used the cuirass with success.

Non-invasive positive pressure ventilators (NIPPVs) administer pressurized air to the lungs through the naso-oropharynx. This allows greater volumes of air to enter the lungs, and as with invasive ventilation, it can halt or even reverse micro-atelectasis. Many varieties of NIPPV exist; however, not all are appropriate for patients with ALS.

Continuous positive airway pressure (CPAP) is commonly used for otherwise healthy patients with sleep apnea, but it is entirely inappropriate for patients with ALS since it applies a constant pressure during both the inspiratory and expiratory phases, thus increasing the work of breathing. In contrast, bi-level positive airway pressure (BIPAP) applies a lighter expiratory pressure than inspiratory pressure, thus reducing the work of breathing. BIPAP may be administered via a mask or nasal pillows and is typically used for 6–8 hours continuously during sleep, although it can be used for longer periods according to patient needs. It is a very effective method of treating the signs and symptoms of chronic hypoventilation in ALS, of increasing oxygen tension and tidal volume and of decreasing carbon dioxide tension. However, a major limitation to BIPAP is that patients with considerable bulbar involvement experience difficulty in learning how to use the device.[20]

Other positive-pressure ventilation methods include intermittent positive vibration (IPV) and insufflation–exsufflation. IPV involves the delivery of pressurized, intermittently vibrating, nebulized saline, bronchodilators, or expectorants through the mouth for 10–15 minutes at a time in order to aid clearing of pulmonary and bronchial secretions and to decrease mucous plugging. The insufflator–exsufflator (or coughalator) delivers air under positive pressure and then sucks the air back out, thereby assisting the patient to cough and decreasing mucous plugging. For patients who are able to use this device without gagging or prolonged coughing, it can be very effective.

When mechanical ventilation is started, a contract should be made between patient, family, and physician agreeing on terms for ultimately withdrawing the ventilator support. This is especially important in invasive ventilator involving trachestomy. ALS patients have the legal and ethical right to refuse to initiate or to continue ventilator support.[44] As ALS continues to progress, patients will eventually become 'locked in'.[45,46] For this reason, an agreement should be reached that ventilation may be discontinued when the patient is no longer able to communicate.

Ventilator withdrawal as a pre-terminal procedure should be done in a manner that considers the physical and emotional comfort of the patient and significant others. The authors recommend a combination of narcotic analgesics and lorazepam or diazepam[47,48] but strongly discourage the use of neuromuscular blocking agents, which may render the patient unable to express pain or distress.[49] In some cases, an antiemetic must be added since narcotics and analgesics can cause nausea.

Pain and pressure sores

Although pain is not generally thought to be a feature of ALS, it is extremely common late in the course of the illness.[45,46] Pain may be due to muscle cramping or secondary joint changes such as adhesive capsulitits or hip dislocation. Pain can also occur when there is prolonged immobility of paralysed limbs or decubiti. Patients should be specifically questioned about pain and pressure sores and symptom-specific intervention, such as physical therapy for painful spasms, should be prescribed when appropriate. Bony prominences should be inspected for decubiti. Furthermore, when indicated, specialized mattresses and seating systems, such as alternating air flow mattresses and air and gel cushions, should be offered.

Mild pain may be alleviated by non-narcotic agents such as non-steroidal anti-inflammatory agents or acetaminophen. In the case of more severe pain, aggressive treatment, including narcotics, should be implemented[13] (see below). Side effects from narcotics may include nausea and constipation, which can be treated with antiemetics, such as prochlorperazine, as well as with the liberal use of laxatives. When possible the oral route of administration is preferred. When patients cannot take medication by mouth and do not have a PEG, medications may be given via an indwelling venous line or a subcutaneous pump. Transdermal routes are often erratic and therefore ineffective, and repeated intramuscular injections are painful; therefore these routes of administration should be avoided.

Terminal management

At some point in the progression of ALS, patients may become tired of the struggle to remain living. Ultimately, many patients reach a level where they feel they can no longer maintain a satisfactory quality of life. At this point the patient's interests shift from extending life to making the remaining days more comfortable.

Home nursing agencies and, in particular, hospice agencies are invaluable when patients find it increasingly difficult to come to the clinic for periodic evaluation. Hospice and home nursing agencies are able to maintain continuity of care, mediating between patient and physician to ensure that the patient's needs are addressed in a timely fashion. Maintaining rapport between the physician and the hospice agencies is crucial in order that the maximum benefit for the patient is realized.

At this point in the disease, the goal is for the patient to be pain-free, to be as alert as possible during the day, and to have a comfortable uninterrupted sleep at night. The principle of dual effect allows a physician to prescribe whatever treatment is necessary to maintain the patient's comfort and relieve suffering, even if it does shorten life.[50] Short-acting anxiolytics such as lorazepam, soporifics such as temazepam, and analgesics, including morphine, should be offered liberally for agitation or pain. Frequently, patients require antiemetic medications such as prochlorperazine, since hypoxia and morphine both cause nausea.

In this advanced stage, family members become more involved in communication with the physician in order that the patient's needs and comforts are assured. The physician should render family support as an extension of good patient care. This is a time when both the patient and family feel frightened and isolated. While home nursing care may be preferable, other settings (e.g. hospice, nursing facilities) can and should be explored at this juncture. Ministers of religion, when the patient is receptive, can provide comfort to both the patient and the family at this stage. In the end, when patient care is managed well, the patient with ALS will become progressively less attentive to the demands of the outside world and more focused on preparing for death. Death should and often can occur in the bosom of family and friends with the patient drifting into a deepening sleep from carbon dioxide narcosis. In this fashion, death is usually viewed as a welcomed end to patient suffering.

Quality of life

Although no one would actively choose to have ALS, patients and families affirm that ALS has brought blessings to their lives as well as many adversities. With candor, patients report new appreciation of family, nature, and life itself. Many patients find the capacity to enjoy life each and every day throughout the course of treatment. Morrie Schwartz reported, 'After you have wept and grieved for your physical losses, cherish the functions and life you have left'.[51] As a physician, it is a privilege to be included in this intimate celebration of living and to witness how ordinary people summon extraordinary faith and courage to accept and succeed in the face of seemingly unbearable adversity. We can become privileged listeners — learning from our exceptional patients, not only about the ALS, but also ultimately about ourselves.

References

1. El Escorial World Federation of Neurology. Criteria for the diagnosis of amyotrophic lateral sclerosis. *J Neurol Sci* 1994; **124 (suppl)**: 96–104.
2. Louwerse ES, Visser CE, Bossuyt PM, Weverling GJ. Amyotrophic lateral sclerosis: mortality risk during the course of disease and prognostic factors. *J Neurol Sci* 1997; **152 (suppl)**: 510–517.
3. Fallat RJ, Norris FH, Holden D et al. Respiratory monitoring and treatment: objective treatments using non-invasive measurements. *Adv Exp Med Biol* 1987; **209**: 191–200.
4. Cedarbaum JM, Stamblers N. Performance of the amyotrophic lateral sclerosis functional rating scale in multicenter clinical trials. *J Neurol Sci* 1997; **152 (suppl)**: 151–159.
5. Gay P, Westbrook PR, Daube JR et al. Effects of alterations in pulmonary function and sleep variables on survival in patients with amyotrophic lateral sclerosis. *Mayo Clin Proc* 1991; **66**: 686–694.
6. Bensimon G, La Comblez L, Meininger V. ALS/Riluzole Study Group: a controlled trial of riluzole in amyotrophic lateral sclerosis. *N Engl J Med* 1994; **330**: 585–591.
7. Lacomblez L, Bensimon G, Leigh PN et al. Dose-ranging study of riluzole in patients with amyotrophic lateral sclerosis. *Lancet* 1996; **347**: 1425–1431.
8. Gurney ME, Cutting FB, Zhai P et al. Benefit of vitamin E, riluzole and gabapetin in a transgenic model of familial amyotrophic lateral sclerosis. *Ann Neurol* 1996; **39**: 147–157.
9. Mendoza M, Rafter E. *Functioning When Your Mobility is Affected. Living with ALS.* Manual Number 4. ALS Association, 1997.
10. Davidoff RA. Pharmacology of spasticity. *Neurology* 1978; **29**: 46–51.
11. Coffey RJ, Cahill D, Steers W et al. Intrathecal baclofen for intractable spasticity of spinal origin: results of a long term multicenter study. *J Neurosurg* 1993; **78**: 226–232.
12. Norris FH, Smith RA, Denys EH. Motor neurone disease: towards better care. *Br Med J* 1985; **291**: 259–262.
13. Marcello N, Ortaggio F. Detection of sleep respiratory disturbances by transcutaneous PCO_2 and PO_2 monitoring in advanced cases of duchenne muscular dystrophy. *Acta Cardiomiol* 1990; **II NI**: 55–66.
14. Flemons WW, Tsai W. Quality of life consequences of sleep disordered breathing. *J Allergy Clin Immunol* 1997; **99**: 750–756.
15. De Wester JN. Recognizing and treating the patient with somatic manifestations of depression. *J Fam Pract* 1996; **43 (suppl)**: S3–S15.
16. Fergusson KA, Ono T, Lowe AA et al. The relationship between obesity and craniofacial

structure in obstructive sleep apnea. *Chest* 1995; **108**: 375–381.

17. Guilleminault C, Stooks R, Clerk A et al. From obstructive sleep apnea syndrome to upper airway resistance syndrome. Consistency of daytime somnolence. *Sleep* 1992; **15**: 513–516.

18. Guilleminault C, Stooks R, Quera-Salva MA. Sleep related obstructive and nonobstructive apneas and neurologic disorders. *Neurology* 1992; **42 (suppl 6)**: 53–60.

19. Glesson K, Zwillich CW, White DP. The influence of increasing ventilatory effort on arousal from sleep. *Am Review Respir Dis* 1990; **142**: 295–300.

20. Aboussouan LS, Khan SU, Meeker DP et al. Effects of noninvasive positive-pressure ventilation on survival in amyotrophic lateral sclerosis. *Ann Intern Med* 1997; **127**: 450–453.

21. Kryger MH. Restrictive Lung Diseases. In: Kryger MH, Roth T, Dement WC, eds. *Principles and Practice of Sleep Medicine* Philadelphia: WB Saunders, 1993.

22. Schiffman PL, Belsh JM. Effect of respiratory resistance and theophylline on respiratory muscle strength in patients with amyotrophic lateral sclerosis. *Am J Respir Dis* 1989; **139**: 1418–1423.

23. Iannocone S, Ferrini-Strambi L. Pharmacologic treatment of emotional lability. *Clin Neuropharmacol* 1996; **19**: 532–535.

24. Schiffer RB, Cash J, Hernon RM. Treatment of emotional lability with low dose tricyclic antidepressants. *Psychosomatics* 1983; **24**: 1094–1096.

25. Neary D, Snowden JS, Mann DMA et al. Frontal lobe dementia and motor neuron disease. *J Neurol Neurosurg Psychiatry* 1990; **53**: 23–32.

26. Charchafflie RJ, Fernandez LB, Perec CJ et al. Functional studies of the parotid and pancrease glands in amyotrophic lateral sclerosis. *J Neurol Neurosurg Psychiatry* 1974; **37**: 863–867.

27. Mandel L, Tamai K. Sialorrhea and gastroesophageal reflux. *J Am Dent Assoc* 1995; **126**: 1537–1541.

28. Stern LM. Preliminary study of glycopyrrolate in the management of drooling. *J Pediatr Child Health* 1997; **33**: 52–54.

29. Newall AR, Orser R, Hunt M. The control of oral secretions in bulbar ALS/MND. *J Neurol*

Sci 1996; **139 (suppl)**: 43–44.

30. Webb K, Raddihough DS, Johnson DH, Bennett CS. Long term outcome of salivary control surgery. *Dev Med Child Neurol* 1995; **37**: 755–762.

31. Hanayama K, Ishikawa Y, Bach JR. Amyotrophic lateral sclerosis: successful treatment of mucous plugging by mechanical insufflation–exsufflation. *Am J Phys Med Rehabil* 1997; **76**: 338–339.

32. Bortolotti M. Laryngospasm and reflex central apnea caused by aspiration of refluxed gastric content in adults. *Gut* 1989; **30**: 233–238.

33. Bauman N, Sandler AD, Schmidt C et al. Reflex laryngospasm induced by stimulation of distal esophageal afferents. *Laryngoscope* 1994; **104**: 209–214.

34. Sartori RB, Trevisian L, Tassinari D et al. Prevention of aspiration pneumonia during long term feeding by percutaneous endoscopy: might cisapride play a role? An open pilot study. *Support Care Cancer* 1994; **2**: 188–190.

35. Bruce ML, Seeman TE, Merrill SS, Blazer DG. The impact of depressive symptomatology on physical disability: MacArthur studies of successful aging. *Am J Public Health* 1994; **84**: 1796–1799.

36. Cunningham LA. Depression and anxiety in the primary care setting. *Compr Ther* 1997; **23**: 400–406.

37. Kazandjan MS. Communication Intervention Communication and Swallowing Solutions for the ALS/MND Community. *(Singular Pub Group)*. 1997, 7–40.

38. Carter G, Miller RG. Comprehensive Management of Amyotrophic Lateral Sclerosis. *Rehabilitation of Neuromuscular Disease* 1997, **9**: 271–284.

39. Matthus-Vliegen LMH, Louwerse LS, Markus MP et al. Percutaneous endoscopic gastrostomy in patients with amyotrophic lateral sclerosis and impaired pulmonary function. *Gastrointest Endosc* 1994; **40**: 463–469.

40. Drickamer MA, Cooney LM. A geriatrician's guide to enteral feeding. *J Am Geriatr Soc* 1993; **41**: 672–679.

41. Louizou LA, Small M, Dalton GA. Cricopharyngeal myotomy in motor neurone disease. *J Neurol Neurosurg Psychiatry* 1980; **43**: 42–45.

42. Moss AH, Casey P, Stocking CB et al. Home

ventilation for amyotrophic lateral sclerosis patients: outcomes, costs and patient, family and physician attitudes. *Neurology* 1993; **43**: 438–443.

43. Cazzoli P, Oppenheimer EA. Home mechanical ventilation for amyotrophic lateral sclerosis: nasal compared to tracheostomy – intermittent positive pressure ventilation. *J Neurol Sci* 1996; **139** (**suppl**): 123–128.

44. Goldblatt D, Greenlaw J. Starting and stopping the ventilator for patients with amyotrophic lateral sclerosis. *Neurol Clin* 1989; **7**: 789–805.

45. Oliver D. The quality and care and symptom control: the effects on the terminal phase of ALS/MND. *J Neurol Sci* 1996; **139**: 134–136.

46. Newrick PG, Langton-Hewer R. Pain in motor neuron disease. *J Neurol Neurosurg Psychiatry* 1985; **48**: 838–840.

47. Campbell MJ, Endersby P. Management of motor neurone disease. *J Neurol Sci* 1984; **64**: 65–71.

48. Wilson WC, Smedira NG, Fink C et al. Ordering and administration of sedatives and analgesics during the withholding and withdrawal of life support from critically ill patients. *J Am Med Assoc* 1992; **267**: 949–953.

49. Truog RD, Burns JP. To breathe or not to breathe. *J Clin Ethics* 1994; **5**: 39–41.

50. Moss AH, Oppenheimer EA, Casey P et al. Patients with amyotrophic lateral sclerosis receiving long term mechanical ventilation. *Chest* 1996; **110**: 249–255.

51. Albom M. Tuesdays with Morrie: An Old Man, A Young Man and the Last Great Lesson. New York. Doubleday Press, 1997.

24

The case for physician-assisted suicide and active euthanasia in amyotrophic lateral sclerosis

Len Doyal

Introduction

There is an inherent moral tension between the duty to protect the life and health of patients and the duty to respect their autonomy. The former proclaims that clinicians should act in what are professionally agreed to be the best interests of patients. The latter demands informed consent, even when this conflicts with the first duty. The tension between these two duties can be illustrated in the treatment of patients with amyotrophic lateral sclerosis (ALS). Sometimes, such patients no longer wish for their lives or health to be protected but instead want the opportunity to organize the circumstances of their deaths. They might wish to exercise such choice through refusing life-saving treatment. Less commonly but increasingly, they may request physician-assisted suicide (PAS) or active euthanasia (AE).[1]

This chapter explores arguments for and against both options. My conclusion is that, with strict regulation, PAS should be legalized now and that this should be followed eventually by the legalization of AE. In so doing, I argue that the most recent renunciation of PAS and AE by the American Academy of Neurology is more a declaration of moral rectitude than a coherent argument.[2] Such affirmations may be comforting for many patients who would never consider PAS or AE. However, in the face of such an apparent professional consensus, some patients (perhaps many) may hide their true feelings and desires. They are, after all, totally dependent on these same doctors for optimal care during the progression of their illness.

Why might some patients with ALS wish for PAS or AE? Should they be allowed to choose how and when they die with the help of their clinicians?

Why is respect for autonomy so important in the practice of medicine?

The moral tension in medicine between the two duties to protect life and health and to respect autonomy is not one that can be arbitrarily resolved simply by declaring greater allegiance to the former. Despite the compelling emotional priority of the duty to save life, it is now widely accepted throughout the medical profession that this should only be done with the informed consent of competent patients who can generally understand, remember, reason about, and believe information that is communicated to them about their condition and treatment. Provided that competent patients are appropriately informed and have not been coerced, they can refuse life-sustaining treatment. This is so even when the refusal causes anguish to the clinicians and relatives involved. Thus, if competent patients with ALS refuse to be ventilated or resuscitated or to receive antibiotics, then failure to respect this is in breach of both established professional guidelines and the law.[3-5] Why should priority be placed on the autonomy of such patients, especially when others who genuinely care for them question the 'rationality' of their decisions?

What makes us morally special as humans is precisely our autonomy—our ability to plan our lives through formulating goals and beliefs about how to achieve them and to set about attempting to do so. Indeed, it is the choices that we are able to exercise as a result of such planning that differentiate us from other animals.[6] If we morally endorse treating animals in ways that we would not deem appropriate for humans then it is their lack of these abilities—and thus their lack of humanity itself—that will probably be one of the moral justifications cited.

It is through the exercise of autonomy in social life that we learn who we are as individuals. We do this through exploring, with the help of others, our capabilities—our special emotional, cognitive and physical characteristics, and skills.[7] Not to respect autonomy challenges the right of individuals to evolve and flourish within their social environment and to obtain the respect of others for the personal attributes that characterize them and no one else. Disrespect for autonomy is therefore a moral affront that is harmful in its own right, even if no physical or emotional injury results.[8] The civil law of battery reflects this fact. If I intentionally touch you without your consent, I am liable for the offence, irrespective of any other personal harm to you that may result.[4] The harm rests in the violation of your autonomy per se.

This is not, however, to suggest that the abuse of individual autonomy cannot also cause harm in other ways. For competent, autonomous humans to be forced to do something that contradicts their deeply held beliefs, goals, and values can also be horrifying. The anger and sense of personal injury felt by patients and research subjects who have been subjected to such intervention without consent is well documented.[9] Thus the only thing that makes surgical interventions or medical research on competent patients morally and legally tolerable is the fact that the patients have consented to them. Similarly, in describing the horror of their experiences, torture victims focus not just on physical pain and emotional distress. Of more importance is the personal impact of being robbed of control over what happens to their bodies. This can dramatically damage the understanding that victims of torture have of themselves—both their self-identity and their self-respect.[10]

The potential demand of ALS victims to control the circumstances of their own death

The moral importance of respect for individual autonomy should inform our understanding of the particular horror that ALS can pose for some victims. It can be intolerable to watch oneself rapidly and increasingly lose control over physical abilities that ordinarily define individual independence and privacy. In such circumstances, to be cared for is a double-edged sword, involving both comfort and indignity. Indeed, most ALS patients know that there will come a point in their physical degeneration when they may be totally dependent, devoid of any physical autonomy even though still intellectually capable of reasoning and emotionally capable of experiencing despair and indignity.

Of course, the threat of such a dramatic reduction in physical autonomy does not affect all sufferers from ALS in the same way. All people do not place the same priority on the expression of physical autonomy in their lives, and the disease usually leaves the cognitive and emotional dimensions of autonomy intact.[11] Yet some people have a much stronger sense of their physical autonomy than others and choose to exercise it in circumstances that might not be deemed appropriate by others. For example, irrespective of the type and degree of their illness, some patients notoriously want more information than others about their diagnoses, prognoses and treatment plans, together with the side effects and risks.[12] Equally, some patients allow relatives and other carers much wider access to otherwise confidential information about their care than other patients do.[13] While both these moral claims are not direct indicators of the importance to individuals of physical autonomy, the desire for information and privacy often go hand in hand with important life goals, about which clinicians and relatives may know nothing but that cannot be achieved in the face of severe physical disability.

It is hardly surprising, therefore, that this reduction in their autonomy may be intolerable for some victims of ALS. The thought of experiencing a death believed to be devoid of dignity is one that can haunt the early stages of the illness and can crushingly dominate its terminal phase.[14,15] Fears about loss of physical function, especially the ability to talk and swallow, can for some be almost like torture, albeit administered arbitrarily by nature rather than deliberately by an enemy. These fears may be exacerbated by the thought of the impact that increasing helplessness, vulnerability, and dependency will produce in family and carers.

Such concerns may generate the desire for either PAS or AE.[1,16] The argument put forward for this would be that the shortened life expectancy and degenerative character of ALS is tragedy enough without victims being placed in a position of experiencing a highly distressing and clinically managed death. In its minimum form, this argument maintains that willing clinicians should be legally able to provide access to the medical means for patients to commit suicide in circumstances of comfort and dignity and in an environment of choice. Maximally, the claim is that it should be legal for ALS patients to receive a lethal injection from willing clinicians when the patients are no longer capable of killing themselves.

Some relatives also support PAS and AE.[17] Apart from their own respect for the autonomy and dignity of the ALS patient, relatives (and friends) can also suffer from having to witness and participate in such a process. To watch someone one loves and respects rapidly lose the very attributes that he or she believes to define his or her own personal identity can be a harrowing experience. Of course, the relatives of many victims would never support PAS or AE. Indeed, some relatives may insist on the continuation of life-preserving treatment even after it has been refused by victims or advised against by clinicians.[18,19] For now, however, the key point is that those with the closest emotional bonds to victims do not necessarily perceive death that is either self-inflicted or physician-inflicted as being in conflict with their love and respect.

Moral arguments in favour of PAS and AE

Having established why sufferers from ALS might wish to have access to the medical means of their own demise or to be killed painlessly in circumstances of their own choosing, we must now examine arguments that purport to provide moral justification for such actions.

Physician-assisted suicide

Let us begin by returning to the wide professional and legal consensus that competent adult patients have the moral and legal right to refuse life-sustaining treatment. This means that if ALS victims state the circumstances under which they wish to be allowed to die without medical intervention then, morally and legally, such intervention should not be forced upon them. Such refusals might be verbal or, if the victim cannot speak or has become incompetent, may take the form of a properly drafted or spoken advance directive.[20] The right to refuse life-sustaining treatment trumps the preferences of others—clinicians or possibly relatives—who may wish for such treatment to be continued despite the declared wishes of victims.

Therefore, in these circumstances, competent adult ALS patients can make decisions to instigate a causal process that will kill them, and these decisions command clinical respect and compliance. These patients are able to foresee one consequence of their action—their own death—and may intend it to the degree that they believe that death is the only way in which they can achieve other intended goals (e.g. the cessation of pain, indignity, or any other form of suffering that they deem to be significant). It can thus be argued that what such victims are really doing is choosing to achieve their desire to die through morally and legally barring others from saving them when they can and ordinarily would do so. In much the same way, competent people can choose to die either through not feeding themselves or through demanding that others not feed them when they become unable to do so themselves.

Provided that there is no reason (e.g. severe mental illness) to question the competence of such persons, and provided also that there is no doubt about their intent to die (i.e. that they have no hope that they will survive the consequences of their actions), we can morally describe their choice to refuse the necessary conditions for life as suicide.[21]

A counter-argument might be that to call competent refusals of life-sustaining care 'suicide' is a misuse of the term: those who make such choices would clearly not do so were it not for their illnesses.[22] They would not otherwise want to die. However, the same point can be made about all competent suicides: life is not perceived as worth living for whatever reason which prompted the action or inaction. Successful action or inaction that has the foreseen and intended consequence of death as the chosen way of resolving that reason, is suicide. The desire of some sufferers from ALS to commit suicide through refusal of treatment is understandable, as is the concurrence of relatives and clinicians who believe that the decision to do so is in the patient's best interests.

Legally, in all of the UK and most of the USA, the competent refusal of life-sustaining treatment is not regarded as suicide for the argument already advanced: that were it not for their medical condition, such patients would not wish to die.[22,23] Despite such apparent legal certainty, however, the moral argument remains that if the intent of the refusal of life-sustaining treatment is death, the fact that it may be motivated by considerations relating to the physical and emotional experience of disease is neither here nor there. The refusal remains an act of suicide and one in which it may be morally appropriate for clinicians to assist through action or inaction—'assisting' in this context being defined as 'foresight of a death almost certainly resulting from the actions or inactions undertaken and one that will occur earlier than it otherwise would'. Clinicians assist suicide in these circumstances, rather than facilitate suicidal behaviour, if they are disappointed when the results of their actions do not lead to a death of the sort desired by the patient.[24] It follows that, morally, such clinicians can be said to be assisting suicide irrespective of whether they withdraw life-sustaining treatment or enable patients who wish to kill themselves to do so through their own action or inaction.

Therefore, if clinicians are already morally and legally aiding and abetting the suicides of patients who intend death as a consequence of their refusal of life-sustaining treatment, why should they not do the same for patients who wish to bring about their own deaths for themselves? For example, suppose that a patient is permanently on a ventilator and unable to switch it off herself. Then assume that she competently refuses further ventilator support because she believes life to be no longer worth living. It is legally accepted that her clinician should switch off the machine on her behalf.[25] Now suppose that the same patient makes it clear that she wants her clinician to devise a mechanical means by which she can disable her ventilator for herself when she wishes to die.[26] If he does so at present, her clinician might be charged with aiding and abetting suicide, provided that he knows of her intent and acts in order to assist her in achieving it.[26] This is so despite the fact that not to respect her autonomy in such circumstances is inconsistent with the very respect for autonomy that morally underwrites the right of patients who wish to refuse life-saving treatment in order to die in circumstances of their own choosing.

Professional acceptance of this argument is particularly important for ALS patients because they too will be physically unable to kill themselves at the end-stage of their illness.

No matter how effective palliative care is, the effects of dying in end-stage ALS without the beneficial effects of life-sustaining care may for some patients be needlessly distressing and undignified.[27] With the exception of Oregon in the USA, PAS is illegal throughout the world, although it is openly tolerated in The Netherlands under highly specific conditions.[28] It should be legalized.

Active euthanasia

Although AE does not yet command the same degree of support outside or within the medical profession as PAS does, this too is changing and the reasons are clear.[29] AE can be justified using similar arguments as for PAS. Clinicians do not just wait for competent patients to request that their deaths be hastened through not being given life-sustaining treatment. Such non-treatment decisions (NTDs) are also made on behalf of incompetent patients who cannot competently decide to refuse such treatment. Because of their pre-existing duty to protect life and health, clinicians must always be able to justify NTDs as either a response to the known wishes of the patient before he or she became incompetent or as being in the best interests of their incompetent patients on other grounds.[30]

AE and incompetent patients
For example, it may be argued that it is not in the best interests of incompetent patients to try to extend their lives when they are imminently and irreversibly close to death or when they are so brain-damaged that they will never again be able to engage in self-directed activity.[31] In the former situation, the patients will die anyway, with potentially increased suffering and indignity, owing to continued medical intervention. In the latter situation, patients will have permanently lost the minimal levels of autonomy that are necessary to engage in

any human activity at all. Whatever levels of discomfort they must endure because of their condition and treatment will remain unintelligible to them and they will never be able to attach value to their lives or do anything at all with them. Therefore, since they no longer have any interest in living, a quick death is either in their interests because of their potential for suffering or certainly not against their interests if they have no such potential (e.g. patients in a persistent vegetative state).

Actions are defined as NTDs with regard to permanently and severely incompetent patients when their clinicians understand that their omission to treat will shorten life. Proponents of AE argue that, since death is foreseen as the eventual and highly probable *effect* of such action (i.e. to be inactive), there is no moral difference between a clinical decision to allow an incompetent patient to die when he or she can be saved and a clinical decision to kill the patient actively.[32] For example, if we stand by and watch someone drown when we could easily save them without risk to ourselves then are we not just as morally responsible for their death as we would be if we actively killed them? This argument applies all the more to clinicians, since their explicit duty of care demands that, in ordinary circumstances, they must protect life and health. Thus a doctor could be charged with murder if he or she allowed an elderly, incompetent patient to die simply because of age rather than because the patient suffered from a clinical condition which meant that accelerated death was in the patient's best interest.

However, despite the apparent moral equivalence between passive and active euthanasia, legally clinicians may not administer a lethal substance in identical clinical circumstances to those in which they can legally omit to provide life-sustaining care. There is no place in the world where such action is legal, although in

The Netherlands AE is judicially tolerated in certain circumstances.[33] Yet, many argue that continuing the illegality of AE is both morally incoherent and cruel. Once the decision is made, perfectly legally, that the deaths of incompetent patients should be accelerated on justifiable grounds then surely should it not be legally possible to kill them painlessly to avoid further suffering and indignity?[34]

AE and competent patients

However, if this argument holds for the active killing of incompetent patients then it holds all the more so for competent adult ALS patients who have decided that life is no longer worth living but who are too physically disabled by their disease to commit suicide with the help of their clinician (were this to be an available option).[35] If they cannot kill themselves then the only way in which they can exert their autonomy is for clinicians to use their skill and privileged access to lethal drugs to agree to kill them—assuming that it is not morally acceptable or practical for non-clinicians to be given such access. It is true that, in these circumstances, such clinicians would be placing more moral priority on respect for autonomy than for the protection of life and health. However, we have seen that this is already accepted to be good moral and legal practice as regards competent patients who refuse life-saving treatment. The same argument holds for competent patients who make a valid advance directive stating that, in certain circumstances, they wish to be killed clinically in specific ways.

Proponents of AE conclude from these arguments that the law should be changed to make AE possible for both incompetent and competent patients.

Arguments against PAS and AE

Opponents of PAS and AE do agree about the appropriateness of NTDs for competent and incompetent patients in some circumstances. However, they reject the view that, because clinicians can foresee the terminal consequences of their NTDs, they are morally responsible (and should be legally responsible) for them. Opponents maintain that it is just as absurd to suggest that we are morally responsible for all of the foreseeable consequences of our inactions as it is to claim that we cause all of those events that we fail to prevent. We may well do nothing to prevent foreseen starvation throughout the world. However, is it not nonsense to claim that we are morally responsible for such starvation when we do not intend for it to happen?[36]

Foreseen consequences and the moral importance of intent

Opponents of PAS and AE emphasize that NTDs have foreseen consequences other than death—the relief of suffering, for example. They argue that NTDs only become the moral equivalent of AE when the intent of clinicians who omit to provide care is death.[37] Opponents of PAS and AE claim that it is never morally acceptable for clinicians to bring about the death of a patient as a conscious clinical goal, either through omission or commission. This is so despite the fact that death may indeed be a foreseen and virtually certain consequence of many NTDs. Only the goals of the relief of suffering or the relief of the burdens of medical care can acceptably reconcile NTDs with the duty of care to act in the patient's best interest. Always assuming that active treatment would indeed prolong life, such decisions should not be made for any other reason. This belief that actions can have

two consequences, the intention of only one of which is morally acceptable, is called the argument from double effect.

The argument from double effect

This same argument from double effect is used morally and legally to justify the sustained and increased administration of potentially lethal doses of morphine to patients who are in extreme pain and distress. As with NTDs, such administration sometimes occurs with the foresight that the effect of palliation will be the inevitable shortening of the life of the patient, through, for example, its aggregate impact on respiration. As long as the effect that is intended is the relief of suffering and not death then opponents of PAS and AE believe that such a programme of palliation is morally acceptable. The argument from double effect that is applied to such palliation gains further endorsement by the law in many jurisdictions.[38,39] Again, the key is the ability of clinicians to argue that their sole intent was the relief of suffering, despite the other potentially terminal consequences of their treatment.

Thus, for opponents of PAS and AE, the very identity of human acts (e.g. mercy versus murder) becomes equivalent to the individual intent accepted as the goal of the act to be identified, as opposed to any unintended further side effects of the achievement of that goal.[37] It is this imputation of moral and legal importance to individual intent that supposedly undermines any claim to change the law in favour of PAS or AE. Once it is accepted that the relief of suffering is the only acceptable intent of NTDs or of potentially lethal palliation, any analogy of the sort already drawn between them and PAS and AE must break down. This is because the intent of PAS and AE is the facilitation or causation of death. Opponents of PAS and AE argue that such actions can no more be morally justified than NTDs motivated by the same intent. Whenever the direct or indirect causation of death is the intent of the clinician, then their actions become criminalized—aiding and abetting suicide at the least, murder at the most. Such intent has no place in a profession that is supposed to be driven by an ethic of care.[40] The law should remain as it is.

Slippery slopes

Thirdly, it is argued that PAS and AE should not be morally or legally tolerated because of the threat that they pose to the medical profession and to vulnerable patients who might be pressurized by their medical advisers, carers, or family into embracing death when they are not ready for it.

As regards the medical profession, successful clinical relationships are predicated on the trust that patients have that clinicians will always act in their best interests. Opponents of PAS and AE argue that this relationship will be undermined if patients believe that clinical consultancy may include evaluations of whether or not they would be better off dead. There may well be a minority of patients with ALS or other conditions who wish to kill themselves or to be killed because of what they perceive to be the poor quality of their lives. Yet whatever distress they may feel through being denied these choices does not outweigh the much greater distress that would result if the majority of other patients felt that they could not trust their clinicians to sustain their life and health for as long as possible.

Such cruelty is amplified by the potential for the abuse and exploitation of the vulnerable that would be created by the legalization of PAS or AE.[41] For example, ALS patients may be sensitive about the burden that they can pose for their primary carers, usually relatives. Were PAS to be legalized, it is likely that some victims would feel pressurized to kill themselves or to be killed before they are ready to die. Equally, relatives may believe that they have good reason to apply such pressure both to patients and their clinicians. Clinicians may accept this, believing that the quality of life of some patients is so poor and the distress that their condition causes is so great that they would be better off dead. These possibilities are not just the object of academic speculation. Opponents of PAS and AE argue that we have witnessed their increasing occurrence since PAS and AE have been legally tolerated in The Netherlands.[42,43] Any form of intentional assisted or direct killing in medicine should remain outlawed.

Criticisms of arguments against PAS and AE

We have seen that all parties to the debate about PAS and AE accept that NTDs and causing death through the deliberate physical administration of a lethal substance have potentially the same moral and legal status. For example, both proponents and opponents agree that if clinicians either allow patients to die or kill them because they do not like their looks, then they can and should be prosecuted for murder. The debate between the proponents and the opponents is focused primarily on the moral status of the argument from double effect: that NTDs and potentially lethal palliations in situations where foreshortened life can be foreseen with a high degree of certainty are acceptable only when the intent is not to kill but to relieve suffering.

Do individual goals exhaust the totality of intention to act?

The difficulty with the argument from double effect is that it identifies the action to be morally and legally evaluated with the individual intent of the person carrying out that action. Yet this equation is no more valid than the suggestion that I am able to determine the meaning of the sentences that I utter simply through a declaration of my goals in uttering them. In everyday life, I act—in the same way that I speak—in an already existing social environment of meaning. I can divorce neither my intent nor the meaning of my actions from this environment if I wish to be linguistically understood or morally accepted as a good citizen.[44] Within this environment of moral relevance, we do not ordinarily pretend to be able to isolate completely individual intention from recognized pre-existing duties or from the foreseen consequences of not carrying out those duties. Both duties and the foreseen consequences of actions associated with them have an objective existence over and above whatever specific goals individuals may claim informed their actions.

Within the practice of medicine, the duty of care (not the professed goal of the clinician) specifies the types of circumstances that clinicians should foresee and avoid in their treatments. Ordinarily, they should act in the best interests of their patients through doing nothing that might knowingly damage their health or threaten their lives. When clinicians apparently neglect this duty through a NTD, their action must also be defended as being in the best interests of their patients. This means that their action must correspond, at least roughly, to the clinical criteria that have been deemed appropriate to regulate such decisions, which define the boundaries of when life-sustaining treatment is no longer to be viewed as of clinical benefit. It is the perceived conformity of the actions of clinicians to their duty in these terms (not just their individual professions of intent in executing these actions) that forms the basis on which their professional practice will be judged to be morally permissible.

Indeed, were declared individual goals the sole defining characteristics of all actions, it would become impossible to blame anyone of a criminal offence who could correctly claim that they did not intend the foreseeable consequences of their action, no matter how certain. Despite their stated intent to the contrary, we regularly impute moral blame to people who cause harm to others because they must have also foreseen the consequences of their actions. Indeed, criminal convictions occur when juries believe that people who carry out an action have ignored their duty to take into account the consequences of that action, again, irrespective of their professed individual goals.[45]

To this degree, in criminal law, real intent is not necessarily identified with declared intent, as opponents of PAS and AE maintain, although to be sure it might be. Rather, as proponents of AE argue, criminal intent may be judged with reference to both the declared goal for the criminal act and the certainty with which the perpetrator foresees the harmful consequences of his or her actions.[46] Even when the goal that informs the criminal act is unclear, a conviction may follow simply from the fact that perpetrators understood (or should have understood) these consequences and yet chose to ignore them.

The moral and legal acceptability of NTDs for incompetent adults should be similarly judged. We have seen that NTDs are acceptable only when certain objective conditions are met (e.g. when a person is so brain-damaged that he or she will never again be able to engage in any form of self-directed activity). This will be so, irrespective of the declared goal of the clinician. Thus the moral and legal responsibility of clinicians who engage in NTDs should be judged with respect to the conformity of the foreseen consequences of their actions and such conditions, not just with respect to their declared goals.

For example, suppose that a doctor allows an indigent, temporarily unconscious but otherwise healthy old woman to die through omitting to treat her life-threatening chest infection. The doctor's stated and believed goal is to relieve the suffering caused by her poverty, unhappiness and old age. Let us also assume that the doctor correctly believes that his or her inaction will foreshorten the patient's life with virtual certainty. Finally, despite this belief, let us accept that the doctor never waivers in keeping his or her declared goal of the relief of suffering at the forefront of his mind. Despite this fact, the real intent embodied in the doctor's action should not be equated with his or her declared goal. This is because the patient does not conform to standards for an acceptable NTD, standards that are independent of that goal. Indeed, in this case, it should be argued that criminal charges of murder be brought against the doctor, again, irrespective of the doctor's stated goal. The doctor's duty of care dictates that in these clinical circumstances, life must be protected rather than placed at such a high risk. The doctor has failed to do his or her duty, despite good intentions.

The argument of double effect and palliative care

Similar arguments apply to the argument from double effect in the context of palliative care. Opponents of PAS and AE attempt to draw support from palliative care for their moral emphasis on the moral and legal priority of declared individual goals. We have seen that if patients are dying and in great suffering, it is legal to administer increasing doses of morphine that are foreseen in aggregate to foreshorten life—grounds for which, in other circumstances, one could be charged with murder.[38] To avoid such a charge, the administering clinician must be able to demonstrate that his or her intent is to relieve suffering rather than to cause death.

We can see, however, that this argument again places more burden on the moral status of declared goals than it can bear. Suppose that as the result of an accident, an otherwise healthy patient is in agonising and difficult-to-control pain and is unable to make competent decisions about his or her situation, although not at obvious risk of death. Equally assume that the patient's attending clinician in the accident and emergency department gives a dramatically increasing regime of morphine which he or she knows may shorten the patient's life. The patient dies and the clinician defends this action through arguing that his or her action is acceptable because the goal was only to relieve the patient's suffering. After all, the patients was screaming for pain relief, and morphine was administered accordingly.

Such a defence would be unacceptable. Against the background of the duty of care and the fact that the temporarily incompetent patient is neither imminently and irreversibly near death nor very severely and permanently brain-damaged, saving the patient's life should have priority over the relief of pain. To do otherwise—to risk shortening the patient's life in the pursuit of pain relief—is both immoral and illegal because it is not in the patient's best interests, whatever the goal of the doctor. Thus, the key moral distinction between situations in which the risk of administering potentially lethal regimes of morphine is and is not acceptable turns on the judgement of whether or not the lives of some patients are worth taking such risks over. It has nothing to do with the stated goals of administering clinicians. Yet, clinicians' stated goals must be to endorse what the opponents of PAS and AE reject: that death is in the interests of some patients more than pain and that some lives are more worth risking saving than others. Hence, the declared goal of relieving suffering is not a sufficient moral justification for the potentially lethal palliation of incompetent patients, any more than it is for NTDs.

One can play this same argument the other way around. Suppose that a decision is made to allow a patient with end-stage ALS who, for some other reason, is also permanently incompetent to die peacefully without further medical intervention. Equally assume that no one on the clinical team objects to this or to the objective grounds concerning the patient's condition on which the decision was made. Just when the patient is peacefully slipping away—in the carefully arranged presence of relatives—the responsible clinician changes his mind and insists on placing the patient on a ventilator, which will extend life. The reason is that the clinician suddenly realizes that the goal has been not the relief of suffering but the death of the patient.

Presumably, despite this pang of conscience, the clinician's action to reverse the NTD ought to be regarded as an act of cruelty rather than kindness, one motivated by his or her moral introspection rather than by concern for the patient's best interests. Therefore, as proponents of PAS and AE argue, the declared goal of the responsible clinician must be of secondary moral and legal concern in relation to decisions and NTDs concerning the end of life. If one looks at the numerous professional guidelines on the circumstances where NTDs are morally and legally acceptable, the declared goals of clinicians are never referred to. What is deemed important by the medical profession are the objective criteria by which the lives of patients can be judged as appropriate or not to be saved. If such lives are deemed

not to be worth living and thus saving, it is difficult morally to understand why opponents of PAS and AE continue to maintain the importance of the declared goal of the relief of suffering, as opposed to actions that do indeed have the foreseeable consequence of bringing about such relief, through death.

Proponents of PAS and AE may still retort that it is just as absurd to hold people morally responsible for the foreseen consequences of their actions, as opposed to their intent, as it would be to argue that they were morally responsible for the terrible occurrences throughout the world that they might choose to prevent but do not. For example, I can foresee that my not intervening to prevent the starvation of some people in sub-Saharan Africa will lead to their death. However it does not follow that I should be held morally responsible for their starvation—so the argument goes—as long as I do not intend them to starve. Hence, the issue of responsibility surely must, therefore, be linked to personal motivation.[36]

Even here, however, the argument collapses against the background of duties of care that have already been established. Suppose that I have such a duty, say as an aid worker in a relevant country, and I neglect it on the grounds that to keep people alive there will just perpetuate their suffering in the long term. Here I will be deemed to be morally responsible for the foreseen consequences of my inaction in precisely the same way that we have seen clinicians are. Indeed, one can develop a strong argument that even without such a recognized duty of care, if we foresee that the basic needs of strangers in other countries are not being satisfied and do nothing to avert this fact then we have blood on our hands. This will be true even if others may have more direct responsibility for the resulting suffering and its alleviation.[7] The fact that we intend no harm through our failure to participate in the prevention of such suffering is morally irrelevant to our culpability for them, always remembering that the imputation of responsibility should not be confused with an evaluation of its degree or the appropriateness of forms of punishment in light of its degree.[47]

The argument from double effect and competent patients

Once the argument from double effect is seen in this light, it becomes clear that clinicians are morally responsible for the deaths of those incompetent patients whose lives they know are being shortened either through the omission or withdrawal of life-sustaining treatment or through the administration of potentially lethal palliation. The issue is not whether or not they are responsible; it is whether or not they have exercised this responsibility acceptably. Thus if competent ALS patients believe that their life is not worth living, why then should they not have the same moral prerogative as clinicians do for incompetent patients—through taking responsibility themselves for obtaining PAS or AE?

The argument from double effect and the law

The moral rejection of the argument from double effect argument must be understood in the context of its legal acceptability with respect both to NTDs and to the administration of potentially lethal palliation. Judges—wrongly according to the moral view argued here—do not wish legally to endorse AE. However, noted legal commentators argue that the legality of the argument from double effect is tantamount to a covert endorsement by the courts of the right of clinicians to do in palliative care what in other circumstances would be murder (i.e. deliberately to shorten

life against the background of their duty of care to save it). Given the horrific consequences of their not being allowed to do so—patients dying in needless physical suffering or self-perceived indignity—judges have made the legality of claims of double effect in such circumstances a matter of public policy rather than coherent jurisprudence.[30] The latter demands the legalization of both PAS and AE.

Back to slippery slopes

The third argument does not depend on either of the preceding two arguments for its force. Whether or not these arguments are correct, the contention is that, in any case, PAS and AE constitute a slippery slope that will both undermine the relationship of trust, which is so crucial for the success of medicine, and lead to the increased suffering and exploitation of ALS patients. There are two problems with such arguments.

On the one hand, there is little evidence to support them. Apart from The Netherlands, where PAS is legally tolerated, and the Northern Territory of Australia, where it was legalized for a short period, PAS is not legal anywhere in the world other than Oregon. Therefore, the first examples of legal PAS have only recently occurred. Attempts have been made to demonstrate that evidence from The Netherlands suggests that the toleration of PAS and AE has led to a significant increase in AE among both competent and incompetent patients.[42,43] Yet others counter-argue that these attempts, among other things, conflate reported instances of AE with NTDs, which occur for the same acceptable professional reasons in The Netherlands as they do elsewhere.[48] At best, the existing evidence is so small and contentious that it should not stand in the way of implementing public policy on the basis of moral coherence rather than unsubstantiated fear. Not to do so in the face of increasing public support for PAS and AE is more of an indication of the political power of pressure groups wedded to doctrines about the sanctity of life than evidence of the inevitability of slippery slopes of distress and exploitation.

Moreover, even if there were clear evidence that the legislation of PAS or AE had already led to abuses of the sorts that its opponents envisage, it would not follow that such abuses were necessary. We have good evidence that it is possible to control the potential dangers of many different types of technology. Thus, if someone argues that existing regulation of AE in The Netherlands is not sufficient to prohibit abuse and has no other hidden moral agenda, the reasonable response is to advocate the significant strengthening of such regulation.[48] However, opponents of PAS and AE never take this line. Can this be because their minds are already made up, along with their confidence about imposing their moral will on others at whatever costs to those who are denied the opportunity to control the circumstances of their own death?

The way forward for patients with ALS

This chapter has attempted to show that none of the arguments against PAS or AE can be sustained. They all collapse into the dogmatic belief that providing ALS patients with either route to self-destruction is just wrong. Almost everywhere, the law also endorses this view, as do the key institutions of the medical profession. There can be no doubt that the illegality and unprofessional status accorded PAS and AE are good reasons for clinicians not to engage in either. Yet we also know that clinicians have helped to end life or have ended life in both ways. Thus clinicians who agree with

the arguments that have been outlined here in favour of PAS and AE should begin more publicly to challenge the moral coherence of the current legal and professional consensus. This could be done in two stages.

The most immediate focus should be on the legalization and professional endorsement of PAS. In many countries, attempted suicide is now legal and more clinicians support PAS than AE.[53–55] For clinicians to provide the pharmaceutical means for suicide can even be consistent with the beliefs of those who oppose AE. The clinician is neither omitting to provide life-sustaining treatment nor involved in actively killing. Indeed, if one excludes the problems outlined with the argument from double effect, the intent of clinicians participating in PAS need not be the death of their patients but simply the respect of the patient's autonomy. The effect of prescribing such drugs to patients is not necessarily foreseen and, as has been indicated, patients may change their mind. When these facts are placed alongside the strong arguments for respecting the right of ALS patients to choose the circumstances of their death, then, with one exception, the force of counter-arguments evaporates.

The exception is the slippery slope argument. Relatives and others may well place pressure on vulnerable patients to kill themselves through PAS. There can be little doubt that some patients will succumb to such pressure or exert it on themselves for fear of being a burden to their family. Therefore, it is essential that if PAS is to be legalized it must be rigorously regulated. Regulations must ensure that:[49]

(a) the patient is competent to make such an important decision;
(b) the decision is not made under coercion;
(c) the decision is the product of sustained deliberation;

(d) the decision is made against the background of a clinical condition that is terminal, though not necessarily imminently so;

(e) the condition is actually or potentially degenerative enough, painful enough, or distressing enough for it to be understandable that the patient may believe that his or her life is demonstrably awful in terms of his or her own stated primary interests.

The thrust of such a legislative or judicial alteration in the law would be to ensure that an ALS patient's decision to end his or her life really is competent, considered, and sustained; otherwise there is too much risk of making a mistake that can never be corrected. For such regulation to be seen by the public to work, it will be necessary for at least three clinicians—one of whom is a neurologist and one a palliative care expert—along with a social worker who is trained for this kind of work, to confirm that the preceding conditions have been met. It will also be important to make it clear that no clinician or social worker would have to participate in PAS if they objected for any reason.

It is probable that when legalization of PAS comes, it will be through alterations in case law rather than through new legislation.[50] It equally seems clear that new legislation will have to be enacted at some point, along with the establishment of a regulatory body to ensure that the preceding conditions are met in practice and to enable patients to appeal if they believe that they or their relatives have been unfairly treated. These are practical proposals that reflect, and go beyond, conditions already in existence in both Oregon and The Netherlands. To the degree that there is growing support for PAS, these proposals should help to increase that support and make clear that ALS patients have everything to gain and nothing to lose from such developments.

The struggle for the legalization of AE is more complex and there can be little doubt that success will be elusive for some time to come. However, the tide of both public and professional opinion is beginning to change. Not only do more and more clinicians support the legalization of AE, they are admitting to having already killed patients in what they believed to be acceptable circumstances.[51-53] Leaving the doctrine of the sanctity of life aside, the concern of many doctors is that their own caring emotions, as well as the trust of their patients, will be corrupted if they engage in active killing.[54] This concern is understandable and commands respect. As we have seen, from a philosophical perspective the most convincing response is that they are already engaged in such killing, albeit through omission and through commission in the case of some programmes of aggressive lethal palliation (e.g. terminal sedation).[55] The fact that these activities may not emotionally feel the same as actively administering a lethal substance is neither here nor there. Emotions can change with increased understanding and regulation can be as tough as is desired—along the lines of, but if necessary even stricter than, those just outlined for PAS.

Yet it takes more than coherent argument to hold sway in matters of public policy. The reality is that emotion can often be a powerful counter to reason. This is why those who wish to see the legalization of PAS and AE should initially focus on the former.[50] As has been shown, the arguments favouring the one can, to a degree, be applied to the other. Most importantly, the successful legalization of PAS could demonstrate that the slippery slopes of 'non-natural' death can be prevented through effective regulation and that the medical profession will not be corrupted by clinicians beginning to respect the right of patients to determine the circumstances of their own deaths in the way in which they now do when they refuse life-sustaining treatment.

Conclusion

This chapter has explored the reasons why some patients with ALS might want to exert maximum control over their own deaths and why they should be allowed to do so. Traditional arguments against PAS and AE have been shown to lack coherence against the background of the right of competent patients to refuse life-saving treatment and the fact that clinicians can now professionally and legally shorten the lives of an incompetent patient when they believe on objective grounds that it is in the patient's best interests. Specific recommendations have been made about how PAS and AE should be regulated in order to avoid the exploitation of vulnerable patients and damage to the moral character of the medical profession. Failure to do so can be argued to be immoral since it forces some patients with ALS to endure a death that for them is unnatural and without human dignity and that, in the small percentage of cases in which palliation is ineffective, may be dominated by pain and distress. Ironically, such an approach lacks the very compassion and concern for human suffering that its proponents so often claim for themselves and their cause.

Acknowledgements

Many thanks to Lesley Doyal, Michael Swash, Ian Kennedy, Celia Wells, and especially Daniel Wilsher.

References

1. Ganzi L, Johnston WS, McFarland BH et al. Attitudes of patients with Amyotrophic lateral sclerosis and their care givers toward assisted suicide. *N Engl J Med* 1998; **339**: 967–973.

2. Ethics and Humanities Subcommittee of the American Academy of Neurology. Assisted suicide, euthanasia and the neurologist. *Neurology* 1998; **50**: 596–598.

3. General Medical Council. *Good Medical Practice*. London: General Medical Council, 1997.

4. Kennedy I. Consent to treatment: the capable person. In: Dyer C, ed. *Doctors, Patients and the Law*. Oxford: Blackwell Scientific, 1992.

5. Meisel A. *The Right to Die*. New York: Wiley, 1995.

6. Carruthers P. *The Animals Issue*. Cambridge: Cambridge University Press, 1992, 122–170.

7. Doyal L, Gough I. *A Theory of Human Need*. London: Macmillan, 1991.

8. Crisp R. Medical negligence, assault, informed consent and autonomy. *J Law Soc* 1990; **17**: 77–89.

9. Doyal L. Journals should not publish research to which patients have not given fully informed consent—with three exceptions. *Br Med J* 1997; **314**: 1107–1111.

10. American College of Physicians. The role of the physician and the medical profession in the prevention of international torture and in the treatment of survivors. *Ann Am Med* 1995; **122**: 607–661.

11. Silverstein MD, Stocking CB, Antel JP. Amyotrophic lateral sclerosis and life sustaining therapy: patients' desires for information, participation in decision making, and life sustaining therapy. *Mayo Clin Proc* 1991; **66**: 906–913.

12. Davis H, Fallowfield L. *Counselling and Communication in Health Care*. London: Wiley, 1991, 3–24.

13. Benson J, Britten N. Respecting the autonomy of cancer patients when talking with their relatives: qualitative analysis of semistructured interviews with patients. *Br Med J* 1996; **313**: 729–773.

14. Dyer C. Woman asks court for peaceful death. *Br Med J* 1997; **314**: 7096.

15. Poenisch C. Merian Frederick's story. *N Engl J Med* 1998; **339**: 996–998.

16. Kluge EH. Doctors, death and Sue Rodriguez. *Can Med Assoc J* 1993; **148**: 1015–1017.

17. Asch DA. The role of critical care nurses in euthanasia and assisted suicide. *N Engl J Med*

1996; **334:** 1374–1379.

18. Brody B. *Life and Death Decision Making.* New York: Oxford University Press, 1988, 100–142.

19. Cranford RE. Helga Wanglie's ventilator. *Hastings Cent Rep* 1992; **21:** 23–24.

20. Sommerville A. Remembrance of conversations past: oral statements about medical treatment. *Br Med J* 1995; **310:** 1663–1665.

21. Tolhurst WE. Suicide, self-sacrifice and coercion. In: Donnelly J, ed. *Suicide: Right or Wrong?* Buffalo: Prometheus Books, 1990, 77–92.

22. *Airedale NHS Trust* v. *Bland* (1993). 12BMLR at 112.

23. Gostin L. Deciding life and death in the courtroom: from Quinlin to Cruzan, Glucksberg, and Vacco—a brief history and analysis of constitutional protection and the 'right to die'. *J Am Med Assoc* 1997; **278:** 1532–1528.

24. Stell LK. Physician assisted suicide: to decriminalize or to legalize, that is the question. In: Battin MP, Rhodes R, Silvers A, eds. *Physician Assisted suicide: Expanding the Debate.* New York: Routledge, 1998, 225–251.

25. Montgomery J. *Health Care Law.* Oxford: Oxford University Press, 1997, 449–451.

26. Thomasma D. The ethics of physician-assisted suicide. In: Humber J, Almeder RF, Kasting G, eds. *Physician-Assisted Death.* Totowa, NJ: Humana Press, 1994, 135–150.

27. Farsidies B. Palliative care: a euthanasia free zone. *J Med Ethics* 1998; **24:** 149–150.

28. Alpers A, Lo B. Physician assisted suicide in Oregon: a bold experiment. *J Am Med Assoc* 1995; **274:** 483–488.

29. Emanuel EJ, Fariclough DL, Daniels ER, Clarridge BR. Euthanasia and physician assisted suicide: attitudes and experiences of oncology patients, oncologists, and the public. *Lancet* 1996; **347:** 1805–1810.

30. Kennedy I, Grubb A. *Medical Law: Text with Materials.* London: Butterworths, 1994, 1203–1210.

31. Doyal L, Wilsher D. Witholding and withdrawing life sustaining treatment from elderly people: towards formal guidelines. *Br Med J* 1994; **308:** 1689–1692.

32. Rachels J. Active and passive euthanasia. In: Steinbock B, Norcross A, eds. *Killing and Letting Die.* New York: Fordham University Press, 1994, 112–119.

33. de Wachter MA. Euthanasia in the Netherlands. *Hastings Cent Rep* 1992; **22:** 23–30.

34. Brock DW. Voluntary active euthanasia. *Hastings Cent Rep* 1992; **22:** 10–22.

35. Orentlicher D. The legalization of physician-assisted suicide. *N Engl J Med* 1996; **335:** 663–666.

36. Finnis J. Misunderstanding the case against euthanasia: response to Harris' first reply. In: Keown J, ed. *Euthanasia Examined.* Cambridge: Cambridge University Press, 1995, 62–71.

37. Finnis J. A philosophical case against euthanasia. In: Keown J, ed. *Euthanasia Examined.* Cambridge: Cambridge University Press, 1995, 23–35.

38. R v. *Bodkin Adams* (1957). Crim. L. R. 773.

39. *Washington* v. *Glucksberg* 117 Sct 2258 (1997).

40. Twycross RG. Where there is hope, there is life: a view from the hospice. In: Keown J, ed. *Euthanasia Examined.* Cambridge: Cambridge University Press, 1995, 141–168.

41. *Report of the Select Committee on Medical Ethics.* London: Her Majesty's Stationary Office, 1994 48–49.

42. Keown J. Euthanasia in the Netherlands: sliding down the slippery slope? In: Keown J, ed. *Euthanasia Explained.* Cambridge: Cambridge University Press, 1995, 261–296.

43. Jochemsen H, Keown J. Voluntary euthanasia under control?: further empirical evidence from the Netherlands. *J Med Ethics* 1999; **25:** 16–21.

44. Doyal L, Harris R. *Empiricism, Explanation and Rationality.* London: Routledge, 1986, 73–89.

45. R v. *Nedrick* (1986) 3 All ER 1; R v. *Woolin* (1988) 4 All ER 102.

46. Clarkson C, Keating H. *Criminal Law: Text and Materials.* London: Sweet and Maxwell, 1994, 134–158.

47. Harris J. *Violence and Responsibility.* London: Routledge, 1980.

48. Battin MP. *Least Worst Death.* New York: Oxford University Press, 1994, 130–181.

49. Quill TE. *Death and Dignity.* New York: WW Norton, 1993, 159–175.

50. Kennedy I. The right to die. In: Mazzoni CM, ed. *A Legal Framework for Bioethics*. Dordrecht: Kluwer Law International, 1998.

51. Back AL, Wallace JI, Starks JE, Pearlman RA. Physician-assisted suicide and euthanasia in Washington state: patient requests and physician responses. *J Am Med Assoc* 1996; **275**: 919–925.

52. Dyer C. Two doctors confess to helping patients to die. *Br Med J* 1997; **315**: 206.

53. Meier DE, Emmons CA, Wallenstein S et al. A national survey of physician-assisted suicide and euthanasia in the United States. *N Engl J Med* 1998; **338**: 1193–1201.

54. Callahan D. When self-determination runs amok. *Hastings Cent Rep* 1992; **22**: 52–55.

55. Quill TE, Lo B, Brock DW. Palliative options of last resort: a comparison of voluntarily stopping eating and drinking, terminal sedation, physician-assisted suicide, and voluntary active euthanasia. *J Am Med Assoc* 1997; **278**: 2099–2104.

25

Terminal care in amyotrophic lateral sclerosis
Isabelle Richard and Joanna Rome

Evolution of amyotrophic lateral sclerosis (ALS) is caracterized by progressive aggravation of motor deficit as a result of increasing loss of motor neurons. The ability to walk, use the upper limbs for daily life activities (DLAs), and feed orally are progressively reduced by the extending paralysis. In the terminal phase, none of these functions can be independently performed and respiratory functions become compromised. At this stage, the physician's concern is no longer centered on diagnostic or curative issues, and terminal care will be entirely planned in terms of limiting functional impairment and providing the best possible quality of life. This requires efficient association of both simple, non-invasive therapeutic measures and sophisticated, potentially expensive, technical means such as environment control devices and assisted ventilation. The effectiveness of high standard terminal care has been proved.[1–3]

High-quality terminal care increases quality of life but also prolongs survival[2,4] and is probably, at least for a number of simple measures, cost-effective.[5] Planned active terminal care remains insufficiently available for ALS patients.[6] Physicians and neurologists may be reluctant to follow these patients up to their death, doubtful that active care will make any difference, unsure that prolongation of life is worthwhile, and finally feel hopeless.[7]

The past decade has been marked by a considerable interest in ALS, and the follow-up of large cohorts, often in the setting of therapeutic trials, has allowed considerable accumulation of knowledge on the evolution of ALS and the practical everyday problems encountered by patients and their families. The recent development of techniques such as computerized environment control, perendoscopic gastrostomy, and non-invasive ventilation provides possible remedies for some of the impairments of ALS patients and allows a very different, active approach to terminal care in ALS.[7] Awareness and optimal use of these therapeutic opportunities gives the medical team the opportunity to offer positive and comprehensive support to the patient and his or her family up to the end and greatly relieves the feeling of hopelessness of both the patient and the caregiver. Leaving aside the ethical problems that are crucial at this stage and are addressed in chapter 24, this chapter reviews the therapeutic measures that are available to substitute for the loss of ambulation and independence in DLAs, and which deals with progressive impairment of swallowing. A large part of the chapter is devoted to indications for and techniques of assisted ventilation, which remains one of the most controversial issues in ALS care.

Loss of ambulation

Loss of ambulation is one of the landmarks in the evolution of ALS and often represents the first step towards total loss of independence. Principles of evaluation and care are similar to those that have been developed for other neuromuscular diseases. Evaluation of the maximum walking distance without fatigue is accurate enough in evaluating lower limb function. The main problem then is that of the prescription of a suitable wheelchair, which will at first be used for long outdoor distances but will progressively become necessary for all displacements. The discussion with the patient and his or her family over the necessity of a wheelchair and whether the independence gained from it is worthwhile often crystallizes the difficulties in communicating over the prognosis of ALS.

The best choice of wheelchair, when affordable, is that of a light, electrically powered wheelchair that will allow non-fatiguing outdoor use and remain useful when upper limb deficit precludes any manual propulsion. Correct adaptation and, when necessary, custom realization of the command interface will be provided as the deficit modifies the possible grip. The wheelchair must be equipped with a cushion to prevent pressure sores. Weakness of the trunk and neck musculature may render sitting uncomfortable or impossible. It is then necessary to turn to reclinable wheelchairs and fit arm rests and head supports. When the patient becomes severely paretic and unable to move the limbs in the full range of movements, passive mobilization is necessary, preferably twice a day, to prevent articular ankylosis. A regular turning-over program should also be scheduled by the caregivers to prevent pressure sores. Contractures caused by upper motor neuron involvement are rarely problematic in terminal ALS.[8] Transfer equipment will be necessary if the patient lives at home.

Impairment of upper limb function and loss of independence in DLAs

The progression of upper limb deficit towards complete quadriplegia interferes with all DLAs. The remaining movement often allows the triggering of a switch, so that the implementation of environment control devices for such patients is fully justified, albeit often difficult. The device should be simple to use and should preferably provide access to both environmental control and communication functions. The user interface must be flexible to allow adaptation to extending motor deficit and so remain useable as long as minimal movement is present. Voice-commanded systems are not suitable. In the future, ALS may represent a very good indication for devices based on the detection of eye movements[9] since extrinsic ocular movements are preserved even at the very terminal stage. Available resources and short life expectancy often limit the opportunity to acquire such devices, and the alternative probably lies in their purchase by ALS patient associations. When the resources do exist the feasibility of the use of environment control and augmentative communication devices has been documented.[10]

Even if technical means may allow some independent control of the environment, complete dependence for DLAs implies the organization of around-the-clock presence of caregivers. Many authors[1,3,7,11] have reported successful organization of homecare when a reliable primary caregiver can be identified in the family (most often the spouse). This alternative tends to be preferred to institutional care, in part because of reduced costs.[5] It may provide better comfort and quality of life for the patient and family.[5] The ability of the family to cope with the high burden imposed on them should nevertheless be carefully evaluated.[12] Homecare is more easily organized if the family can be supported by a multidisciplinary team and offered respite by hospitalizing the patient for short periods if necessary.

Impairment of swallowing and management of enteral feeding

Bulbar involvement sooner or later compromises swallowing and speech, and the inability to eat is another landmark in the evolution of ALS. The occurrence of aspiration is a life-threatening event and is often one of the major concerns and the greatest fears of both patients and families.[13] Correct evaluation and decision making regarding dysphagia and nutrition are of major importance and can greatly improve both the quality of life and the duration of survival.[2] ALS interferes mainly with the oral and pharyngeal phase of swallowing.[14]

The oral phase of swallowing includes holding the food in the mouth by contraction of the lips, masticating, gathering the food against the anterior palate and propelling it backwards by contraction of the anterior tongue, obstructing the nasal fossa by contraction of the soft palate. Deficit in the oral phase first results in an increase in the duration of meal time. The simple question, 'How long do you take to eat lunch?' is a good evaluation of swallowing impairment. The patient may drool first during meals, with an increasing use of napkins, and then permanently. Examination shows the presence of bits of food behind the teeth, owing to insufficient lingual gathering and propulsion. A predominant deficit in

soft palate muscles may result in nasal regurgitation of liquids, but this is often not the case since the deficit of lingual propulsion is usually associated.

The pharyngeal phase of swallowing begins with the contraction of the posterior third of the tongue and the pharyngeal wall, which propels the food downwards. Contraction of the hyoid muscles then brings the larynx forwards and the epiglottis folds down to obstruct the airway. Weakness of the pharyngeal and hyoid muscles results in choking and aspiration. Thorough examination of the face, tongue, and pharynx is necessary. Routine examination at every follow-up visit must include evaluation of the ability to swallow a spoonful of water.

Some simple non-invasive measures may help to maintain safe swallowing when the deficit is still moderate.[14] Modification of the consistency of food, which should be soft and slightly gelified to 'hold together' (for instance, by adding gravy to mashed vegetables) helps. The main problem is usually the swallowing of liquids. Chilled, tasty liquids (for instance cold sodas) will be more easily managed than water at room temperature. Jellies and sorbets may provide valuable liquid intake. Flexion of the neck while swallowing helps to bring the larynx anteriorly and may limit the occurrence of aspiration. The patient may also be taught the double swallowing technique. Indeed, when aspiration of food occurs, the patient will tend to take a deep inspiration in order to cough. This inspiration contributes to the routing of bits of food into the airway. Double swallowing consists of a sequence of inspiration, holding of the inspired air, swallowing, coughing, and swallowing again. This technique helps some patients, but it is rarely automatic enough to be efficient.

Careful attention to the nutritional and hydration status remains the main guide to adequate management of swallowing impairment. If eating becomes tedious or makes the patient and his family anxious, or if weight loss exceeds 5%, enteral feeding should be discussed before acute complications such as deshydration or aspiration pneumonia occur. All authors[1-3,13-15] agree that the best technique for ALS patients is percutaneous endoscopic gastrostomy (PEG). PEG is possible in 85% of ALS patients, the main contraindications being anatomic abnormalities or previous abdominal surgery.[15] PEG is preferably performed in patients who are in good general condition and properly hydrated and who have a vital capacity above 50% of the predicted value. In these conditions, the complication rate is below 10% and hospital stay may be limited to 24–48 hours. It is thus important to propose PEG early enough before the nutritional status suffers and dehydration occurs.

Adaptations of the PEG technique for ALS patients have been described.[15] Pre-medication is avoided when possible and the volume of insufflated air is reduced to avoid excessive reduction of the vital capacity. When possible, PEG should be performed by a team that is familiar with ALS patients. The use of PEG for enteral feeding is simple and easily learned by the patients themselves if upper limb function is preserved, or else by the caregivers. Enteral feeding may be started after 24 hours, first with water and then with home-made or commercially available preparations. Although it may be difficult to persuade patients to undergo PEG, especially when oral alimentation is still possible, 90% are satisfied with the procedure and find it simple to use.[16] The effect of PEG and enteral feeding on the nutritional status and ultimately on the duration of survival has been documented.[2] PEG does not, of course, preclude maintaining oral alimentation; rather, it helps to ensure that eating remains a pleasure. The patient is free to choose to eat what he or she enjoys and can rely on enteral feeding for caloric and liquid intake.

If PEG is technically impossible, surgical gastrostomy may be performed. Nasogastric tube feeding may be necessary either for temporary hydration (e.g. in preparation for PEG) or because PEG has been refused or postponed until restriction of the vital capacity makes it hazardous, but it is a much less comfortable solution and should be avoided.

Impairment of ventilation and assisted ventilation

Deficit of the respiratory muscles, resulting in severe restrictive deficit, is universal in the terminal phase of ALS but may occur sooner in the evolution of the disease. Pulmonary complications and respiratory failure account for at least 84% of mortality of ALS patients.[10] The fear of death by suffocation is a major source of anxiety for patients, families, caregivers, and medical teams. Thus, regular evaluation and timely decisions regarding respiratory management are crucial to cope with the terminal phase of ALS.

Respiratory impairment in ALS is managed on physiopathological grounds.[17] As motor neuron loss progresses, all respiratory muscles become weaker.[18] Weakening of inspiratory muscles (the diaphragm and the accessory inspiratory muscles) reduces the vital capacity. Microatelectasia appear and lead to a reduction in the pulmonary compliance, which in turn increases the work of the deficient inspiratory muscles. Clinical evaluation reveals superficial breathing and orthopnea. Spirometry can evaluate the reduction of the vital capacity. The deficit is often asymptomatic until the vital capacity is below 50% of the predicted value. When the deficit progresses and reduces the vital capacity to below 30%, clinical signs of hypoxia and hypercapnia occur. These consist of headaches, mood disorders, and daytime sleepiness.[19,20] Alterations in blood gases are delayed and only shortly precede acute respiratory failure. Regular follow-up of transcutaneous oxygen saturation, especially by nocturnal monitoring, is a better and more reliable marker of the evolution of the ventilation deficit. Control of expiratory and inspiratory mouth pressures is also an easy and reliable means of evaluating the progression of respiratory impairment.[18]

Active expiration is also affected, owing to the deficits in the abdominal and intercostal muscles. This induces a reduction in maximum expiratory flow during coughing and reduces the effectiveness of pulmonary toilet, leading to bronchial mucus plugging.[21] Acceleration of expiratory flows also requires proper closing and explosive opening of the glottus. Thus, expiratory flow and, finally, the efficiency of coughing are also affected by the bulbar deficit. The combination of expiratory muscle deficits and bulbar deficits places the patient at high risk of aspiration, reduced pulmonary toilet, and finally atelectasia and pneumonia.

Clinical and spirometric evaluation should clearly distinguish between hypoventilation, which is due primarily to deficient inspiratory muscles, and bronchial mucus plugging, which is due to the combination of weak expiratory muscles and bulbar impairment. Both may of course be associated, in variable proportions, in the same patient.

Treatment of hypoventilation

Incitative spirometry[20] or drug treatment such as theophylline[22] have been considered in the treatment of inspiratory muscle weakness, but there is no absolute evidence that they influence the rate of progression of the restrictive deficit. Anxiolytic and hypnotic drugs are generally contraindicated and may lead to acute respiratory failure. In the terminal phase the only alternative is substitution of the deficient inspiratory muscles by assisted ventilation. Placing a patient under assisted ventilation is one of the most difficult and controversial decisions in ALS care.[6,23]

The effect of ventilation has been demonstrated.[4,10,24] Ventilation normalizes arterial blood gases, and symptoms that are caused by hypoxia or hypercapnia, such as disrupted sleep, daytime sleepiness, and headaches, disappear. It is therefore reasonable to consider that ventilation is likely to improve the comfort and quality of life. This has not yet been documented in well-conducted studies, which are difficult to design for both ethical and practical reasons. Some authors have evaluated the satisfaction rate of ALS ventilated patients, and 80% have been found to be glad to be alive and ventilated.[6,25] The satisfaction rate is higher when patients have been active in the decision to start ventilation.[6] Ventilation also prolongs survival. This has been clearly demonstrated by several studies.[4,10,24] Some patients may live on ventilation for as long as 15 years,[19] with a mean survival in a series by Bach[10] of 4.5 years. Pinto,[4] in a series of 20 patients who had comparable respiratory parameters at inclusion showed a very significant difference in the survival rate at 3 years — 87% in the ventilated group versus 22% in the non-ventilated group. Despite this body of evidence that ventilation does prolong survival and may, at least at the beginning, improve the quality of life, many physicians and neurologists remain very reluctant[6] and less than 10% of ALS patients are offered ventilation. The main argument against assisted ventilation is that it will lead to unacceptable survival conditions as the deficit progresses and the patient becomes quadriplegic and unable to communicate.

Thus, assisted ventilation is often not discussed and not offered. When acute failure occurs, the decision is sometimes taken to intubate the patient and the family and medical team are then faced with the difficult decision of stopping (and not starting) assisted ventilation. The only way of avoiding such situations and offering the patient a real choice as to whether ventilation will be started or not is to discuss it openly early enough.[16] The difficult correlate is also to discuss the circumstances in which the patient wishes ventilation to be discontinued.[5]

A number of practical considerations may help in this difficult decision-making process. When a patient has any of the following items, there is a risk of acute respiratory failure and the decision as to whether or not to propose assisted ventilation should be taken:[26–28]

(a) vital capacity below 40%;
(b) frequent aspiration;
(c) previous episode of acute respiratory failure;
(d) clinical signs of hypoxia or hypercapnia;
(e) alteration in arterial blood gases; or
(f) nocturnal episodes of desaturation.

If the patient and the medical team consider the opportunity of assisted ventilation, it should be started when any of the previous situations occur, *without* waiting for acute respiratory failure. If clinical and spirometric expertise show mainly hypoventilation, with little occurrence of aspiration, it is probable that non-invasive ventilation will be successful at least for some time.[26] Although it may slightly improve the function of respiratory muscles by temporary rest and improved lung compliance,[24] ventilation does not greatly modify the evolution of the deficit itself. Thus, as the disease progresses, the duration of ventilation required to maintain adequate oxygenation will increase. If some patients start

off with nocturnal ventilation only, most will require round-the-clock ventilation within a few months.[10,26,28]

If the patient decides not to undergo ventilation, the evolution of hypoventilation will be that of progressive hypoxia and hypercapnia and the patient will progressively become comatose. Acute failure may occur, caused for instance by infection, and it is then logical not to intubate a patient who had previously decided not to undergo ventilation.

If the decision is taken to start assisted ventilation the next step is to choose between non-invasive and invasive ventilation.

Non-invasive ventilation

Non-invasive ventilation has developed during the past decade and is the first choice type of ventilation for ALS patients with hypoventilation and preserved bulbar function. It should be instituted and managed by a team that is familiar with the use of this technique in patients with neuromuscular diseases. Practical management of non-invasive ventilation implies the choice of a ventilator and of a patient–ventilator interface and the adaptation of the environment and of the caregivers to the technique.

Choice of the type of ventilator

Non-invasive ventilation can be achieved by body ventilators or positive-pressure ventilators. Body ventilators were developed in the 1950s for the treatment of poliomyelitis and have been successfully used in other conditions, such as spinal cord injury.[29] Exsufflation belts exert a pressure on the abdominal wall, causing the diaphragm to rise and creating active expiration. Inspiration is passive when the diaphragm returns to its rest position. Exsufflation belts may be used only when sitting. They have been used in ALS patients.[10] Negative-pressure body ventilators create active inspiration by extending the thorax by active external depression. They have become more acceptable for long-term ventilation with the development of devices such as 'punchos' or 'pulmowraps'.[30]

Positive-pressure ventilators are by far the most commonly used ventilators for non-invasive ventilation in all indications and may be volume-cycled or pressure-cycled. In volume-cycled ventilators, the volume is set and the peak airway pressures vary depending on ventilator-delivered volumes, insufflation and interface leakage, and lung impedance. In pressure-cycled ventilators, the pressure is set and the ventilator adapts the volume to compensate for leakage. Increased airway resistance results in a decrease in the delivered volume. Bi-level intermittent positive air pressure (BIPAP) ventilators triggered by the patient are the most easily and commonly used ventilators. Most of the available data concerning the ventilation of ALS patients have been obtained with BIPAP ventilators.[4,28]

Choice of the interface

The patient–ventilator interface is of considerable importance for the efficacity and tolerance of non-invasive ventilation. The most widely used interfaces are nasal masks that are analogous to those used in other indications, such as sleep apoea.[21,24] If the ventilator is volume-cycled the control of leakage is crucial and custom-molded masks are recommended. They are also better tolerated. For pressure-cycled ventilators, commercially available nasal masks may be sufficient, but the tolerance of the skin must be carefully checked. Alternating use of two slightly different masks may help to prevent pressure sores. Facial masks may be used if nasal masks are inefficient, especially because of mouth opening at night. They are not recommended if the patient is unable to remove the mask unaided.

The use of mouthpieces in ALS patients is usually limited by the deficit of the lips.[10]

Environment considerations and education of the patient and caregivers

Multidisciplinary follow-up, including by neurologists, physiatrists, and respiratory physicians, in close co-operation with the family physician, offers the best context to discuss, plan, and initiate non-invasive ventilation. Starting non-invasive ventilation requires a few days' hospital stay in a unit specialized in respiratory rehabilitation. The choice of the ventilator and the adaptation of the interface and of the ventilation parameters rely on the arterial blood gases measured at the end of a period of ventilation. Closer monitoring can also be achieved by measuring transcutaneous oxygen saturation. The patient can then return home. In a population survey by Moss and Colleagues,[6] 50% of ventilated patients live at home. The acceptance of non-invasive ventilation by hospice services is also better than that of invasive ventilation. In all cases, the organization of care should be carefully planned before the decision to use non-invasive ventilation is taken. Some authors consider that non-invasive ventilation may be continued with as little as 15 minutes' autonomous breathing,[10] whereas most authors consider that invasive ventilation should be considered when autonomy is reduced to less than 1 hour.[19]

The cost of non-invasive ventilation is relatively low compared to the global cost of taking care of a quadriplegic, dependent patient. It has been estimated at around $US500 per month.[31] In some countries, associations have organized the purchase, installation, and maintenance of non-invasive ventilation devices.[32]

Education of the patient and caregivers should include awareness of the clinical signs of hypoxia and hypercapnia, manipulation of the interface and ventilator and, if the patient's autonomy is reduced, knowledge of how to use a manual ventilation device. Providing the patient with a trancutaneous oxymeter is very useful, both for caregivers and for the family physician. The patient should be instructed to refer to the rehabilitation unit if the oxygen saturation falls below 85%. The existence of an ALS 'hotline' that can keep the patient, family, and family physician in contact with the specialized team is probably the best guarantee of the feasibility of long-term ventilation.

Invasive ventilation

Invasive ventilation by tracheotomy allows ventilation with reduced dead space and easy suction of bronchic secretions. It may be considered in ALS patients for one of several reasons. When bulbar impairment is such that intractable aspiration occurs despite correct management by gastrostomy, tracheotomy and the use of a cuffed tube is the only way of both ventilating the patient and protecting the airway from aspiration. Thus, invasive ventilation may be the first choice in an ALS patient who wishes to be ventilated and presents such bulbar impairment that non-invasive ventilation is unlikely to be efficient. Nevertheless, even in such patients, some authors have described the successful use of non-invasive ventilation,[4] and it is probably worthwhile trying non-invasive ventilation if the decision is made early enough to have some time to evaluate the results.

Some patients are unsuccessful in using non-invasive ventilation because of difficulties in adapting the interface, and invasive ventilation should be considered in these patients if they are motivated.

In most patients using non-invasive ventilation, the question of turning to invasive ventilation will eventually occur, either because they have become completely dependent or because

bulbar deficit has progressed, leading to aspiration. Again, this question should be discussed in advance with the patient, and the decision as to whether tracheotomy will or will not be performed should be taken with the patient.

The last reason for performing tracheotomy and starting invasive ventilation is when acute respiratory failure develops in a patient with whom the question of assisted ventilation has never been discussed. This eventuality remains frequent,[5] leads to impossible ethical dilemmas 'solved' in the emergency ward by the neurology resident, and should be avoided.

Implementation of invasive ventilation again requires choosing a ventilator and a cannula and training the caregivers. Many simple-to-use volume-cycled ventilators may be used for invasive ventilation. The ventilator should be equipped with both a high-pressure alarm and a low-pressure alarm to detect airway obstruction and leakage or unplugging of the system. The inspired air must be humidified. A back-up ventilator is necessary if the patient's autonomy is reduced. Portable ventilators may be fixed on electrical wheelchairs.

The choice of the cannula depends on the risk of aspiration and the residual phonation capacities of the patient.[20] If phonation is possible and the risk of aspiration is low, uncuffed tubes or deflated cuff tubes are preferable. The insufflated volume must of course be increased to compensate for leakage. Protection of the airway requires the use of cuffed tubes, and cylindric cuffs may offer better protection than ovoid cuffs. Phonation may be partially preserved by deflating the cuff when the patient is off ventilation and by using fenestrated inner cannulas. If autonomy is very reduced and cuff deflation is poorly tolerated, 'talking-trach' tubes[30] may be used. These cannulas provide an extra air line above the tracheostomy balloon, which allows a flow of air through the vocal cords for phonation.

Implementation of invasive ventilation should be considered in a specialized unit. Home discharge of ventilated patients is possible, but this requires the intervention of a specialized nurse once or twice a week to change the tracheotomy cannula.[33] The inner cannula can be changed every day by non-specialized caregivers. The tracheal wound should also be carefully cleaned every day. Regular contacts and follow-up with the specialized team are again necessary. Tracheostomy per se carries the risk of a number of complications: infections, drying of secretions, tracheal mucosa injury with the risk of stenosis and malacia[34] and accidental decannulation. Invasive ventilation is probably less comfortable than non-invasive ventilation, although no data comparing the quality of life with the two types of ventilation appear to be available. Certainly, invasive ventilation is more difficult to manage and requires intervention of specialized caregivers. Finally, invasive ventilation, even more than non-invasive ventilation, makes the patient ineligible for most nursing facilities. Invasive ventilation should thus be strictly restricted to patients in whom non-invasive ventilation is not or is no longer possible, if and only if they wish to undergo tracheostomy and invasive ventilation. In these circumstances, most of the patients who have chosen invasive ventilation are satisfied with it.[6,25] The possibility of discontinuing invasive ventilation if the patient no longer desires it should also be clearly stated.

Treatment of bronchial mucus plugging

Mucus plugging increases hypoxia and carries the risk of atelectasia and acute respiratory failure. It is caused by the combination of weakness of active expiration and aspiration. A number of simple measures may decrease obstruction by bronchial secretions. Drainage postures help to clear the secretions. Physiotherapy should include manual assisted expiration, which should be performed by trained physiotherapists. Mechanical assisted expiration by insufflation–exsufflation devices has been used in ALS patients and may be efficient.[35] In bulbar impairment it may be impossible for the patient to hold the insufflated air because of deficiency of glottal closing. In the case of acute aspiration and atelectasia, fibroaspiration may be performed. When the disease progresses and aspiration becomes intractable despite enteral feeding, tracheotomy may be the only alternative to ensure pulmonary toilet.

Conclusion

Although there is no curative treatment available at the terminal stage of ALS, patients should be carefully followed by multidisciplinary teams up to the time of their death. There is a considerable body of evidence that planned and active care is worthwhile and does make a difference both in terms of quality of life and length of survival. The first effect of implementing structured terminal care programs is to relieve the anxiety of both patients and caregivers and restore a positive relationship between the patient and the medical team. The effect of correct management of physiological impairments such as swallowing and respiratory disorders is demonstrated with a dramatic increase in survival. In combination with the attempts to slow the evolution of the disease by medical treatment reviewed elsewhere, the development of substitutive techniques at all stages may progressively change ALS from being a short-term, lethal illness to being a possibly chronic condition. Moral, ethical, and economic questions as to what type of program should be offered should then be considered in the same terms as for any other chronic disabling condition.

References

1. Hudson AJ. Outpatient management of amyotrophic lateral sclerosis. *Semin Neurol* 1987; **74:** 344–351.

2. Mazzini L, Corrà T, Zaccala M et al. Percutaneous endoscopic gastrostomy and enteral nutrition in amyotrophic lateral sclerosis. *J Neurol* 1995; **242:** 695–698.

3. Janiszewski DW, Caroscio JT, Wisham LH. Amyotrophic lateral sclerosis: a comprehensive rehabilitation approach. *Arch Phys Med Rehabil* 1983; **64:** 304–307.

4. Pinto AC, Evangelista T, Carvalho M et al. Respiratory assistance with non invasive ventilator (Bipap) in MND/ALS patients: survival rates in a controlled trial. *J Neurol Sci* 1995; **129 (suppl 1)**; 19–26.

5. Moss AH, Oppenheimer EA, Casey P et al. Patients with amyotrophic lateral sclerosis receiving long term mechanical ventilation. Advanced care and outcome. *Chest* 1996; **110:** 249–255.

6. Moss AH, Casey P, Stocking CB et al. Home ventilation for amyotrophic lateral sclerosis patients: outcomes, costs, and patient, family, and physician attitudes. *Neurology* 1993; **43:** 438–443.

7. Norris FH, Holden D, Kandal K, Stanley E. Homenursing care by families for severely paralyzed ALS patients. *Arch Exp Med Biol* 1987; **209:** 191–200.

8. Johnson ER, Fowler WM, Lieberman JS. Contractures in neuromuscular disease. *Arch Phys Med Rehabil* 1992; **73:** 807–810.

9. Thoumie P, Charlier JR, Alecki M et al. Clinical and functional evaluation of a gaze controlled system for the severely handicapped. *Spinal Cord* 1998; **36:** 104–109.

10. Bach JR. Amyotrophic lateral sclerosis. Communication status and survival with ventilatory support. *Am J Phys Med Rehabil* 1993; **72:** 343–349.

11. Kirisits H, Reisecker F. Ambulante Intensivtherapie bei bulbärer Form des amyotrophen Lateralsklerose. *Wien Med Wochenschr* 1996; **146:** 202–203.

12. DJ Callaghan. Families as care givers: the limits of morality. *Arch Phys Med Rehabil* 1988; **69:** 323–327.

13. Hillel AD, Miller R. Bulbar amyotrophic lateral sclerosis: patterns of progression and clinical management. *Head Neck* 1989; **11:** 51–59.

14. Hillel AD, Miller RM. Management of bulbar symptoms in amyotrophic lateral sclerosis. *Adv Exp Med Biol* 1987; **209:** 201–221.

15. Mathus-Vliegen LM, Louwerse LS, Merkus MP et al. Percutaneous endoscopic gastrostomy in patients with lateral sclerosis and impaired pulmonary function. *Gastrointest Endosc* 1994; **40:** 463–469.

16. Meininger V. Breaking bad news in amyotrophic lateral sclerosis. *Palliat Med* 1993; **7 (suppl 2):** 37–40.

17. Vitacca M, Clini E, Facchetti D et al. Breathing pattern and respiratory mechanics in patients with amyotrophic lateral sclerosis. *Eur Respir J* 1997; **10:** 1614–1621.

18. Schiffman PL, Belsh JM. Pulmonary function at diagnosis of amyotrophic lateral sclerosis. Rate of deterioration. *Chest* 1993; **103:** 508–513.

19. Oppenheimer EA. Amyotrophic lateral sclerosis. *Eur Respir Rev* 1992; **2:** 323–329.

20. Fallat RJ, Norris FH, Holden D et al. Respiratory monitoring and treatment: objective treatments using non invasive measurements. *Arch Exp Med Biol* 1987; **209:** 191–200.

21. Bach JR, Saporito LR. Indications and criteria for decannulation and transition from invasive to non invasive ventilatory support. *Respir Care* 1994; **39:** 515–531.

22. Schiffman PL, Belsh JM. Effect of inspiratory resistance and theophylline on respiratory muscle strength in patients with amyotrophic lateral sclerosis. *Chest* 1989; **139:** 1418–1423.

23. Oppenheimer EA. Decision-making in the respiratory care of amyotrophic lateral sclerosis: should home mechanical ventilation be used? *Palliat Med* 1993; **7:** 49–64.

24. Hill NS. Non invasive ventilation. Does it work, for whom, and how. *Am Rev Respir Dis* 1993; **147:** 1050–1055.

25. McDonald ER. Evaluation of the psychological status of ventilatory supported patients with ALS/MND. *Palliat Med* 1996; **10:** 35–41.

26. Bach JR. Amyotrophic lateral sclerosis: predictors for prolongation of life by noninvasive respiratory aids. *Arch Phys Med Rehabil* 1995; **76:** 828–832.

27. Hopkins LC, Tatrain GT, Pianta TF. Manage-

ment of ALS: respiratory care. *Neurology* 1996; **47** (**suppl 2**): S123–S125.

28. Cazzolli PA, Oppenheimer EA. Home mechanical ventilation for amyotrophic lateral sclerosis: nasal compared to tracheostomy intermittent positive pressure ventilation. *J Neurol Sci* 1996; **139**: 123–128.

29. Bach JR. *Pulmonary Rehabilitation. The Obstructive and Paralytic Condition*. Philadelphia: Hanley and Delfus, 1996.

30. Schermann RS, Paz HL. Review of respiratory care of the patient with amyotrophic lateral sclerosis. *Respiration* 1994; **61**: 61–67.

31. Klein LM, Forshew DA. The economic impact of ALS. *Neurology* 1996; **47** (**suppl 2**): S126–S129.

32. Raphael JC. Ventilation à domicile dans les maladies neurologiques. *Rev Neurol* 1997; **153**: 626–628.

33. Muir JF. Home mechanical ventilation. *Thorax* 1993; **48**: 1264–1273.

34. Richard I, Giraud M, Perrouin-Verbe B et al. Laryngotracheal stenosis after intubation or tracheostomy in neurological patients. *Arch Phys Med Rehabil* 1996; **77**: 493–496.

35. Hanayama K, Ishikawa Y, Bach JR. Amyotrophic lateral sclerosis: successful treatment of mucous plugging by mechanical insufflation–exsufflation. *Am J Phys Med Rehabil* 1997; **76**: 338–339.

26

The role of the lay associations
George Levvy

The starting point

Most readers of this book will have some knowledge of how amyotrophic lateral sclerosis (ALS) manifests. Many will have witnessed the progression of the disease in someone they have known. They will have felt the shock and helplessness most of us feel in the face of the disease. To some degree, they will have been able to identify with the experiences of the person with ALS and those of his or her family in the face of relentless cumulative loss: of physical capability, of earning ability, of social contact, of possibilities of all sorts, and of hopes and dreams.

However, few readers will be aware of the way that the quality of life of those affected by ALS is so largely determined by the responses of their environment, in particular those of the system of which they — the professionals — are part.

The lay associations start from the experiences and wishes of people affected by ALS. They seek to ensure that those experiences and wishes guide the work of all those involved in improving their quality of life or developing treatments. This chapter, therefore, begins from the perspective of those who live with ALS, as revealed in studies undertaken by two of the lay associations. It then describes the approach of the lay associations and their activities. Finally, it describes the International

Alliance of ALS/MND Associations, the organisation that brings together and represents associations from different countries.

What people affected by ALS say

Two studies, one carried out by the Motor Neurone Disease Association[1] (the organization serving England, Wales and Northern Ireland) and the other by Motor Neurone Disease Association of Victoria, Australia,[2] give an overview of the experiences and concerns of people affected by ALS. Because these studies were carried out in countries with advanced health and social care delivery systems, the priorities that they identify may not be the same as the ones that surveys in less developed nations would. Moreover, because health and social care systems vary between countries, the emphases might be different if these studies were repeated in different places. However, informal feedback makes it clear that people affected by ALS in any developed country would identify very similar issues.

Research

For people affected by ALS, research equates with hope. Even those who know they are unlikely to benefit from current research find hope in the prospect that effective treatments will be found. Both patients and carers in the UK placed 'more research' as their top priority among changes they would most want to see.[1]

Information

Every individual contact with those affected by ALS, as well as both studies,[1,2] reconfirms the importance of clear, simple information on everything to do with the disease. From the moment at which they learn they have ALS until they are able to access useful information, people are pitched into a bewildering and totally unknown world in which they are at the mercy of every part of the health and social care system. For the majority of people, comprehensible information of any sort is desperately hard to find, unless and until they make contact with one of the lay associations, which almost always prove to be their only dependable source of understandable and useful information.[1]

Professional ignorance

The relatively low prevalence of ALS means that the majority of health and social care professionals have little or no experience of caring for people with the diagnosis. In the UK, it is estimated that on average a general practitioner (GP) can expect to see one case of ALS in his or her working life.[3] And — in the UK at least — it is GPs' lack of knowledge that represents the greatest obstacle of all.[1]

The consequences of this are manifold. GPs' failure to recognize that the symptoms might be neurological in origin produces great delay in obtaining the diagnosis. One study (*From First Symptoms to Diagnosis*, an ongoing research project sponsored by Rhone–Poulenc Rorer) has found that the time from first symptom to diagnosis is as much as 17 months, many patients being referred to one or two consultants in other specialties before

seeing a neurologist. Given the importance of having a diagnostic label, both in order to access health and social care and benefits and in order to make personal adjustments, this delay is far too great — especially in the light of a study in Scotland that showed that 50% survival from the time of diagnosis was only 14 months.[4]

At the time of diagnosis itself, professional inexperience shows itself again in the insensitive manner in which the diagnosis is too often communicated. The stories of people being told in corridors or in curtained-off cubicles where everyone else can hear are still myriad. The consequences of such thoughtlessness go far beyond causing more distress than is necessary. The trauma caused by the manner in which the diagnosis was communicated is felt and expressed by many people with ALS and their carers long after the event. There is evidence that this has consequences throughout the remainder of the patient's life,[5] quite apart from the damage done to the patient's confidence in the clinician and indeed in the profession of which he or she is part.

Not surprisingly, professionals' lack of experience in managing the disease affects the quality of the services provided from the time of diagnosis to death. Professionals who know too little or who understandably feel impotent in the face of the disease prevent people from obtaining services that could dramatically improve their quality of life, be it speech therapy, palliative care, or any other of the many services people with ALS need access to.[1] Equally, failure to apply current understanding of effective multidisciplinary, patient-centred practice can make the services provided as much a burden as a help for those with ALS.

Access to specialist centres

Patients who do not have access to a medical centre with expertise in the management of ALS believe that they would benefit in a range of ways if they had. Those who are fortunate enough to visit such centres seem to confirm that these anticipated benefits do materialize.[1]

Importance of lay associations and of family and friends

Both the UK[1] and the Australian[2] studies make it clear how large a part is played by the lay associations in giving information and emotional support, overcoming isolation, and providing time to talk as well as direct support services such as loan of specialist equipment. In the UK study, patients with ALS and their carers listed 'family and friends' and the 'MND Association' as the top two things that had 'gone well for them' in enabling them to live with the disease.

Carers' situations

As with any health problem, the needs of the carers are often neglected. As a group, they generally put their needs second to those of the person with ALS, often at great cost to themselves; and they can find it hard to accept help.[1] However, it is evident that their needs are often forgotten by health and social care professionals (e.g. around the time that the diagnosis is given,[1] when they have a crucial role to play in supporting the patient and ensuring good understanding but also have specific needs that differ from those of the patient).

The lay associations
Overall approach

Although the lay associations differ in many respects they have a few features in common:

(a) nearly all have a primary focus on improving the quality of life of people affected by ALS (i.e. they address the 'care' services that are available);

(b) they were formed in response to the — generally poor — experiences of people living with ALS;

(c) they base their activities on the expressed experiences and needs of people living with ALS;

(d) they aim to empower people living with ALS to determine for themselves how they live.

Many associations also fund research; a few have only this role, although such associations usually exist only because the law of their country requires the establishment of a separate charity for this purpose. As discussed above, promotion of research is itself a response to the wishes of those living with the disease and contributes to their quality of life through the hope it gives.

Activities of the lay associations

The activities of the lay associations vary, but all will undertake some or all of those listed in *Table 26.1*. Of these, a number warrant further comment.

Provision of information

The most important factors in enabling patients and carers affected by ALS to achieve the best possible quality of life is the availability of clear and appropriate information and the expertise of the professionals on whom they depend. Conversely, their lack are the greatest obstacles. All the lay associations therefore consider provision of information to be a central part of their work — not only for those affected by the disease but also for researchers, health and social care professionals, health and social care planners, govern-

Providing information — leaflets, helplines, videos, meetings, magazines
Professional education
Scientific meetings
Care services (e.g. equipment loan, financial support)
Awareness raising
Fundraising
Political campaigning and lobbying
Advocacy
Funding of research (e.g. project grants, studentships, fellowships)
Commissioning research on management issues
Personal support through professional staff, support groups, and volunteers
Counselling
Setting standards for management of ALS

Table 26.1
Activities undertaken by lay associations.

ment, and the media. Their effectiveness is demonstrated by the reports of those affected by ALS of their dependence on the associations for information.[1,2]

In its minimum form, provision of information comprises publication of leaflets tailored to the needs and understanding of those recently diagnosed and the availability of people at the end of a phone. Those associations with larger resources develop a more sophisticated range of materials that are targeted at the needs and situations of specific audiences. Some associations have established professionally managed helplines.

Many associations also demonstrate great skill and innovation in this area. A booklet and leaflet explaining about ALS and the resources available to help those affected by ALS have been prepared jointly by the MND

Association of Australia and the Australian Neurology Association. These materials are available to all neurologists in Australia for patients at diagnosis.[6,7] A booklet first published by the MND Association in 1996,[8] which provides GPs with a complete guide to the disease in a brief and easily accessible format, has been enthusiastically received by all professional groups. A revised edition was produced in 1998 in response to the demand for an updated version. It has now been adapted for use in several other countries.

Some of the associations extend information provision into the territory of professional education. Many health and social care professionals involved in the management of a case of ALS will be encountering the disease for the first time. Several associations employ staff drawn from these professions specifically to be an educational resource for them and hence ensure the quality of the service they provide, while training seminars run for health and social care professionals by the associations are increasingly in demand.

Care services

Even in the richest countries, there is a gap between what could be done and what is done to help people affected by ALS. As discussed above, much of this results from lack of information and professional lack of experience of the disease. The rest is largely due to service planners' and providers' failings, whether through resource limitations or their lack of understanding of the nature of the disease and the needs it creates.

Many associations step into this gap by providing services themselves, such as loan of equipment or financial support for respite care, house alteration, or equipment purchases. As might be expected, these services contrast with those of publicly funded providers in the priority that they give to speed of response to requests.

Research

The lay associations are vital players in the world-wide research effort. Two of the largest funders of research into ALS in the world are the ALS Association and Muscular Dystrophy Association in the USA. Several of the other associations around the world provide significant research funding, and they are the only means by which a meaningful level of ALS research expertise is maintained in their respective countries.

The other major contribution is the International Symposium on ALS/MND, organized by the Motor Neurone Disease Association in cooperation with the International Alliance of ALS/MND Associations. The first symposium was held in 1990, when approximately 50 delegates attended; it is now established as the most important research forum on ALS and MND in the world and attracts over 600 participants each year.

Speaking out

One of the greatest concerns of those affected by ALS and one of the major obstacles to improving their lot is the lack of awareness and understanding of the disease among the public and key decision makers. Even within the circles of those concerned with the disease, the perspective of those living with it is often unknown or ignored. Changing this situation may be the biggest challenge of all those facing the lay associations, which tackle it in a wide range of ways, the most basic of which is to make accurate, reliable and understandable information available.

In the face of limited resources, the associations have to decide which audiences they are most concerned with and able to influence. Against these criteria, most associations give priority to those with the power to shape service provision (i.e. governments and service providers and planners) and to health and social care practitioners, whose individual actions directly affect the quality of life of those with the disease.

Thus, many associations undertake 'advocacy' on behalf of individuals, helping them obtain the services they need from providers. Some undertake political campaigning at some level. The ALS Association in the USA, for example, has been successful in getting a bill before both Houses of Congress that would give all ALS patients in the USA who qualify a reduction in the eligibility waiting time for medical services, more funding for research, and payment for medications.

Recently, there have been initiatives to set standards for the care and support that people affected by ALS should be able to obtain. The

Management of the disease determined by the needs and wishes of the person with ALS and the family and carers
Flexibility and speed in response to referral
Continuity of care throughout the progression of the disease
Co-ordination and co-operation between service providers
Regular monitoring and review

Table 26.2
The key principles that underpin care of people with ALS. From Motor Neurone Disease Association.[9]

Motor Neurone Disease Association has published a standards of care[9] (*Table 26.2*) that defines reasonable service expectations throughout the course of the illness from the onset of symptoms. The International Alliance of ALS/MND Associations is developing a baseline services standard (unpublished), which will be applicable in all health and social care provision environments. Initiatives are under way to audit delivery against each of these standards in several countries. The evidence generated will strengthen the associations' arguments to influence service provision.

The unique capabilities of the lay associations

It could be argued that the individual activities described in the previous section could be carried out by other organizations — and hence that the associations are, in theory at least, not essential. There is, for example, no absolute reason why health and social care providers should not become effective providers of information as well. Moreover, good research does not care where the money comes from, as long as it does come. In reality, of course, the lay associations are a response to a need that is felt urgently by people all round the world.

Yet there are aspects of the lay associations that go beyond any single activity and that represent a unique, irreplaceable contribution in the fight against ALS. The basis of this unique quality is the fact that the associations are of and for those affected by the disease. ALS, like other diseases, too frequently becomes the 'property' of other groups — the researchers, the neurologists, the service providers, even the lay associations if they become distanced from their 'customers'. Thankfully, most of the associations remain very close to those living with the disease and base their actions on ongoing and direct feedback on their needs and wishes. They therefore have the great authority of speaking for those affected by the disease. At a time when most health and social care is still shaped on the basis of 'doctor knows best', the presence of an effective voice for those with the disease is vital if they are to take charge of the decisions that shape their lives.

The lay associations are also unique in the expertise that they build through meeting and knowing more people living with ALS than any other group of people. The expertise that this establishes is about the care and support needed by people who are affected by the disease and is complementary to that of the health and social care professionals in provider organizations.

Finally, it is important to recognize one element of the associations' work that is often undervalued: the work of volunteers in supporting people living with ALS. Volunteers make a unique and irreplaceable contribution to the lives of those affected by ALS through the time, understanding, and companionship that they give. The despair and isolation experienced through the disease would be immeasurably greater without that gift, for which no amount of professionals' time could substitute.

The International Alliance of ALS/MND Associations

The relatively low prevalence of ALS and the general low awareness of the disease mean that most lay associations are small and have very little money. Many are staffed entirely by volunteers. The majority of lay associations have an income of less than £50,000.

As a result, many associations struggle with a sense of isolation as their country's health and social care providers seem not to understand or to prioritize the needs of people with ALS. The support they are able to provide, which may be the only help that those with the disease receive, is far less than is needed. Even in richer countries, demands exceed the associations' capacities, and the associations struggle to be heard among the clamour of health issues, many of them representing much larger constituencies.

The formation of the International Alliance of ALS/MND Associations in 1992 is one response to these problems. Membership can counter the sense of isolation by providing both direct contact with other associations facing similar battles and regular information on developments around the world. Ideas exchanged at and between annual meetings enable members to increase their effectiveness by using methods that have been successfully employed elsewhere.

The Alliance also gives people affected by ALS greater influence through the creation of an international 'voice' for their needs and views. This can help the efforts of a single association that is trying to influence events domestically, as well as providing a medium for those with ALS to be heard in international forums, such as those organized by the World Federation of Neurology Subcommittee on Motor Neurone Diseases.

Membership of the Alliance grows annually and in 1998 stood at 26 associations (*Table 26.3*).

Conclusion

Although most of the lay ALS associations are less than 25 years old, they make a major and vital contribution both to the quality of life of those living with the disease and to the funding and promotion of research. In representing the interests of those affected by ALS, they see health and social care professionals as key customers, providing them with a source of information, education, and support. At a broader level, they play a unique role in speaking for those with the disease to governments, health and social care organizations, and professional groups.

In an environment in which the wishes of users, quality of life, and rationing of treatments on the basis of evidence of cost-effectiveness are being given increasing priority, it is as well that the lay associations have established a level of expertise in so many areas. They will be essential partners with other groups — investigators, clinicians, care planners and providers, and care professionals — in bringing about meaningful change in the experience of ALS in the next decade.

MND Association of Australia

ALS Support Group (Belgium)

ALS Society of Canada

Union of Muscular Dystrophy Societies (Croatia)

Muskelvindfonden (Denmark)

Association pour la Récherche Sclérose Latérale Amyotrophique (France)

Association Lutte et Soutien Maladies du Motoneurone (France)

Deutsche Gesellschaft für Muskelkranke (DGM, Germany)

MND Society of Iceland

MND Association of India

Irish MND Association

Israeli Association of ALS/MND (ATLAS)

Associatione Italiano Sclerosi Laterale Amiotrofia (AISLA, Italy)

Japan ALS Association

Vereniging Spierziekten Nederland (VSN, Netherlands)

MND Association of New Zealand

Scottish MND Association

MND Association of South Africa

Associación Española de ELA (ADELA, Spain)

Taiwan MND Association

Association of Muscular Dystrophy (Turkey)

MND Association (England, Wales, and Northern Ireland)

Associación Nacional para la Lucha contra las Enfermadedes Motorneuronales o Esclerosis Lateral Amiotrófica (MONDELA, Uruguay)

Les Turner ALS Foundation (USA)

Forbes H Norris ALS Research Center (USA)

Yugoslavia MND Association

Table 26.3
Members of the International Alliance of ALS/MND Associations.

References

1. Birch P, Ferlie E, Gritzner C. *Report on the Views and Experiences of People Affected by Motor Neurone Disease*. Northampton: Motor Neurone Disease Association, 1995.

2. Sach J. *People Living with Motor Neurone Disease in Victoria — Profiles and Strategies: with Applications to Other Neurological Conditions*. Melbourne: Motor Neurone Disease Association of Victoria, 1995.

3. Cochrane GM. *The Management of Motor Neurone Disease*. Edinburgh: Churchill Livingston, 1987.

4. Chancellor AM, Slattery JM, Fraser H et al. The prognosis of adult-onset motor neuron disease: a prospective study based on the Scottish Motor Neuron Disease Register. *J Neurol* 1993; **240**: 339–346.

5. Johnston M, Earll L, Mitchell E et al. Communicating the diagnosis of motor neurone disease. *Palliat Med* 1996; **10**: 23–34.

6. *Motor Neurone Disease — Some Facts*. Melbourne: Motor Neurone Disease Association of Australia, 1996.

7. *Motor Neurone Disease — More Facts*. Melbourne: Motor Neurone Disease Association of Australia, 1996.

8. *Motor Neurone Disease: a Problem Solving Approach, for General Practitioners and the Primary Care Health Team*. Northampton: Motor Neurone Disease Association, 1998.

9. *Standards of Care to Achieve Quality of Life for People Affected by Motor Neurone Disease*. Northampton: Motor Neurone Disease Association, 1998.

Index

Page numbers in *italic* refer to the illustrations

New peer-review quarterly journal

Amyotrophic Lateral Sclerosis
and other motor neuron disorders

Editor: M Swash

Martin Dunitz Publishers are pleased to announce the launch of a new quarterly journal covering all aspects of the diagnosis and management of ALS (Lou Gehrig's disease), primary lateral sclerosis, spinal muscular atrophy and related motor neuron disorders. The aim of this journal is to disseminate information on new developments in the management of motor neuron diseases, and enhance awareness of these devastating and often under-recognised disorders. The journal will be the official publication of the World Federation of Neurology Committee on Motor Neuron Disease. The first issue is planned for publication in November 1999.

Each issue will feature reviews, original research, case reports and other short reports on all aspects of ALS, including new treatments, basic science, clinical trials, care issues, ethics and legal issues and reports from ALS centres.

Information on subscribing and manuscript submission is available from Ian Mellor, Journals Manager, Martin Dunitz Ltd, The Livery House, 7–9 Pratt Street, London NW1 0AE (tel +44 (0)171 482 2202; fax +44(0)171 482 7088; e-mail als@dunitzco.globalnet.co.uk).

Contents of early issues will include

Reviews
How can physicians and their patients with ALS decide to use the newly-available treatments to slow disease progression?
Gastrointestinal dysfunction in ALS
Nutritional assessment and survival in ALS patients
The skin in ALS
MR imaging in ALS
Current status of SOD1 mutations in familial ALS
Cognitive impairment in ALS
Ubiquitinated intracytoplasmic neuronal inclusions in the hippocampus of ALS presenting with dementia

Original Research
Abnormalities of visual search behavior in ALS patients detected with event-related brain potentials
GDNF is trophic for mouse motoneurons that express a mutant SOD-1 gene

Evidence for the validity and reliability of the ALS assessment questionnaire: the ALSAQ-40
Quantitative proton MR spectroscopy of the subcortical white matter in MND
Motor neuron disease – classification and nomenclature
Fibrillation and sharp-waves: do we need them to diagnose ALS?

Case Reports
Distinct hyperintense MRI signal changes in a patient with motor neuron disease

Short Report
ALS Database – Database of SOD1 and other gene mutations in ALS on the Internet

ALS Centre Reports
Eleanor and Lou Gehrig MND/ALS Center
King's MND Care and Research Centre

Historical vignettes
ALS diagnostic criteria, El Escorial and Philip II of Spain: a historial perspective